Synopsis of
Clinical Oncology

Synopsis of Clinical Oncology

EDITED BY

Michael D. Stubblefield, MD

Assistant Attending Physiatrist
Rehabilitation Medicine Service
Department of Neurology
Memorial Sloan-Kettering Cancer Center
Assistant Professor of Rehabilitation Medicine
Weill Cornell Medical College of Cornell University
New York, New York

Michael W. O'Dell, MD

Chief of Clinical Services
Department of Rehabilitation Medicine
New York-Presbyterian Hospital
Weill Cornell Medical Center
Professor of Clinical Rehabilitation Medicine
Weill Cornell Medical College of Cornell University
New York, New York

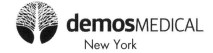

demosMEDICAL

New York

Acquisitions Editor: Beth Barry
Cover Design: Joe Tenerelli
Copyediting, Indexing, and Composition: Newgen North America
Printer: Offset Paperback Manufacturing

Visit our website at www.demosmedpub.com

The material contained herein appeared in *Cancer Rehabilitation: Principles and Practice*, edited by Michael D. Stubblefield and Michael W. O'Dell, Demos Medical Publishing, New York, 2009.

Library of Congress Cataloging-in-Publication Data

Synopsis of clinical oncology / edited by Michael D. Stubblefield, Michael W. O'Dell.
    p. ; cm.
  Abridged version of: Cancer rehabilitation principles and practice / edited by Michael D. Stubblefield, Michael W. O'Dell. c2009.
  Includes bibliographical references and index.
  ISBN 978-1-936287-00-0
  1. Cancer—Handbooks, manuals, etc. 2. Oncology—Handbooks, manuals, etc.
I. Stubblefield, Michael D. II. O'Dell, Michael W. III. Cancer rehabilitation principles and practice.
  [DNLM: 1. Neoplasms—therapy. 2. Neoplasms—diagnosis. QZ 266 S993 2010]
  RC262.5.S96   2010
  616.99'4—dc22   2010002638

Special discounts on bulk quantities of Demos Medical Publishing books are available to corporations, professional associations, pharmaceutical companies, health care organizations, and other qualifying groups. For details, please contact:

Special Sales Department
Demos Medical Publishing
11 W. 42nd Street
New York, NY 10036
Phone: 800–532–8663 or 212–683–0072
Fax: 212–941–7842
Email: rsantana@demosmedpub.com

Made in the United States of America

10 11 12 13   5 4 3 2 1

Contents

Preface

The material presented in this book was originally published in *Cancer Rehabilitation: Principles and Practice* (© 2009 Demos Medical Publishing). We believe that the foundation for successful rehabilitation of cancer patients begins with a working understanding of the diseases and their treatments. To this end, the "principles" section, authored by some of the world's leading cancer experts from wide-ranging disciplines including oncology, radiation oncology, neurosurgery, orthopedic surgery, and radiology, provides state-of-the-art primer level overviews of the various cancer types, their evaluation, and treatment. The success of the original textbook and the overwhelmingly positive response to the inclusion of the "principles of oncology" section highlighted the need to make this material available to those whose primary interest is not the rehabilitation of cancer patients.

Synopsis of Clinical Oncology is intended to serve as a valuable reference for students, residents, and other trainees and practitioners from diverse disciplines such as internal medicine, primary care, emergency medicine, surgery, and nursing just to name a few. Each chapter is concise but highlights the basic tenets health care professionals working with cancer patients need to know to understand the diseases and current treatment options. To facilitate review, Key Points are boxed in each chapter to summarize important clinical information and concepts at a glance. This book represents a synthesis of information from some of the top physicians in oncology that is not as easily accessed anywhere else.

Michael D. Stubblefield, MD
Michael W. O'Dell, MD

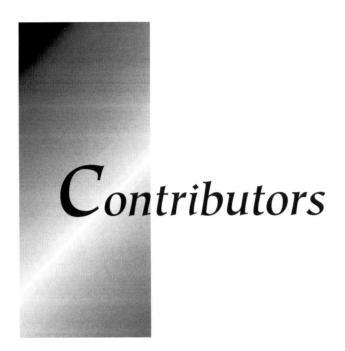

Contributors

Mark H. Bilsky, MD
Associate Attending Surgeon
Department of Neurosurgery
Memorial Sloan-Kettering Cancer Center
Associate Professor
Department of Neurological Surgery
Weill Cornell Medical College
New York, New York

Patrick J. Boland, MD
Attending Orthopaedic Surgeon
Orthopaedic Service
Department of Surgery
Memorial Sloan-Kettering Medical Center
New York, New York

Melissa M. Center, MPH
Epidemiologist
Surveillance and Health Policy Research
American Cancer Society
Atlanta, Georgia

Dennis S. Chi, MD
Gynecology Service
Department of Surgery
Memorial Sloan-Kettering Cancer Center
New York, New York

Lisa M. DeAngelis, MD
Chair
Department of Neurology
Memorial Sloan-Kettering Cancer Center
New York, New York

Joseph J. Disa, MD
Associate Attending Surgeon
Plastic and Reconstructive Surgery Service
Memorial Sloan-Kettering Cancer Center
New York, New York

Austin G. Duffy, MD
Clinical Fellow
Medical Oncology Branch
National Cancer Institute
Bethesda, Maryland

Mark G. Frattini, Md, PhD
Assistant Member
Department of Medicine
Memorial Sloan-Kettering Medical Center
New York, New York

Jorge E. Gomez, MD
Assistant Professor of Medicine
UM Sylvester Comprehensive Cancer Center
Miller School of Medicine
University of Miami
Miami, Florida

Sean A. Grimm, MD
Assistant Professor of Neurology
Feinberg School of Medicine
Northwestern University
Chicago, Illinois

Clifford A. Hudis, MD
Chief, Breast Cancer Medicine Service
Department of Medicine
Memorial Sloan-Kettering Cancer Center
New York, New York

Ahmedin Jemal, DVM, PhD
Department of Epidemiology and Surveillance
   Research
American Cancer Society
Atlanta, Georgia

Tari A. King, MD
Assistant Attending Surgeon
Breast Service
Department of Surgery
Jeanne A. Petnek Junior Faculty Chair
Memorial Sloan-Kettering Cancer Center
New York, New York

Guenther Koehne, MD, PhD
Attending Physician
Allogeneic Bone Marrow Transplantation Service
Department of Medicine
Memorial Sloan-Kettering Cancer Center
Assistant Professor
Weill Cornell Medical College of Cornell University
New York, New York

George Krol, MD
Attending Neuroradiologist
Department of Radiology
Neuroradiology Service
Memorial Sloan-Kettering Cancer Center
Professor of Clinical Radiology
Weill Cornell Medical College of Cornell University
New York, New York

Heather J. Landau, MD
Assistant Attending
Hematology Service
Department of Medicine
Memorial Sloan-Kettering Cancer Center
New York, New York

Rebecca Leboeuf, MD
Assistant Professor of Medicine
Assistant Attending Physician
Endocrinology Service
Department of Medicine
Memorial Sloan-Kettering Cancer Center
New York, New York

Jon Lewis, MD
Neuroradiology Fellow
Department of Radiology
Neuroradiology Service
New York-Presbyterian Medical Center
Memorial Sloan-Kettering Cancer Center
New York, New York

Su Hsien Lim, MD
Medical Oncology and Hematology, PC
Yale-New Haven Shoreline Medical Center
Guilford, Connecticut

Eric Lis, MD
Associate Attending Neuroradiologist
Director of Neurointerventional Radiology
Department of Radiology
Neuroradiology Service
Memorial Sloan-Kettering Cancer Center
New York, New York

Laura Locati, MD
Instituto Nazionale Tumori
Department of Medical Oncology
Milan, Italy

Robert G. Maki, MD, PhD
Associate Member and Co-Director
Adult Sarcoma Program
Department of Medicine
Memorial Sloan-Kettering Cancer Center
New York, New York

Vicky Makker
Assistant Member
Gynecologic Medical Oncology Service
Department of Medicine
Memorial Sloan-Kettering Cancer Center
New York, New York

Enrica Marchi, MD
Herbert Irving Comprehensive Cancer Center
New York, New York

Christopher Mazzone
Neuroradiology Research Assistant
Department of Radiology
Neuroradiology Service
Memorial Sloan-Kettering Cancer Center
New York, New York

Heather L. McArthur, MD, MPH
Clinical Research Fellow
Breast Cancer Medicine Service
Department of Medicine
Memorial Sloan-Kettering Cancer Center
New York, New York

Colleen M. McCarthy, MD, MS
Assistant Attending Surgeon
Plastic and Reconstructive Service
Department of Surgery
Memorial Sloan-Kettering Cancer Center
New York, New York

Sarah A. McLaughlin, MD
Assistant Professor of Surgery
Department of Surgery
Mayo Clinic
Jacksonville, Florida

Alexei Morozov, MD, PhD
Fellow, Hermatology-Oncology
Department of Medicine
Memorial Sloan-Kettering Cancer Center
New York, New York

Carol D. Morris, MD, MS
Associate Attending Surgeon
Orthopedic Surgery Service
Department of Surgery
Memorial Sloan-Kettering Cancer Center
New York, New York

Stephen D. Nimer, MD
Chief, Hematology Service
Vice Chair, Faculty Development
Department of Medicine
Alfred Sloan Chair
Memorial Sloan-Kettering Cancer Center
New York, New York

Owen A. O'Connor, MD, PhD
Director
Lymphoid Development and Malignancy Program
Herbert Irving Comprehensive Cancer Center
Chief, Lymphoma Service
College of Physicians and Surgeons
New York-Presbyterian Hospital
Columbia University
New York, New York

Kristen M. O'Dwyer, MD
Leukemia Service
Department of Medicine
Memorial Sloan-Kettering Cancer Center
New York, New York

Gary C. O'Toole, BSc, MCh, FRCS
Consultant, Orthopaedic Surgeon
St. Vincent's University Hospital
Cappagh National Orthopaedic Hospital
Dublin, Ireland

Meena J. Palayekar, MD
Department of Obstetrics and Gynecology
Saint Peter's University Hospital
New Brunswick, New Jersey

Snehal Patel, MD
Attending Surgeon
Head and Neck Service
Department of Surgery
Memorial Sloan-Kettering Cancer Center
New York, New York

David G. Pfister, MD
Member and Attending Physician
Chief, Head and Neck Medical Oncology
Co-leader, Head and Neck Cancer Disease
    Management Team
Memorial Sloan-Kettering Cancer Center
New York, New York

Corey Rothrock, MD
Clinical Instructor, Orthopedic Surgery
Musculoskeletal Oncology
Norton Cancer Institute
University of Louisville
Louisville, Kentucky

Yvonne Saenger, MD
Assistant Professor
Department of Medicine, Hematology and
    Medical Oncology
Mount Sinai School of Medicine
New York, New York

Leonard B. Saltz, MD
Attending Oncologist
Gastrointestinal Oncology Service
Department of Medicine
Memorial Sloan-Kettering Cancer Center
Professor of Medicine
Weill Cornell Medical College of Cornell University
New York, New York

Susan F. Slovin, MD, PhD
Associate Attending Oncologist
Genitourinary Oncology Service
Department of Medicine
Memorial Sloan-Kettering Cancer Center
New York, New York

David Spriggs, MD
Head, Division of Solid Tumor Oncology
Winthrop Rockefeller Chair in Medical Oncology
Memorial Sloan-Kettering Cancer Center
New York, New York

Robert Michael Tuttle, MD
Professor of Medicine
Attending Physician
Endocrinology Service
Department of Medicine
Memorial Sloan-Kettering Cancer Center
New York, New York

Jedd D. Wolchok, MD, PhD
Associate Attending
Melanoma and Sarcoma Service
Department of Medicine
Memorial Sloan-Kettering Cancer Center
New York, New York

Yoshiya Yamada, MD, FRCPC
Assistant Attending Radiation Oncologist
Department of Radiation Oncology
Memorial Sloan-Kettering Cancer Center
New York, New York

Jasmine Zain, MD
Assistant Clinical Professor
Columbia University Medical Center
New York, New York

I

PRINCIPLES OF CANCER AND CANCER TREATMENT

Principles of Neoplasia

Kristen M. O'Dwyer
Mark G. Frattini

Decades of cancer research have revealed that human cancer is a multistep process involving acquired genetic mutations, each of which imparts a particular type of growth advantage to the cell and ultimately leads to the development of the malignant phenotype. The consequences of the mutations in the tumor cells include alterations in cell signaling pathways that result in uncontrolled cellular proliferation, insensitivity to growth inhibition signals, resistance to apoptosis, development of cellular immortality, angiogenesis, and tissue invasion and metastasis (1). Here we address the fundamental principles of cancer genetics, cell cycle control, and invasion and metastasis. Due to limitations in space and given the complexity of the subject matter and the many excellent textbooks and review articles that are available for each topic, we will highlight the most important principles. A list of historical and current references will be provided for the interested reader.

CANCER GENETICS

The idea that human cancer is a result of multiple mutations in the deoxyribonucleic acid (DNA) sequence of a cell has developed during the past 30 years. A mutation is any change in the primary nucleotide sequence of DNA, and the mutation may or may not have a functional consequence. The field of cancer genetics emerged to study the different types of mutations, as well as the consequences of the mutations in tumor cells. Bert Vogelstein and Ken Kinzler provide the most thoroughly studied example of a human cancer that illustrates this multistep process. Their research of families with rare inherited colon cancer syndromes demonstrated that multiple somatic mutation events (5 to 10) are required for the progression from normal colonic epithelium to the development of carcinoma in situ. The mechanisms through which the mutations in the DNA occur are varied and include imprecise DNA repair processes, random replication errors, splicing errors, messenger ribonucleic acid (mRNA) processing errors, exposure to carcinogens such as radiation or chemotherapy, or incorporation of exogenous DNA into the genome such as viral DNA or RNA (2).

CLASSES OF CANCER GENES— ONCOGENES, TUMOR SUPRESSOR GENES, AND GATEKEEPER GENES

The specific genes that are mutated in the cancer cell have been described as falling into two general functional classes. The first class of genes directly regulates the processes of cell growth and includes the oncogenes and tumor suppressor genes. The second class of genes that are mutated in the cancer cell is the so-called "caretaker" genes. These genes are involved in processes of maintaining the integrity of the genome.

KEY POINTS

- Cancer is a multistep process involving acquired genetic mutations, each of which imparts a particular type of growth advantage to the cell and ultimately leads to the development of the malignant phenotype.
- The specific genes that are mutated in the cancer cell have been described as falling into two general functional classes. The first class of genes directly regulates the processes of cell growth and includes the oncogenes and tumor suppressor genes. The second class of genes that are mutated in the cancer cell is the so-called "caretaker" genes. These genes are involved in processes of maintaining the integrity of the genome.
- While the majority of cancers develop as a result of acquired somatic mutations in the genome, a small percentage (5%–10%) of cancer syndromes develop as a result of inherited mutations.

- Certain viruses are true etiologic agents of human cancers, including human papillomavirus (cervical carcinoma), hepatitis B and C viruses (hepatocellular carcinoma), Epstein-Barr virus (Burkitt lymphoma), and human T-cell leukemia virus type I (T-cell leukemia).
- Cancer metastasis is a complex multistep process and requires multiple genetic changes in the tumor cell in order for it to acquire all of the capabilities necessary to colonize a distant organ.
- It is important to realize that the single cells that form the tumor metastasis can grow fast and take over the organ quickly; in other cases, the metastatic tumors remain small and dormant for months to years. This latency is referred to as metastatic dormancy.
- Metastatic cancer of any origin is generally not curable, and complications from metastasis account for 90% of deaths from solid tumors.

Oncogenes

The study of human retroviruses in the 1970s and the discovery of reverse transcriptase (3,4) led to the finding of the first human oncogenes (5). Oncogenes are mutated forms of normal cellular genes called proto-oncogenes. Proto-oncogenes include several classes of genes involved in mitogenic signaling and growth control, typically encoding proteins such as extracellular cytokines and growth factors, transmembrane growth factor receptors, transcription factors, and proteins that control DNA replication. Importantly, all of the proteins encoded by proto-oncogenes control critical steps in intracellular signaling pathways of the cell cycle, cell division, and cellular differentiation. To date, more than 75 different proto-oncogenes have been identified (6).

In human cancer, the mutation event in the proto-oncogene typically occurs in a single allele of the gene and imitates an autosomal dominant mode of inheritance (ie, mutations in a single allele are sufficient to cause disease), producing a gain-of-function phenotype. The mutations that activate the proto-oncogene to the oncogene include point mutations, DNA amplification, and chromosomal rearrangements.

Examples of point mutations are found in three major Ras family members of proteins (HRAS, KRAS, NRAS). Briefly, Ras proteins are membrane-associated guanine nucleotide exchange proteins. Their downstream targets control diverse processes such as cell proliferation, cellular differentiation, and apoptosis. The activating mutations in the RAS genes involve

codons 12, 13, and 61 and result in an amino acid substitution in the phosphate binding domain of the protein. The functional consequence is a Ras protein that is "locked" in an active guanosine triphosphate (GTP) bound state, resulting in a constitutively active Ras-signaling pathway that now can impart a growth advantage to the cell via uncontrolled cellular proliferation and evasion of apoptosis (7).

The activating mutations in the Ras proteins have been identified in 30% of human tumors (8), though certain tumor types have a particularly high incidence of RAS mutations and include 95% of pancreatic cancers, 50% of colorectal cancers, and 30% of lung carcinomas. While Ras proteins are ubiquitously expressed in human cells, it is unclear why certain tumor types have a higher incidence of mutations.

DNA amplification is the second mechanism of activation of a proto-oncogene. Though the exact mechanism is unknown, DNA amplification results in an increase in DNA copy number of the cellular proto-oncogene. The increase in gene copy number can lead to characteristic chromosomal changes that can be identified with traditional cytogenetic studies used to asses the karyotype. These include extrachromosomal double-minute chromatin bodies (dmins) and homogeneously staining regions in which the amplified sequences are integrated into the chromosomes. The functional result is an increase in the gene expression levels and the corresponding RNA and protein levels.

The first proto-oncogene found to be amplified in a human cancer was MYC when it was identified in the HL-60 human promyelocytic leukemia cell line (9,10). MYC is a member of the basic helix-loop-helix leucine zipper family of transcription factors and regulates multiple cellular processes, including cell growth and differentiation, cell-cycle progression, apoptosis, and cell motility (11,12). MYC is frequently amplified in solid tumors, including small cell lung carcinoma (18%–31%), neuroblastoma (25%), and sarcomas, and the increased gene copy number results in concordant increases in the Myc protein level, leading to unregulated cell growth and division. An important clinical correlation is that in childhood neuroblastoma, an MYC family member, N-MYC, is amplified in approximately 40% of advanced pediatric neuroblastomas and has prognostic significance. Children with neuroblastoma and minimal or no N-MYC amplification have a very good prognosis, while children with >10 copies of N-MYC have a significantly poorer prognosis and shorter survival (13).

Another important gene that is commonly amplified in human cancer, specifically breast, ovarian, and lung cancers, is the c-erbB2/HER-2 gene. The c-erbB2/HER-2 gene encodes a transmembrane receptor of the epidermal growth factor receptor (EGFR) family with associated tyrosine-kinase activity (14,15). The signal transduction pathways that are activated control epithelial cell growth and differentiation. Amplification of the c-erbB2/HER-2 gene is correlated with an increased expression of the Her2 protein. It is estimated that HER2 is amplified in 18%–20% of breast tumors and it, too, carries prognostic value. Slamon et al. demonstrated that DNA amplification of more than five copies of HER2 per cancer cell were found to correlate with a decreased survival in patients with breast cancer (16).

Chromosomal rearrangement is the third mechanism of activation of a proto-oncogene. The mechanism of the rearrangements can be gain and loss of chromosomes that are usually seen in human solid tumors, as well as chromosome translocations, such as those seen in human leukemias, lymphomas, and sarcomas. Because proto-oncogenes are often located at or near chromosomal breakpoints, they are susceptible to mutation. The result is a structural rearrangement that juxtaposes two different chromosomal regions and typically produces a chimeric gene that encodes a fusion protein (17,18).

One of the most studied chromosomal translocations in human cancer came from the study of leukemia cells by Peter Nowell, David Hungerford, and Janet Rowley. In 1960, Hungerford observed a characteristic small chromosome in the leukemia cells of two patients with chronic myelogenous leukemia (CML) (19). At that time, the technology was such that the specific chromosome could not be identified, and so it was designated the Philadelphia chromosome (Ph), as both Hungerford and Nowell resided in Philadelphia. The development of cytogenetic banding in the 1970s was the technologic breakthrough that ultimately led Janet Rowley to identify the Philadelphia chromosome and that, in fact, the Philadelphia chromosome resulted from a translocation of a small portion of chromosome 22 being displaced to chromosome 9 (20). The next advance in this field came in 1984 when Gerard Grosveld and his colleagues cloned the 9;22 translocation and identified the Abelson leukemia (ABL) gene on chromosome 9 and the breakpoint cluster region (BCR) gene on chromosome 22, the two genes that, when joined, expressed an in-frame fusion protein and resulted in a constitutively active ABL tyrosine kinase (21). It is the unregulated BCR-ABL tyrosine-kinase activity that is the transforming event leading to the development of CML. In 2001, Brian Drucker and colleagues published the first report of a specific inhibitor of the BCR-ABL tyrosine kinase, imatinib mesylate, that is active in patients with CML (22). Imatinib mesylate is currently the first-line treatment for all patients with CML and represents one of the first examples of molecularly targeted therapy.

The identification of the Philadelphia chromosome popularized the concept that specific chromosomal rearrangements were linked to cancer. Prior to her studies in CML, Janet Rowley and colleagues had discovered the first reciprocal chromosome rearrangement between chromosomes 8 and 21 in patients with acute myeloid leukemia (AML) (23,24). In this subtype of AML, the AML1 gene (also called CBFα2 for core binding factor or PEBP2αB) on the distal long arm of chromosome 21 becomes fused to the ETO gene (eight, twenty-one gene) on chromosome 8 (24). The consequence of expression of the AML1-ETO gene rearrangement is a new fusion protein that interferes with normal transcription of a number of genes critical for hematopoietic cell development, function, and differentiation (25).

In 1977, Janet Rowley and her colleagues also discovered the 15;17 translocation that characterizes acute promyelocytic leukemia (APL) (26). In this subtype of acute leukemia, a portion of the promyelocytic leukemia (PML) gene on chromosome 15 is fused with a portion of the retinoic acid receptor alpha (RARα) gene on chromosome 17. The resulting PML-RARα fusion protein inhibits differentiation of the myeloid cell, leading to arrested differentiation in the promyelocyte stage. Additionally, the PML-RARα fusion protein acquires antiapoptotic activity that allows the malignant clone to survive under conditions of growth-factor deprivation. In the past, this type of AML was among the most fatal due to the associated coagulopathic state in patients with APL, but with the use of all-trans-retinoic acid (ATRA) and arsenic trioxide in combination with standard chemotherapy, it is now curable in the majority of patients (27), as the use of ATRA and arsenic trioxide allow for differentiation and subsequent apoptotic cell death of the malignant clone.

Tumor Suppressor Genes

Tumor suppressor genes regulate diverse cellular processes in normal cells, including cell-cycle checkpoint responses, DNA repair, protein ubiquitination and degradation, mitogenic signaling, cell specification, differentiation and migration, and tumor angiogenesis.

In human cancers, the mutation event in a tumor suppressor gene in sporadic cancers must occur in both alleles, ie, "two-hit hypothesis" to inactivate the function of the gene, producing a recessive loss-of-function phenotype (28,29). In contrast to the familial cancer syndromes, a germline inheritance of a mutant allele of a tumor suppressor gene requires only one somatic mutation to inactivate the wild-type allele, and the development of the cancer phenotype is thereby greatly accelerated. Also, the tumor suppressor gene identified in a familial syndrome must be found to be mutated in sporadic cancer in order for it to be classified as a tumor suppressor.

There are different types of mutations that inactivate tumor suppressor genes. A point mutation can lead to an amino acid substitution if it occurs in the coding region, or it can introduce a premature stop codon and, therefore, result in a truncated protein. Large deletions of nucleotide sequence of DNA may affect a portion of a gene or the entire arm of a chromosome, causing loss of heterozygosity (LOH) in the tumor DNA. The retinoblastoma gene (RB) is mutated by this mechanism and results in a large deletion in chromosome 13q14 (30).

There are epigenetic mechanisms that can inactivate tumor suppressor genes and contribute to the development of malignancy. The term *epigenetic* refers to the inheritance of genetic information on the basis of gene expression levels, and these changes are employed by mechanisms other than mutations in the primary nucleotide sequence of the DNA. The epigenetic mechanisms that modify gene expression levels include methylation of clusters of cytosine and guanine residues, known as CpG-islands, in the promoter regions of genes, histone modification, and chromatin remodeling (31,32). As the molecular evidence emerged that DNA methylation was a powerful mechanism for inactivating tumor suppressor genes and that it was a potentially reversible process, there has been significant clinical interest in developing inhibitors of DNA methylation as novel therapeutic agents. Recently, with regard to the myelodysplastic syndromes (MDS), the U.S. Food and Drug Administration approved azacitidine as the first in a new class of drugs, the demethylating agents, for the treatment of MDS, and a recent large randomized clinical trial shows improved survival (33).

To date, more than 20 tumor suppressor genes have been identified (6). The first tumor suppressor gene to be identified was the retinoblastoma (RB1) tumor suppressor gene (34). The RB1 gene, together with p107 and p130, corepress transcription of genes that regulate signal transduction pathways that govern cell-cycle progression, apoptosis, and differentiation (35). The RB1 gene product (pRb) utilizes a complex array of protein interactions to govern these processes. More than 100 proteins have been reported to interact with pRb, though the most-studied protein partners have been the E2F transcription factors and various viral oncoproteins, including the Large T antigen of simian virus 40 (SV40) and the E7 protein encoded by the oncogenic human papillomaviruses (36). Germline inactivation of RB1 causes the familial pediatric cancer retinoblastoma, and somatic loss of RB1 is common in many types of human cancer, including breast cancer and sarcomas (37–39). In addition, work from a number of laboratories has demonstrated that the key proteins in the pRb regulatory pathway may be mutated in almost 100% of human tumors (40–43). The p53 tumor suppressor gene will be discussed in the cell cycle portion of this chapter.

Caretaker Genes

The caretaker genes are involved in preserving DNA repair mechanisms and thereby protecting the genome from the various environmental and chemical compounds that cause damage to the nucleotide bases, sugars, and phosphate groups of the DNA. When the caretaker genes are mutated, all of the genes in the cell have an increased rate of mutation, including the proto-oncogenes and tumor suppressor genes. Hereditary nonpolyposis colorectal cancer (HNPCC) is an autosomal-dominant colon cancer syndrome. The mutation event in HNPCC is an inactivating germline mutation in one of the DNA mismatch repair (MMR) genes. Patients who inherit the germline mutation are at increased risk for colorectal cancers, uterine and ovarian cancers, gastric cancers, urinary tract cancers, and some brain tumors (44). Other examples of human disorders that involve a mutation in a caretaker gene and result in instability of the genome are Fanconi anemia, ataxia telangiectasia, Bloom syndrome, and xeroderma pigmentosum.

TABLE 1.1
Common Familial Cancer Syndromes and the Inherited Affected Gene

INHERITED GENE	FAMILIAL SYNDROME
Rb1	Retinoblastoma and osteosarcoma
TP53	Li-Fraumeni syndrome
WT1	Wilms tumor
VHL	Von-Hippel Lindau syndrome—renal cell carcinoma
BRCA1 and BRCA2	Breast cancer and ovarian cancer
APC	Familial adenomatous polyposis; colorectal tumors
MMR	Hereditary nonpolyposis-colorectal cancer
NF1	Von Recklinghausen disease; neurofibromatosis type1; schwannoma and glioma
NF2	Neurofibromatosis type 2; acoustic neuroma and meningiomas

FAMILIAL CANCER SYNDROMES

While the majority of cancers develop as a result of acquired somatic mutations in the genome, a small percentage (5%–10%) of cancer syndromes develop as a result of inherited mutations. Typically, a specific organ is affected, and the patient develops the cancer at a much younger age than the general population. Some of the common familial cancer syndromes are listed in Table 1.1 with the corresponding affected gene.

RNA AND DNA TUMOR VIRUSES

DNA and RNA viruses were studied extensively in the 1970s, as they were thought to be the key agents that caused cancer (45,46). Ultimately, research revealed that only a minority of cancers is caused by viruses; however, the study of RNA and DNA viruses exposed the machinations of cellular growth control pathways and led to the current concepts of the genetic basis of cancer. Though the mechanism of action of these various viruses are different in regard to how they infect a human cell and integrate into the genome, the end result is either activation of a growth-promoting pathway or inhibition of a tumor suppressor. We know now that certain viruses are true etiologic agents of human cancers, including human papillomavirus (cervical carcinoma), hepatitis B and C viruses (hepatocellular carcinoma), Epstein-Barr virus (Burkitt lymphoma), and human T-cell leukemia virus type I (T-cell leukemia).

GENOMIC TECHNOLOGY TO STUDY HUMAN CANCER

High-density complementary DNA (cDNA) microarrays for "profiling" gene expression allow for the simultaneous analysis of thousands of known human genes from a biologic specimen in a single experiment (47–49). In fact, with the present technology, the gene expression levels of the entire human genome can be represented in a single experiment. This technology has been utilized by nearly all fields of cancer research, as it has provided a more comprehensive analysis of the genetic changes that occur in cancer cells and identified novel disease genes for many cancer types and cancer mechanisms. In addition, this technology has been used to classify several common cancer types at the molecular level. Current studies in many laboratories around the world are using these novel classification models to predict clinical outcomes and to propose new molecular targets for therapy (50–58). The first randomized clinical trials [The Trial Assigning IndividuaLized Options for Treatment (TAILORx) and Microarray In Node-negative Disease may Avoid ChemoTherapy (MINDACT)] using the gene expression data to make treatment decisions for patients with breast cancer are underway in the United States, Canada, and Europe (59,60).

Gene expression profiling using cDNA microarray technology is one method to obtain a more comprehensive view of the consequences of genetic changes in the cancer cell. Currently, many other microarray platforms have been developed, including oligonucleotide microarrays (61,62), microarrays of bacterial artificial chromosome (BAC) clones (63), comparative genomic hybridization (CGH) to examine high-resolution DNA copy number, and oligonucleotide single-nucleotide polymorphism (SNP) arrays that report both copy number and genotype in the same hybridization (64–66), but the principle for all of these types of microarrays is essentially the same.

A brief description of gene expression profiling is described next and is illustrated in Figure 1.1, as it is the most utilized of the genomic technologies. Gene expression profiling uses RNA from a sample of interest (tumor specimen) and a common reference source of RNA. The RNA is differentially labeled using a single round of reverse transcription and incorporating fluorescently labeled nucleotides. The fluorescently labeled reference cDNA and tumor cDNA is pooled and hybridized to the clones, or probes, on the microarray (the glass slide—Fig. 1.1A). Each clone is derived from a specific sequence of an individual human gene and located at a unique position on the array surface. The glass slide is scanned with a confocal laser microscope

A
Prepare cDNA Probe   Prepare Microarray

B

C
Tumors

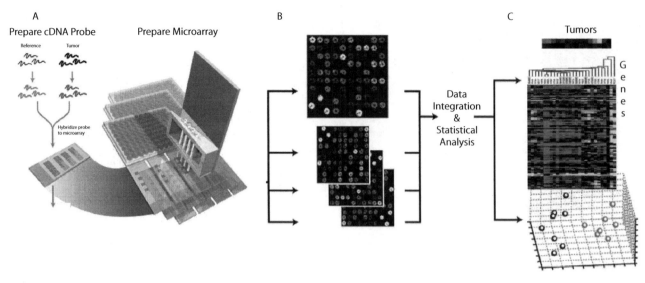

FIGURE 1.1

Gene expression profiling technology. A: Total RNA from the reference source and the tumor is fluorescently labeled with either Cye-3 or Cye-5-dUTP using a single round of reverse transcription. The fluorescently labeled cDNAs are pooled and allowed to hybridize to the clones on the array. B: The slide is then scanned with a confocal laser–scanning microscope to measure the fluorescence pattern, monochrome images from the scanner are imported into specialized software, and the images are colored and merged for each hybridization with RNA from the tumor and reference cells. C: Several statistical methods are used to visualize the expression patterns between tumor samples.

to measure the fluorescence ratio of each gene. The data from a single hybridization experiment represents the abundance of each specific gene transcript, and is viewed as a normalized ratio of each gene in each sample enumerated as either a ratio to a reference sample or as an absolute intensity value. Normalization is required for proper data analysis because differences exist in labeling and detection efficiencies of the fluorescent labels and differences exist in the quantity of RNA from the various samples. Once the ratios have been normalized, the experiment can be examined for differential gene expression. The data is then imported into statistical software programs, and the information that comes from the array is exhibited as a pseudocolor image (Fig. 1.1B). Typically, genes overexpressed in the tumor are shown in red and genes with decreased expression in the tumor are shown in green. Visualization tools are common methods used to represent the data generated from microarray experiments. Because many genes with many different expression patterns are being assayed in each experiment, these visualization tools are helpful for representing the data in a format that can produce biologic input. Two-dimensional hierarchical clustering dendograms are a frequently used method for viewing gene expression data (Fig. 1.1C). In general, the dendogram is a two-dimensional matrix where the tumor samples constitute the columns and the genes constitute the rows. The matrix makes it possible to quickly recognize the areas where highly corre-

lated expression sets of genes differentiate the sample types.

CELL CYCLE CONTROL

Cell division is tightly controlled through the complex interaction of multiple proteins to ensure the faithful reproduction of each component of the cell cycle—cell growth, chromosome replication, and mitosis. To guarantee the fidelity of the process, safeguards exist to prevent errors or to correct them when they occur. Genetic mutations that modify proteins that control cell-cycle regulation can weaken the safeguards, and, over time, as mutations accumulate, can result in genomic instability and ultimately lead to malignant transformation and unrestrained cell growth.

The cell cycle is separated into four phases: G_1 (gap 1), S (synthetic), G_2 (gap 2), and M (mitotic) or mitosis (67). During S phase, DNA synthesis occurs, and in M phase, the mother cell is divided into two daughter cells. The intervening gap phases, G_1 and G_2, allow for cell growth and regulatory inputs. Specifically, these gap phases of the cell cycle integrate complex signals in order to determine whether the cell should proceed into S phase and M phase, respectively, allowing the cell to make a decision to stop within the gap phases and therefore not interrupt chromosome replication and/or chromosome segregation.

Work from a number of laboratories utilizing various experimental model systems has significantly advanced our understanding of cell-cycle control by identifying many of the genes and signaling pathways that regulate the cell cycle (68,69). Exploiting the budding yeast *Saccharomyces cerevisiae* as a model system and creating conditional mutations (termed *cell division cycle*, or cdc mutations) that impaired specific phases of the cell cycle, Lee Hartwell and colleagues discovered the majority of genes that were required for regulating cell-cycle progression (68). The significance of this finding was that it demonstrated for the first time that the cell cycle is organized through a series of dependent reactions, and in order for its accurate execution, the completion of one event is required for the beginning of the next. A key finding extending from these studies was the discovery of the Cdc2 protein kinase by Nurse and colleagues (70,71). This kinase was first identified in the fission yeast *Schizosaccharomyces pombe* and later in budding yeast and was found to be the key regulator of the G_1/S and G_2/M phase transition points (72–76). This work provided the cornerstone for an entire field of molecular biology and genetics, and highlighted the role of Cdc2 in each of the major cell-cycle transitions. The next breakthrough in cell-cycle biology came with the discovery of a family of proteins in metazoans that were homologous to the yeast Cdc2, the cyclin-dependent kinases (Cdk) (77). Like Cdc2, the primary function of the Cdks is to provide information to the cell, allowing for successful passage through the cell cycle, ie, the G_1/S-phase transition, as well as the G_2/M transition (78). In fact, each phase of the cell cycle has a corresponding unique pattern of Cdk activity. The Cdks consist of a catalytic subunit (the Cdk) and a regulatory activating subunit (the cyclin). The catalytic Cdk subunit is without intrinsic enzymatic activity and thus requires the binding of the cyclin subunit in a heterodimeric conformation for full activation of the protein kinase domain. The kinase activity of the Cdk is further regulated through phosphorylation and dephosphorylation of conserved amino acid residues (usually serine or threonine) and through the binding of specific inhibitory proteins (Cdk-inhibitory proteins), specifically the INK4 proteins (p15, p16, p18, p19) and Cip/Kip proteins (p21, p27, p57).

As mentioned, safeguard mechanisms exist to regulate the timing of the cell cycle, specifically at the transition points, and to suspend progression of the cell cycle in order to remove and repair DNA damage when it occurs in order to eliminate genetic mutations during cell division and preserve genomic integrity. These biochemical regulatory pathways are termed *cell-cycle checkpoints* (79–81). Disabling the checkpoint pathways through mutations in key genes is thought to bring about the genomic instability seen in cancer cells.

The enzymes that mediate DNA replication and the segregation of chromosomes during mitosis are mostly responsible for the accurate transmission of genetic information. Though these enzymes work with great precision, they have an intrinsic error rate and cause genetic mistakes. Additionally, metabolic byproducts or exogenous exposure to certain chemicals or radiation can lead to DNA damage. Depending on the phase of the cell cycle that DNA damage occurs and is sensed, cell-cycle progression can be blocked at multiple points: prior to S-phase (G_1 DNA damage checkpoint response), during S-phase (intra-S phase DNA damage checkpoint response or DNA replication checkpoint), and prior to M-phase entry (G_2 DNA damage checkpoint response or the mitotic spindle integrity checkpoint). Otherwise, unrepaired DNA damage causes physical barriers (ie, chemical adducts and/or double-stranded breaks) to DNA replication forks, leading to replication that is predisposed to errors and followed by segregation of abnormal chromosomes during mitosis.

Though the precise molecular mechanisms for all of the checkpoint pathways are not completely understood, the G_1 DNA damage checkpoint is the best studied. Several mammalian genes regulate the DNA damage checkpoint: mutated in ataxia telangiectasia (ATM), ataxia telangiectasia and Rad-3 related (ATR), TP53, and p21. Of these, the tumor suppressor gene, TP53, is the most thoroughly studied, as well as the most commonly mutated gene in sporadically occurring human tumors (82). The human TP53 gene is located on the short arm of human chromosome 17 band 13, and the gene expressed encodes a transcription factor that is activated in response to DNA damage, such as nucleotide mismatches and double-stranded breaks. Specifically, accumulation of the p53 protein causes the cells to undergo G_1 arrest and prevents cells from entering S-phase and replicating a damaged chromosome (83). TP53 also mediates apoptosis and regulates the cellular response to DNA damage caused by ultraviolet irradiation, g-irradiation, and some chemotherapeutic agents. As mentioned, inactivating mutations of the TP53 gene have been observed in most human tumors, including osteosarcomas, soft-tissue sarcomas, rhabdomyosarcomas, leukemias, brain tumors, and lung and breast carcinomas. Germline mutations of the TP53 gene account for the majority of cases of the autosomal dominant disorder the Li-Fraumeni syndrome.

THE BIOLOGY OF HUMAN CANCER METASTASIS

Cancer metastasis is a complex multistep process and requires multiple genetic changes in the tumor cell in order for it to acquire all of the capabilities necessary to colonize a distant organ (84,85). In addition, new data is emerging that identifies genetic changes in the tumor stroma that assists in the survival of the invading tumor cell and helps to ensure stability in the distant organ (86). Though the exact genetic mutations that are necessary for the metastatic phenotype are mostly unknown, the general pathways that are involved have been studied intensely (87).

The traditional model of cancer metastasis involves the following basic steps: The cancer cell in the epithelium detaches from its neighboring cells, usually through the loss of E-cadherin, a member of the cadherin family of cell-cell adhesion molecules (88), and acquires motility to cross the basal lamina, typically by activating the signal transduction pathways that are mediated by the integrins (89). At this point, the tumor cell must also recruit new blood vessel formation, the process of angiogenesis (90). The tumor cells accomplish angiogenesis by producing powerful angiogenic factors, such as fibroblast growth factor (FGF) and vascular endothelial growth factor (VEGF). Angiogenesis creates a vascular system around the tumor and allows the tumor to grow to a larger size. The newly formed vascular system also provides a way for tumor cells to migrate into the bloodstream and subsequently to penetrate through them, a process termed intravasation. Intravasation is thought to be mediated by the microenvironment of the bloodstream, such as oxygen tension, blood pH, or a chemotactic gradient, and possibly augmented by the transcription factor Twist (91). The tumor cells circulating in the bloodstream must evade immune surveillance. Eventually the circulating tumor cells then arrest in the capillary bed and are able to grow intravascularly. The presence of the tumor cells in the blood vessels are thought to cause a physical disruption of the vessels and lead to penetration of the tumor cells out of the vessels and into the organ parenchyma, a process referred to as extravasation (92). Recently, some molecular mechanisms of extravasation have been uncovered (93–98). Lastly, there is colonization of the distant organ. This step alone is a complex process and involves not only the genetic transformation of the cancer cell, but it is thought that the cancer cell also sets in motion specific adaptations of the distant tissue stroma that will come to house the metastatic tumor cells.

This distant coordination of the stroma by the primary tumor cell may help to explain the clinical observation that certain tumor types have a preference for specific metastatic target organs. For example, in breast cancer, the bone is a significant site for metastasis and causes osteolytic lesions. The preference of breast cancer cells to metastasize to the bone is thought to be mediated by specific factors (parathyroid hormone-related protein, TNF-α, IL-1, IL6, IL8, and IL11) secreted by the tumor cells that activate osteoclasts and degrade the bone matrix. Then, once the invading tumor cells degrade the bone matrix, growth factors, such as transforming growth factor-β (TGF-β), are secreted from the bone matrix and further stimulate proliferation of the tumor cells (99–101). Similarly, prostate cancer has a tendency towards bone metastasis, though in this case, the cancer cells result in osteoblastic bone lesions. Though the precise genes that regulate prostate cancer metastasis are unknown, the proposed mechanism of regulation is similar to that described for breast cancer metastasis: The prostate tumor cells secrete paracrine factors that stimulate the osteoblasts to proliferate and cause bone remodeling, and the osteoblasts make factors that further fuel the growth of prostate tumor cells (102).

The lung, liver, and brain are other common target organs of metastasis for many solid tumors. Though extensive animal models have been developed, the mechanisms for the organ-selective metastasis are not yet thoroughly understood at the molecular level. Recent data from gene expression analysis is beginning to identify novel genes that are thought to be responsible for organ-selective metastasis in breast cancer (103,104).

It is important to realize that the single cells that form the tumor metastasis can grow fast and take over the organ quickly; in other cases, the metastatic tumors remain small and dormant for months to years. This latency is referred to as *metastatic dormancy*. Eventually, however, the metastatic tumor will expand and cause the death of the patient. In fact, metastatic cancer of any origin is generally not curable and complications from metastasis account for 90% of deaths from solid tumors. More importantly, however, the metastatic cascade offers multiple targets for therapeutic attack. For example, the angiogenesis inhibitor bevacizumab, a recombinant monoclonal antibody that targets the activity of the VEGF, when used in combination with standard chemotherapy in patients with metastatic colon cancer, has improved overall survival (105). At the root of the complexity of the metastatic cascade lies the interplay between the unique tumor microenvironment and genetic predisposition. Current research by many investigators in the field of metastasis involves developing a new paradigm that would reconcile the traditional model with recent genetic data (98).

References

1. Hanahan D, Weinberg RA. The hallmarks of cancer. *Cell.* 2000;100(1):57–70.
2. Vogelstein B, Kinzler KW. The multistep nature of cancer. *Trends Genet.* 1993;9(4):138–141.

3. Temin HM, Mizutani S. RNA-dependent DNA polymerase in virions of Rous sarcoma virus. *Nature.* 1970;226(5252):1211–1213.

4. Baltimore D. RNA-dependent DNA polymerase in virions of RNA tumour viruses. *Nature.* 1970;226(5252):1209–1211.

5. Stehelin D, Varmus HE, Bishop JM, Vogt PK. DNA related to the transforming gene(s) of avian sarcoma viruses is present in normal avian DNA. *Nature.* 1976;260(5547):170–173.

6. Hesketh. *The Oncogene and Tumor Suppressor Gene Facts Book*, 2nd ed. San Diego: Academic Press; 1997.

7. Downward J. Targeting RAS signalling pathways in cancer therapy. *Nature Rev.* 2003;3(1):11–22.

8. Bos JL. Ras oncogenes in human cancer: a review. *Cancer Res.* 1989;49(17):4682–4689.

9. Collins S, Groudine M. Amplification of endogenous myc-related DNA sequences in a human myeloid leukaemia cell line. *Nature.* 1982;298(5875):679–681.

10. Dalla-Favera R, Wong-Staal F, Gallo RC. Onc gene amplification in promyelocytic leukaemia cell line HL-60 and primary leukaemic cells of the same patient. *Nature.* 1982;299(5878):61–63.

11. Cole MD. The myc oncogene: its role in transformation and differentiation. *Annu Rev Genet.* 1986;20:361–384.

12. Henriksson M, Luscher B. Proteins of the Myc network: essential regulators of cell growth and differentiation. *Adv Cancer Res.* 1996;68:109–182.

13. Schmidt ML, Lukens JN, Seeger RC, et al. Biologic factors determine prognosis in infants with stage IV neuroblastoma: a prospective Children's Cancer Group study. *J Clin Oncol.* 2000;18(6):1260–1268.

14. Yang-Feng TL, Schechter AL, Weinberg RA, Francke U. Oncogene from rat neuro/glioblastomas (human gene symbol NGL) is located on the proximal long arm of human chromosome 17 and EGFR is confirmed at 7p13-q11.2 (Abstract). *Cytogenet Cell Genet.* 1985;40:784.

15. Coussens L, Yang-Feng TL, Liao YC, et al. Tyrosine kinase receptor with extensive homology to EGF receptor shares chromosomal location with neu oncogene. *Science.* 1985;230(4730):1132–1139.

16. Slamon DJ, Clark GM, Wong SG, Levin WJ, Ullrich A, McGuire WL. Human breast cancer: correlation of relapse and survival with amplification of the HER-2/neu oncogene. *Science.* 1987;235(4785):177–182.

17. Rowley JD. The critical role of chromosome translocations in human leukemias. *Annu Rev Genet.* 1998;32:495–519.

18. Rabbitts TH. Perspective: chromosomal translocations can affect genes controlling gene expression and differentiation—why are these functions targeted? *J Path.* 1999;187(1):39–42.

19. Nowell PC, Hungerford D. A minute chromosome in human chronic granulocytic leukemia [abstract]. *Science.* 1960;132:1497.

20. Rowley JD. Letter: a new consistent chromosomal abnormality in chronic myelogenous leukaemia identified by quinacrine fluorescence and Giemsa staining. *Nature.* 1973;243(5405):290–293.

21. Heisterkamp N, Stephenson JR, Groffen J, et al. Localization of the c-ab1 oncogene adjacent to a translocation break point in chronic myelocytic leukaemia. *Nature.* 1983;306(5940):239–242.

22. Druker BJ, Talpaz M, Resta DJ, et al. Efficacy and safety of a specific inhibitor of the BCR-ABL tyrosine kinase in chronic myeloid leukemia. *New Eng J Med.* 2001;344(14):1031–1037.

23. Rowley JD. Identification of a translocation with quinacrine fluorescence in a patient with acute leukemia. *Annales de genetique.* 1973;16(2):109–112.

24. Nucifora G, Rowley JD. AML1 and the 8;21 and 3;21 translocations in acute and chronic myeloid leukemia. *Blood.* 1995;86(1):1–14.

25. Tenen DG, Hromas R, Licht JD, Zhang DE. Transcription factors, normal myeloid development, and leukemia. *Blood.* 1997;90(2):489–519.

26. Rowley JD, Golomb HM, Dougherty C. 15/17 translocation, a consistent chromosomal change in acute promyelocytic leukaemia. *Lancet.* 1977;1(8010):549–550.

27. Warrell RP, Jr., Frankel SR, Miller WH, Jr., et al. Differentiation therapy of acute promyelocytic leukemia with tretinoin (all-trans-retinoic acid). *N Engl J Med.* 1991;324(20):1385–1393.

28. Knudson AG, Jr. Mutation and cancer: statistical study of retinoblastoma. *Proc Natl Acad Sci USA.* 1971;68(4):820–823.

29. Comings DE. A general theory of carcinogenesis. *Proc Natl Acad Sci USA.* 1973;70(12):3324–3328.

30. Dryja TP, Rapaport JM, Joyce JM, Petersen RA. Molecular detection of deletions involving band q14 of chromosome 13 in retinoblastomas. *Proc Natl Acad Sci USA.* 1986;83(19):7391–7394.

31. Feinberg AP. Epigenetics at the epicenter of modern medicine. *JAMA.* 2008;299(11):1345–1350.

32. Gal-Yam EN, Saito Y, Egger G, Jones PA. Cancer epigenetics: modifications, screening, and therapy. *Annu Rev Med.* 2008;59:267–280.

33. Kaminskas E, Farrell A, Abraham S, et al. Approval summary: azacitidine for treatment of myelodysplastic syndrome subtypes. *Clin Cancer Res.* 2005;11(10):3604–3608.

34. Whyte P, Buchkovich KJ, Horowitz JM, et al. Association between an oncogene and an anti-oncogene: the adenovirus E1A proteins bind to the retinoblastoma gene product. *Nature.* 1988;334(6178):124–129.

35. Weinberg RA. The retinoblastoma protein and cell cycle control. *Cell.* 1995;81(3):323–330.

36. Morris EJ, Dyson NJ. Retinoblastoma protein partners. *Adv Cancer Res.* 2001;82:1–54.

37. Friend SH, Bernards R, Rogelj S, et al. A human DNA segment with properties of the gene that predisposes to retinoblastoma and osteosarcoma. *Nature.* 1986;323(6089):643–646.

38. Friend SH, Horowitz JM, Gerber MR, et al. Deletions of a DNA sequence in retinoblastomas and mesenchymal tumors: organization of the sequence and its encoded protein. *Proc Natl Acad Sci USA.* 1987;84(24):9059–9063.

39. Horowitz JM, Park SH, Bogenmann E, et al. Frequent inactivation of the retinoblastoma anti-oncogene is restricted to a subset of human tumor cells. *Proc Natl Acad Sci USA.* 1990;87(7):2775–2779.

40. Jiang W, Zhang YJ, Kahn SM, et al. Altered expression of the cyclin D1 and retinoblastoma genes in human esophageal cancer. *Proc Natl Acad Sci USA.* 1993;90(19):9026–9030.

41. Lee EY, To H, Shew JY, Bookstein R, Scully P, Lee WH. Inactivation of the retinoblastoma susceptibility gene in human breast cancers. *Science (New York, NY).* 1988;241(4862):218–221.

42. Mori T, Miura K, Aoki T, Nishihira T, Mori S, Nakamura Y. Frequent somatic mutation of the MTS1/CDK4I (multiple tumor suppressor/cyclin-dependent kinase 4 inhibitor) gene in esophageal squamous cell carcinoma. *Cancer Res.* 1994;54(13):3396–3397.

43. Kamb A, Gruis NA, Weaver-Feldhaus J, et al. A cell cycle regulator potentially involved in genesis of many tumor types. *Science (New York, NY).* 1994;264(5157):436–440.

44. Vogelstein B, Kinzler KW. *The Genetic Basis of Human Cancer*, 2nd ed. New York. McGraw Hill Companies, Inc; 2002.

45. Ellermann V, Bang O. Experimentelle Leukaamie bei Huhnern. *Zentralb Bakteriol.* 1908;46:595–609.

46. Rous P. A transmissible avian neoplasm: sarcoma of the common fowl. *J Exp Med.* 1910;12:696–705.

47. Augenlicht LH, Wahrman MZ, Halsey H, Anderson L, Taylor J, Lipkin M. Expression of cloned sequences in biopsies of human colonic tissue and in colonic carcinoma cells induced to differentiate in vitro. *Cancer Res.* 1987;47(22):6017–6021.

48. Schena M, Shalon D, Davis RW, Brown PO. Quantitative monitoring of gene expression patterns with a complementary DNA microarray. *Science (New York, NY).* 1995;270(5235):467–470.

49. DeRisi J, Penland L, Brown PO, et al. Use of a cDNA microarray to analyse gene expression patterns in human cancer. *Nat Genet.* 1996;14(4):457–460.

50. Alizadeh AA, Eisen MB, Davis RE, et al. Distinct types of diffuse large B-cell lymphoma identified by gene expression profiling. *Nature.* 2000;403(6769):503–511.

51. Dhanasekaran SM, Barrette TR, Ghosh D, et al. Delineation of prognostic biomarkers in prostate cancer. *Nature*. 2001;412(6849):822–826.

52. Khan J, Wei JS, Ringner M, et al. Classification and diagnostic prediction of cancers using gene expression profiling and artificial neural networks. *Nat Med*. 2001;7(6):673–679.

53. MacDonald TJ, Brown KM, LaFleur B, et al. Expression profiling of medulloblastoma: PDGFRA and the RAS/MAPK pathway as therapeutic targets for metastatic disease. *Nat Genet*. 2001;29(2):143–152.

54. Rosenwald A, Wright G, Chan WC, et al. The use of molecular profiling to predict survival after chemotherapy for diffuse large-B-cell lymphoma. *N Engl J Med*. 2002;346(25):1937–1947.

55. Shipp MA, Ross KN, Tamayo P, et al. Diffuse large B-cell lymphoma outcome prediction by gene-expression profiling and supervised machine learning. *Nat Med*. 2002;8(1):68–74.

56. Sorlie T, Perou CM, Tibshirani R, et al. Gene expression patterns of breast carcinomas distinguish tumor subclasses with clinical implications. *Proc Natl Acad Sci USA*. 2001;98(19):10869–10874.

57. van 't Veer LJ, Dai H, van de Vijver MJ, et al. Gene expression profiling predicts clinical outcome of breast cancer. *Nature*. 2002;415(6871):530–536.

58. van de Vijver MJ, He YD, van't Veer LJ, et al. A gene-expression signature as a predictor of survival in breast cancer. *N Engl J Med*. 2002;347(25):1999–2009.

59. TAILORx. http://www.cancer.gov/clinicaltrials/digestpage/TAILORx.

60. MINDACT. http://www.eortc.be/services/unit/mindact/MINDACT_websiteii.asp.

61. Lucito R, Healy J, Alexander J, et al. Representational oligonucleotide microarray analysis: a high-resolution method to detect genome copy number variation. *Genome Res*. 2003;13(10):2291–2305.

62. Carvalho B, Ouwerkerk E, Meijer GA, Ylstra B. High resolution microarray comparative genomic hybridisation analysis using spotted oligonucleotides. *J Clin Pathol*. 2004;57(6):644–646.

63. Pinkel D, Segraves R, Sudar D, et al. High resolution analysis of DNA copy number variation using comparative genomic hybridization to microarrays. *Nat Genet*. 1998;20(2):207–211.

64. Bignell GR, Huang J, Greshock J, et al. High-resolution analysis of DNA copy number using oligonucleotide microarrays. *Genome Res*. 2004;14(2):287–295.

65. Huang J, Wei W, Zhang J, et al. Whole genome DNA copy number changes identified by high density oligonucleotide arrays. *Hum Genomics*. 2004;1(4):287–299.

66. Zhao X, Li C, Paez JG, et al. An integrated view of copy number and allelic alterations in the cancer genome using single nucleotide polymorphism arrays. *Cancer Res*. 2004;64(9):3060–3071.

67. Howard A, Pelc SR. Nuclear incorporation of p32 as demonstrated by autoradiographs. *Exp Cell Res*. 1951;2(2):178–187.

68. Hartwell LH, Mortimer RK, Culotti J, Culotti M. Genetic control of the cell division cycle in yeast: V. Genetic Analysis of cdc Mutants. *Genetics*. 1973;74(2):267–286.

69. Nurse P. Universal control mechanism regulating onset of M-phase. *Nature*. 1990;344(6266):503–508.

70. Lee MG, Nurse P. Complementation used to clone a human homologue of the fission yeast cell cycle control gene cdc2. *Nature*. 1987;327(6117):31–35.

71. Nurse P, Bissett Y. Gene required in G1 for commitment to cell cycle and in G2 for control of mitosis in fission yeast. *Nature*. 1981;292(5823):558–560.

72. Hindley J, Phear GA. Sequence of the cell division gene CDC2 from Schizosaccharomyces pombe; patterns of splicing and homology to protein kinases. *Gene*. 1984;31(1–3):129–134.

73. Nurse P. Genetic control of cell size at cell division in yeast. *Nature*. 1975;256(5518):547–551.

74. Beach D, Durkacz B, Nurse P. Functionally homologous cell cycle control genes in budding and fission yeast. *Nature*. 1982;300(5894):706–709.

75. Reed SI, Wittenberg C. Mitotic role for the Cdc28 protein kinase of Saccharomyces cerevisiae. *Proc Natl Acad Sci USA*. 1990;87(15):5697–5701.

76. Piggott JR, Rai R, Carter BL. A bifunctional gene product involved in two phases of the yeast cell cycle. *Nature*. 1982;298(5872):391–393.

77. Meyerson M, Enders GH, Wu CL, et al. A family of human cdc2-related protein kinases. *EMBO J*. 1992;11(8):2909–2917.

78. Harper JW, Adams PD. Cyclin-dependent kinases. *Chem Rev*. 2001;101(8):2511–2526.

79. Hartwell L, Weinert T, Kadyk L, Garvik B. Cell cycle checkpoints, genomic integrity, and cancer. *Cold Spring Harb Symp Quant Biol*. 1994;59:259–263.

80. Elledge SJ, Harper JW. Cdk inhibitors: on the threshold of checkpoints and development. *Curr Opin Cell Biol*. 1994;6(6):847–852.

81. Weinert T, Hartwell L. Control of G2 delay by the rad9 gene of Saccharomyces cerevisiae. *J Cell Sci*. 1989;12:145–148.

82. Hollstein M, Sidransky D, Vogelstein B, Harris CC. p53 mutations in human cancers. *Science (New York, NY)*. 1991;253(5015):49–53.

83. Kuerbitz SJ, Plunkett BS, Walsh WV, Kastan MB. Wild-type p53 is a cell cycle checkpoint determinant following irradiation. *Proc Natl Acad Sci USA*. 1992;89(16):7491–7495.

84. Fidler IJ. The pathogenesis of cancer metastasis: the "seed and soil" hypothesis revisited. *Nat Rev*. 2003;3(6):453–458.

85. Chambers AF, Groom AC, MacDonald IC. Dissemination and growth of cancer cells in metastatic sites. *Nat Rev*. 2002;2(8):563–572.

86. Gupta GP, Nguyen DX, Chiang AC, et al. Mediators of vascular remodelling co-opted for sequential steps in lung metastasis. *Nature*. 2007;446(7137):765–770.

87. Pantel K, Brakenhoff RH. Dissecting the metastatic cascade. *Nat Rev*. 2004;4(6):448–456.

88. Christofori G. New signals from the invasive front. *Nature*. 2006;441(7092):444–450.

89. Guo W, Giancotti FG. Integrin signalling during tumour progression. *Nat Rev Mol Cell Biol*. 2004;5(10):816–826.

90. Hanahan D, Folkman J. Patterns and emerging mechanisms of the angiogenic switch during tumorigenesis. *Cell*. 1996;86(3):353–364.

91. Yang J, Mani SA, Donaher JL, et al. Twist, a master regulator of morphogenesis, plays an essential role in tumor metastasis. *Cell*. 2004;117(7):927–939.

92. Al-Mehdi AB, Tozawa K, Fisher AB, Shientag L, Lee A, Muschel RJ. Intravascular origin of metastasis from the proliferation of endothelium-attached tumor cells: a new model for metastasis. *Nat Med*. 2000;6(1):100–102.

93. Kim YJ, Borsig L, Varki NM, Varki A. P-selection deficiency attenuates tumor growth and metastasis. *Proc Natl Acad Sci USA*. 1998;95(16):9325–9330.

94. Khanna C, Wan X, Bose S, et al. The membrane-cytoskeleton linker ezrin is necessary for osteosarcoma metastasis. *Nat Med*. 2004;10(2):182–186.

95. Yu Y, Khan J, Khanna C, Helman L, Meltzer PS, Merlino G. Expression profiling identifies the cytoskeletal organizer ezrin and the developmental homeoprotein Six-1 as key metastatic regulators. *Nat Med*. 2004;10(2):175–181.

96. Criscuoli ML, Nguyen M, Eliceiri BP. Tumor metastasis but not tumor growth is dependent on Src-mediated vascular permeability. *Blood*. 2005;105(4):1508–1514.

97. Muller A, Homey B, Soto H, et al. Involvement of chemokine receptors in breast cancer metastasis. *Nature*. 2001;410(6824):50–56.

98. Gupta GP, Massague J. Cancer metastasis: building a framework. *Cell*. 2006;127(4):679–695.

99. Mundy GR. Metastasis to bone: causes, consequences and therapeutic opportunities. *Nat Rev*. 2002;2(8):584–593.

100. Boyle WJ, Simonet WS, Lacey DL. Osteoclast differentiation and activation. *Nature*. 2003;423(6937):337–342.

101. Kang Y, Siegel PM, Shu W, et al. A multigenic program mediating breast cancer metastasis to bone. *Cancer Cell.* 2003;3(6):537–549.

102. Logothetis CJ, Lin SH. Osteoblasts in prostate cancer metastasis to bone. *Nat Rev.* 2005;5(1):21–28.

103. Minn AJ, Gupta GP, Siegel PM, et al. Genes that mediate breast cancer metastasis to lung. *Nature.* 2005;436(7050):518–524.

104. Saha S, Bardelli A, Buckhaults P, et al. A phosphatase associated with metastasis of colorectal cancer. *Science (New York, NY).* 2001;294(5545):1343–1346.

105. Hurwitz HI, Fehrenbacher L, Hainsworth JD, et al. Bevacizumab in combination with fluorouracil and leucovorin: an active regimen for first-line metastatic colorectal cancer. *J Clin Oncol.* 2005;23(15):3502–3508.

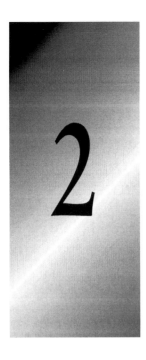

Principles of Chemotherapy

2

Vicky Makker
David Spriggs

Over the last two decades, there has been a steady improvement in the survival statistics for nearly all cancers due in large part to earlier detection and advances in surgery, radiation, and chemotherapy. In particular, chemotherapy has changed profoundly. While the entire discipline of medical oncology was founded on the management of serious toxicity, most of the newer agents that have been introduced into practice have had modified toxicity profiles with preserved efficacy (Table 2.1). Carboplatin has replaced cisplatin in many cancers, and the introduction of pegylated liposomal doxorubicin promises to do the same for anthracyclines. Nonetheless, the longer survival of patients with cancer has led to an increase in the chronic long-term toxicities associated with chemotherapy. The entire field is now increasingly focused on the problems of cancer survivors, and we are likely to see an expanding role for rehabilitation medicine in cancer centers and their programs.

In this chapter, we have focused primarily on the subacute and chronic toxicities associated with chemotherapy treatment. The acute toxicities, like myelosuppression and acute allergic reactions, are primarily the responsibility of the chemotherapist and unlikely to be treated by rehabilitation specialists. Rehabilitation practitioners, however, should be familiar with these acute toxicities. We have linked the characteristic organ toxicities to specific agents, both in the text and in tables, which should provide ready access to an

extensive literature. Clearly, the huge numbers of drug entities in clinical development will continue to cause novel toxicities that are not anticipated in this chapter, which focuses on approved drugs.

CARDIAC TOXICITY

Cardiomyopathy

Anthracyclines include daunorubicin, doxorubicin, epirubicin, and idarubicin, and are utilized in the treatment of breast cancer, ovarian cancer, endometrial cancer, soft tissue sarcomas, Hodgkin and non-Hodgkin lymphoma, non-small cell lung cancer (NSCLC) and small cell lung cancer (SCLC), hepatomas, thyroid cancer, and gastric cancer. The incidence of anthracycline-induced cardiotoxicity is related to the cumulative dose administered. The risk is increased in patients with underlying heart disease, when anthracyclines are used concurrently with other cardiotoxic agents or radiation, and in patients undergoing hematopoietic cell transplantation. Cardiovascular complications can arise acutely (during administration), early (several days to months following administration), or years to decades following exposure (Table 2.2).

Anthracyclines intercalate into deoxyribonucleic acid (DNA) of replicating cells, resulting in inhibition of DNA synthesis and inhibition of transcription

KEY POINTS

- Over the last two decades, there has been a steady improvement in the survival statistics for nearly all cancers due in large part to earlier detection and advances in surgery, radiation, and chemotherapy.
- Longer survival of patients with cancer has led to an increase in the chronic long-term toxicities associated with chemotherapy.
- Anthracycline-induced cardiovascular complications can arise acutely (during administration), early (several days to months following administration), or years to decades following exposure.
- Bleomycin therapy can result in life-threatening interstitial pulmonary fibrosis in up to 10% of patients.
- Cisplatin is used to treat testicular, ovarian, bladder, esophageal, and head and neck cancers, as well as non-small cell lung cancer (NSCLC), small cell lung cancer (SCLC), non-Hodgkin lymphoma, and trophoblastic disease, and is commonly associated with peripheral neuropathy and ototoxicity.
- Lhermitte sign is a shocklike, nonpainful sensation

of paresthesias radiating from the back to the feet during neck flexion, can develop in patients receiving cisplatin, and typically occurs after weeks or months of treatment.
- Taxane-induced motor and sensory neuropathies are cumulative and dose- and schedule-dependent.
- A peripheral neuropathy develops in approximately 75% of patients who receive prolonged thalidomide treatment.
- The dose-limiting toxicity of vincristine is an axonal neuropathy, which results from disruption of the microtubules within axons and interference with axonal transport.
- Chemotherapeutic agents can affect the glomerulus, tubules, interstitium, or the renal microvasculature, with clinical manifestations that range from an asymptomatic elevation of serum creatinine to acute renal failure requiring dialysis.
- Almost any chemotherapeutic agent can result in post-chemotherapy rheumatism, and this is a fairly common clinical phenomenon.

through inhibition of DNA-dependent ribonucleic acid (RNA) polymerase. These agents also inhibit topoisomerase II, which results in DNA fragmentation, and form cytotoxic free radicals, which result in single- and double-stranded DNA breaks with subsequent inhibition of DNA synthesis. Myocyte injury has been attributed to the production of toxic oxygen free radicals and an increase in oxidative stress, which cause lipid peroxidation of membranes. This, in turn, leads to vacuolation and myocyte replacement by fibrous tissue (1). Doxorubicin is also associated with a decrease of endogenous antioxidant enzymes, such as glutathione peroxidase, which are responsible for the scavenging of free radicals (2,3).

The strongest predictor of anthracycline-induced cardiotoxicity is cumulative dose administered, but age over 70, prior irradiation, concomitant administration of other chemotherapeutic agents (particularly paclitaxel and trastuzumab), concurrent chest irradiation, and underlying heart disease are also important factors (4–6). In addition, female gender has been demonstrated to be an independent risk factor (7).

Early reports in adults showed that with cumulative doxorubicin doses of 400, 550, and 700 mg/m^2 the percentage of patients who developed cardiotoxicity was 3%, 7%, and 18%, respectively (6). Subsequent series suggested that the incidence of

doxorubicin-related cardiotoxicity was underestimated in these studies. A report that included 630 patients treated with doxorubicin alone in three controlled trials estimated that as many as 26% of patients receiving a cumulative doxorubicin dose of 550 mg/m^2 would develop doxorubicin-related heart failure (8). The use of a single threshold dose has been replaced by monitoring for early evidence of cardiotoxicity using better surveillance techniques. Therapy thus should be stopped at a lower cumulative dose if there is evidence of cardiotoxicity.

Age extremes predispose to cardiotoxicity at lower cumulative anthracycline doses (8). In older patients, it is not clear whether preexisting heart disease increases susceptibility to anthracycline-induced damage or whether there is less functional reserve to tolerate additional myocardial damage. Prior mediastinal irradiation may increase the susceptibility to anthracycline-induced cardiotoxicity by inducing endothelial cell damage and compromising coronary artery blood flow. The magnitude of increased risk may depend upon the anthracycline dose. The administration of nonanthracycline agents that also cause cardiotoxicity may result in synergistic toxicity when anthracyclines are given concurrently, and the most important agents in this regard are the taxanes (paclitaxel and docetaxel) and trastuzumab.

TABLE 2.1

Alphabetical List of Common Chemotherapy Agents

GENERIC NAME	TRADE NAME	CLASSIFICATION
Albumin-bound paclitaxel	Abraxane	Taxane
Aldesleukin	Proleukin, Interleukin-2, IL-2	Biological response modifier
Alemtuzumab	Campath, Hexalen, Hexamethylmelamine, HMM	Anti-CD 52 monoclonal antibody altretamine, alkylating agent
Amifostine	Ethyol	Organic thiophosphate analog
Anastrozole	Arimidex, Trisonex	Nonsteroidal aromatase inhibitor arsenic trioxide antineoplastic differentiating agent
Asparaginase	Elspar, L-Asparaginase	Antitumor antibiotic
Bacillus Calmette-Guerin (BCG)	Immucyst, Oncotice	Biological response modifier
Bevacizumab	Avastin	Anti-VEGF monoclonal antibody
Bicalutamide	Casodex	Nonsteroidal antihormone
Bleomycin	Blenoxane	Antitumor antibiotic
Bortezomib	Velcade	Reversible inhibitor of 26S proteosome, cytotoxic
Busulfan	Myleran, Busulfex	Alkylating agent
Capecitabine	Xeloda	Antimetabolite, cytotoxic
Carboplatin	Paraplatin, CBDCA	Platinum
Carmustine	BCNU, Bischloronitrosurea, BICNU	Alkylating agent
Cetuximab	Erbitux	EGF-R tyrosine kinase inhibitor
Chlorambucil	Leukeran	Alkylating agent
Cisplatin	Platinol, CDDP, CIS-Diamminedichloroplatinum	Platinum
Cladribine	Leustatin, 2-Chlorodeoxy-adenosine, 2-CDA	Antimetabolite
Clofarabine	Clolar	Antimetabolite
Cyclophosphamide	Cytoxan, CTX	Alkylating agent
Cytarabine	Cytosar U, Cytosine-arabinoside, ARA-C	Antimetabolite
Dacarbazine	DTIC-DOME Carboxamide, DIC, Imidazole, Carboxamide	Alkylating agent
Dactinomycin	Cosmegen, Actinomycin-D	Antitumor antibiotic
Dasatinib	Sprycel	Signal transduction inhibitor
Daunorubicin	Cerubidine, Daunomycin, Ruidomycin	Anthracycline
Daunorubicin Liposome	Daunoxomed	Anthracycline
Decitabine	Dacogen, 5-AZA-2-Deoxycytidine	Antimetabolite
Denileukin Diftitox	Ontak	Biologic response modifier
Dexrazoxane	Zinccard	Cardioprotectant
Docetaxel	Taxotere	Taxane
Doxorubicin	Adriamycin	Anthracycline
Doxorubicin Liposome	Doxil	Anthracycline

(Continued)

TABLE 2.1 *Alphabetical List of Common Chemotherapy Agents, Continued*

GENERIC NAME	TRADE NAME	CLASSIFICATION
Epirubicin	Ellence, 4 Epidoxorubicin	Anthracycline
Erlotnib	Tarceva	ERF-R tyrosine kinase inhibitor
Estramustine	EMCYT, Estracyte	Alkylating agent
Etoposide	Vepesid, VP-16	Topoisomerase II inhibitor
Exemestane	AROMASIN	Aromatase inhibitor
Filgrastim	Neupogen, G-CSF 5-Fluro-2-deoxyuridine, FUDR	Recombinant human granulocyte colony-stimulating factor floxuridine, antimetabolite
Fludarabine	Fludara, 2-Furo-ARA-AMP	Antimetabolite
5-Flurouracil	Efudex, 5-FU	Antimetabolite
Flutamide	Eulexine	Nonsteroidal antiandrogen
Fulvestrant	Faslodex	Estrogen receptor antagonist
Gefitinib	Iressa	EGF-R tyrosine kinase inhibitor
Gemcitabine	Gemzar	Antimetabolite
Gemtuzumab Ozogamicin	Mylotarg	Anti-CD33 monoclonal antibody
Goserelin	Zoladex	Gonadotropin-releasing hormone analog
Hydroxyurea	Hydrea	Alkylating agent
Ibritumomab	Zevalin	Radiopharmaceutical monoclonal
Idarubicin	Idamycin, 4-Demethoxydaunorubicin	Anthracycline
Ifosfamide	IFEX, Isophosphamide	Alkylating agent
Imatinib	Gleevec	Bcr-Abl tyrosine kinase inhibitor
Interferon alfa	-Intron-A	Biologic response modifier
Irinotecan	Camptosar, CPT-II	Topoisomerase I inhibitor
Lenalidomide	Revlimid	Antiangiogenesis agent
Letrozole	Femara	Aromatase inhibitor
Leukovorin	Lederle Leukovorin	Folic acid metabolite
Leuprolide	Lupron	Gonadotropin-releasing hormone analog
Lomustine	CCNU, Bischloronitrosoure	Alkylating agent
Mechlorethamine	Mustargen, Nitrogen mustard	Alkylating agent
Megestrol	Megace	Synthetic progestin
Melphalan	Alkeran	Alkylating agent
Mercaptopurine	Purinethol, 6-MP	Antimetabolite
Mesna	Mesnex	Chemoprotective agent
Methotrexate	MTX, Amethopterin	Antimetabolite
Mitomycin-C	Mutamycin, mitomycin	Antitumor antibiotic
Mitotane	Lysodren	Adrenolytic agent
Mitoxantrone	Novantrone	Antitumor antibiotic
Nilutamide	Nilandron	Antiandrogen
Octreotide	Sandostatin	Somatostatin analog
Oxaliplatin	Eloxatin, dach-platinum, diaminocyclohexane platinum	Platinum

(Continued)

TABLE 2.1 *Alphabetical List of Common Chemotherapy Agents, Continued*

GENERIC NAME	TRADE NAME	CLASSIFICATION
Paclitaxel	Taxol	Antimicrotubule agent, taxane
Pamidronate	Aredia	Bisphosphonate
Panitumumab	Vectibix	Anti-EGFR monoclonal antibody
Pegylated filgrastim	Neulasta	Recombinant human granulocyte colony-stimulating factor
Pemetrexed	Alimta	Antifolate antimetabolite
Pentostatin NIPENT, Antimetabolite	2-deoxycoformycin, DCF	
Procarbazine	Matulane, N-methylhydrazine	Alkylating agent
Rituximab	Rituxan	Anti CD-20 monoclonal antibody
Sorafenib	Nexavar	Multitarget tyrosine kinase inhibitor
Streptozocin	Zanosar	Antitumor antibiotic
Sunitinib	Sutent	Multitarget tyrosine kinase inhibitor
Tamoxifen	Nolvadex	Antiestrogen
Temozolomide	Temodar	Alkylating agent
Thalidomide	Thalomid	Immunomodulator, antiangiogenesis factor
Thioguanine	6-thioguanine, 6-TG	Antimetabolite
Thiotepa	Thioplex	Alkylating agent
Topotecan	Hycamtin	Topoisomerase I inhibitor
Toremifene	Fareston	Antiestrogen
Tositumomab	Bexxar	Radiolabeled monoclonal antibody
Trastuzumab	Herceptin	Her2Neu monoclonal antibody
Tretinoin	Atra	Retinoid
Vinblastine	Velban	Vinca alkaloid
Vincristine	Oncovin	Vinca alkaloid
Vindesine	Eldisine	Vinca alkaloid
Vinorelbine	Navelbine	Vinca alkaloid

Three stages of anthracycline cardiotoxicity have been identified: acute, subacute, and late.

In acute toxicity, electrocardiographic abnormalities, ventricular dysfunction, an increase in plasma brain natriuretic peptide, and a pericarditis-myocarditis syndrome have been reported during or immediately after the administration of anthracyclines (9). These events are rare and seldom of clinical importance since they usually resolve within a week (10). The relationship between acute toxicity and the subsequent development of early and late cardiotoxicity is unclear.

In subacute toxicity, the appearance of heart failure can occur from days to months after the last anthracycline dose. The peak time for the appearance of clinical heart failure is three months after the last anthracycline dose, and mortality has been reported as high as 60% (5,6). More recently, survival in patients who develop heart failure has improved due to more aggressive medical management with medications such as angiotensin-converting enzyme (ACE) inhibitors and beta blockers.

In late toxicity, the onset of symptomatic heart failure can occur from 5 years to more than a decade after the last anthracycline dose. Serious arrhythmias, including ventricular tachycardia, ventricular fibrillation, and sudden cardiac death, have been identified in both symptomatic and asymptomatic patients with late cardiotoxicity. Late toxicity is primarily of concern where anthracyclines are used as part of a curative or adjuvant regimen. Late toxicity is most common in survivors of childhood malignancy, in whom late heart failure is due to a nonischemic dilated cardiomyopathy.

TABLE 2.2
Chemotherapy-Induced Cardiotoxicity

TOXICITY TYPE	AGENT	REFERENCES
Cardiomyopathy	Doxorubicin	(5,6,8,9)
	Epirubicin	(241)
	Trastuzumab	(13–16, 18, 19)
	Rituximab	(17)
	Bevacizumab	(7, 20)
	Cyclophosphamide	(11)
	Mitomycin	(242)
	Interferon-alfa	(25, 26)
	Sorafenib	(243)
	Sunitinib	(244)
	Imatinib	(245)
	Cisplatin	(246)
Rhythm disturbance	Paclitaxel	(27)
	Docetaxel	(247)
	Trastuzumab	(12)
	Ifosfamide	(11)
	Cisplatin	(246)
	Interferon-alfa	(22, 23)
	Methotrexate	(248)
	Cytarabine	(249)
	Interleukin-2	(34, 35)
	Arsenic Trioxide	(60)
	Alemtuzumab	(250)
	Rituximab	(17)
QT prolongation	Arsenic Trioxide	(48)
Vascular complications	Bleomycin	(251)
	Etoposide	(252)
	5-flurouracil	(39, 40)
	Capecitabine	(43)
	Vinca Alkaloids	(253, 254)
	Methotrexate	(248)
	Interleukin-2	(33)
	All-trans-retinoic acid	(255)
Hypertension	Bevacizumab	(44, 256)
	Sorafenib	(45)
	Sunitinib	(47)

In adults, other causes of heart failure must be excluded if delayed symptoms develop.

Approaches aimed at reducing the risk of anthracycline-induced cardiotoxicity have included the use of alternative administration schedules, the development of structural analogs (mitoxantrone, daunorubicin, idarubicin, and epirubicin), liposome encapsulation of the anthracycline molecule (liposomal doxorubicin), and the use of adjunctive cardioprotective agents (dexrazoxane).

The inability to develop safe ways to administer large doses of anthracyclines has made monitoring for the earliest evidence of cardiotoxicity necessary. Echocardiography and radionuclide angiography are the standard approaches for noninvasive monitoring. The prognosis in adults appears to be related to the severity of cardiac symptoms when cardiotoxicity is first diagnosed. Patients who present with clinical symptoms have a worse prognosis than those diagnosed with an asymptomatic decrease in left ventricular ejection fraction (LVEF).

Cyclophosphamide is a cell-cycle–nonspecific alkylating agent that is activated by the liver p450 cytochrome system and forms cross-links with DNA, resulting in inhibition of DNA synthesis. Cyclophosphamide is used for the treatment of breast cancer, non-Hodgkin lymphoma, chronic lymphocytic leukemia, ovarian cancer, bone and soft tissue sarcomas, and rhabdomyosarcoma, and has been associated with an acute cardiomyopathy. The incidence of cardiotoxicity may be particularly high in patients receiving cyclophosphamide as part of a high-dose chemotherapy program followed by autologous stem cell rescue. Other complications include hemorrhagic myopericarditis resulting in pericardial effusions, tamponade, and death, typically within the first week after treatment (11).

Trastuzumab is a recombinant humanized monoclonal antibody directed against the extracellular domain of the HER2/new human epidermal growth factor receptor, which down-regulates expression of HER2/new receptors and inhibits HER2/new intracellular signaling pathways. This receptor is overexpressed in 25%–30% of breast cancers, and in patients whose tumors overexpress HER2/neu, trastuzumab is effective, both as monotherapy and in combination with cytotoxic chemotherapy in the treatment of metastatic disease and in the adjuvant setting in combination with cytotoxic chemotherapy.

Trastuzumab-induced cardiomyopathy is most commonly manifested by an asymptomatic decrease in the LVEF and less often by clinical heart failure (11), though arrhythmias may also occur (12). The risk of any cardiac problem (asymptomatic decrease in LVEF or clinical heart failure) in patients receiving trastuzumab alone for metastatic breast cancer is between 2%–7% (13,14). The mechanism of trastuzumab-associated cardiac dysfunction is not fully understood, but data suggest that it is neither immune-mediated nor due to effects outside of the heart and that it does not result solely from exacerbation of anthracycline-induced cardiac dysfunction.

In a 2002 review of seven phase 2 and 3 trials of trastuzumab monotherapy involving 1,219 women, the incidence of cardiac dysfunction was between 3%–7%. The incidence of cardiomyopathy for patients receiving trastuzumab concurrently with chemotherapy was markedly higher in those receiving trastuzumab plus doxorubicin and cyclophosphamide (AC) than with AC alone (27% vs 8%, respectively). When trastuzumab was combined with paclitaxel, the increased risk of cardiomyopathy was substantially lower (13% vs 1% with paclitaxel alone). The incidence of moderate to severe heart failure (New York Heart Association [NYHA] class III to IV) was only 2%–4% with trastuzumab alone, 2% with paclitaxel plus trastuzumab (compared to 1% for paclitaxel alone), and 16% with AC plus trastuzumab (compared to 4% for AC alone) (14).

In randomized trials comparing chemotherapy plus trastuzumab with chemotherapy alone, a significant benefit for the addition of trastuzumab to adjuvant anthracycline-containing chemotherapy has been observed (15–18). In these trials, trastuzumab was administered sequentially after anthracyclines when anthracyclines were a component of the chemotherapy regimen due to concerns for increased cardiotoxicity. All trials included serial assessment of cardiac function at baseline, during, and after completion of treatment. Results suggest that approximately 5% of all patients treated with adjuvant trastuzumab, anthracycline, and taxane-containing therapy will develop some degree of cardiac dysfunction, 2% will develop symptomatic heart failure, and approximately 1% will develop NYHA class III or IV heart failure (19). These rates are substantially higher than those in control patients who did not receive trastuzumab.

In contrast to anthracycline-induced cardiotoxicity, trastuzumab-induced cardiotoxicity does not appear to be dose-related and usually responds to medical treatment for heart failure. Also, it may simply resolve with the discontinuation of trastuzumab (13,15). Continuation of trastuzumab therapy or resumption of treatment after resolution of cardiac abnormalities may be safe in some women with metastatic breast cancer who develop evidence of cardiac dysfunction (13,15). In the pivotal trial in women with metastatic breast cancer, 33 patients continued trastuzumab after developing cardiac dysfunction; of these, 21 (64%) had no further decrease in cardiac function (18).

Rituximab is a chimeric anti-CD 20 monoclonal antibody directed against the CD 20 antigen on malignant B lymphocytes. Rituximab is used to treat relapsed and/or refractory low-grade or follicular lymphoma and low-, intermediate- and high-grade non-Hodgkin lymphoma. Arrhythmias and angina have been reported during ≤1% of infusions, and acute infusion-related deaths occurring within 24th have a reported incidence of ≤0.1%. These deaths appear to be related to an infusion-related complex of hypoxia, pulmonary infiltrates, adult respiratory distress syndrome, myocardial infarction, ventricular fibrillation, and cardiogenic shock (17). Caution should be exercised when rituximab is used in patients with preexisting heart disease, as there is an increased risk of cardiotoxicity. Long-term cardiac toxicity has not been reported with rituximab administration.

Bevacizumab is a recombinant humanized monoclonal antibody directed against vascular endothelial growth factor (VEGF), blocking its activity. VEGF is a proangiogenic growth factor that is overexpressed in a myriad of solid-tumor malignancies. Bevacizumab is approved by the Food and Drug Administration (FDA) for the treatment of metastatic colorectal cancer and NSCLC, and is also used for the treatment of breast and ovarian cancers. Bevacizumab-induced cardiotoxicity includes angina, myocardial infarction, heart failure, hypertension, stroke, and arterial thromboembolic events. Grade 2 to 4 left ventricular dysfunction can occur in 2% of patients receiving treatment with single-agent bevacizumab. Concurrent use of anthracycline is associated with a 14% risk of heart failure, while prior anthracycline use is associated with an intermediate level of risk (7,20). Patients with an age >65 years and those with previous arterial thromboembolic events are at increased risk (7,20).

The interferons are a family of biologic response modifiers and are composed of interferon alpha (IFN β), interferon beta (IFN α), and interferon gamma (IFN γ). Cardiotoxicity of these agents appears to be a class effect, with IFN α being the most widely studied interferon in phase 1 and 2 trials. IFN α induces 2'5'-oligoadenylate synthetase and protein kinase, leading to decreased translation and inhibition of tumor cell protein synthesis, induction of differentiation, and modulation of oncogene expression. IFN α also causes indirect induction of host antitumor mechanisms mediated by cytotoxic T cells, helper T cells, natural killer (NK) cells, and macrophages. IFN α is used in the treatment of melanoma and renal cell carcinoma (RCC), and cardiotoxic effects of IFN α include myocardial ischemia and infarction, which are generally related to a prior history of coronary artery disease. These may be due to increased fever or associated flulike symptoms that increase myocardial oxygen requirements (21). Atrial and ventricular arrhythmias have reported in up to 20% of cases (22,23)and two cases of sudden death

have been reported (24). Prolonged administration of IFN α has been associated with cardiomyopathy, manifested by a depressed ejection fraction and heart failure, and is reversible upon cessation of IFN α infusion in some but not all cases (25,26).

Dysrhythmias

Paclitaxel is a cell-cycle–specific (active in M phase of the cell cycle) antimicrotubule agent that is used in the treatment of ovarian cancer, breast cancer, NSCLC, head and neck cancer, esophageal cancer, prostate cancer, bladder cancer, and AIDS-related Kaposi sarcoma. Paclitaxel has been associated with bradycardia and heart block, as reported in a phase 2 series of 140 women with ovarian cancer in whom transient asymptomatic bradycardia occurred in 29%. Serious cardiotoxicity (atrioventricular conduction block, ventricular tachycardia, cardiac ischemia) was reported in 5% (27). The risk of cardiotoxicity is higher when paclitaxel is combined with doxorubicin, and heart failure has developed in up to 20% of patients treated with this combination (28). The development of heart failure may occur at cumulative doxorubicin doses much lower than would be expected with doxorubicin alone (29,30).

Albumin-bound paclitaxel is a nano-particle (about 130 nm) form of paclitaxel, and is FDA-approved for treatment of advanced breast cancer, and has the same cardiac toxicity profile as non-albumin–bound paclitaxel. Asymptomatic electrocardiogram (ECG) changes, including nonspecific changes, sinus bradycardia, and sinus tachycardia, are most common (31).

Docetaxel is also an M-phase–specific antimicrotubule agent that is FDA-approved for the treatment of breast cancer and NSCLC, and is also indicated for the treatment of SCLC, head and neck cancer, gastric cancer, refractory ovarian cancer, and bladder cancer. Docetaxel has been associated with conduction abnormalities, cardiovascular collapse, and angina (37). Similar to paclitaxel, docetaxel appears to potentiate the cardiotoxicity of anthracyclines. This was illustrated in a trial of 50 women with stage III breast cancer who received neoadjuvant and adjuvant therapy with docetaxel and doxorubicin (32). In this study, congestive heart failure developed in 8%, with a mean decrease in ejection fraction of 20%, and total doxorubicin dose was <400 mg/m² in all patients.

Vascular Complications

Interleukin-2 (IL-2) is a biologic response modifier that has been used for the treatment of RCC, and is associated with capillary leak syndrome, manifested by increased vascular permeability and hypotension and a cardiovascular profile similar to septic shock. IL-2 has also been associated with direct myocardial toxicity, and in patients with underlying coronary artery disease, ischemia, myocardial infarction, arrhythmias, and death have been reported (33). Ventricular and supraventricular arrhythmias have been reported in 6%–21% of patients (34,35).

All-trans-retinoic acid (ATRA) is a derivative of vitamin A and differentiates leukemic promyelocytes into mature cells. ATRA is used to treat acute promyelocytic leukemia (APL), and approximately 10%–15% of patients develop the retinoic acid syndrome, which is marked by fever, weight gain, pulmonary infiltrates, pleural and pericardial effusions, myocardial ischemia/infarction (20), hypotension, and renal failure. The majority of patients make a complete and rapid recovery if the syndrome is recognized early and ATRA is withdrawn.

5-fluorouracil (5-FU) is a fluorinated pyrimidine that impairs DNA synthesis by inhibiting thymidylate synthetase that is used to treat colorectal cancer, breast cancer, various gastrointestinal (GI) malignancies, and head and neck cancer, and is the second most common cause of chemotherapy-related cardiotoxicity, after anthracyclines (36). Chest pain, which can be nonspecific or anginal in nature, is the most common 5-FU–induced cardiotoxicity. Other cardiac manifestations can include arrhythmias (including atrial fibrillation, ventricular tachycardia, and ventricular fibrillation) and acute pulmonary edema due to ventricular dysfunction. Cardiogenic shock and sudden cardiac death have also been reported (20). The incidence of 5-FU–induced cardiotoxicity ranges from 1%–19% (36–38), although most series report a risk of ≤8% (20). Risk may be associated with the method of 5-FU administration, the presence of coronary artery disease, and the use of concurrent radiation or anthracyclines.

The underlying mechanism of toxicity is thought to be coronary artery vasospasm. However, other mechanisms, including myocarditis and a thrombogenic effect due to endothelial cytotoxicity, have also been postulated (39,40). Cardiac symptoms usually resolve with termination of 5-FU treatment and/or administration of nitrates or calcium channel blockers. Rechallenging patients who have had 5-FU–induced cardiotoxicity is controversial. If rechallenge is attempted, patients should be followed carefully during drug infusion, and in some instances changing from infusional to bolus 5-FU may allow treatment to be successfully resumed (41,42).

Capecitabine is a fluoropyrimidine that is metabolized in the liver and tissues to form 5-FU, which is the active moiety, and is FDA-approved to treat advanced breast and colorectal cancers. Capecitabine-induced cardiotoxicity profile is similar to that of infusional 5-FU. In clinical studies, reported cardiac complications have included angina, atrial fibrillation, myocarditis, myocardial infarction, and ventricular fibrillation (20,43).

Hypertension

Hypertension has emerged as one of the most common adverse effects of therapy with angiogenesis inhibitors such as bevacizumab, sorafenib, and sunitinib. Sorafenib is a signal transduction inhibitor that inhibits Raf kinase, VEGF receptor, and platelet-derived growth factor (PDGF) receptor, and is FDA-approved for the treatment of advanced RCC. Sunitinib is also a signal transduction inhibitor and inhibits VEGF receptor, PDGF receptor, stem cell receptor (KIT), Fms-like tyrosine kinse-3 (FLT-3), colony-stimulating factor receptor type 1 (CSF-IR), and glial cell line-derived neurotrophic factor receptor (RET), and is FDA-approved for the treatment of gastrointestinal stromal tumors (GIST) and advanced RCC.

Hypertension was observed in 22.4% of patients (11% with grade 3 hypertension) in a phase 3 trial of bevacizumab, irinotecan, fluorouracil, and leucovorin patients with colon cancer (51). In another study of renal cell carcinoma patients who were treated with high-dose bevacizumab, hypertension was reported in 36% (44).

A recent study evaluating the incidence of hypertension in patients with metastatic solid-tumor malignancies who were treated with sorafenib found that 75% of patients experienced an increase of ≥10 mmHg in systolic blood pressure and 60% of patients experienced an increase of ≥20 mmHg in systolic blood pressure (45). In a recent phase 3 trial of sorafenib in patients with advanced renal cell carcinoma, 17% of patients developed hypertension. Ten percent of patients experienced grade 2 hypertension, and 4% experienced grade 3 or 4 hypertension (46). A phase 1 trial of sunitinib revealed that at the maximum-tolerated dose, the most common side effects were grade 3 fatigue, grade 3 hypertension, and grade 2 bullous toxicity (47).

QT Prolongation

Arsenic trioxide induces differentiation of APL cells by degrading the chimeric PML/RAR-α protein, and is used to treat relapsed acute promyelocytic leukemia. Arsenic trioxide treatment can result in fluid retention, the "APL differentiation syndrome," which is similar to ATRA syndrome; QT prolongation (>500 msec) (48); complete atrioventricular block; and sudden death (49).

Management of Complications

Animal studies have suggested that the beta blocker carvedilol may protect against the cardiotoxicity of anthracyclines (50,51). Further support comes from a randomized trial of 50 patients undergoing anthracycline chemotherapy for a variety of malignancies. Patients were randomly assigned to carvedilol, 12.5 mg daily, or placebo. All patients underwent echocardiography prior to and six months after chemotherapy. Among the patients assigned to carvedilol, there was no change in the mean LVEF after chemotherapy (70% before and after therapy). In contrast, patients assigned to placebo had a statistically significant absolute reduction in LVEF of 17% (69% to 52%) (52).

ACE inhibitors have been shown to slow disease progression in patients with left ventricular systolic dysfunction due to a variety of causes. The potential protective effect of ACE inhibitors in patients with elevated serum cardiac troponin following chemotherapy was evaluated in a randomized trial (53). Of 473 patients treated with a variety of high-dose chemotherapy regimens, 114 patients with an elevated troponin T were randomly assigned to one year of treatment with the ACE inhibitor enalapril (2.5 mg daily, titrated to a maximum of 20 mg daily) or to no enalapril. After one year, an absolute reduction in LVEF of ≥10% was found in 43% of the untreated patients, but in none of the patients treated with enalapril.

Hence, if patients undergoing treatment with cardiotoxic chemotherapeutic agents develop a decline in cardiac function, initiation of beta blockers and ACE inhibitors is encouraged. Additionally, management of overt congestive heart failure may require diuretics (eg, furosemide) and/or spironolactone.

Dexrazoxane is an FDA-approved, EDTA-like iron chelator, which may prevent anthracycline-induced cardiotoxicity by stripping iron from the doxorubicin-iron complex, thereby preventing free radical formation (54). In a meta-analysis of 1,013 adult and pediatric patients, dexrazoxane, initiated either with the start of anthracycline treatment or after a cumulative dose of 300 mg/m^2 had been attained, significantly reduced the incidence of congestive heart failure (relative risk = 0.28, 95% CI 0.18–0.42) (55). The cardioprotective effect of dexrazoxane is observed whether the drug is started initially or after 300 mg/m^2 of doxorubicin.

PULMONARY TOXICITY

Bleomycin is an antitumor antibiotic that contains a DNA-binding region and an iron-binding region at opposite ends of the molecule (Table 2.3). Cytotoxic effects result from the generation of an activated oxygen free-radical species, which causes single- and double-strand DNA breaks and eventual cell death. Bleomycin is used to treat cancers of the head and neck, cervix, and esophagus; germ cell tumors; and both Hodgkin and non-Hodgkin lymphoma. Bleomycin therapy can

TABLE 2.3
Chemotherapy-Induced Pulmonary Toxicity

TOXICITY TYPE	AGENT	REFERENCES
Acute toxicity	Gemcitabine	(114–116)
	Gefitinib	(110)
	Mitomycin C	(87,88)
	Cyclophosphamide	(107,108)
	Paclitaxel	(239,257)
	Docetaxel	(258,259)
Chronic toxicity	Bleomycin	(61)
	Methotrexate	(68,70,71)
	Chlorambucil	(81)
	Mitomycin C	(87,88)
	Carmustine, lomustine,	(96, 97)
	Cyclophosphamide	(107,109)

result in life-threatening interstitial pulmonary fibrosis in up to 10% of patients (56,57). Other, less common forms of pulmonary toxicity include hypersensitivity pneumonitis and nodular pulmonary densities.

Patient age; drug dose; renal function; severity of the underlying malignancy at presentation; and concomitant use of oxygen, radiation therapy, or other chemotherapeutic agents may influence the risk of developing bleomycin-induced pulmonary toxicity (57). Administration of higher doses of bleomycin increases the risk of lung injury, but damage can occur at doses less than 50 mg. Rapid intravenous infusion may also increase the risk of toxicity.

High concentrations of inspired oxygen increase the risk of developing bleomycin-induced pulmonary toxicity, whereas low oxygen concentrations substantially decrease the risk. Administration of high inspired fractions of oxygen may even result in pulmonary toxicity several years after bleomycin treatment (58). Thoracic irradiation increases the risk of bleomycin-induced pulmonary toxicity, whether it is administered prior to or simultaneously with bleomycin. It is not known whether a long interval between irradiation and administration of bleomycin eliminates the increased risk of pulmonary toxicity (59). Greater than 80% of bleomycin is eliminated by the kidneys, and renal insufficiency is a risk factor for bleomycin-induced toxicity (56,60).

Symptoms, physical signs, and pulmonary function abnormalities of bleomycin-induced pulmonary fibrosis are nonspecific and usually develop subacutely between one and six months after bleomycin treatment. Findings include nonproductive cough, dyspnea, pleuritic or substernal chest pain, fever, tachypnea, rales, lung restriction, and hypoxemia. Pneumothorax and/or pneumomediastinum are rare complications (61). Bleomycin-induced hypersensitivity pneumonitis may present with rapidly progressive symptoms. During bleomycin infusion, an acute chest pain syndrome arises in approximately 1% of patients, but does not predict the development of pulmonary fibrosis (62). Early radiographic findings can include bibasilar subpleural opacification with blunting of the costophrenic angles and fine nodular densities, and late findings can include progressive consolidation and honeycombing. Sputum analysis to rule out infection should be performed, and bronchoalveolar lavage (BAL) is encouraged in patients unable to expectorate sputum.

Bleomycin should be discontinued in patients with documented or suspected bleomycin-induced pulmonary toxicity. Reinitiation of treatment is contraindicated in patients with pulmonary fibrosis, but may be attempted in patients with hypersensitivity pneumonitis. Corticosteroid treatment of bleomycin-induced hypersensitivity pneumonitis usually results in a rapid response. Case reports have also described substantial recovery when a significant inflammatory pneumonitis is present. Short-term improvement in symptoms may be followed by recurrence of symptoms when therapy is tapered. Also, pulmonary function abnormalities may revert over a period of four to five years, even in patients with an initially positive response to corticosteroids (63).

Methotrexate is a cell-cycle–specific antifolate analog, which is active in the S phase of the cell cycle, and competitively inhibits the enzyme dihydrofolate reductase and blocks the conversion of dihydrofolate to tetrahydrofolate. This results in depletion off folate and in impaired synthesis of thymidine, DNA, and RNA, and ultimately in reduced cellular proliferation. Methotrexate is used to treat breast cancer, head and neck cancer, gestational trophoblastic disease, meningeal leukemia and carcinomatous meningitis, bladder cancer, non-Hodgkin lymphoma, and osteogenic sarcoma.

Methotrexate-induced pulmonary toxicity may be classified as inflammatory, infectious, and possibly neoplastic. There is conflicting data regarding the influence of methotrexate on the development of malignancy (64).

Although the most common methotrexate-induced pulmonary toxicity is hypersensitivity pneumonitis, bronchiolitis obliterans with organizing pneumonia (BOOP), acute lung injury with noncardiogenic pulmonary edema, pulmonary fibrosis, and bronchitis have also been associated with methotrexate treatment (65,66). Both low- and high-dose methotrexate treatment and a variety of routes of administration can result in pulmonary toxicity. None of the proposed mechanisms of toxicity account for the observation that pulmonary toxicity may remit despite continued therapy and may not occur upon rechallenge (65,66). Hence, the mechanisms of methotrexate pulmonary toxicity are unresolved and may be multiple.

Methotrexate treatment may increase the risk for opportunistic infections by *Pneumocystis jiroveci*, cytomegalovirus, varicella-zoster virus, *Nocardia*, mycobacteria, or fungi (67). *Pneumocystis* is the most commonly reported pathogen, and has accounted for up to 40% of the infectious complications in some series (68,69).

Methotrexate-induced pulmonary toxicity may present in an acute, subacute, or chronic form. Subacute presentations are most common. The majority of patients who develop methotrexate pulmonary toxicity do so within the first year of therapy; cases have been reported as early as 12 days and as late as 18 years after the drug was initiated (68,70,71).

Acute methotrexate pneumonitis is generally nonspecific and progressive over several weeks, and is marked by fever, chills, malaise, cough, dyspnea, and chest pain (72,73). Rapid decompensation to respiratory failure may occur (65,66). Subacute pneumonitis is marked by dyspnea, nonproductive cough, fever, crackles, and cyanosis (74), and progression to pulmonary fibrosis is observed in approximately 10% of patients. Pleural effusions are uncommon, but can occur, with or without parenchymal involvement (75).

Pulmonary function testing reveals a restrictive pattern with a decrease in carbon monoxide diffusing capacity (DLCO), hypoxemia, and an increased alveolar-arterial (A-a) gradient (65,66). However, the majority of patients display no clinically significant deterioration of pulmonary function (76,77). BAL and lung biopsy are the primary modalities by which to establish diagnosis of methotrexate-induced lung disease, but are not necessary in all patients. BAL may be helpful in ruling out an infectious etiology of pneumonitis and in supporting the diagnosis of methotrexate pneumonitis.

Methotrexate-induced adverse reactions, including stomatitis and gastrointestinal and hematologic toxicity, can be alleviated or prevented by folic acid supplementation without altering the efficacy of methotrexate. Repletion of folate stores, however, does not reduce the risk for methotrexate-induced pulmonary or hepatic toxicity, suggesting that mechanisms other than folate depletion are involved in their pathogenesis (78,79).

Discontinuation of methotrexate is the initial step in management. Clinical improvement generally occurs within days of stopping the drug (75). Rechallenge with methotrexate is not recommended despite reports of successful rechallenge and even regression of pulmonary toxicity despite continued therapy (65,66). Exclusion of an infectious etiology and empiric antimicrobial therapy may be indicated while definitive procedures are performed. There have not been any prospective, randomized, placebo-controlled trials to support the use of corticosteroids in methotrexate-induced pulmonary toxicity, but anecdotal reports support this approach.

Chlorambucil is an alkylating cytotoxic agent used in the treatment of chronic lymphocytic leukemia, lymphomas, polycythemia vera, and amyloidosis. Chlorambucil-induced toxicity includes nausea, vomiting, hepatotoxicity, hallucinations, bone marrow suppression, and pulmonary toxicity. The incidence of chlorambucil-induced pulmonary toxicity is estimated at <1% (80).

The most common presentation of chlorambucil-induced pulmonary toxicity is chronic interstitial pneumonitis, and onset of symptoms varies from 5 months to 10 years (81). Patients present with insidious onset of nonproductive cough, dyspnea, weight loss, and fever,

and physical examination often reveals bilateral inspiratory crackles.

The diagnosis of chlorambucil-induced pulmonary toxicity is one of exclusion, and specific markers or diagnostic clinical features are absent. Supporting signs include development of new pulmonary symptoms after beginning treatment, new chest radiograph abnormalities, a decrease in total lung capacity (TLC) or in DLCO, marked CD8+ lymphocytosis in BAL fluid, no evidence of infection, improvement in lung manifestations following withdrawal of the drug, and recurrence of interstitial pneumonia upon retreatment. Once chlorambucil-induced interstitial pneumonia is suspected, cessation of treatment should occur. Generally, patients improve within a few days of stopping treatment, but corticosteroid treatment is recommended in patients who do not improve rapidly after drug cessation and in those who develop acute respiratory failure (82,83).

Mitomycin C (MMC) is a cell-cycle–specific alkylating agent that cross-links DNA and results in inhibition of DNA synthesis and subsequent transcription by targeting DNA-dependent RNA polymerase. MMC is used to treat gastric, pancreatic, breast, cervical, bladder, head and neck, and NSCLCs. Adverse effects of MMC are dose-related, and include myelosuppression (most common) (84), nausea, vomiting, diarrhea, stomatitis, dementia, and alopecia (85,86). The frequency of pulmonary toxicity is between 3%–12%, and includes bronchospasm, acute pneumonitis, hemolytic uremiclike syndrome with acute lung injury, chronic pneumonitis manifested by the development of diffuse parenchymal, and pleural disease (87,88).

MMC-associated bronchospasm occurs at a frequency of 4%–6%, and most cases involve the concomitant use of vindesine and MMC (89,90). Bronchospasm typically develops within a few hours of treatment and resolves within 12–24 hours, either spontaneously or with bronchodilator administration (90). MMC-associated acute interstitial pneumonitis is characterized by sudden onset of dyspnea occurring on a day when a vinca alkaloid is administered. In a study of 387 patients with advanced NSCLC, there was a 6% incidence of acute dyspnea following treatment with mitomycin and vindesine or vinblastine (91). Significant improvement in dyspnea occurred over 24 hours, but approximately 60% experienced chronic respiratory impairment that only partially resolved with corticosteroid therapy.

MMC-induced thrombotic microangiopathy is similar to hemolytic uremic syndrome (HUS), but in 50% of cases is also associated with acute respiratory failure. This syndrome generally occurs during or shortly after treatment, and is characterized by microangiopathic hemolytic anemia, thrombocytopenia, renal insufficiency due to thrombotic occlusion of glomerular capillaries, and acute lung injury. The incidence of thrombotic microangiopathy is directly related to the total dose of drug administered, and prior blood transfusions or 5-FU treatment may increase the risk of developing this syndrome (102). In a review of 39 cases of MMC-associated thrombotic microangiopathy, 75% of patients developed the syndrome 6–12 months after starting chemotherapy. Approximately 50% of patients developed associated acute respiratory distress syndrome (ARDS) and had a significantly higher mortality rate, compared with patients who did not develop ARDS (95% vs 50%) (92).

MMC-associated interstitial fibrosis is marked dyspnea, nonproductive cough, tachypnea, and rales, and appears to be a dose-related condition that is unusual below a cumulative dose of 30 mg/m² (93). Chest radiograph may reveal bilateral diffuse reticular opacities with occasional fine nodularity, and pulmonary function testing reveals a restrictive pattern with a decrease in DLCO (94,95). Treatment with corticosteroids may result in rapid improvement of dyspnea and interstitial opacities, and abrupt cessation or early withdrawal of corticosteroids can result in a relapse of dyspnea and pulmonary opacities (94).

Pleural disease, characterized by exudative effusions, fibrinous exudates, and fibrosis over the pleural surfaces with occasional aggregates of lymphocytes and eosinophils, has been reported. Pleural effusion is often associated with underlying MMC-associated parenchymal lung disease (80,86).

The nitrosourea drugs include carmustine (BCNU), lomustine (CCNU), and semustine (methyl CCNU), and are a class of cell-cycle–nonspecific, DNA-alkylating agents. Nitrosourea drugs are used to treat Hodgkin and non-Hodgkin lymphoma, multiple myeloma, brain tumors, melanoma, and other solid tumors, including breast cancer. Carmustine is the most widely used nitrosourea, and can induce both acute and chronic pulmonary toxicity. Semustine has been associated with pulmonary fibrosis following treatment.

Although most patients develop pulmonary fibrosis within three years of carmustine treatment, some patients can present with fibrosis decades after exposure (96,97). The reported incidence of carmustine-induced pulmonary toxicity has ranged from 1% to 20%–30% (109). When carmustine is part of a preparative regimen for stem cell transplantation, the incidence of interstitial pneumonitis or idiopathic pneumonia has been reported to be 2%–23% (98,99). Lung fibrosis is most likely with very high doses, concurrent administration of other agents known to cause pulmonary toxicity, preexisting lung disease, localized chest wall radiotherapy, or atopy (98).

Patients with early-onset carmustine-induced lung fibrosis usually present with dry cough, breathlessness, and bilateral inspiratory crackles within weeks to months of treatment. Others may present with a fulminant disease similar to ARDS, and many others may have subclinical disease detected by pulmonary function testing (24,96,100). Radiographic imaging may reveal bilateral diffuse infiltrates or nodules, localized consolidation, localized or diffuse interstitial fibrotic changes, or ARDS. Apical pleural thickening, spontaneous pneumothoraces, and fibrotic stranding have also been described (101). Pulmonary function testing reveals decreased vital capacity (VC) and TLC, as well as reduced DLCO (96,102).

Corticosteroids have been beneficial in some studies if given early based upon symptoms or a fall in DLCO (24,100), but have been shown to be minimally effective in other reports (103,104). Patients with mild disease, and especially those who received low doses of carmustine or responded to steroid treatment, usually survive. However, these individuals may be at increased risk of late pulmonary fibrosis. Carmustine should be discontinued if lung fibrosis is suspected.

Patients with late-onset carmustine-induced lung fibrosis often have no symptoms for several years, although chest radiographs and lung function studies can reveal evidence of lung fibrosis (105). Severe fibrosis can result in breathlessness and sometimes cough at late stage of the disease. Radiographic changes can include upper-zone patchy linear opacities and volume loss due to apical pleural thickening. Pulmonary function testing reveals restricted lung volumes and reduced DLCO.

No treatment has proven to be efficacious in the management of late-onset carmustine-induced lung injury. Corticosteroids are not effective, and lung transplantation offers the best hope of long-term survival for severely debilitated patients. Prognosis is the worst for patients treated below the age of seven years, and patients who are treated beyond puberty appear to have the slowest rate of decline in pulmonary function (106).

Cyclophosphamide is cell-cycle–nonspecific alkylating agent that is used to treat breast and ovarian cancer, non-Hodgkin lymphoma, chronic lymphocytic leukemia, bone and soft tissue sarcomas, and rhabdomyosarcoma. The toxicity profile of cyclophosphamide includes leukopenia, hemorrhagic cystitis, infertility, the development of secondary malignancies, and pulmonary toxicity.

Cyclophosphamide-induced pulmonary toxicity is rare, but the risk may be increased by the concomitant administration of radiation, oxygen therapy, or other drugs with potential pulmonary toxicity. Two distinct patterns of pulmonary toxicity are associated with cyclophosphamide: an acute pneumonitis that occurs early in the course of treatment and a chronic, progressive, fibrotic process that may occur after prolonged therapy (107).

In acute pulmonary toxicity, patients present with cough, dyspnea, fatigue, and occasionally fever within one to six months after the onset of therapy. Radiographic imaging can show interstitial inflammation and/or a ground-glass appearance. Discontinuation of the drug and institution of corticosteroids usually result in complete resolution of symptoms (107,108).

Late-onset pulmonary toxicity typically develops in patients who have received treatment over several months to years with relatively low doses of cyclophosphamide (107,109), and is marked by progressive lung fibrosis. Symptoms arise insidiously and include slowly progressive dyspnea and nonproductive cough. Discontinuation of treatment and initiation of corticosteroids are minimally effective, and late-onset pneumonitis and fibrosis invariably lead to terminal respiratory failure. Radiographic imaging reveals bilateral reticular or nodular diffuse opacities with a fibrotic appearance. Bilateral pleural thickening of the mid- and upper lung zones is also a common feature (107). Pulmonary function testing typically displays a restrictive pattern with a reduced DLCO.

Gefitinib is an orally active selective epidermal growth factor receptor (EGFR) tyrosine kinase inhibitor, which is FDA-approved for the treatment of pancreatic cancer, NSCLC, breast cancer, and ovarian cancer, and is also used to treat bladder cancer and soft tissue sarcomas, and rarely results in dyspnea and interstitial lung disease (110,111). In a multi-institutional randomized phase 2 trial of gefitinib for previously treated patients with advanced NSCLC, 2 out of 106 patients experienced interstitial pneumonia and pneumonitis (112). In a recent retrospective analysis of 325 patients with NSCLC, 22 patients (6%) developed interstitial lung disease (ILD) after gefitinib treatment. The median toxicity grade of ILD was 3 (range 2–4), and 10 (3.1%) patients died. The median time to ILD after initiation of gefitinib treatment was 18 days (range 3–123), and half of the patients developing ILD manifested acute onset of dyspnea. Radiographic findings were characterized predominantly by diffuse ground-glass opacities. Statistically significant factors affecting the occurrence of ILD by multivariate analysis were the presence of pulmonary fibrosis prior to gefitinib therapy and poor functional status. (113).

Limited evidence suggests that the combination of gemcitabine, an S phase cell cycle–specific antimetabolite, and taxanes may also lead to pulmonary toxicity. In one series, 4 of 12 patients with NSCLC who were treated with the combination of paclitaxel and gemcitabine developed pneumonitis (114), which was marked by increasing exertional dyspnea, a dry cough, malaise, and low-grade pyrexia that developed and progressed over a few days. None of the patients had received thoracic radiotherapy at any time during the course of their illness. Severe pulmonary toxicity has also been documented in patients receiving docetaxel in combination with gemcitabine for treatment of transitional cell bladder cancer (115,116).

Management of Complications

Management of chemotherapy-induced pulmonary toxicity involves prompt discontinuation of the offending chemotherapeutic agent and initiation of corticosteroids (as detailed previously). Oftentimes, there is a rapid improvement in pulmonary function with these measures, but depending on the agent, long-term pulmonary fibrosis and restricted pulmonary function can occur. In some instances, supplemental oxygen and referral to a pulmonary medicine specialist may be necessary. Pulmonary opportunistic infections should be managed with early judicious use of appropriate antibiotics.

NEUROTOXICITY

The platinum agents covalently bind to DNA and produce intrastrand (>90%) and interstrand (<5%) crosslinks, which result in inhibition of DNA synthesis and inhibition of transcription (Table 2.4). Cisplatin is used to treat testicular, ovarian, bladder, esophageal, and head and neck cancers, as well as NSCLC, SCLC, non-Hodgkin lymphoma, and trophoblastic disease, and is commonly associated with peripheral neuropathy and ototoxicity. Cisplatin induces an axonal neuropathy that predominantly affects large myelinated sensory fibers with damage occurring at dorsal root ganglion (primarily) and peripheral nerves (117–120). This leads to the subacute development of numbness, paresthesias, and occasionally pain, which begins in the toes and fingers and spreads proximally to affect the legs and arms, and also results in impairment of proprioception and loss of reflexes. Pinprick, temperature sensation, and power are usually spared. Nerve conduction studies reveal decreased amplitude of sensory action potentials and prolonged sensory latencies, consistent with a sensory axonopathy, and sural nerve biopsy reveals both demyelination and axonal loss. Cisplatin-induced neuropathy is usually generalized, but focal and autonomic neuropathies can rarely occur (121).

Patients with mild neuropathy can continue to receive full-dose cisplatin, but if the neuropathy interferes with neurologic function, the risk of potentially disabling neurotoxicity must be weighed against the

TABLE 2.4
Chemotherapy-Induced Neurotoxicity

TOXICITY TYPE	AGENT	REFERENCES
Central	Methotrexate	(130–133)
	Cytarabine	(155,156)
	5-flurouracil	(157)
	Ifosfamide	(162,163)
	Nitrosoureas	(167)
	Procarbazine	(168,169)
	Interferon alpha	(170,171)
	Interleukin-2	(177,178)
	Bevacizumab	(180, 181)
	Busulfan	(182)
	All-trans-retinoic acid	(184)
	Fludarabine	(186)
	Cladribine	(185)
	Pentostatin	(163, 185)
Vascular	Carboplatin	(120)
	Bevacizumab	(180,181)
Peripheral	Cisplatin	(180,181)
	Carboplatin	(180,181)
	Oxaliplatin	(126–128)
	Paclitaxel	(134–137)
	Docetaxel	(140,141)
	Thalidomide	(142)
	Vincristine (and, less frequently, other vinca alkaloids, such as vinorelbine, vinblastine, and vindesine)	(147–150)
	Cytarabine	(155,157)
	5-flurouracil	(159)
	Bortezomib	(146)
	Interferon alpha	(173,174)
	Interleukin-2	(179)
	Gemcitabine	(182)
	All-trans-retinoic acid	(186)

benefit of continued treatment. Alternatives include cisplatin dose reduction or replacement of cisplatin with a less neurotoxic agent, such as carboplatin. In 30% of patients, the neuropathy continues to deteriorate for up to several months even after cisplatin is discontinued (121), and in some cases, neuropathy may even begin after therapy is discontinued. Cessation of cisplatin use eventually results in improvement of neuropathy in most patients, although recovery is often incomplete.

Cisplatin-induced ototoxicity is characterized by a dose-dependent, high-frequency sensorineural hearing loss with tinnitus (122). Although symptomatic hearing loss affects only 15%–20% of patients receiving cisplatin, audiometric evidence of hearing impairment occurs in >75% of patients. Radiotherapy to the normal cochlea or cranial nerve VIII can result in sensorineural hearing loss, and concurrent administration of cisplatin results in synergistic ototoxicity, especially in the high-frequency speech range (123).

Lhermitte's sign is a shocklike, nonpainful sensation of paresthesias radiating from the back to the feet during neck flexion. It can develop in patients receiving cisplatin, and typically occurs after weeks or months of treatment. It has also been reported in patients receiving high cumulative doses of oxaliplatin (121).

Carboplatin is used to treat ovarian, endometrial, bladder, and head and neck cancers, as well as NSCLC, SCLC, germ cell tumors, and relapsed and refractory acute leukemia. Carboplatin is rarely associated with peripheral neuropathy and central nervous system (CNS) toxicity when given at conventional doses. However, a severe neuropathy can develop with higher-than-standard doses, as used in the setting of high-dose therapy with stem cell transplantation (124). Other neurotoxic manifestations include a microangiopathic hemolytic anemia resulting in progressive neurologic impairment and death (118), and retinal toxicity following intra-arterial administration to patients with brain tumors (125).

Oxaliplatin is a third-generation platinum complex that is FDA-approved for treatment of early-stage and advanced colorectal cancer and for the treatment of pancreatic and gastric cancers. The main dose-limiting toxicity of oxaliplatin is neuropathy. Oxaliplatin has been associated with two distinct syndromes: an acute neurosensory complex, which can appear during or shortly after the first few infusions; and a cumulative sensory neuropathy, with distal loss of sensation and dysesthesias. Ototoxicity is rarely associated with oxaliplatin. Infrequently, a neuromyotonialike hyperexcitability syndrome can occur, which can be marked by eyelid twitching, ptosis, visual field changes, teeth jittering, jaw stiffness, voice changes, dysarthria, hand shaking, and dysesthesias of the hands and feet. Acute transient neurotoxicity occurs in about 85%–95% of patients (126) and appears to be due to hyperexcitability of the peripheral nerves (127,128). Unusual pharyngolaryngeal dysesthesias, which can cause a feeling of difficulty in breathing or swallowing, have been described in 1%–2% of patients. Symptoms can be induced or aggravated by exposure to cold (126).

The dose-limiting cumulative sensory neuropathy develops in 10%–15 % of patients after a cumulative dose of 780–850 mg/m² (126). In about 75% of patients, the sensory neuropathy is reversible, with a median time to recovery of 13 weeks after treatment cessation (129).

Methotrexate (MTX)-induced neurotoxicity can be manifested as aseptic meningitis, transverse myelopathy, acute and subacute encephalopathy, and leukoencephalopathy. Aseptic meningitis is the most common neurotoxic effect of intrathecal (IT) MTX (130), and is characterized by headache, nuchal rigidity, back pain, nausea, vomiting, fever, and lethargy. Approximately 10% of patients are affected, but incidence rates as high as 50% have been reported. Symptoms usually begin 2–4 hours after drug injection, and may last for 12–72 hours (131). Cerebrospinal fluid (CSF) analysis usually demonstrates a pleocytosis with elevated protein content. Symptoms are usually self-limited, and treatment is usually not required. Some patients who develop aseptic meningitis can be subsequently retreated with MTX without further toxicity.

Transverse myelopathy is an uncommon complication of IT MTX manifested by isolated spinal cord dysfunction, which develops over hours to days in the absence of a compressive lesion. Transverse myelopathy is associated with IT MTX and is generally seen in patients receiving concurrent radiotherapy (RT) or frequent IT MTX injections. Affected patients typically develop back or leg pain followed by paraplegia, sensory loss, and sphincter dysfunction. The onset is usually between 30 minutes and 48 hours after treatment, but can occur up to two weeks later. The majority of cases show clinical improvement, but the extent of recovery is variable (132), and further administration of IT MTX is contraindicated.

Acute neurotoxicity is most frequently seen after high-dose MTX and is characterized by somnolence, confusion, and seizures within 24 hours of treatment. Symptoms usually resolve spontaneously without sequelae, and retreatment is often possible (131). Weekly or biweekly administration of high-dose MTX may produce a subacute "strokelike" syndrome, characterized by transient focal neurologic deficits, confusion, and occasionally seizures. Symptoms develop approximately six days after drug administration, last from 15 minutes to 72 hours, and then resolve spontaneously without sequelae. CSF analysis is usually normal, but the electroencephalogram (EEG) may show diffuse slowing and diffusion-weighted images may be abnormal. Subsequent administration of high-dose MTX may be accomplished without recurrent subacute encephalopathy (133).

The major delayed complication of MTX is leukoencephalopathy, which is dependent upon dose and route of administration (131). Although this syndrome may be produced by MTX alone, it is more common in the setting of concurrent or past RT. The mechanism is unknown, but it is possible that cranial irradiation either potentiates the toxic effects of MTX or disrupts the blood-brain barrier, allowing high concentrations of MTX to reach the brain.

The characteristic feature of leukoencephalopathy is a gradual impairment of cognitive function months to years following treatment with MTX. Clinical manifestations range from mild learning disability to severe progressive dementia accompanied by somnolence, seizures, ataxia, and hemiparesis. Many patients stabilize or improve following discontinuation of MTX, but the course is progressive in others and may be fatal. No effective treatment is available. The diagnosis is supported by cranial computed tomography (CT) and magnetic resonance imaging (MRI), which typically show cerebral atrophy and diffuse white-matter lesions. CT reveals characteristic hypodense nonenhancing lesions, while MRI reveals areas of high signal intensity on T2-weighted images.

Taxane-induced motor and sensory neuropathies are cumulative and dose- and schedule-dependent. Paclitaxel induces a neuropathy that involves sensory nerve fibers. The major manifestations include burning paresthesias of the hands and feet and loss of reflexes. Paclitaxel also causes a motor neuropathy, which predominantly affects proximal muscles (134). The incidence of grade 3 or 4 motor neuropathy is between 2%–10% (135). Other, less common manifestations include perioral numbness, autonomic neuropathies, severe myalgias and arthralgias, phantom limb pain, transient encephalopathies, and seizures (136,137).

Paclitaxel-induced neuropathies often do not progress even if treatment is continued, and there are reports of symptomatic improvement despite continued therapy. After completing treatment, approximately 50% of patients improve over a period of months (138). Additionally, the neurotoxicity of paclitaxel is synergistic with the concurrent platinum administration (139).

Docetaxel causes both sensory and motor neuropathies, although both of these occur less frequently than with paclitaxel. Any neuropathy occurs in less than 15% of patients, and grade 3 or 4 neuropathies occur in less than 5% (140). Lhermitte's sign has also been associated with docetaxel use (141).

Thalidomide is an antiangiogenic agent that is used in the treatment of multiple myeloma. A peripheral neuropathy develops in approximately 75% of patients who receive prolonged thalidomide treatment (142). This neuropathy is only partially reversible, and dose reduction or cessation of treatment is required in up to 60% of patients. Somnolence is also common, affecting 43%–55% of patients, and decreases in many patients after two or three weeks of continued therapy

(143). Other reported manifestations of neurotoxicity include tremor and dizziness (142) and, rarely, seizures (144). Lenalidomide, a thalidomide derivative, appears to be substantially less neurotoxic. In a phase 2 study in 70 patients with refractory or relapsed myeloma, significant peripheral neuropathy was seen in only two patients (145). Bortezomib is proteosome inhibitor that is used in the treatment of multiple myeloma, and has been associated with a sensory neuropathy. In a phase 2 study of 202 patients, 31% of patients developed a peripheral sensory neuropathy, in which 12% experienced grade 3 neuropathy (146).

Vincristine is a vinca-alkaloid used in the treatment of acute lymphoblastic leukemia, Hodgkin and non-Hodgkin lymphoma, multiple myeloma, rhabdomyosarcoma, neuroblastoma, Ewing sarcoma, chronic leukemias, thyroid cancer, brain malignancies, and trophoblastic neoplasms, whose dose-limiting toxicity is an axonal neuropathy, which results from disruption of the microtubules within axons and interference with axonal transport. The neuropathy involves both sensory and motor fibers, although small sensory fibers are especially affected (147). The earliest symptoms are usually paresthesias in the fingertips and feet, with or without muscle cramps. These symptoms often develop after several weeks of treatment, but can occur after the first dose. Also, symptoms may appear after the drug has been discontinued and progress for several months before improving (148).

Initially, in comparison to subjective complaints, objective sensory findings tend to be relatively minor, but loss of ankle jerks is common. Occasionally, there may be profound weakness, with bilateral foot drop, wrist drop, and loss of all sensory modalities. Neurophysiologic studies reveal a primarily axonal neuropathy (149). Patients with mild neuropathy can usually continue to receive full doses of vincristine, but progressive symptoms require dose reduction or discontinuation of drug. Discontinuation of treatment results in gradual improvement, which may take up to several months (150).

Vincristine can also cause autonomic neuropathies manifested by colicky abdominal pain and constipation, which can occur in almost 50% of patients, and rarely a paralytic ileus may result (150). Hence, patients receiving vincristine should take prophylactic stool softeners and/or laxatives. Less commonly, patients may develop impotence, postural hypotension, or an atonic bladder.

Vincristine may also cause focal neuropathies involving the cranial nerves (121). Most commonly, this affects the oculomotor nerve, but the recurrent laryngeal nerve, optic nerve, facial nerve, and auditory nerve may also be involved. Vincristine may also cause retinal damage and night blindness, and some patients may experience jaw and parotid pain during treatment.

Rarely, vincristine may cause syndrome of inappropriate antidiuretic hormone secretion (SIADH), resulting in hyponatremia, confusion, and seizures (151). Other rare CNS complications (unrelated to SIADH) include seizures, encephalopathy, transient cortical blindness, ataxia, athetosis, and parkinsonism (152).

Vindesine, vinblastine, and vinorelbine are associated with less neurotoxicity and have less affinity for neural tissue. Vinorelbine is associated with mild paresthesias in only about 20% of patients (153), and severe neuropathy is rare, occurring most often in patients with prior paclitaxel exposure (154).

Cytarabine is a pyrimidine analogue that is used to treat leukemias, lymphomas, and intrathecally for neoplastic meningitis. Conventional doses are associated with little neurotoxicity. However, high doses (3 g/m^2 every 12 hours) cause an acute cerebellar syndrome in 10%–25% of patients (155,156). Patients over the age of 40 who have abnormal liver or renal function, underlying neurologic dysfunction, or who receive a total dose of >30 g are particularly likely to develop cerebellar toxicity. The characteristic syndrome begins with somnolence and occasionally an encephalopathy that develops two to five days after beginning treatment. Immediately thereafter, cerebellar signs are noted on physical examination; symptoms range from mild ataxia to an inability to sit or walk unassisted. Rarely, seizures can occur.

High-dose cytarabine infrequently causes peripheral neuropathies resembling Guillain-Barré syndrome, brachial plexopathy, encephalopathy, lateral rectus palsy, or an extrapyramidal syndrome (155,157). Rarely, IT cytarabine can cause a transverse myelitis that is similar to that seen with IT MTX (157). IT cytarabine has also been associated with aseptic meningitis, encephalopathy, headaches, and seizures (121).

5-fluorouracil (5-FU) is rarely associated with an acute cerebellar syndrome (157) that is manifested by acute onset of ataxia, dysmetria, dysarthria, and nystagmus, and develops weeks to months after beginning treatment. 5-FU should be discontinued in any patient who develops cerebellar toxicity; over time, symptoms usually resolve completely. Other rarer neurologic side effects include encephalopathy, an optic neuropathy, eye movement abnormalities, focal dystonia, cerebrovascular disorders, a parkinsonian syndrome (152,158), peripheral neuropathy (159), or seizures (160). 5-FU derivatives doxifluridine, carmofur, and ftorafur have also been reported to rarely cause encephalopathies and cerebellar syndromes (152,161).

Ifosfamide is an analog of cyclophosphamide, and is used to treat recurrent germ cell tumors, soft tissue sarcomas, non-Hodgkin lymphoma, Hodgkin lymphoma, NSCLC and SCLC, bladder cancer, head and neck cancer, cervical cancer, and Ewing sarcoma. Ifosfamide had a systemic toxicity similar to cyclophosphamide, but unlike cyclophosphamide, about 10%–20% of patients treated with ifosfamide develop an encephalopathy. Patients at increased risk include those with a prior history of ifosfamide-related encephalopathy, renal dysfunction, low serum albumin, or prior cisplatin treatment (162,163). Other rare ifosfamide-associated neurologic toxicities include seizures, ataxia, weakness, cranial nerve dysfunction, neuropathies (147), or an extrapyramidal syndrome (164).

The nitrosoureas are lipid-soluble alkylating agents that rapidly cross the blood-brain barrier. High-dose intravenous (IV) carmustine, as used in the setting of hematopoietic cell transplantation, can cause an encephalomyelopathy and seizures, and these symptoms typically develop over a period of weeks to months following drug administration. Intra-arterial administration of carmustine produces ocular toxicity and neurotoxicity in 30%–48% of patients (165,166). Patients often complain of headache, eye, and facial pain. Confusion, seizures, retinopathy, and blindness also may occur. Concurrent radiotherapy increases the neurotoxicity of intracarotid carmustine (167).

Procarbazine is an alkylating agent that is used to treat Hodgkin lymphoma, non-Hodgkin lymphoma, cutaneous T-cell lymphoma, and brain tumors. At conventional doses, procarbazine can cause a mild reversible encephalopathy and neuropathy, and rarely psychosis and stupor (121,152). The incidence of encephalopathy may be higher in patients receiving higher doses of procarbazine, such as in the treatment of malignant gliomas (168). The combination of intravenous and intra-arterial procarbazine produces a severe encephalopathy (169). Procarbazine also potentiates the sedative effects of opiates, phenothiazines, and barbiturates. Concurrent use of alcohol or tyramine containing food with procarbazine can result in nausea, vomiting, CNS depression, hypertensive crisis, visual disturbances, and headache. Concurrent use of procarbazine with tricyclic antidepressants can result in CNS excitation, tremors, palpitations, hypertensive crisis, and/or angina.

IFN α is associated with dose-related neurotoxicity that is generally mild when low doses are used, as in the adjuvant treatment of malignant melanoma. In a study of 37 such patients treated with IFN α, the most frequent neurotoxicity observed in 22% of patients was tremor (170). At higher doses, IFN α can cause confusion, lethargy, hallucinations, and seizures (171). Although these effects are usually reversible, a permanent dementia or persistent vegetative state may result (172). Rarely, IFN α has been associated with oculomotor palsy, sensorimotor neuropathy (173), myasthenia gravis (188), brachial plexopathy, and polyradiculopathy (174).

IFN α-2a has been associated with depression and suicidal behavior/ideation (:15%), dizziness (21%), irritability (15%), insomnia (14%), vertigo (19%), and mental status changes (12%). Somnolence, lethargy, confusion, and mental impairment may also occur. Motor weakness may be seen at high doses, and usually reverses within a few days. Although IFN α-2b is associated with neurologic side effects similar to IFN α-2a, a particularly high incidence of neuropsychiatric toxicity has been noted in patients with CML treated with recombinant IFN α-2b. In one study of 91 patients, 25% experienced grade 3 or 4 neuropsychiatric toxicity that affected daily functioning. All patients recovered upon withdrawal of IFN α (175).

Intrathecal administration of IFN α has been evaluated for the treatment of meningeal and brain tumors and progressive multifocal leukoencephalopathy. An acute reaction (within hours of the first injection) consists of headache, nausea, vomiting, fever, and dizziness; these usually resolve over 12–24 hours. A severe dose-dependent encephalopathy develops in a significant number of patients within several days of the onset of treatment (176), and is worse in patients who have received cranial radiation (174).

Interferon beta and gamma have neurotoxicities that are similar to IFN α, although interferon beta appears to be better tolerated in general. Hypertonia and myasthenia have been reported with interferon beta (174).

IL-2 has been associated with neuropsychiatric complications in up to 30%–50% of patients, and these include cognitive changes, delusions, hallucinations, and depression (177). Transient focal neurologic deficits (178), acute leukoencephalopathy, carpal tunnel syndrome, and brachial neuritis (179) have been reported with IL-2.

Bevacizumab has been associated with a significant increase in the risk of serious arterial thromboembolic events (including transient ischemic attack, cerebrovascular accident, angina, and myocardial infarction). The incidence of such events is approximately 5%. Reversible posterior leukoencephalopathy syndrome (RPLS) occurs in ≤0.1% of patients (180,181), and symptoms can include headache, seizure, lethargy, confusion, blindness, and other visual and neurologic disturbances. The onset may occur from 16 hours to 1 year after initiation of therapy. Symptoms usually resolve with discontinuation of bevacizumab and control of any associated hypertension.

Other rare causes of neurotoxicity include the following chemotherapeutic agents. High-dose busulfan is a cell-cycle–nonspecific alkylating agent that is used in the treatment of chronic myelogenous leukemia (CML), and is also used in stem cell preparative regimens for refractory leukemia and lymphoma. Busulfan therapy, as used in the setting of hematopoietic stem cell transplantation, can cause seizures. Gemcitabine can cause mild paresthesias in up to 10% of patients. Occasionally, more severe peripheral and autonomic neuropathies can occur (182). An acute inflammatory myopathy has been reported following chemotherapy with gemcitabine and docetaxel, presenting as a symmetrical, painful, proximal muscle weakness (183). ATRA can rarely cause pseudotumor cerebri (184) and multiple mononeuropathies (164).

Fludarabine is a purine analog that is used to treat chronic lymphocytic leukemia (CLL) and indolent lymphomas, and can cause headache, somnolence, confusion, and paresthesias at low doses (185). A delayed progressive encephalopathy with seizures, cortical blindness, paralysis, and coma is more common at high doses, and rarely, a progressive multifocal leukoencephalopathy has been reported (186). Cladribine is also a purine analog, and is used to treat hairy cell leukemia, CLL, and Waldenström macroglobulinemia, and is associated with little neurotoxicity at conventional doses, but can produce a paraparesis or quadriplegia at high doses (185). Pentostatin, another purine analog, is used to treat hairy cell leukemia, cutaneous T-cell lymphomas, and CLL. At low doses, lethargy and fatigue are common, and at higher doses, severe encephalopathy, seizures, and coma can occur (146,185).

Management of Complications

Central toxicity induced by chemotherapeutic agents is managed with cessation of chemotherapy. Often this results in rapid improvement of toxicity. Peripheral symptoms such as numbness and pins-and-needles or burning paresthesias also often improve with drug cessation. In some patients, however, peripheral neuropathy often persists, and symptoms can be severe enough to affect quality of life. In these instances, agents such as gabapentin (Neurontin; Pfizer, Inc., New York, New York), pregabalin (Lyrica; Pfizer, Inc., New York, New York), amifostine (Ethyol; Medimmune, Gaithersburg, Maryland), acetyl L-carnitine, calcium and magnesium infusions, tricyclic antidepressants (amitriptyline), duloxetine (Cymbalta; Eli Lilly and Co.; Indianapolis, Indiana), venlafaxine (Effexor; Wyeth Pharmaceuticals, Philadelphia, Pennsylvania), and selective serotonin reuptake inhibitors (SSRIs) may be beneficial.

Gabapentin is an anticonvulsant, which is taken three times a day and can be quite effective for peripheral neuropathy, such as that induced by diabetes. However, in a recent phase 3 trial evaluating the efficacy of gabapentin in the management of chemotherapy-induced peripheral neuropathy (CIPN), 115 patients were randomly assigned to treatment with gabapentin or to the control arm. This study found that changes in symptom severity were statistically similar between the two groups and concluded that gabapentin was not effective in treating symptoms of CIPN (187).

Carbamazepine use has revealed conflicting results. In one study of oxaliplatin and capecitabine, 25 patients received detailed neurologic evaluation, including electromyography (EMG) and nerve conduction studies. Twelve of these patients were treated with carbamazepine during the second cycle of therapy, and all 12 patients had neurologic studies that included EMG and nerve conduction studies at baseline and after one cycle of therapy. Eleven patients were also evaluated after the second cycle of therapy. There was no evidence of nerve abnormalities at baseline in any patient. Abnormal EMG results were noted in 11 of 12 patients, and abnormal nerve conduction studies were reported in 8 of 12 patients after the first course of therapy (without carbamazepine). Carbamazepine was administered for five days before administration of oxaliplatin and continued for two days afterward. One of nine evaluated patients reported some reduction of cold-induced paresthesias. EMG and nerve conduction studies indicated no benefit from carbamazepine. Adverse effects associated with carbamazepine included ataxia, memory loss, dizziness, somnolence, fatigue, and unsteady gait (128).

In another trial of 40 patients treated with oxaliplatin, fluorouracil and leucovorin (FOLFOX), 10 patients received carbamazepine beginning one week before oxaliplatin administration. There were no cases of grade 2 or 3 neuropathy by World Health Organization (WHO) criteria after an average cumulative oxaliplatin dose of 722 mg/m^2. This was contrasted with a set of historical controls that received a cumulative dose of 510 mg/m^2 and experienced grade 2–4 neuropathy at a rate of 30% (188).

Pregabalin, a newer anticonvulsant, is titrated to three times a day dosing, with a maximum daily dose of 600 mg. Somnolence, dizziness, and ataxia can occur, but in general, pregabalin is well tolerated. In a report of a patient with stage IIB pancreatic cancer, pregabalin was successfully used to treat oxaliplatin-induced hyperexcitability syndrome with 72 hours of treatment (189). Randomized studies to further characterize the benefit of pregabalin are warranted.

Amifostine is an organic thiophosphate analog, and in a recent phase 2 trial of amifostine in the first-line treatment of advanced ovarian cancer with carboplatin/paclitaxel chemotherapy, a significant improvement in sensory neuropathy in accordance with National Cancer Institute Common Toxicity Criteria (NCI-CTC) was found ($P = 0.0046$), but amifostine failed to significantly improve the "global health status quality of life" score (190). Hypotension, nausea, and vomiting have been associated with intravenous amifostine, and these can largely be ameliorated with the use of the subcutaneous formulation (191).

Acetyl L-carnitine is an acetyl ester of L-carnitine, a naturally occurring compound that is synthesized from lysine and methionine amino acids. The effect of acetyl L-carnitine in paclitaxel- and cisplatin-induced peripheral neuropathy was evaluated in a study of 26 patients, and at least one WHO grade improvement in peripheral neuropathy was shown in 73% of patients (192).

The role of calcium and magnesium infusions was evaluated in patients with advanced colorectal cancer receiving FOLFOX. Fourteen patients were treated with infusions of calcium gluconate and magnesium sulfate before and after oxaliplatin treatment. Sensory neuropathy was noted in 57.1% of patients after four cycles of therapy. Hence, calcium and magnesium infusions may decrease acute oxaliplatin-induced neurotoxicity (193).

Tricyclic antidepressants, such as amitriptyline, may be effective in some patients, but their use has largely been replaced by SSRIs, venlafaxine (Effexor), and duloxetine (Cymbalta), due to significant side effects, including orthostatic hypotension, ECG changes, atrioventricular (AV) conduction delays, insomnia, sedation, ataxia, cognitive impairment, weight gain, and SIADH. In one report, venlafaxine at a 50-mg dose was effective in the management of oxaliplatin-induced peripheral neuropathy (194).

NEPHROTOXICITY

Chemotherapeutic agents can affect the glomerulus, tubules, interstitium, or the renal microvasculature, with clinical manifestations that range from an asymptomatic elevation of serum creatinine to acute renal failure requiring dialysis. The kidneys are one of the major elimination pathways for many antineoplastic drugs and their metabolites, further enhancing their potential for nephrotoxicity. Delayed drug excretion can result in increased systemic toxicity and is a major concern in patients with renal impairment. Many drugs, including azathioprine, bleomycin, carboplatin, cisplatin, cyclophosphamide, high-dose cytarabine, etoposide, hydroxyurea, ifosfamide, melphalan, methotrexate, mitomycin C, and topotecan, require dose adjustment when administered in the setting of renal insufficiency (Table 2.5).

Several factors can potentiate renal dysfunction and contribute to the nephrotoxic potential of antineoplastic drugs. These include intravascular volume

TABLE 2.5
Chemotherapy-Induced Nephrotoxicity

AGENT	TOXICITY	MANAGEMENT	REFERENCES
Cisplatin	Renal failure, renal tubular acidosis, hypomagnesemia	Vigorous saline hydration and diuresis	(195,196,198)
Carboplatin	Hypomagnesemia, renal salt wasting	Close laboratory monitoring and electrolyte replacement	(198,200)
Oxaliplatin	Renal tubular necrosis	Drug cessation and hydration	(202)
Cyclophosphamide	Hyponatremia and hemorrhagic cystitis	Hydration and mesna	(197,203)
Ifosfamide	Renal tubular acidosis, hemorrhagic cystitis, nephrogenic diabetes insipidus, Fanconi syndrome	Hydration and mesna	(209)
Nitrosoureas	Chronic interstitial nephritis and renal failure	Drug cessation	(204,205)
Mitomycin C	Hemolytic uremic syndrome	Drug cessation	(206,207)
Vinca alkaloids	SIADH	Drug cessation	(213)
Bevacizumab Sorafenib Sunitinib	Albuminuria and nephritic syndrome	Dose reduction or drug cessation	(217)
Interleukin-2	Capillary leak and resulting prerenal azotemia	Vigorous hydration and diuresis and urine alkalinization	(218)
Interferon-alpha	Minimal change nephropathy and massive proteinuria	Drug cessation	(219)
Methotrexate	Nonoliguric renal failure	Vigorous hydration and diuresis and urine alkalinization	(210,211)

depletion, either due to external losses or fluid sequestration (ascites or edema). The concomitant use of nonchemotherapeutic nephrotoxic drugs or radiographic ionic contrast media in patients with or without preexisting renal dysfunction can also potentiate renal dysfunction. Also, urinary tract obstruction secondary to underlying tumor and intrinsic idiopathic renal disease that is related to other comorbidities or to the cancer itself can also result in increased risk of renal dysfunction.

Cisplatin is a potent renal tubular toxin, and approximately 25%–42% of patients administered cisplatin will develop a mild and partially reversible decline in renal function after the first course of therapy (195). The incidence and severity of renal failure increases with subsequent courses, eventually becoming partially irreversible. Vigorous saline hydration with forced diuresis is the mainstay for preventing cisplatin-induced nephrotoxicity, along with the avoidance of

concomitant use of other nephrotoxic drugs. Discontinuation of therapy is generally indicated when a progressive rise in the plasma creatinine concentration is noted. In addition to the rise in the plasma creatinine concentration, potentially irreversible hypomagnesemia due to urinary magnesium wasting may occur in >50% of cases (196). Treatment generally consists of magnesium supplementation, and high doses may be required since raising the plasma magnesium concentration will increase the degree of magnesium wasting.

Cisplatin may also be associated with thrombotic microangiopathy with features of the hemolytic uremic syndrome or thrombotic thrombocytopenic purpura when combined with bleomycin (197). The onset of renal failure may be abrupt or insidious, and in the latter setting can develop months after treatment has been discontinued. The diagnosis of this form of nephrotoxicity is suggested by the concurrent presence of a microangiopathic hemolytic anemia and thrombocytopenia. Direct tubular injury leading to acute tubular necrosis is the primary mechanism. A less common renal side effect is renal salt wasting (198).

Carboplatin is significantly less nephrotoxic than cisplatin (199), and hypomagnesemia is the most common manifestation of nephrotoxicity, although it occurs less often than with cisplatin (200). Acute renal failure has been reported, particularly in patients previously treated with several courses of cisplatin (199). Direct tubular injury leading to acute tubular necrosis (ATN) is the primary mechanism. A less common renal side effect is renal salt wasting (198). Oxaliplatin has rarely been associated with ATN, (201), and limited data suggest that oxaliplatin does not cause exacerbation of preexisting mild renal impairment during treatment (202).

Cyclophosphamide is primarily associated with hemorrhagic cystitis, and the primary renal effect of cyclophosphamide is hyponatremia, which is due to an increased effect of antidiuretic hormone (ADH), impairing the kidney's ability to excrete water (203). Chemotherapy-induced nausea may also play a contributory role, since nausea is a potent stimulus for ADH release. Hyponatremia is usually seen in patients receiving high doses of intravenous cyclophosphamide (eg, 30–50 mg/kg or 6 g/m^2 in the setting of hematopoietic stem cell transplantation), and typically occurs acutely and resolves within approximately 24 hours after discontinuation of the drug. Hyponatremia poses a particular problem for patients undergoing high-dose intravenous cyclophosphamide treatment, who are often fluid-loaded to prevent hemorrhagic cystitis (197). The combination of increased ADH effect and enhanced water intake can lead to severe, occasionally fatal, hyponatremia within 24 hours.

The predominant urinary toxicity of ifosfamide is hemorrhagic cystitis. However, nephrotoxicity is more likely with ifosfamide than with cyclophosphamide. Ifosfamide-induced nephrotoxicity affects the proximal renal tubule, and is characterized by metabolic acidosis with a normal anion gap (hyperchloremic acidosis) due to type 1 (distal) or type 2 (proximal) renal tubular acidosis. Other toxicities include hypophosphatemia induced by decreased proximal phosphate reabsorption, renal glucosuria, aminoaciduria, and a marked increase in fl2-microglobulin excretion, all from generalized proximal dysfunction, polyuria due to nephrogenic diabetes insipidus, and hypokalemia resulting from increased urinary potassium losses. Preexisting renal disease is a risk factor for ifosfamide nephrotoxicity, and dose adjustments are recommended based upon renal function.

Prolonged therapy with the nitrosoureas can induce a slowly progressive, chronic interstitial nephritis that is generally irreversible (204). Although the exact mechanism of nephrotoxicity is not completely elucidated, these agents may produce nephrotoxicity by alkylation of tubular cell proteins. Their metabolites, which are thought to be responsible for nephrotoxicity, persist in the urine for up to 72 hours following administration (205).

MMC is associated with thrombotic thrombocytopenic purpura/hemolytic uremic syndrome (TTP-HUS) and resulting renal failure and microangiopathic hemolytic anemia (206). It most commonly occurs after at least six months of therapy, and the overall incidence is related to cumulative dose. Direct endothelial injury is the initiating event (207). Affected patients typically present with slowly progressive renal failure, hypertension, and relatively bland urine sediment, often occurring in the absence of clinically apparent tumor. MMC can be administered to patients with renal insufficiency, with close monitoring for signs and symptoms of TTP-HUS. Some guidelines suggest a 50% dose reduction for serum creatinine 1.6–2.4 mg/dL and avoidance of the drug for creatinine values >2.4 mg/dL (208). However, others note that urinary elimination accounts for only 20% of an administered dose and recommend dose reduction of 25% only for patients with creatinine clearance.

Low-dose methotrexate treatment (≤ 0.5–1.0 g/m^2) is usually not associated with renal toxicity unless underlying renal dysfunction is present. High-dose intravenous methotrexate (1–15 g/m^2) can precipitate in the tubules and induce tubular injury. Patients who are volume-depleted and those who excrete acidic urine are at particular risk. Maintenance of adequate urinary output and alkalinization will lessen the probability of methotrexate precipitation. Methotrexate can also produce a transient decrease in glomerular filtration rate (GFR), with complete recovery within six to eight hours of discontinuing the drug. The mechanism responsible for this functional renal impairment involves afferent arteriolar constriction or mesangial cell constriction that produces reduced glomerular capillary surface area and diminished glomerular capillary perfusion and pressure (210). In patients with renal insufficiency, methotrexate excretion is decreased and more significant bone marrow and gastrointestinal toxicity may result (211). Patients with ileal conduits and those with third-space fluid collections (eg, ascites, pleural effusion) may experience greater methotrexate toxicity, particularly if their creatinine clearance is low (212).

Vincristine, vinblastine, and vinorelbine are associated with SIADH (213). Topotecan is not associated with renal toxicity, but is predominantly cleared by the kidneys, and increased toxicity may result in patients with moderate renal insufficiency (214). Approximately 20%–40% of etoposide is excreted in the urine, and the dose should be reduced by 25% in patients with creatinine clearance 10–50 mL/min and by 50%

for clearance Bevacizumab, sunitinib, and sorafenib produce albuminuria in 10%–25% of patients and occasionally result in nephrotic syndrome (217). This toxicity appears to be an effect common to all agents targeted at the VEGF pathway, but the factors associated with occurrence and severity of the proteinuria are unknown. If clinically significant, decreasing the dose or discontinuation of drug is recommended.

IL-2 can induce a relatively severe capillary leak syndrome, leading to edema, plasma volume depletion, and a reversible fall in glomerular filtration rate (218). Patients with normal renal function before treatment usually recover within the first week after discontinuing therapy. Patients with underlying renal dysfunction may take longer to recover from the renal failure. Therapy for renal failure secondary to IL-2 treatment is supportive. Interferon alfa and gamma have both been associated with renal insufficiency. Interferon alpha can cause massive proteinuria as a result of minimal-change nephropathy (219). Thrombotic microangiopathy is a rare complication, seen mostly in patients with chronic myelogenous leukemia treated with high doses of alpha interferon over a long time period (220). Interferon gamma has been associated with acute tubular necrosis when used for the treatment of acute lymphoblastic leukemia (221).

Management of Complications

Numerous chemotherapeutic agents can induce nephrotoxicity in a myriad of ways, and clinical manifestations can vary from asymptomatic elevation in creatinine to renal failure requiring dialysis. Hence, clinicians must follow renal function trends very carefully during chemotherapy treatment. It is also imperative to ensure that patients are not intravascularly depleted as a result of dehydration or third spacing of fluid (ie, ascites or peripheral edema). Concomitant use of nonchemotherapeutic nephrotoxic drugs (eg, nonsteroidal anti-inflammatory drugs [NSAIDs] and certain antibiotics), and contrast media should be minimized in the setting of even mild renal insufficiency. Also, extrinsic and intrinsic urinary obstruction and idiopathic renal disease (acute interstitial nephritis and glomerulonephritis) should be ruled out, and medical comorbidities (hypertension and diabetes) should be optimized. Referral to nephrology should be considered early should renal function not rapidly normalize with the previously described interventions.

AUTOIMMUNE TOXICITY

Autoimmune complications, including autoimmune hemolytic anemia (AIHA) and autoimmune thrombo-

cytopenia, have been reported with the use of purine analogs (fludarabine, cladribine, pentostatin). One report described 24 patients with CLL who developed fludarabine-associated autoimmune hemolytic anemia (FA-AIHA) (241). Seventy-one percent of patients developed AIHA during the first three cycles of therapy, and one case occurred after six cycles. In six cases, AIHA was also associated with autoimmune thrombocytopenia (AITP). There are a myriad of case reports of AIHA in CLL or other lymphoproliferative disorders triggered by therapy with cladribine (242,243) or pentostatin (244). The two most important risk factors for developing AIHA are a positive direct antiglobulin test (Coomb test) and a prior history of AIHA. CLL patients are also at increased risk of acquiring AITP. The exact incidence of AITP is unknown, but is thought to be less frequent than AIHA (222).

IL-2 has been associated with a syndrome mimicking painless thyroiditis. In one study of 130 patients receiving IL-2–based immunotherapy, primary hypothyroidism occurred in 12% of patients before, 38% during, and 23% after immunotherapy. Hyperthyroidism occurred in 1%, 4%, and 7% of patients at those time intervals. Among patients initially euthyroid ($n = 111$), primary hypothyroidism developed in 32% during and 14% after immunotherapy, persisting a median of 54 days, and three patients required levothyroxine treatment. Hyperthyroidism developed in 2% of patients during immunotherapy and 6% after. Thyroid dysfunction was not a function of gender, diagnosis, type of treatment, or response to immunotherapy. Elevated titers of antithyroglobulin and antithyroid microsomal antibodies were detected after treatment in 9% and 7%, respectively (223).

In another study designed to evaluate the incidence and risk factors of this adverse autoimmune response, triiodothyronine, thyroxine, and thyrotropin levels were measured serially in 146 consecutive patients treated with IL-2 for refractory solid tumor (77 patients) or malignant hemopathy (69 patients). IL-2 was administered intravenously alone in 79 cases or in combination with autologous bone marrow transplantation in 26 cases, with interferon-gamma in 37 cases, with tumor necrosis factor-alpha in 13, and with cyclophosphamide in 5 cases. Some patients underwent more than one therapeutic treatment. Peripheral hypothyroidism was present upon entry in nine (6.2%) patients. Thyroid dysfunction appeared or worsened during IL-2 therapy in 24 (16.4%) patients. Sixteen (10.9%) patients exhibited peripheral hypothyroidism, out of which four exhibited biphasic thyroiditis. Another five (3.4%) patients developed transient hyperthyroidism. Thyroid dysfunction appeared early after one or two cycles, and all surviving patients recovered. Only gender and presence of antithyroid antibody were correlated significantly with IL-2–induced thyroid abnormalities. Antithyroid antibodies were detected in 60.9% of patients, and thyroid-stimulating antibodies were never detected (224).

Sunitinib-induced hypothyroidism has also been described. In one study of patients with metastatic renal cell carcinoma (RCC), 85% of patients had abnormalities in their thyroid function tests and 84% experienced symptoms related to hypothyroidism (225). In another study, 62% of patients had an abnormal level of thyroid-stimulating hormone (TSH) and 36% had hypothyroidism with sunitinib therapy for GISTs (226). However, in this study, 10% of patients were noted to have an elevated TSH before initiating sunitinib treatment and an additional 12% were being treated with L-thyroxine prior to enrollment. It has been theorized that increased thyroid function testing in patients treated with sunitinib may lead to increased detection of abnormalities in the absence of symptoms, a finding that may not necessarily have clinical consequences.

Management of Complications

AIHA treatment includes cessation of drugs and initiation of corticosteroids. In corticosteroid-resistant cases, immunosuppressive agents, such as cyclosporine A and azathioprine, may be utilized. Other agents, such as rituximab and intravenous immune globulin (IVIG), may also be efficacious (227,228). Splenectomy is considered for patients whose autoimmune disorder has proven refractory to the previously described treatments. Treatment of AITP is generally not indicated until platelet counts are <20,000 or bleeding occurs, and treatment is similar to that of AIHA (228, 229).

Thyroiditis treatment generally includes initiation of thyroid replacement therapy with L-thyroxine and frequent monitoring of thyroid function tests while on replacement therapy. It is also important to delineate whether symptoms of fatigue are due to sunitinib therapy (independent of thyroid dysfunction), underlying cancer itself, or due to clinical hypothyroidism, for, as stated, not all thyroid function derangements warrant treatment.

RHEUMATIC TOXICITY

Almost any chemotherapeutic agent can result in postchemotherapy rheumatism, and this is a fairly common clinical phenomenon. In one study of eight breast cancer patients receiving cyclophosphamide and 5-fluorouracil containing adjuvant combination chemotherapy, patients (ages 41–53) developed rheumatic symptoms (myalgias, arthralgias, joint stiffness, generalized musculoskeletal achiness, and periarticular tenderness) between one and four months after (one patient developed symptoms during treatment) chemotherapy treatment. Symptoms resolved between 2 and >16 months after completion of chemotherapy, and in all cases, recurrent cancer and rheumatic disorders (polymyositis, cancer-associated arthritis, systemic lupus erythematosus, polymyalgia rheumatica, and fibromyalgia) were ruled out as possible etiologies. In this study, NSAIDs were generally not beneficial, and one patient experienced prompt resolution of symptoms after initiation of low-dose oral corticosteroids (230).

Aromatase inhibitors (AIs) (anastrozole [Arimidex], letrozole [Femara], and exemestane [Aromasin]) are oral antiestrogen agents that are widely used as adjuvant endocrine treatment in postmenopausal women with early-stage breast cancer. AI-associated arthralgias are highly variable, and usually include bilateral symmetrical pain/soreness in the hands, knees, hips, lower back, shoulders, and/or feet, along with early-morning stiffness and difficulty sleeping. Typical onset is within two months of treatment initiation, and some patients develop more severe symptoms over time. Spontaneous symptom resolution is rare during treatment, but common after cessation of therapy (231). In the Arimidex and Tamoxifen Alone or in Combination (ATAC) trial, which had the longest median follow-up time, the incidence of musculoskeletal disorders was 30% with Arimidex and 23.7% with tamoxifen ($P < 0.001$). The incidence of arthralgia was 35.6% versus 29.4% ($P < 0.001$) with Arimidex versus tamoxifen, and the incidence of fractures was 11.0% versus 7.7% ($P < 0.001$) with Arimidex versus tamoxifen (232). The risk of important long-term skeletal problems, including osteoporosis, may increase with the use of aromatase inhibitors. The maintenance of bone density depends in part on estrogen, and aromatase inhibitors may enhance bone loss by lowering circulating estrogen levels. Short-term use of letrozole has been shown to be associated with an increase in bone-resorption markers in plasma and urine. However, it is possible that osteopenia might be prevented or modified with concurrent use of bisphosphonates (233).

Paclitaxel and docetaxel can also cause myalgias and arthralgias that are sometimes severe and can impair both physical function and quality of life. The incidence of these side effects is not known, although it has been reported to occur in up to 75% of patients (234–239). This still poorly understood process usually develops 24–48 hours following the completion of a paclitaxel infusion and may persist for 3–5 days. Occasionally, the symptoms of achiness and pain in the muscles and joints may last for a week or longer.

Management of Complications

There are no formal studies of treatment for chemotherapy-induced arthralgia syndrome. The most commonly prescribed treatment are NSAIDs, but chronic use of NSAIDs such as ibuprofen can contribute to adverse effects on the GI tract, heart, and kidneys. More potent NSAIDs, such as nabumetone, have also been prescribed in conjunction with a proton pump inhibitor in an effort to control GI side effects. Combinations of NSAIDs and other analgesics (both narcotic and non-narcotic) are also often used, but it is not clear to what extent these treatments improve chemotherapy-induced arthralgias. Cyclooxygenase 2 (COX-2) inhibitors had also been proposed as treatment of this syndrome, but have recently fallen out of favor due to their association with adverse cardiovascular events. Some data suggests that gabapentin may beneficial in the treatment of this syndrome (240). Gentle exercise may also be beneficial. The use of bisphosphonates to counter AI-induced bone loss is also recommended.

References

1. Singal PK, Deally CM, Weinberg LE. Subcellular effects of adriamycin in the heart: A concise review. *J Mol Cell Cardiol.* 1987;19(8):817–828.
2. Li T, Singal PK. Adriamycin-induced early changes in myocardial antioxidant enzymes and their modulation by probucol. *Circulation.* 2000;102(17):2105–2110.
3. Singal PK, et al. Adriamycin cardiomyopathy: pathophysiology and prevention. *FASEB J.* 1997;11(12):931–936.
4. Singal PK, Iliskovic N. Doxorubicin-induced cardiomyopathy. *N Engl J Med.* 1998;339(13):900–905.
5. Von Hoff DD, et al. Risk factors for doxorubicin-induced congestive heart failure. *Ann Intern Med.* 1979;91(5):710–717.
6. Von Hoff DD, et al. Daunomycin-induced cardiotoxicity in children and adults. A review of 110 cases. *Am J Med.* 1977;62(2):200–208.
7. Miller KD, et al. Randomized phase III trial of capecitabine compared with bevacizumab plus capecitabine in patients with previously treated metastatic breast cancer. *J Clin Oncol.* 2005;23(4):792–799.
8. Swain SM, Whaley FS, Ewer MS. Congestive heart failure in patients treated with doxorubicin: A retrospective analysis of three trials. *Cancer.* 2003;97(11):2869–2879.
9. Isner JM, et al. Clinical and morphologic cardiac findings after anthracycline chemotherapy. Analysis of 64 patients studied at necropsy. *Am J Cardiol.* 1983;51(7):1167–1174.
10. Lefrak EA, et al. A clinicopathologic analysis of adriamycin cardiotoxicity. *Cancer.* 1973;32(2):302–314.
11. Appelbaum F, et al. Acute lethal carditis caused by high-dose combination chemotherapy. A unique clinical and pathological entity. *Lancet.* 1976;1(7950):58–62.
12. Ferguson C, Clarke J, Herity NA. Ventricular tachycardia associated with trastuzumab. *N Engl J Med.*, 2006;354(6):648–649.
13. Keefe DL. Trastuzumab-associated cardiotoxicity. *Cancer.* 2002;95(7):1592–1600.
14. Seidman A, et al. Cardiac dysfunction in the trastuzumab clinical trials experience. *J Clin Oncol.* 2002;20(5):1215–1221.
15. Perez EA, Rodeheffer R. Clinical cardiac tolerability of trastuzumab. *J Clin Oncol.* 2004;22(2):322–329.
16. Esteva FJ, et al. Phase II study of weekly docetaxel and trastuzumab for patients with HER-2-overexpressing metastatic breast cancer. *J Clin Oncol.* 2002;20(7):1800–1808.
17. Millward PM, et al. Cardiogenic shock complicates successful treatment of refractory thrombotic thrombocytopenia purpura with rituximab. *Transfusion.* 2005;45(9):1481–1486.
18. Slamon DJ, et al. Use of chemotherapy plus a monoclonal antibody against HER2 for metastatic breast cancer that overexpresses HER2. *N Engl J Med.* 2001l;344(11):783–792.
19. Slamon D, Eiermann W, Robert N, et al. Phase III trial comparing AC-T with AC-TH and with TCH in the adjuvant treatment of HER2 positive early breast cancer: First planned interim efficacy analysis (abstract 1). In San Antonio Breast Cancer Symposium. 2005. San Antonio, TX.
20. Floyd JD, et al. Cardiotoxicity of cancer therapy. *J Clin Oncol.* 2005;23(30):7685–7896.
21. Sonnenblick M, Rosin A. Cardiotoxicity of interferon. A review of 44 cases. *Chest.* 1991;99(3):557–561.
22. Budd GT, et al. Phase-I trial of Ultrapure human leukocyte interferon in human malignancy. *Cancer Chemother Pharmacol.* 1984;12(1):39–42.
23. Martino S, et al. Reversible arrhythmias observed in patients treated with recombinant alpha 2 interferon. *J Cancer Res Clin Oncol.* 1987;113(4):376–378.
24. Chap L, et al. Pulmonary toxicity of high-dose chemotherapy for breast cancer: A non-invasive approach to diagnosis and treatment. *Bone Marrow Transplant.* 1997;20(12):1063–1067. Bone Marrow Transplant
25. Cohen MC, Huberman MS, Nesto RW. Recombinant alpha 2 interferon-related cardiomyopathy. *Am J Med.* 1988;85(4):549–551.
26. Sonnenblick M, Rosenmann D, Rosin A. Reversible cardiomyopathy induced by interferon. *BMJ.* 1990;300(6733):1174–1175.
27. Rowinsky EK, et al. Cardiac disturbances during the administration of Taxol. *J Clin Oncol.* 1991;9(9):1704–1712.
28. Gianni L, et al. Paclitaxel by 3-hour infusion in combination with bolus doxorubicin in women with untreated metastatic breast cancer: High antitumor efficacy and cardiac effects in a dose-finding and sequence-finding study. *J Clin Oncol.* 1995;13(11):2688–2699.
29. Biganzoli L, et al. Doxorubicin-paclitaxel: a safe regimen in terms of cardiac toxicity in metastatic breast carcinoma patients. Results from a European Organization for Research and Treatment of Cancer multicenter trial. *Cancer.* 2003;97(1):40–45.
30. Giordano SH, et al. A detailed evaluation of cardiac toxicity: A phase II study of doxorubicin and one- or three-hour-infusion paclitaxel in patients with metastatic breast cancer. *Clin Cancer Res.* 2002;8(11):3360–3368.
31. Abi 007. *Drugs R D,* 2004. 5(3): p. 155-9.
32. Malhotra V, et al. Neoadjuvant and adjuvant chemotherapy with doxorubicin and docetaxel in locally advanced breast cancer. *Clin Breast Cancer.* 2004;5(5):377–384.
33. Margolin KA, et al. Interleukin-2 and lymphokine-activated killer cell therapy of solid tumors: Analysis of toxicity and management guidelines. *J Clin Oncol.* 1989;7(4):486–498.
34. Crum E. Biological-response modifier—induced emergencies. *Semin Oncol.* 1989;16(6):579–587.
35. White RL, Jr. et al. Cardiopulmonary toxicity of treatment with high dose interleukin-2 in 199 consecutive patients with metastatic melanoma or renal cell carcinoma. *Cancer.* 1994;74(12):3212–3222.
36. Akhtar SS, Salim KP, Bano ZA. Symptomatic cardiotoxicity with high-dose 5-fluorouracil infusion: A prospective study. *Oncology.* 1993;50(5):441–444.
37. de Forni M, et al. Cardiotoxicity of high-dose continuous infusion fluorouracil: A prospective clinical study. *J Clin Oncol.* 1992;10(11):1795–1801.
38. Wacker A, et al. High incidence of angina pectoris in patients treated with 5-fluorouracil. A planned surveillance study with 102 patients. *Oncology.* 2003;65(2):108–112.

39. Kuropkat C, et al. Severe cardiotoxicity during 5-fluorouracil chemotherapy: A case and literature report. *Am J Clin Oncol.* 1999;22(5):466–470.

40. Sasson Z, et al. 5-Fluorouracil related toxic myocarditis: Case reports and pathological confirmation. *Can J Cardiol.* 1994;10(8):861–864.

41. Cianci G, et al. Prophylactic options in patients with 5-fluorouracil-associated cardiotoxicity. *Br J Cancer.* 2003;88(10):1507–1509.

42. Eskilsson J, Albertsson M. Failure of preventing 5-fluorouracil cardiotoxicity by prophylactic treatment with verapamil. *Acta Oncol.* 1990;29(8): 1001–1003.

43. Ng M, Cunningham D, Norman AR. The frequency and pattern of cardiotoxicity observed with capecitabine used in conjunction with oxaliplatin in patients treated for advanced colorectal cancer (CRC). *Eur J Cancer.* 2005;41(11): 1542–1546.

44. Hurwitz H, et al. Bevacizumab plus irinotecan, fluorouracil, and leucovorin for metastatic colorectal cancer. *N Engl J Med.* 2004;350(23):2335–2342.

45. Veronese ML, et al. Mechanisms of hypertension associated with BAY 43 9006. *J Clin Oncol.* 2006;24(9):1363–1369.

46. Escudier B, et al. Sorafenib in advanced clear-cell renal-cell carcinoma. *N Engl J Med.* 2007;356(2):125–134.

47. Faivre S, et al. Safety, pharmacokinetic, and antitumor activity of SU11248, a novel oral multitarget tyrosine kinase inhibitor, in patients with cancer. *J Clin Oncol.* 2006;24(1):25–35.

48. Chiang CE, et al. Prolongation of cardiac repolarization by arsenic trioxide. *Blood.* 2002;100(6):2249–2252.

49. Westervelt P, et al. Sudden death among patients with acute promyelocytic leukemia treated with arsenic trioxide. *Blood.* 2001;98(2):266–271.

50. Matsui H, et al. Protective effects of carvedilol against doxorubicin-induced cardiomyopathy in rats. *Life Sci.* 1999;65(12):1265–1274.

51. Santos DL, et al. Carvedilol protects against doxorubicin-induced mitochondrial cardiomyopathy. *Toxicol Appl Pharmacol.* 2002;185(3):218–227.

52. Kalay N, et al. Protective effects of carvedilol against anthracycline-induced cardiomyopathy. *J Am Coll Cardiol.* 2006;48(11):2258–2262.

53. Cardinale D, et al. Prevention of high-dose chemotherapy-induced cardiotoxicity in high-risk patients by angiotensin-converting enzyme inhibition. *Circulation.* 2006;114(23): 2474–2481.

54. Seifert CF, Nesser ME, Thompson DF. Dexrazoxane in the prevention of doxorubicin-induced cardiotoxicity. *Ann Pharmacother.* 1994;28(9):1063–1072.

55. van Dalen EC, et al. Cardioprotective interventions for cancer patients receiving anthracyclines. *Cochrane Database Syst Rev.* 2005;(1):CD003917.

56. O'Sullivan JM, et al. Predicting the risk of bleomycin lung toxicity in patients with germ-cell tumours. *Ann Oncol.* 2003;14(1):91–96.

57. Sleijfer S. Bleomycin-induced pneumonitis. *Chest.* 2001;120(2):617–624.

58. Blum RH, Carter SK, Agre K. A clinical review of bleomycin— a new antineoplastic agent. *Cancer.* 1973;31(4):903–914.

59. Berend N. Protective effect of hypoxia on bleomycin lung toxicity in the rat. *Am Rev Respir Dis.* 1984;130(2):307–308.

60. Kawai K, et al. Serum creatinine level during chemotherapy for testicular cancer as a possible predictor of bleomycin-induced pulmonary toxicity. *Jpn J Clin Oncol.* 1998;28(9): 546–550.

61. Sikdar T, MacVicar D, Husband JE. Pneumomediastinum complicating bleomycin related lung damage. *Br J Radiol.* 1998;71(851):1202–1204.

62. White DA, et al. Acute chest pain syndrome during bleomycin infusions. *Cancer.* 1987;59(9):1582–1585.

63. Maher J, Daly PA. Severe bleomycin lung toxicity: reversal with high dose corticosteroids. *Thorax.* 1993;48(1):92–94.

64. Conaghan PG, et al. Hazards of low dose methotrexate. *Aust N Z J Med.* 1995;25(6):670–673.

65. Cronstein BN, Molecular therapeutics. Methotrexate and its mechanism of action. *Arthritis Rheum.* 1996;39(12):1951–1960.

66. Lynch JP, 3rd, McCune WJ. Immunosuppressive and cytotoxic pharmacotherapy for pulmonary disorders. *Am J Respir Crit Care Med.* 1997;155(2):395–420.

67. Morice AH, Lai WK. Fatal varicella zoster infection in a severe steroid dependent asthmatic patient receiving methotrexate. *Thorax.* 1995;50(11):1221–1222.

68. Hilliquin P, et al. Occurrence of pulmonary complications during methotrexate therapy in rheumatoid arthritis. *Br J Rheumatol.* 1996;35(5):441–445.

69. Weinblatt ME. Methotrexate in rheumatoid arthritis: toxicity issues. *Br J Rheumatol.* 1996;35(5):403–405.

70. Golden MR, et al. The relationship of preexisting lung disease to the development of methotrexate pneumonitis in patients with rheumatoid arthritis. *J Rheumatol.* 1995;22(6):1043–1047.

71. Kremer JM, et al. Clinical, laboratory, radiographic, and histopathologic features of methotrexate-associated lung injury in patients with rheumatoid arthritis: A multicenter study with literature review. *Arthritis Rheum.* 1997;40(10):1829–1837.

72. Carroll GJ, et al. Incidence, prevalence and possible risk factors for pneumonitis in patients with rheumatoid arthritis receiving methotrexate. *J Rheumatol.* 1994;21(1):51–54.

73. Hassell A, Dawes P. Serious problems with methotrexate? *Br J Rheumatol.* 1994;33(11):1001–1002.

74. St Clair EW, Rice JR, Snyderman R. Pneumonitis complicating low-dose methotrexate therapy in rheumatoid arthritis. *Arch Intern Med.* 1985;145(11):2035–2038.

75. Searles G, McKendry RJ. Methotrexate pneumonitis in rheumatoid arthritis: Potential risk factors. Four case reports and a review of the literature. *J Rheumatol.* 1987;14(6):1164–1171.

76. Beyeler C, et al. Pulmonary function in rheumatoid arthritis treated with low-dose methotrexate: A longitudinal study. *Br J Rheumatol.* 1996;35(5):446–452.

77. Wall MA, et al. Lung function in adolescents receiving high-dose methotrexate. *Pediatrics.* 1979;63(5):741–746.

78. Dijkmans BA. Folate supplementation and methotrexate. *Br J Rheumatol.* 1995;34(12):1172–1174.

79. Morgan SL, et al. Supplementation with folic acid during methotrexate therapy for rheumatoid arthritis. A double-blind, placebo-controlled trial. *Ann Intern Med.* 1994;121(11):833–841.

80. Lane SD, et al. Fatal interstitial pneumonitis following high-dose intermittent chlorambucil therapy for chronic lymphocyte leukemia. *Cancer.* 1981;47(1):32–36.

81. Rosner V, et al. Contribution of bronchoalveolar lavage and transbronchial biopsy to diagnosis and prognosis of drug-induced pneumopathies. *Rev Pneumol Clin.* 1995;51(5): 269–274.

82. Crestani B, et al. Chlorambucil-associated pneumonitis. *Chest.* 1994;105(2):634–636.

83. Tomlinson J, et al. Interstitial pneumonitis following mitoxantrone, chlorambucil and prednisolone (MCP) chemotherapy. *Clin Oncol (R Coll Radiol).* 1999;11(3):184–186.

84. Verweij J, Pinedo HM. Mitomycin C: Mechanism of action, usefulness and limitations. *Anticancer Drugs.* 1990;1(1):5–13.

85. Folman RS. Experience with mitomycin in the treatment of non-small cell lung cancer. *Oncology.* 1993;50(Suppl 1):24–30.

86. Orwoll ES, Kiessling PJ, Patterson JR. Interstitial pneumonia from mitomycin. *Ann Intern Med.* 1978;89(3):352–355.

87. Castro M, et al. A prospective study of pulmonary function in patients receiving mitomycin. *Chest.* 1996;109(4):939–944.

88. Linette DC, McGee KH, McFarland JA. Mitomycin-induced pulmonary toxicity: Case report and review of the literature. *Ann Pharmacother.* 1992;26(4):481–484.

89. Kris MG, et al. Dyspnea following vinblastine or vindesine administration in patients receiving mitomycin plus vinca alkaloid combination therapy. *Cancer Treat Rep.* 1984;68 (7–8):1029–1031.

90. Luedke D, et al. Mitomycin C and vindesine associated pulmonary toxicity with variable clinical expression. *Cancer.* 1985;55(3):542–545.

91. Rivera MP, et al. Syndrome of acute dyspnea related to combined mitomycin plus vinca alkaloid chemotherapy. *Am J Clin Oncol.* 1995;18(3):245–250.

92. McCarthy JT, Staats BA. Pulmonary hypertension, hemolytic anemia, and renal failure. A mitomycin-associated syndrome. *Chest.* 1986;89(4):608–611.

93. Verweij J, et al. Prospective study on the dose relationship of mitomycin C-induced interstitial pneumonitis. *Cancer.* 1987;60(4):756–761.

94. Chang AY, et al. Pulmonary toxicity induced by mitomycin C is highly responsive to glucocorticoids. *Cancer.* 1986;57(12):2285–2290.

95. Okuno SH, Frytak S. Mitomycin lung toxicity. Acute and chronic phases. *Am J Clin Oncol.* 1997;20(3):282–284.

96. Selker RG, et al. 1,3-Bis(2-chloroethyl)-1-nitrosourea (BCNU)-induced pulmonary fibrosis. *Neurosurgery.* 1980;7(6):560–565.

97. Weiss RB, Poster DS, Penta JS. The nitrosoureas and pulmonary toxicity. *Cancer Treat Rev.* 1981;8(2):111–125.

98. Frankovich J, et al. High-dose therapy and autologous hematopoietic cell transplantation in children with primary refractory and relapsed Hodgkin's disease: Atopy predicts idiopathic diffuse lung injury syndromes. *Biol Blood Marrow Transplant.* 2001;7(1):49–57.

99. Wong R, et al. Idiopathic pneumonia syndrome after high-dose chemotherapy and autologous hematopoietic stem cell transplantation for high-risk breast cancer. *Bone Marrow Transplant.* 2003;31(12):1157–1163.

100. Cao TM, et al. Pulmonary toxicity syndrome in breast cancer patients undergoing BCNU-containing high-dose chemotherapy and autologous hematopoietic cell transplantation. *Biol Blood Marrow Transplant.* 2000;6(4):387–394.

101. Parish JM, Muhm JR, Leslie KO. Upper lobe pulmonary fibrosis associated with high-dose chemotherapy containing BCNU for bone marrow transplantation. *Mayo Clin Proc.* 2003;78(5):630–634.

102. Lind PA, et al. Predictors for pneumonitis during locoregional radiotherapy in high-risk patients with breast carcinoma treated with high-dose chemotherapy and stem-cell rescue. *Cancer.* 2002;94(11):2821–2829.

103. Rubio C, et al. Idiopathic pneumonia syndrome after high-dose chemotherapy for relapsed Hodgkin's disease. *Br J Cancer.* 1997;75(7):1044–1048.

104. Schmitz N, Diehl V. Carmustine and the lungs. *Lancet.* 1997;349(9067):1712–1713.

105. O'Driscoll BR, et al. Active lung fibrosis up to 17 years after chemotherapy with carmustine (BCNU) in childhood. *N Engl J Med.* 1990;323(6):378–382.

106. O'Driscoll BR, et al. Late carmustine lung fibrosis. Age at treatment may influence severity and survival. *Chest.* 1995;107(5):1355–1357.

107. Malik SW, et al. Lung toxicity associated with cyclophosphamide use. Two distinct patterns. *Am J Respir Crit Care Med.* 1996;154(6 Pt 1):1851–1856.

108. Segura A, et al. Pulmonary fibrosis induced by cyclophosphamide. *Ann Pharmacother.* 2001;35(7–8):894–897.

109. Hamada K, et al. Cyclophosphamide-induced late-onset lung disease. *Intern Med.* 2003;42(1):82–87.

110. Cohen EE, et al. Phase II trial of ZD1839 in recurrent or metastatic squamous cell carcinoma of the head and neck. *J Clin Oncol.* 2003;21(10):1980–1987.

111. Culy CR, Faulds D. Gefitinib. *Drugs.* 2002;62(15):2237–2248; discussion 2249–2250.

112. Fukuoka M, et al. Multi-institutional randomized phase II trial of gefitinib for previously treated patients with advanced non-small-cell lung cancer (The IDEAL 1 Trial) (corrected). *J Clin Oncol.* 2003;21(12):2237–2246.

113. Hotta K, et al. Interstitial lung disease in Japanese patients with non-small cell lung cancer receiving gefitinib: An analysis of risk factors and treatment outcomes in Okayama Lung Cancer Study Group. *Cancer J.* 2005;11(5):417–424.

114. Thomas AL, et al. Gemcitabine and paclitaxel associated pneumonitis in non-small cell lung cancer: Report of a phase I/II dose-escalating study. *Eur J Cancer.* 2000;36(18):2329–2334.

115. Androulakis N, et al. Salvage treatment with paclitaxel and gemcitabine for patients with non-small-cell lung cancer after cisplatin- or docetaxel-based chemotherapy: a multicenter phase II study. *Ann Oncol.* 1998;9(10):1127–1130.

116. Dunsford ML, et al. Severe pulmonary toxicity in patients treated with a combination of docetaxel and gemcitabine for metastatic transitional cell carcinoma. *Ann Oncol.* 1999;10(8):943–947.

117. Mollman JE, et al. Cisplatin neuropathy. Risk factors, prognosis, and protection by WR-2721. *Cancer.* 1988;61(11):2192–2195.

118. Siegal T, Haim N. Cisplatin-induced peripheral neuropathy. Frequent off-therapy deterioration, demyelinating syndromes, and muscle cramps. *Cancer.* 1990;66(6):1117–1123.

119. van der Hoop RG, et al. Prevention of cisplatin neurotoxicity with an ACTH(4-9) analogue in patients with ovarian cancer. *N Engl J Med.* 1990;322(2):89–94.

120. von Schlippe M, Fowler CJ, Harland SJ. Cisplatin neurotoxicity in the treatment of metastatic germ cell tumour: Time course and prognosis. *Br J Cancer.* 2001;85(6):823–826.

121. Posner JB. *Side Effects of Chemotherapy; Neurologic Complications of Cancer.* Philadelphia: FA Davis; 1995.

122. Rademaker-Lakhai JM, et al. Relationship between cisplatin administration and the development of ototoxicity. *J Clin Oncol.* 2006;24(6):918–924.

123. Low WK, et al. Sensorineural hearing loss after radiotherapy and chemoradiotherapy: A single, blinded, randomized study. *J Clin Oncol.* 2006;24(12):1904–1909.

124. Heinzlef O, Lotz JP, Roullet E. Severe neuropathy after high dose carboplatin in three patients receiving multidrug chemotherapy. *J Neurol Neurosurg Psychiatry.* 1998;64(5):667–669.

125. Stewart DJ, et al. Phase I study of intracarotid administration of carboplatin. *Neurosurgery.* 1992;30(4):512–516; discussion 516–517.

126. Gamelin E, et al. Clinical aspects and molecular basis of oxaliplatin neurotoxicity: Current management and development of preventive measures. *Semin Oncol.* 2002;29(5 Suppl 15):21–33.

127. Lehky TJ, et al. Oxaliplatin-induced neurotoxicity: acute hyperexcitability and chronic neuropathy. *Muscle Nerve.* 2004;29(3):387–392.

128. Wilson RH, et al. Acute oxaliplatin-induced peripheral nerve hyperexcitability. *J Clin Oncol.* 2002;20(7):1767–1774.

129. Cassidy J, Misset JL. Oxaliplatin-related side effects: characteristics and management. *Semin Oncol.* 2002;29(5 Suppl 15):11–20.

130. Geiser CF, et al. Adverse effects of intrathecal methotrexate in children with acute leukemia in remission. *Blood.* 1975;45(2):189–195.

131. Phillips PC. Methotrexate toxicity. In: Rottenberg DA, ed. *Neurological Complications of Cancer Treatment.* Boston: Butterworth-Heinmann; 1991.

132. Gagliano RG, Costanzi JJ. Paraplegia following intrathecal methotrexate: Report of a case and review of the literature. *Cancer.* 1976;37(4):1663–1668.

133. Walker RW, et al. Transient cerebral dysfunction secondary to high-dose methotrexate. *J Clin Oncol.* 1986;4(12):1845–1850.

134. Freilich RJ, et al. Motor neuropathy due to docetaxel and paclitaxel. *Neurology.* 1996;47(1):115–118.

135. Lee JJ, Swain SM. Peripheral neuropathy induced by microtubule-stabilizing agents. *J Clin Oncol.* 2006;24(10):1633–1642.

136. Akerley W, 3rd. Paclitaxel in advanced non-small cell lung cancer: An alternative high-dose weekly schedule. *Chest.* 2000;117(4 Suppl 1):152S–155S.

137. Perry JR, Warner E. Transient encephalopathy after paclitaxel (Taxol) infusion. *Neurology.* 1996;46(6):1596–1599.

138. Postma TJ, et al. Paclitaxel-induced neuropathy. *Ann Oncol.* 1995;6(5):489–494.

139. Piccart MJ, et al. Randomized intergroup trial of cisplatin-paclitaxel versus cisplatin-cyclophosphamide in women with advanced epithelial ovarian cancer: Three-year results. *J Natl Cancer Inst.* 2000;92(9):699–708.

140. Smith A, Rosenfeld S, Dropcho E, et al. High-dose thiotepa with hematopoietic reconstitution for recurrent aggressive oligodendroglioma (abstract). *Am Soc Clin Oncol.* 1997.

141. van den Bent MJ, et al. Lhermitte's sign following chemotherapy with docetaxel. *Neurology.* 1998;50(2):563–564.

142. Tosi P, et al. Neurological toxicity of long-term (>1 yr) thalidomide therapy in patients with multiple myeloma. *Eur J Haematol.* 2005;74(3):212–216.

143. Isoardo G, et al. Thalidomide neuropathy: clinical, electrophysiological and neuroradiological features. *Acta Neurol Scand.* 2004;109(3):188–193.

144. Clark TE, et al. Thalomid (Thalidomide) capsules: a review of the first 18 months of spontaneous postmarketing adverse event surveillance, including off-label prescribing. *Drug Saf.* 2001;24(2):87–117.

145. Richardson PG, et al. A randomized phase 2 study of lenalidomide therapy for patients with relapsed or relapsed and refractory multiple myeloma. *Blood.* 2006;108(10):3458–3464.

146. Richardson PG, et al. A phase 2 study of bortezomib in relapsed, refractory myeloma. *N Engl J Med.* 2003;348(26):2609–2617.

147. Postma TJ, Heimans JJ. Chemotherapy-induced peripheral neuropathy. In: Vecht CJ, ed. *Handbook of Clinical Neurology.* Amsterdam: Elsevier Science; 1998:459.

148. Verstappen CC, et al. Dose-related vincristine-induced peripheral neuropathy with unexpected off-therapy worsening. *Neurology.* 2005;64(6):1076–1077.

149. McLeod JG, Penny R. Vincristine neuropathy: An electrophysiological and histological study. *J Neurol Neurosurg Psychiatry.* 1969;32(4):297–304.

150. Legha SS. Vincristine neurotoxicity. Pathophysiology and management. *Med Toxicol.* 1986;1(6):421–427.

151. Robertson GL, Bhoopalam N, Zelkowitz LJ. Vincristine neurotoxicity and abnormal secretion of antidiuretic hormone. *Arch Intern Med.* 1973;132(5):717–720.

152. Forsyth PA, Cascino TL. Neurologic complications of chemotherapy. In: Wiley RG, ed. *Neurologic Complications of Cancer.* New York: Marcel Dekker; 1995.

153. Paleologos N. Complications of chemotherapy. In: Biller J, ed. *Iatrogenic Neurology.* Boston: Butterworth-Heinemann; 1998:241.

154. Fazeny B, et al. Vinorelbine-induced neurotoxicity in patients with advanced breast cancer pretreated with paclitaxel—a phase II study. *Cancer Chemother Pharmacol.* 1996;39 (1–2):150–156.

155. Phillips PC, Reinhard CS. Antipyrimidene neurotoxicity: Cytosine arabinoside and 5-fluorouracil. In: Rottenberg DA, et al., eds. *Neurological Complications of Cancer Treatment.* Boston: Butterworth-Heinemann; 1991:97.

156. Smith GA, et al. High-dose cytarabine dose modification reduces the incidence of neurotoxicity in patients with renal insufficiency. *J Clin Oncol.* 1997;15(2):833–839.

157. Dunton SF, et al. Progressive ascending paralysis following administration of intrathecal and intravenous cytosine arabinoside. A Pediatric Oncology Group study. *Cancer.* 1986;57(6):1083–1088.

158. Brashear A, Siemers E. Focal dystonia after chemotherapy: A case series. *J Neurooncol.* 1997;34(2):163–167.

159. Stein ME, et al. A rare event of 5-fluorouracil-associated peripheral neuropathy: A report of two patients. *Am J Clin Oncol.* 1998;21(3):248–249.

160. Pirzada NA, Ali II, Dafer RM. Fluorouracil-induced neurotoxicity. *Ann Pharmacother.* 2000;34(1):35–38.

161. Ohara S, et al. Leukoencephalopathy induced by chemotherapy with tegafur, a 5-fluorouracil derivative. *Acta Neuropathol (Berl).* 1998;96(5):527–531.

162. Meanwell CA, et al. Prediction of ifosfamide/mesna associated encephalopathy. *Eur J Cancer Clin Oncol.* 1986;22(7):815–819.

163. Pratt CB, et al. Ifosfamide neurotoxicity is related to previous cisplatin treatment for pediatric solid tumors. *J Clin Oncol.* 1990;8(8):1399–1401.

164. Yamaji S, et al. All-trans retinoic acid-induced multiple mononeuropathies. *Am J Hematol.* 1999;60(4):311.

165. Shapiro WR, Green SB. Reevaluating the efficacy of intra-arterial BCNU. *J Neurosurg.* 1987;66(2):313–315.

166. Shapiro WR, et al. A randomized comparison of intra-arterial versus intravenous BCNU, with or without intravenous 5-fluorouracil, for newly diagnosed patients with malignant glioma. *J Neurosurg.* 1992;76(5):772–781.

167. Rosenblum MK, et al. Fatal necrotizing encephalopathy complicating treatment of malignant gliomas with intra-arterial BCNU and irradiation: a pathological study. *J Neurooncol.* 1989;7(3):269–281.

168. Postma TJ, et al. Neurotoxicity of combination chemotherapy with procarbazine, CCNU and vincristine (PCV) for recurrent glioma. *J Neurooncol.* 1998;38(1):69–75.

169. Macdonald DR. Neurologic complications of chemotherapy. *Neurol Clin.* 1991;9(4):955–967.

170. Caraceni A, et al. Neurotoxicity of interferon-alpha in melanoma therapy: Results from a randomized controlled trial. *Cancer.* 1998;83(3):482–489.

171. Rohatiner AZ, et al. Central nervous system toxicity of interferon. *Br J Cancer.* 1983;47(3):419–422.

172. Meyers CA, Scheibel RS, Forman AD. Persistent neurotoxicity of systemically administered interferon-alpha. *Neurology.* 1991;41(5):672–676.

173. Rutkove SB. An unusual axonal polyneuropathy induced by low-dose interferon alfa-2a. *Arch Neurol.* 1997;54(7):907–908.

174. Delattre J, Vega F, Chen Q. Neurologic complications of immunotherapy. In: Wiley RG, ed. *Neurologic Complications of Cancer.* Marcel Dekker; 1995.

175. Hensley ML, et al. Risk factors for severe neuropsychiatric toxicity in patients receiving interferon alfa-2b and low-dose cytarabine for chronic myelogenous leukemia: Analysis of Cancer and Leukemia Group B 9013. *J Clin Oncol.* 2000;18(6):1301–1308.

176. Meyers CA, et al. Neurotoxicity of intraventricularly administered alpha-interferon for leptomeningeal disease. *Cancer.* 1991;68(1):88–92.

177. Denicoff KD, et al. The neuropsychiatric effects of treatment with interleukin-2 and lymphokine-activated killer cells. *Ann Intern Med.* 1987;107(3):293–300.

178. Bernard JT, et al. Transient focal neurologic deficits complicating interleukin-2 therapy. *Neurology.* 1990;40(1):154–155.

179. Loh FL, et al. Brachial plexopathy associated with interleukin-2 therapy. *Neurology.* 1992;42(2):462–463.

180. Allen JA, Adlakha A, Bergethon PR. Reversible posterior leukoencephalopathy syndrome after bevacizumab/FOLFIRI regimen for metastatic colon cancer. *Arch Neurol.* 2006;63(10):1475–1478.

181. Ozcan C, Wong SJ, Hari P. Reversible posterior leukoencephalopathy syndrome and bevacizumab. *N Engl J Med.* 2006;354(9):980–982; discussion 980–982.

182. Dormann AJ, et al. Gemcitabine-associated autonomic neuropathy. *Lancet.* 1998;351(9103):644.

183. Ardavanis AS, Ioannidis GN, Rigatos GA. Acute myopathy in a patient with lung adenocarcinoma treated with gemcitabine and docetaxel. *Anticancer Res.* 2005;25(1B):523–525.

184. Selleri C, et al. All-trans-retinoic acid (ATRA) responsive skin relapses of acute promyelocytic leukaemia followed by ATRA-induced pseudotumour cerebri. *Br J Haematol.* 1996;92(4):937–940.

185. Cheson BD, et al. Neurotoxicity of purine analogs: a review. *J Clin Oncol.* 1994;12(10):2216–2228.

186. Gonzalez H, et al. Progressive multifocal leukoencephalitis (PML) in three patients treated with standard-dose fludarabine (FAMP). *Hematol Cell Ther.* 1999;41(4):183–186.

187. Rao RD, et al. Efficacy of gabapentin in the management of chemotherapy-induced peripheral neuropathy: A phase 3

randomized, double-blind, placebo-controlled, crossover trial (N00C3). *Cancer.* 2007;110(9):2110–2118.

188. Lersch C, et al. Prevention of oxaliplatin-induced peripheral sensory neuropathy by carbamazepine in patients with advanced colorectal cancer. *Clin Colorectal Cancer.* 2002;2(1):54–58.

189. Saif MW, Hashmi S. Successful amelioration of oxaliplatin-induced hyperexcitability syndrome with the antiepileptic pregabalin in a patient with pancreatic cancer. *Cancer Chemother Pharmacol.* 2007.

190. Hilpert F, et al. Neuroprotection with amifostine in the first-line treatment of advanced ovarian cancer in patients with carboplatin/paclitaxel-based chemotherapy—a double-blind, placebo-controlled, randomized phase II study from the Arbeitsgemeinschaft Gynakologische Onkologoie (AGO) Ovarian Cancer Study Group. *Support Care Cancer.* 2005;13(10):797–805.

191. Penz M, et al. Subcutaneous administration of amifostine: A promising therapeutic option in patients with oxaliplatin-related peripheral sensitive neuropathy. *Ann Oncol.* 2001;12(3):421–422.

192. Maestri A, et al. A pilot study on the effect of acetyl-L-carnitine in paclitaxel- and cisplatin-induced peripheral neuropathy. *Tumori.* 2005;91(2):135–138.

193. Muto O, et al. Reduction of oxaliplatin-related neurotoxicity by calcium and magnesium infusions. *Gan To Kagaku Ryoho.* 2007;34(4):579–581.

194. Durand JP, Brezault C, Goldwasser F. Protection against oxaliplatin acute neurosensory toxicity by venlafaxine. *Anticancer Drugs.* 2003;14(6):423–425.

195. Ettinger LJ, et al. A phase II study of carboplatin in children with recurrent or progressive solid tumors. A report from the Children's Cancer Group. *Cancer.* 1994;73(4):1297–1301.

196. Ekhart C, et al. Flat dosing of carboplatin is justified in adult patients with normal renal function. *Clin Cancer Res.* 2006;12(21):6502–6508.

197. Bressler RB, Huston DP. Water intoxication following moderate-dose intravenous cyclophosphamide. *Arch Intern Med.* 1985;145(3):548–549.

198. Tscherning C, et al. Recurrent renal salt wasting in a child treated with carboplatin and etoposide. *Cancer.* 1994;73(6):1761–1763.

199. McDonald BR, et al. Acute renal failure associated with the use of intraperitoneal carboplatin: A report of two cases and review of the literature. *Am J Med.* 1991;90(3):386–391.

200. Vogelzang NJ. Nephrotoxicity from chemotherapy: prevention and management. *Oncology (Williston Park).* 1991;5(10):97–102, 105; discussion: 105, 109–111.

201. Levi F, et al. Oxaliplatin: Pharmacokinetics and chronopharmacological aspects. *Clin Pharmacokinet.* 2000;38(1):1–21.

202. Chollet P, et al. Single agent activity of oxaliplatin in heavily pretreated advanced epithelial ovarian cancer. *Ann Oncol.* 1996;7(10):1065–1070.

203. DeFronzo RA, et al. Proceedings: Cyclophosphamide and the kidney. *Cancer.* 1974;33(2):483–491.

204. Harmon WE, et al. Chronic renal failure in children treated with methyl CCNU. *N Engl J Med.* 1979;300(21):1200–1203.

205. Sponzo RW, DeVita VT, Oliverio VT. Physiologic disposition of 1-(2-chloroethyl)-3-cyclohexyl-1-nitrosourea (CCNU) and 1-(2-chloroethyl)-3-(4-methyl cyclohexyl)-1-nitrosourea (Me CCNU) in man. *Cancer.* 1973;31(5):1154–1156.

206. Price TM, et al. Renal failure and hemolytic anemia associated with mitomycin C. A case report. *Cancer,* 1985;55(1):51–56.

207. Groff JA, et al. Endotheliopathy: A continuum of hemolytic uremic syndrome due to mitomycin therapy. *Am J Kidney Dis.* 1997;29(2):280–284.

208. Chang AY, et al. Phase II evaluation of a combination of mitomycin C, vincristine, and cisplatin in advanced non-small cell lung cancer. *Cancer.* 1986;57(1):54–59.

209. Aronoff GM, et al. *Drug Prescribing in Renal Failure: Dosing Guidelines for Adults.* 4th ed. American College of Physicians; 2002.

210. Howell SB, Carmody J. Changes in glomerular filtration rate associated with high-dose methotrexate therapy in adults. *Cancer Treat Rep.* 1977;61(7):1389–1391.

211. Schilsky R. Renal and metabolic toxicities of cancer treatment. In: Perry M, Yarbro JW, eds. *Toxicity of Chemotherapy.* Grune & Stratton; 1984.

212. Bowyer GW, Davies TW. Methotrexate toxicity associated with an ileal conduit. *Br J Urol.* 1987;60(6):592.

213. Cutting HO. Inappropriate secretion of antidiuretic hormone secondary to vincristine therapy. *Am J Med.* 1971;51(2):269–271.

214. O'Reilly S, et al. Phase I and pharmacologic study of topotecan in patients with impaired renal function. *J Clin Oncol.* 1996;14(12):3062–3073.

215. Furuya Y, et al. Pharmacokinetics of paclitaxel and carboplatin in a hemodialysis patient with metastatic urothelial carcinoma—a case report. *Gan To Kagaku Ryoho.* 2003;30(7):1017–1020.

216. Menconboni M, et al. Docetaxel pharmacokinetics with pre- and post-dialysis administration in a hemodyalized patient. *Chemotherapy.* 2006;52(3):147–150.

217. Sandler AB, Johnson DH, Herbst RS. Anti-vascular endothelial growth factor monoclonals in non-small cell lung cancer. *Clin Cancer Res.* 2004;10(12 Pt 2):4258s–4262s.

218. Belldegrun A, et al. Effects of interleukin-2 on renal function in patients receiving immunotherapy for advanced cancer. *Ann Intern Med.* 1987;106(6):817–822.

219. Selby P, et al. Nephrotic syndrome during treatment with interferon. *Br Med J (Clin Res Ed).* 1985;290(6476):1180.

220. Zuber J, et al. Alpha-interferon-associated thrombotic microangiopathy: A clinicopathologic study of 8 patients and review of the literature. *Medicine (Baltimore).* 2002;81(4):321–331.

221. Ault BH, et al. Acute renal failure during therapy with recombinant human gamma interferon. *N Engl J Med.* 1988;319(21):1397–1400.

222. Hamblin T. Disease and its management in chronic lymphocytic leukemia. In: Cheson B, ed. *Chronic Lymphoid Leukemias.* New York: Marcel Dekker; 2001.

223. Schwartzentruber DJ, et al. Thyroid dysfunction associated with immunotherapy for patients with cancer. *Cancer.* 1991;68(11):2384–2390.

224. Vialettes B, et al. Incidence rate and risk factors for thyroid dysfunction during recombinant interleukin-2 therapy in advanced malignancies. *Acta Endocrinol (Copenh).* 1993;129(1):31–38.

225. Rini BI, et al. Hypothyroidism in patients with metastatic renal cell carcinoma treated with sunitinib. *J Natl Cancer Inst.* 2007;99(1):81–83.

226. Desai J, et al. Hypothyroidism after sunitinib treatment for patients with gastrointestinal stromal tumors. *Ann Intern Med.* 2006;145(9):660–664.

227. Bussel JB, Cunningham-Rundles C, Abraham C. Intravenous treatment of autoimmune hemolytic anemia with very high dose gammaglobulin. *Vox Sang.* 1986;51(4):264–269.

228. Del Poeta G, et al. The addition of rituximab to fludarabine improves clinical outcome in untreated patients with ZAP-70-negative chronic lymphocytic leukemia. *Cancer.* 2005;104(12):2743–2752.

229. Hegde UP, et al. Rituximab treatment of refractory fludarabine-associated immune thrombocytopenia in chronic lymphocytic leukemia. *Blood.* 2002;100(6):2260–2262.

230. Loprinzi CL, Duffy J, Ingle JN. Postchemotherapy rheumatism. *J Clin Oncol.* 1993;11(4):768–770.

231. Donnellan PP, et al. Aromatase inhibitors and arthralgia. *J Clin Oncol.* 2001;19(10):2767.

232. Howell A, et al. Results of the ATAC (Arimidex, Tamoxifen, Alone or in Combination) trial after completion of 5 years' adjuvant treatment for breast cancer. *Lancet.* 2005;365(9453):60–62.

233. Smith IE, Dowsett M. Aromatase inhibitors in breast cancer. *N Engl J Med.* 2003;348(24):2431–2442.

234. Eisenhauer EA, et al. European-Canadian randomized trial of paclitaxel in relapsed ovarian cancer: High-dose versus low-dose and long versus short infusion. *J Clin Oncol.* 1994;12(12):2654–2666.

235. Garrison JA, et al. Myalgias and arthralgias associated with paclitaxel. *Oncology (Williston Park)*. 2003;17(2):271–277; discussion 281–282, 286–288.

236. Gelmon K. The taxoids: paclitaxel and docetaxel. *Lancet*. 1994;344(8932):1267–1272.

237. McGuire WP, et al. Taxol: A Unique Antineoplastic Agent with Significant Activity in Advanced Ovarian Epithelial Neoplasms. *Ann Intern Med*. 1989;111(4):273–279.

238. Rowinsky EK, et al. Phase I and pharmacologic study of paclitaxel and cisplatin with granulocyte colony-stimulating factor: Neuromuscular toxicity is dose-limiting. *J Clin Oncol*. 1993;11(10):2010–2020.

239. Rowinsky EK, Donehower RC. Paclitaxel (Taxol). *N Engl J Med*. 1995;332(15):1004–1014.

240. Nguyen VH, Lawrence HJ. Use of gabapentin in the prevention of taxane-induced arthralgias and myalgias. *J Clin Oncol*. 2004;22(9):1767–1769.

241. Ryberg M, et al. Epirubicin cardiotoxicity: An analysis of 469 patients with metastatic breast cancer. *J Clin Oncol*. 1998;16(11):3502–3508.

242. Ravry MJ. Cardiotoxicity of mitomycin C in man and animals. *Cancer Treat Rep*. 1979;63(4):555.

243. Clinical Trial and prescribing information. (cited; Available from: www.fda.gov/cder/foi/label/2005/021923lbl.pdf.

244. Motzer RJ, et al. Activity of SU11248, a multitargeted inhibitor of vascular endothelial growth factor receptor and platelet-derived growth factor receptor, in patients with metastatic renal cell carcinoma. *J Clin Oncol*. 2006;24(1):16–24.

245. Kerkela R, et al. Cardiotoxicity of the cancer therapeutic agent imatinib mesylate. *Nat Med*. 2006;12(8):908–916.

246. Mortimer JE, et al. A phase II randomized study comparing sequential and combined intraarterial cisplatin and radiation therapy in primary brain tumors. A Southwest Oncology Group study. *Cancer*. 1992;69(5):1220–1223.

247. Fossella FV, et al. Phase II study of docetaxel for recurrent or metastatic non-small-cell lung cancer. *J Clin Oncol*. 1994;12(6):1238–1244.

248. Gasser AB, Tieche M, Brunner KW. Neurologic and cardiac toxicity following iv application of methotrexate. *Cancer Treat Rep*. 1982;66(7):1561–1562.

249. Hermans C, et al. Pericarditis induced by high-dose cytosine arabinoside chemotherapy. *Ann Hematol*. 1997;75(1–2):55–57.

250. Lenihan DJ, et al. Cardiac toxicity of alemtuzumab in patients with mycosis fungoides/Sezary syndrome. *Blood*. 2004;104(3):655–658.

251. House KW, Simon SR, Pugh RP. Chemotherapy-induced myocardial infarction in a young man with Hodgkin's disease. *Clin Cardiol*. 1992;15(2):122–125.

252. Schwarzer S, et al. Non-Q-wave myocardial infarction associated with bleomycin and etoposide chemotherapy. *Eur Heart J*. 1991;12(6):748–750.

253. Harris AL, Wong C. Myocardial ischaemia, radiotherapy, and vinblastine. *Lancet*. 1981;1(8223):787.

254. Kantor AF, et al. Are vinca alkaloids associated with myocardial infarction? *Lancet*. 1981;1(8229):1111.

255. Warrell RP, Jr, et al. Acute promyelocytic leukemia. *N Engl J Med*. 1993;329(3):177–189.

256. Yang JC, et al. A randomized trial of bevacizumab, an anti-vascular endothelial growth factor antibody, for metastatic renal cancer. *N Engl J Med*. 2003;349(5):427–434.

257. Weiss RB, et al. Hypersensitivity reactions from Taxol. *J Clin Oncol*. 1990;8(7):1263–1268.

258. Read WL, Mortimer JE, Picus J. Severe interstitial pneumonitis associated with docetaxel administration. *Cancer*. 2002;94(3):847–853.

259. Wang GS, Yang KY, Perng RP. Life-threatening hypersensitivity pneumonitis induced by docetaxel (taxotere). *Br J Cancer*. 2001;85(9):1247–1250.

Principles of Immunotherapy

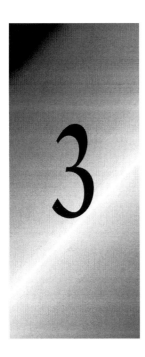

Guenther Koehne

The induction of a humoral and/or cellular immune response to antigens specifically expressed on malignant cells has been the ultimate goal in the approach to curing cancer or preventing its recurrence or development in patients at risk.

Historically, cancer therapy has included surgery, chemotherapy, and/or radiotherapy, either as a single-treatment approach or in combined treatment modalities. Complete surgical removal with negative margins remains a potentially curative approach for localized solid cancers. Also, a variety of solid tumors and hematologic malignancies can be cured by systemic cytotoxic chemotherapy. Adjuvant chemotherapy is the standard of care for breast cancer, colon cancer, and sarcomas, and chemotherapy is commonly given in combination with radiation therapy. High doses of chemotherapy for improved anticancer activity have been introduced, and require autologous stem cell support to shorten the interval of immune reconstitution afterward (1–4). This approach remains a treatment option for patients with relapsed indolent or diffuse large B-cell non-Hodgkin lymphoma (5–7) and relapsed Hodgkin disease, provided the tumor cells remain sensitive to chemotherapy at the time of relapse (8–10). This treatment of relapsed or refractory multiple myeloma has also resulted in an improved response rate and prolonged response duration (11–13).

After a high-dose myeloablative preparative regimen, allogeneic stem cell transplantations were traditionally performed for malignant hematologic malignancies in order to replace diseased bone marrow with stem cells from a healthy related or unrelated donor. Relapse rates following allogeneic stem cell transplantation were lower when acute or chronic graft-versus-host disease (GVHD) developed, and were greater when a syngeneic donor was used or T-cell depleted marrow transplantation was performed. This was evidence of an immunotherapeutic effect from allogeneic T lymphocytes that were transfused with the transplant or that developed after the engraftment occurred (14,15).

Significant progress in the development of cellular immunotherapeutic approaches occurred with patients who relapsed following allogeneic marrow transplant of chronic myelogenous leukemia using infusions of lymphocytes derived from the bone marrow donor (16–20) Consequently, improved laboratory-based methods permitted selective targeting of antigens that are expressed or overexpressed on malignant cell populations. Donor-derived antigen-specific T lymphocytes were generated for adoptive immunotherapeutic approaches in the treatment of minimal residual disease and relapse following an allogeneic marrow transplantation (21). Treatment of viral complications developing after an allograft, such as Epstein-Barr virus (EBV),-induced post-transplantation lymphoproliferative disorders (PTLDs), and cytomegalovirus (CMV) infections, refined the use and logistics of generating donor-derived, antigen-specific T lymphocytes for treatment of these diseases without inducing GVHD (22–24).

KEY POINTS

- Immunotherapies are rapidly evolving and will be increasingly integrated with standard therapies for the treatment of solid tumors and hematologic malignancies.
- The first proof of a graft-versus-leukemia effect resulted from the pioneering findings of Kolb, who demonstrated that patients who developed relapses of chronic myelogenous leukemia following an allogeneic marrow transplant were induced into durable molecular remissions by high doses of peripheral blood mononuclear cells derived from the original HLA-matched transplant.

- It is anticipated that natural killer cell–mediated immunotherapeutic approaches will be further developed and integrated into clinical trials to improve the outcome of hematological malignancies by allogeneic bone marrow transplantations.
- Monoclonal antibody-based therapies have emerged over the past decade for the treatment of hematological malignancies and solid tumors.
- The CD20 antigen is expressed on mature B cells and, therefore, on hematological malignancies derived from B lymphocytes, which can be targeted using rituximab as a single agent or in combination with chemotherapy.

Recently the immunotherapeutic effect of natural killer (NK) cells was advanced with the description of inhibitory and activating receptors (25,26). NK cells, mismatched for immunoglobulinlike receptors (KIRs) that are distinctly expressed on these cells, and HLA-class I molecules presented by recipient cells demonstrated NK-cell–mediated alloreactivity and enhanced NK-cell–mediated lysis of the recipient leukemic cell population. This resulted in improved overall survival in patients following haplotype mismatched and unrelated bone marrow transplantation (26–28). Results will soon be available from clinical trials integrating the NK-cell–mediated immune effect to improve marrow transplantation by use of KIR mismatched donors.

Monoclonal antibody-based therapy has increasingly played a role in the treatment of malignancies. The production of chimeric and humanized monoclonal antibodies has helped to overcome the generation of human antimouse antibodies, which resulted in rapid clearing and the need for multiple infusions of murine monoclonal antibodies. The anti-CD20 monoclonal antibody rituximab is administered as a single agent or in combination with systemic chemotherapy for the treatment of hematological malignancies (29,30). Radioimmunoconjugates of anti-CD20 monoclonal antibodies labeled with yttrium-90 or iodine-131 are being given for relapsed or refractory non-Hodgkin lymphomas (31–33). The CD33 antigen is expressed on myeloid cells and by the leukemic blasts of at least 90% of patients with acute myelogenous leukemia. Several trials targeting the antigen by humanized anti-CD33 monoclonal antibodies that are either unmodified or conjugated to radioisotopes, such as iodine-131 or yttrium-90, or the cell toxin calicheamicin, have been initiated to treat acute

myeloid leukemias or are integrated into a myeloablative conditioning regimen for allogeneic marrow transplants (34–37).

Advances in the identification of tumor-associated antigens and their conjugation to adjuvants have led to cancer vaccines with the potential to induce both cellular and/or humoral immune responses. Pioneering work by Levy et al. established the principle of generating specific immune responses against unique tumor-derived antigens after subcutaneous injections of custom-made vaccines. In these studies, the immunoglobulin idiotype, a unique amino acid sequence contained within the variable region of the immunoglobulin of B-cell non-Hodgkin lymphoma, was identified and complexed with adjuvant before injection to successfully induce anti-idiotype antibody responses (38–40). Advances in utilizing deoxyribonucleic acid (DNA) vaccines or cell based-vaccine strategies have led to clinical trials to assess the immune responses and potential clinical benefits in hematological malignancies and solid tumors (41–43). The enhancement of immune responses from administration of cancer vaccines is currently being addressed following immune manipulation with the blockade of cytotoxic T-lymphocyte–associated antigen (CTLA)-4, which is expressed on the cell surface of T lymphocytes with increased activation (44,45). Studies of the selective depletion of T regulatory cells, which have a capacity for inhibiting T-cell–mediated antitumor effects, are under way in order to improve cancer vaccine–induced immune responses (46).

This chapter describes current immunotherapeutic approaches for the treatment of malignancies. It does not claim to describe all experimental studies under investigation or to provide a complete overview of completed or currently ongoing clinical trials.

PRINCIPLES OF CELLULAR IMMUNE THERAPY

Adoptive Transfer of Donor Lymphocytes

First proof of a graft-versus-leukemia (GVL) effect resulted from the pioneering findings of Kolb et al. (16) and was later confirmed by several centers (17–20). Patients who developed relapses of chronic myelogenous leukemia (CML) following an allogeneic marrow transplant were induced into durable molecular remissions by high doses of peripheral blood mononuclear cells derived from the original HLA-matched transplant. These studies provided the first evidence that enhanced resistance to leukemia, accrued through a marrow allograft by comparisons of relapse rates following syngeneic vs HLA-matched allogeneic transplants, was indeed mediated by cells in the donor graft (14,47). The fact that more than 70% of patients with relapsed chronic myelogenous leukemia could be induced into remission by this approach altered the field of allogeneic bone marrow transplantation (17,48). While the specific effector cells that induced these remissions and the chronic myelogenous leukemia cells targeted by these cells remain only partially characterized, increasing evidence implicates alloreactive donor T cells as the principal mediators of adoptively transferred resistance to CML. More than 75% of the patients responding to these donor leukocyte infusions (DLIs) also developed GVHD. This was initially taken as evidence of the antileukemic effects of GVHD, which had also been proposed to explain the lower relapse rates among patients with acute or chronic GVHD following marrow allografts (15). Evidence of a separate GVL effect mediated by donor-derived, leukemia-specific T lymphocytes was provided by Falkenburg et al. (21). This study generated CD4+ T-cell clones on the basis of their capacity to lyse host leukemic cells and to inhibit the growth of (Philadelphia) Ph+CD34+ host CML precursors, and treated patients with CML relapse in the accelerated post-transplant phase who had failed to respond to donor leukocyte infusions. Three infusions providing a total of 3.2×10^9 total T cells from these T-cell lines induced molecular remission and reestablished complete donor chimerism (21).

Donor leukocyte infusions have also been attempted for AML relapses following allogeneic marrow transplants. Antileukemic effects of DLI have been less consistently observed and are often less durable than those in patients treated for CML. Results of donor leukocyte infusions at centers in the European Organization for Research and Treatment of Cancer (EORTC) (17) and other centers in the United States (14) were reported, with only 20%–29% of patients treated for AML relapses and 30% treated for recurrences of myelodysplastic syndrome (MDS) achieving complete remissions. While the majority of patients achieving remission also developed GVHD, a proportion of patients who developed clinically significant GVHD after DLI have not achieved AML remissions. Even patients with AML in relapse after initial treatment with chemotherapy to decrease tumor load, and who were subsequently treated with donor leukocyte infusions, achieved only marginally better response rates. In addition, most patients who achieved remissions following DLI relapsed within one to two years after treatment (49).

Apparent differences in sensitivity to DLI manifested by AML or acute lymphoblastic leukemia (ALL) and CML have been explained by quantitative differences in tumor load, the number of clonogenic AML or ALL blasts vs clonogenic Ph+ progenitors of chronic-phase CML present at clinical relapse, and differences in the expansion rate of these cells (49). Expansion of AML blasts appears to be rapid, and could outnumber the expansion rate of leukemia-reactive effector cells administered in the infusions of $1–5 \times 10^8$ donor T cells/ kg. In addition, clinical responses are rarely observed before 8–12 weeks after infusion in CML post-DLI, and other features of AML may limit the capacity of these cells to induce a significant donor T-cell response. A characteristic feature of human AMLs and ALLs is their failure to express the costimulatory molecules B7.1 and B7.2, therefore likely limiting their capacity to elicit an immune response. Cardoso et al. (50) and others (51) showed that such B7.1 neg AML and ALL cells are incapable of inducing a proliferative or cytotoxic T-cell response in mixed leukocyte cultures with autologous HLA-matched or fully allogeneic T cells. The T cells emerging after sensitization with these B7.1 leukemic blasts appear to be anergized, are relatively refractory to restimulation, and are therefore incapable of mounting a significant antileukemic response.

Several groups have explored strategies to enhance the capacity of leukemic cells to present leukemia-associated antigens to autologous T cells and thereby to stimulate an antileukemic response. Choudhury et al. (52), confirmed by Smit et al. (53), described that Ph+CD34+ CML progenitor cells can be induced by granulocyte-microphage colony-stimulating factor (GM-CSF), tumor necrosis factor (TNF), and IL-4 to differentiate into dendritic cells capable of presenting antigens and eliciting an autologous leukemia-specific CD8+ T-cell–mediated cytotoxic response. Subsequent studies suggested that AML blasts and Ph+ B-ALL blasts may also be induced to form dendritic cells bearing appropriate costimulatory molecules for induction of a T-cell response (54,55). The direct modification of the antigen-presenting capacity of acute leukemic blasts has been evaluated by Dunussi-Joannnopoulos et al. (56) and Mutis et al. (57), describing that transient transfection of B7.1⁻ murine and human AML cells with a gene encoding human B7.1 permits the generation of T cells reactive against B7.1⁻ unmodified leukemic cells. In addition, culturing of human B7.1⁻ ALL cells on monolayers of murine 3T3 fibroblasts transduced to express CD40 ligand induced the expression of B7.1 on leukemic cells. Sensitization of either allogeneic or autologous T cells with the B7.1-expressing ALL cells elicits a specific proliferative and cytotoxic T-cell response (58). Based on information from these studies and refined laboratory methodologies of cell cultures and cell expansion, the generation of polyclonal antigen-specific T cells and T-cell clones for adoptive transfer rapidly evolved.

Immunotherapeutic Approaches with Donor-Derived, Antigen-Specific T Lymphocytes

Adoptive immunotherapeutic approaches with donor-derived, antigen-specific T lymphocytes were established by the treatment of Epstein-Barr virus (EBV) post-transplantation proliferative disorders (PTLD), and cytomegalovirus (CMV) infections complicating allogeneic marrow transplantation (59–61). EBV-associated lymphomas grow rapidly—a potentially lethal complication of marrow and organ allografts, and the majority of EBV-PTLD are of donor origin. The risk of developing an EBV lymphoma increases in recipients of HLA-disparate related or unrelated unmodified marrow grafts receiving prolonged immunosuppression or T-cell depleted marrow transplants. In 1994, it was reported that infusions of small numbers of peripheral blood mononuclear cells (PBMC) derived from a seropositive marrow donor could induce durable and complete regression of EBV lymphomas as a complication of related or unrelated T-cell–depleted marrow grafts, but infusions of donor-derived peripheral blood mononuclear cells, even in small numbers, also transferred alloreactive T cells sufficient to cause severe or even lethal GVHD, particularly if the donor and host differ at one or more HLA alleles (61–63). Rooney et al. reported the successful treatment of patients with EBV lymphoma in recipients of HLA-mismatched allografts using infusions of donor-derived, EBV-specific cytotoxic lymphocytes without inducing GVHD (23,64). In a follow-up study, 39 recipients of unrelated bone marrows were treated with the prophylactic administration of donor-derived, EBV-specific T cells. None of these patients developed a lymphoproliferative disorder, and only one patient experienced mild worsening of a preexisting GVHD (24).

In allogeneic bone marrow transplants, reactivation of latent CMV remains a major cause of morbidity and mortality (60). The contribution of virus-specific CD8⁺ cytotoxic T cells to control CMV infections has been suggested by the correlation between the reconstitution of CMV virus-specific CD8⁺ cytotoxic T cells and protection of the transplanted host from infection.

The generation, selection, and adoptive transfer of viral-antigen–specific T-cell clones for cytomegalovirus reactivation after allogeneic transplant, as shown by Riddell et al. (22,65) by extended culture in vitro, can markedly reduce or eliminate the risk of GVHD following adoptive T-cell transfer, even in HLA-disparate hosts. Other groups have tested donor-derived T cells sensitized with autologous monocyte-derived dendritic cells loaded with a commercially produced lysate of CMV infection. First, Peggs et al. (66) reported on 16 patients who had developed CMV viremia detected by quantitative polymerase chain reaction (PCR)-based analysis of blood for CMV DNA, who were then treated with donor T cells sensitized with autologous monocyte-derived dendritic cells generated by culturing PBMC with GM-CSF, IL-4, and thereafter TNF-α, which were loaded with a CMV lysate. No toxicities were observed following single infusions of 1×10^5 T cells/kg. Three patients were noted to have grade 1 skin GVHD, which cleared with topical steroid treatment. Of the 16 patients, all 16 cleared CMV viremia, 8 without concurrent treatment with ganciclovir. A second series reported by Einsele et al. (67) described a group of 8 patients with CMV viremia, detected by reverse transcription (RT)-PCR analysis, that persisted despite treatment with ganciclovir. These patients were treated with donor-derived T cells sensitized with CMV cell lysate and expanded with CMV antigen. Despite the resistance to antiviral therapy, five out of seven evaluable patients cleared the viral infection after transfusion of $10^7/m^2$ CMV-specific T cells and remained negative thereafter by RT-PCR analyses.

Clinical trials incorporating adoptive immunotherapeutic approaches are emerging for the treatment of minimal residual diseases and relapse following allogeneic grafts. Strategies for generating leukemia-reactive T cells for adoptive therapy have focused on the generation of T cells specific for peptides encoded by genes uniquely or differentially expressed on leukemic cells. The Wilms tumor gene (WT-1) is such a gene of interest, initially identified as a gene mutated in a Wilms tumor of the kidney in children. The WT-1 gene is a tumor-suppressor gene encoding a zinc finger transcription factor, which binds early growth-factor gene promoters, such as platelet-derived growth factor A chain, colony-stimulating factor-1, transforming growth factor-b1, and insulinlike growth factor II (68,69). The expression of the WT-1 gene is restricted to a limited number of normal tissues, including fetal kidney, ovary, testis, spleen, hematopoietic precursors, and the mesothelial cell lining of visceral organs (70,71). The WT-1 gene is overexpressed in 70%–80% of adult and pediatric AML as well as Ph⁺ ALL and CML in blast crisis, and recent studies indicate that peptides derived from WT-1 proteins are immunogenic (72–74). Initial studies have shown that specific WT-1 encoded peptides have a high affinity for HLA-A*2401 and HLA-A*0201. These peptides can stimulate WT-1-specific HLA-A*2401 or HLA-A*0201–restricted cytotoxic T-lymphocytes, with the capacity to kill WT-1–expressing leukemic cell lines in the context of the appropriate HLA-class I molecule in vitro (75,76). In one study, a WT-1 peptide-specific T-cell clone lysed WT-1, expressing HLA-A*0201 leukemic cell lines, but did not lyse normal HLA-A*0201$^+$ CD34$^+$ progenitor cells (77). In these studies, T-cell responses were generated against the WT-1-derived nonamers $_{126-134}$RMF-PNAPYL and $_{187-195}$SLGEQQYSV. The authors' group demonstrated that human lymphocytes sensitized to HLA-A*0201 and HLA-A*2402–binding WT-1 peptides, loaded on autologous cytokine-activated monocytes or EBV-transformed B cells, yielded HLA-restricted, WT-1 peptide-specific cytotoxic T cells that lysed primary WT-1$^+$ leukemic cells in vitro and in vivo. These WT-1 peptide-specific T cells also homed to and induced regression of WT-1$^+$ leukemic xenografts bearing the appropriate restricting HLA alleles (78).

Proteinase-3 is a myeloid tissue-restricted 26 kDa protease expressed in azurophilic granules in normal myeloid cells but overexpressed in leukemia cells (79,80). Molldrem et al. demonstrated that cytotoxic T-cell lines could be generated against an HLA-A*0201–restricted proteinase 3-derived nonamer, PR1. These PR1-specific T cells induced specific lysis of CML cells and inhibited CML progenitors (81,82). Using HLA-A*0201-PR1–restricted major histocompatibility complex (MHC) tetramers, these investigators illustrated the presence of circulating PR1-specific cytotoxic T lymphocytes in 11 out of 12 patients who responded to IFN-α2b therapy, whereas nonresponders as well as healthy HLA-A*0201$^+$ individuals did not show any peptide-specific T cells (83). Subsequently, a correlation between the presence of PR1-specific T cells and clinical responses after IFN-α2b therapy and allogeneic bone marrow transplantation provided further evidence of the involvement of T-cell immunity in the remission of chronic myelogenous leukemia (82). As a consequence of these observations, early clinical trials to vaccinate patients with myeloid leukemia or myelodysplastic syndrome against PR-1 and/or WT-1 have been initiated. Most of these trials are ongoing, and only limited results have been published (84,85).

Minor histocompatibility antigens (mHA) are derived from normal cellular proteins and are the result of normal genetic variations of the human genome in single nucleotide polymorphisms (SNPs), leading to differences in amino acid sequences of proteins between donor and host cells (86). The mHA are presented by self major histocompatibility complexes (MHC), and can trigger allogeneic T lymphocytes to recognize these peptides as foreign, despite a complete MHC match after allogeneic transplantation (87–89). The recognition of mHA by donor T lymphocytes can induce severe GVHD (87,90), which becomes relevant in the HLA-identical but sex-mismatched transplant from a female donor to a male recipient (91). Several mHAs (eg, SMCY, UTY) are encoded by genes of the Y chromosome, which can trigger a T-cell response from a female donor. Allogeneic transplants from a female donor to a male recipient have been associated with a higher rate of GVHD, but also with a reduced rate of leukemia relapse (91). Conversely, transplantation from a male into a female recipient was recently demonstrated to be associated with increased graft rejection (92). Several minor alloantigens, such as HA-1 and HA-2, are selectively expressed on hematopoietic cells (including leukemia cells) and their immunogenic peptides sequenced (93–97). These mHAs offer ideal targets for adoptive immunotherapeutic approaches, and clinical trials targeting the peptides by mHA-specific donor T lymphocytes have been initiated (98). The diallelic HA-1 minor alloantigens presented by HLA-A*0201 and selectively expressed on hematopoietic cells, including leukemia cells, have been described by den Haan et al. (90) Approximately 8%–13% of patients undergoing a marrow allograft would bear HLA-A*0201 and express an HA-1 disparity that could be recognized by a matched sibling donor (99,100). Disparities for HA-1 alleles have been correlated with GVHD by Goulmy et al. (93) and Tseng et al. (94) High frequencies of T cells binding HLA-A2 tetramers complexed with HA-1 peptides have been detected in HA-1-disparate, HLA-matched marrow graft recipients who develop GVHD (101). Results by Dickinson et al. and Marjit et al. (102,103) confirmed that mHA-specific cytotoxic T cells targeting antigens predominantly expressed on hematopoietic cells can induce complete remissions without inducing GVHD. Additional studies after allogeneic marrow transplantation demonstrated a high percentage of leukemia-reactive T cells targeting HA-1 or HA-2 expressed on the leukemic cell population following treatment with donor lymphocyte infusion (104). Genotyping of minor histocompatibility antigens may be included in the pre-transplantation evaluation of the donor and recipient, and considered in the decision of donor selection to maximize the immunotherapeutic effect of allogeneic transplantations (97,105).

Immunotherapy with Natural Killer Cells

Natural killer (NK) cells are critical effector cells of the innate immune system. They have a capacity for direct lysis of virally infected cells and tumor cells in addition to mediating cellular cytotoxicity through their CD16 receptor that binds to the Fc portion of immunoglobulin G (106). NK cells are derived from CD34+ progenitor cells and are characterized by expression of CD56 and the absence of CD3. Early trials to stimulate antitumor effects of NK cells with differing concentrations of interleukin-2 (IL-2) have been disappointing (107–109), but the exploitation of NK cells for immunotherapeutic effect has gained interest with the description of inhibitory and activating receptors on CD56+CD3− effector cells (110–112). In contrast to the ability of alloreactive T lymphocytes to recognize antigens by presentation of minor or major histocompatibility complexes shared by normal tissue cells and tumor cells resulting in tumor cell killing and/or GVHD, the function of NK cells can be inhibited by the normal expression of matched MHC class I molecules binding to unique receptors, which are expressed on the NK cells. Killer cell immunoglobulinlike receptors (KIRs) are distinctly expressed on NK cells, and can be inhibitory or activating, although it appears that inhibitory KIRs have a greater affinity to MHC class I than the activating KIRs (25). NK-cell–mediated lysis is therefore inhibited when the inhibitory receptor expressed on the NK cell binds to the corresponding HLA-class I molecule. In contrast, mismatching of KIRs and HLA class I molecules would prevent the NK cell inhibition and could, therefore, be utilized for targeted NK-cell–mediated lysis (26). This principle has been explored by Ruggeri and Aversa et al., demonstrating a potent graft-versus-leukemia effect through uninhibited NK cell activity in recipients of HLA haplotype-mismatched transplants (27). When the donor NK cells could not encounter their inhibiting MHC allele, also not expressed in the leukemia cell population, the NK alloreactivity was primarily directed against the leukemia blasts, which led to a reduced leukemia relapse rate in the absence of GVHD (28,113). The NK alloreactivity was completely absent when the donors' KIR repertoire was found to match the corresponding HLA despite HLA haplotype-mismatched transplants. In these studies, patients undergoing haplotype-mismatched transplantations for acute myelogenous leukemia (AML) experienced a 79% five-year risk of relapse in the presence of KIR/HLA match, but only a 17% risk when the KIR repertoire was mismatched with the recipient's HLA allele (28,113). A study comparing KIR/HLA mismatches in 20 recipients of unrelated bone marrow transplants reported an improved 4½-year survival of 87% versus 39% for transplant recipients in which KIR repertoire and HLA matched (114). Analyses of the donors' KIR repertoire and the recipients' HLA also demonstrated a decreased relapse rate and improved overall survival in patients undergoing T-cell–depleted transplants from HLA-identical siblings for AML, in which donor KIRs were mismatched

with the corresponding HLA allele required for NK-cell inhibition (115). The decreased relapse rate could not be attributed to the effect of donor T lymphocytes in these T-cell–depleted transplantations. This outcome also confirms the feasibility of KIR/HLA mismatches despite HLA-matched sibling or matched unrelated transplantations because the KIR genotype, encoded on chromosome 19, is independently segregated from chromosome 6, which encodes the HLA genes (116). In all of these studies, however, the alloreactivity and NK-cell–mediated lysis was restricted to patients with AML, and no antileukemic effect of NK cells could be demonstrated against ALL. The differences in these outcomes are currently unexplained and may be multifactorial, such as varying susceptibility to NK-cell–mediated lysis or different expressions of activating receptors on NK cells. The lack of lymphocyte function antigen 1 (LFA-1) expression on ALL cells has been associated with reduced NK-cell–mediated lysis, indicating that additional factors may play a role in the activation of alloreactive NK cells (113). It is anticipated that NK-cell–mediated immunotherapeutic approaches will be further developed and integrated into clinical trials to improve the outcome of hematological malignancies by allogeneic bone marrow transplantations.

PRINCIPLES OF HUMORAL IMMUNE THERAPY

Monoclonal Antibody Therapy

Monoclonal antibody-based therapies have emerged over the past decade for the treatment of hematological malignancies and solid tumors. The limitations with murine monoclonal antibodies, such as the development of human antimouse monoclonal antibodies with rapid clearing from the body resulting in multiple administrations, could be overcome by chimeric and humanized antibodies. The anti-CD20 monoclonal antibody rituximab is a chimeric antibody with reduced immunogenicity and can be safely administered without the development of human antimouse antibodies. The CD20 antigen is expressed on mature B cells and, therefore, on hematological malignancies derived from B lymphocytes, which can be targeted using rituximab as a single agent or in combination with chemotherapy. Initial phase 2 studies administering the maximum tolerated rituximab dose of 375 mg/m² as a single agent to patients with indolent non-Hodgkin lymphoma (NHL) have demonstrated a 46%–48% response rate (29,30). Rituximab was subsequently evaluated for the treatment of relapsed and refractory diffuse large B-cell lymphoma (DLCBL) in combination with cyclophosphamide, doxorubicin, vincristine, and prednisone

(CHOP) chemotherapy (30,117), and is currently also administered for Epstein-Barr virus–associated lymphoproliferative disorder (EBV-PTLD) (118,119) and chronic GVHD (120,121). Only limited activity in the treatment of chronic lymphocytic leukemia (CLL) was demonstrated (122), which may be explained by the lower antigen density of CD20 expressed on CLL cells compared with the expression level on NHL or EBV-PTLD (123). In addition, circulating CLL cells may bind the monoclonal antibodies and, therefore, act as a sink, resulting in rapid clearance of the drug (124).

Campath-1 and the humanized monoclonal antibody Campath-1H (alemtuzumab) have specificity for CD52, a glycoprotein expressed on B and T lymphocytes that is highly expressed on CLL cells. Clinical trials with single-agent alemtuzumab have demonstrated activity in fludarabine-refractory patients with CLL (125–128). Campath-1H has been evaluated as front-line therapy for CLL as a single agent, with complete remissions of 19%–22% and overall remissions of 85%–87% (129,130). Treatment with alemtuzumab was associated with increased rates of opportunistic infections, particularly CMV reactivation.

CD33 is a 67-kD cell surface glycoprotein whose expression is largely restricted to cells of the monocytic/myeloid lineage (131,132). It is detected on promonocytes and monocytes in the monocytic lineage, on myeloblasts and promyelocytes, and on a proportion of metamyelocytes in the myeloid lineage. CD33 is expressed by the leukemic blasts of at least 90% of patients with acute myelogenous leukemia, but not by acute lymphocytic leukemia. Importantly, the expression is absent from mature granulocytes and primitive pluripotential stem cells, and may, therefore, be an interesting antigen for targeted immunotherapy (131–133). Unmodified antibodies used in the initial studies were limited in their activity against acute leukemia, largely because binding of the antibodies did not induce intracellular signaling and, therefore, did not induce cell death of the leukemic blasts (134). Furthermore, murine antibodies were not well recognized by human antigen-presenting cells, and induced only a weak, antibody-dependent cellular cytotoxicity (135). The humanized mouse IgG1, termed HuM195, was developed as a consequence and studied in a phase 1/2 trial (136). In this study, 60 patients with refractory or relapsed myeloid leukemia were treated with 12–36 mg/m^2 of HuM195 daily for four days, two weeks apart. Decreases in blast counts were observed, but only three complete remissions were obtained (137,138). The conclusion of that study was that unlabeled antibodies demonstrated clinical efficacy in patients with low tumor load and therefore might be most effective in patients with minimal residual disease. Since acute promyelocytic leukemia (APL) is strongly positive for CD33, in subsequent studies, HuM195 was given for consolidation or maintenance therapy in 31 patients with APL who were in complete remission and who had already been treated with all-trans-retinoic acid (ATRA) (139). In this trial, HuM195 was given twice a week for three weeks, followed by consolidation chemotherapy with idarubicin and cytarabine, followed by six months of maintenance therapy with HuM195 given twice a week every four weeks. Of the patients treated with ATRA and/or chemotherapy induction, 2 of 27 became PCR-negative. After treatment with HuM195, 12 of 24 evaluable patients (50%) were PCR-negative, and the probability of disease-free survival after a median follow-up of five years was 93%, compared with 73% obtained after treatment with ATRA and consolidation chemotherapy but without administration of HuM195 in the previous study (139,140).

In order to increase the antitumor effects of the native antibodies, drugs and bacterial toxins have been conjugated to the MoAbs. Sievers et al. studied a conjugate of the antitumor antibiotic, calicheamicin and the humanized anti-CD33 antibody, CMA-676, also known as gemtuzumab ozogamicin or Mylotarg (37). Binding of CD33 antigen causes internalization of the anti-CD33 and calicheamicin conjugate, and upon the release of the drug, causes DNA double-strand breaks and subsequently cell death via apoptosis (141). In an initial phase 1 trial, 40 patients with relapsed or refractory AML were treated with escalating doses of gemtuzumab. In 8 of the 40 patients (20%), leukemic blasts were eliminated and blood counts normalized in 8% of the patients (37). In a subsequent open-label multicenter phase 2 trial, 277 patients with CD33-positive AML in first relapse were treated with gemtuzumab at 9 mg/m^2 intravenously (IV) every two weeks for two doses. In this trial, 26% of patients achieved complete remission, characterized by no blasts in the peripheral blood and <5% in the bone marrow, neutrophils >1,500/mm^3, and independence from platelet infusion for one week. The median recurrence-free survival was 6.4 months for patients who achieved complete remission (142). Hyperbilirubinemia developed in 29% of patients, and hepatic veno-occlusive disease developed in 9% in this study who did not undergo subsequent stem cell transplantation.

The principal adverse effect from conjugated anti-CD33 monoclonal antibodies is myelosuppression. Grade 3–4 neutropenia (98%) and thrombocytopenia (99%) occurred in almost all patients in the postinfusion period. Other common adverse effects were fever, chills, gastrointestinal symptoms, dyspnea, epistaxis, and anorexia. Mucositis, sepsis (17%), and pneumonia (8%) were reported (142). Additional reports also describe evidence of hepatotoxicity induced by gemtuzumab ozogamicin (143,144). However, in some of these studies, the majority of the patients received gemtuzumab in combination with other investigational drugs (145).

Radioimmunotherapy

An alternative approach to enhance the antitumor activity of the anti-CD33 antibody was explored by conjugation with radioisotopes such as iodine-131 (^{131}I) or yttrium 90 (^{90}Y). In an initial phase 1 trial, 24 patients with relapsed or refractory myeloid leukemias were treated with escalating doses of ^{131}I-M195 (34). Twenty-two of the 24 patients had a reduction in leukemic burden, and gamma camera imaging demonstrated targeting to areas of leukemic involvement, such as vertebrae, pelvis, and long bones, as well as liver and spleen. Profound myelosuppression occurred at ^{131}I doses of 135 mCi/m^2 or greater, requiring bone marrow transplantation in eight patients. As in the initial trial with unconjugated murine M195 antibodies, 37% of the patients in this trial developed human antimouse antibodies. Subsequently, myeloablative doses of ^{131}I-M195 and ^{131}I-HuM195 (122–437 mCi) were studied in combination with busulfan (16 mg/kg) and cyclophosphamide (90 or 120 mg/kg) as a conditioning regimen for allogeneic bone marrow transplantation in 31 patients with relapsed or refractory AML, accelerated or blastic CML, or advanced MDS. These studies demonstrated that ^{131}I-M195 and ^{131}I-HuM195 have activity in myeloid leukemia, and can be used with standard chemotherapeutic agents without inducing additional toxicities (35).

Yttrium 90 offers several advantages over ^{131}I for myeloablation. ^{90}Y is a pure β-emitter with a half-life of 64 hours, compared with the 8 days half-life of ^{131}I, which is a β- and γ-emitter. Therefore, larger doses of ^{90}Y can be given safely in an outpatient setting. A phase 1 trial with ^{90}Y-HuM195 for patients with relapsed or refractory AML was performed. Nineteen patients were treated with escalating doses of ^{90}Y-HuM195 (0.1–0.3 mCi/kg) given as a single infusion. Myelosuppression lasted 9–62 days at a maximum tolerated dose of 0.275 mCi/kg, and 13 patients had reduction of bone marrow blasts. One patient achieved complete remission lasting five months (140). The inclusion of ^{90}Y-HuM195 in a reduced-intensity preparative regimen for allogeneic bone marrow transplantation in patients with CD33-expressing myeloid leukemia is currently under investigation (36).

CD45 is a pan-leukocyte antigen, and ^{131}I-labeled anti-CD45 has been investigated in a phase 1 trial in 44 patients with advanced leukemia or MDS (146). Thirty-four evaluable patients received escalating doses of ^{131}I-labeled anti-CD45 (76–612 mCi) followed by total body irradiation, cyclophosphamide, and allogeneic or autologous transplantation. Seven of 25 patients with AML or MDS remained alive and disease-free at 65-month follow-up, and 3 out of 9 patients with ALL remained in remission for 19, 54, and 66 months. A phase 1/2 trial was subsequently initiated combining ^{131}I-labeled anti-CD45 with busulfan and cyclophosphamide as a conditioning regimen in patients with AML in first remission (135).

The conjugation of radioisotope to anti-CD20 monoclonal antibodies has improved the activity induced by targeted radiation of CD20-expressing tumor cells. Anti-CD20 antibodies have been approved as radioimmunoconjugates, labeled with yttrium-90, Zevalin (ibritumomab) or iodine-131 Bexxar (tositumomab), for the treatment of relapsed or refractory low-grade or transformed NHL (33,147). The safety profile of these agents has been well characterized, with the principal side effect being reversible myelosuppression from the radiation. Durable responses have been obtained in patients who were proven resistant to chemotherapy (31,148–150). In addition, long-lasting responses were induced in patients refractory to previous treatments with the unlabeled anti-CD20 antibody (151,152). These results led to a phase 2 study to determine the effect of tositumomab in previously untreated patients with indolent lymphoma. Ninety patients with advanced-stage follicular lymphoma were treated with CHOP chemotherapy followed by I-131 tositumomab. An overall response rate of 90% with a complete remission of 67% was achieved, and treatment was well tolerated (32). In a five-year follow-up of this study, an overall survival of 87% and progression-free survival rate of 67% were recently reported, which compares favorably to CHOP chemotherapy alone (153). Chemotherapy in combination with radioimmunotherapy continues to be evaluated in ongoing clinical trials (154,155).

Monoclonal antibodies targeting epidermal growth factor receptor (EGFR) or blocking the binding of vascular endothelial growth factor (VEGF) to its receptor for the treatment of solid tumors are currently being evaluated in clinical trials.

PRINCIPLES OF CANCER VACCINES

The induction of a humoral and/or cellular immune response to antigens specifically expressed on malignant cells has been the ultimate goal in the approach to curing cancer or preventing its recurrence or development in patients at risk. For a cancer vaccine to be effective, the patient with a tumor or the healthy individual at risk has to mount a robust tumor-antigen–specific immune response after therapeutic or prophylactic vaccination. However, tumor cells are derived from host cells, and tumor antigens represent or are derived from normal self-antigens. The tumor antigen may not be expressed on the cell surface, therefore limiting the recognition of self-derived epitopes or the accessibility of the tumor-associated antigens to a potential immune response. Ideally, for a cancer vaccine to be effective, the targeted tumor-associated antigen would be exclusively expressed on the tumor cells, and the vaccination should overcome tolerance and permit induction of an immune response against the epitope. To modify the intensity of the immune response generated against a potential tumor-associated antigen, adjuvants are complexed with the antigen. A variety of adjuvants, such as lipopolysaccharide (LPS) derived from Gram-negative bacteria, aluminum salts-derived, emulsifier-derived, synthetic adjuvants or cytokines such as GM-CSF, have elicited an enhanced immune response (41–43,156,157). The adjuvants can have selective capacities for induction of specific immune responses, and therefore the appropriate choice of the adjuvant may be crucial in order to achieve the desired immune reaction. These immune reactions are believed to be the consequence of processing and presentation of tumor-associated antigens by antigen-presenting cells (APCs) through their major histocompatibility class I and/or class II molecules to CD8[+] or CD4[+] lymphocytes. The activated CD4[+] cells enhance the function of the CD8[+] cytotoxic T cells, support monoclonal antibody production, and promote survival of B lymphocytes. A humoral immune response and activation of CD8[+] cytotoxic lymphocytes can also be a directly induced immune response after tumor-associated antigen administration.

Anti-idiotype Antibody Vaccines

Anti-idiotype antibody vaccines and DNA vaccines derived from tumor-associated antigens complexed with adjuvants have demonstrated the capacity to induce specific immune responses, and a variety of clinical trials are under way. Immunoglobulin on the surface of B-cell lymphomas contains unique amino acid sequences within the variable region of its heavy and light chains (immunoglobulin idiotype) expressed in low-grade lymphomas, which can be specifically targeted by monoclonal antibodies recognizing the idiotype (anti-idiotype antibodies) (39). Pioneered by Levy et al. (38,40) the description of unique idiotypes on low-grade lymphoma prompted the development of vaccine strategies for patients with low-grade lymphomas who had minimal residual disease or complete remission following chemotherapy. In an initial clinical trial reported by Kwak et al. the immunoglobulin-idiotype protein derived from the tumor cells was conjugated to a protein carrier, mixed with an adjuvant, and the individually custom-made vaccines were injected in

nine patients (158). In seven of the nine, anti-idiotype–specific immune responses were observed. Two patients developed anti-idiotype–specific monoclonal antibody responses, four developed a cellular-mediated response, and one patient developed both a cellular-mediated and a humoral immune response against the idiotype. The two patients with minimal residual but measurable disease in this trial regressed completely, and the vaccine was well tolerated overall. These encouraging results led to a larger trial. Of 41 patients with low-grade lymphoma who received vaccination against the unique idiotype, 50% developed a humoral anti-idiotype antibody response (159). In a subsequent phase 2 clinical trial, previously untreated patients with follicular lymphoma were vaccinated with five monthly subcutaneous injections of the idiotype in combination with adjuvant Keyhole limpet hemocyanin (KLH). In this trial, GM-CSF was also injected subcutaneously near the vaccine site for five days to enhance the immune response. This study demonstrated the induction of tumor-specific CD8[+] and CD4[+] T-cell responses. In this trial, humoral immune responses were also observed in the majority of patients, and three patients developed a molecular remission with detectable antibody response, suggesting that an antibody response was not required to maintain molecular remissions. A sustained molecular remission was obtained in 8 of 11 treated patients who had detectable translocations in the blood by PCR after the completion of chemotherapy (160). A multicenter phase 3 clinical trial is under way for patients with follicular lymphoma in first complete remission, evaluating the clinical benefit of idiotype + KLH vaccine in combination with GM-CSF injections (161). In additional reports from these trials, Davis et al. described low levels of residual lymphomas as assessed by polymerase chain reactions for clonal rearrangement of immunoglobulin sequences in patients who had been in clinical remission for up to eight years. This suggests long-term control of the disease despite the persistence of residual malignancy (38). Weng et al. reported their observations in patients who developed an anti-idiotype antibody response with a longer progression-free survival after their last chemotherapy compared with those patients who did not have an antibody response. In contrast, the development of a cellular immune response did not lead to significant progression-free survival at five years after chemotherapy compared with patients without a cellular response (162). Further analyses of these studies demonstrated an association of clinical response to the vaccine and the IgG Fc receptor (FcγR) polymorphism. Anti-idiotype monoclonal antibodies binding to their respective lymphoma cell are usually recognized by effector cells (such as NK cells) via FcγR and mediate antibody-dependent cellular cytotoxicity (ADCC). Favorable

FcγR polymorphisms have higher affinities to the Fc fraction of the bound antibody, resulting in stronger activation of the effector cells and consequently more potent ADCC. Weng et al. clearly demonstrated a longer progression-free survival in patients with a FcγRIIIa 158 valine/valine genotype compared with the heterozygous valine/phenylalanine or homozygous phenylalanine/phenylalanine FcγRIIIa genotypes (162). The beneficial clinical outcome in patients receiving the vaccine who developed an anti-idiotype antibody production and those with a favorable FcγRIIIa 158 valine/valine genotype proved to be independent of partial or complete remission to induction chemotherapy (163).

Carcinoembryonic antigen (CEA) is a well-characterized, tumor-associated antigen expressed on neoplasms derived from gastrointestinal tract or other adenocarcinomas (164). Vaccination approaches to induce immune responses against this tumor-associated antigen have been initiated for patients with resected colon cancer. To overcome the limitations of anti-idiotype antibody responses against this self-antigen, a unique approach, described by Lindemann and Jerne as the network hypothesis (165,166), was explored by Foon et al. (167) The network hypothesis postulated that immunization with a tumor-associated antigen will induce monoclonal antibody production against this antigen, termed Ab1. Some of the anti-idiotype antibodies, Ab2, generated against the Ab1 antibodies, mimic the structure of the original carcinoembryonic antigen. Vaccinations with these anti-idiotypes, termed Ab2β, can induce immune responses, anti-anti–idiotype antibodies (Ab3), against the original antigen. This approach utilizes an anti-idiotype antibody vaccine to break immune tolerance and permit induction of immune response against the self-derived tumor-associated antigen. In a clinical phase 1 trial, Foon et al. vaccinated a total of 32 patients, 29 with resected Dukes B, C, and D and three with incompletely resected Dukes D disease, using the anti-idiotype antibody vaccine called CeaVac. They assessed the specific immune response against CEA. Four injections of 2 mg CeaVac were administered intracutaneously every other week and then monthly until disease progression. In addition, the impact of concurrent chemotherapy with 5-fluorouracil (5-FU) on the immune response was assessed in 14 patients. All 32 patients developed an antibody response, and 80% of the patients also developed a T-cell proliferative response against CEA, irrespective of concurrent 5-FU treatment, demonstrating the ability to overcome immune tolerance with this approach (167). Although some patients reportedly experienced prolonged progression-free survival, this study was not designed to draw clinical conclusions based on the results of individual patients, and a phase 3 study is required to capture beneficial outcome in these patients.

The principle of inducing anti-anti–idiotype antibodies is currently being tested against other tumor-associated antigens, such as anti-GD-2 (168,169), ACA125 (170), or anti-GD-3 (171).

DNA Vaccines

DNA vaccines consist of a plasmid DNA containing one or multiple genes. The DNA is typically administered intradermally or intramuscularly by needle injection or by use of a gene gun, which propels gold beads coated with plasmid DNA into the skin (172,173). The DNA is translated into the encoded proteins, then processed and presented by APCs, eliciting the vaccine-specific immune response. A variety of DNA vaccines are currently being tested in preclinical and early clinical trials, and only a limited selection of these trials have been included in this chapter to describe the principal approach of DNA immunization.

DNA vaccination against melanoma differentiation antigens has been intensively studied by Houghton et al. (174). The initial immunizations with the melanoma-derived tyrosine-kinase–related proteins TRP-2 and TYRP1 were complicated by development of autoimmunity, resulting in severe vitiligo (hypopigmentation) of the skin (175,176), whereas DNA immunizations against melanoma-derived antigen gp100 induced strong CD8$^+$ T-cell responses with only minimal vitiligo (177). To overcome the poor immunogenicity of the self-antigen gp100, xenogeneic (mouse-derived) DNA vaccines were explored, demonstrating that antibody and T-cell responses induced by the xenogeneic DNA can cross-react with the original syngeneic DNA and induce effective immunity in a preclinical model (175–177). In addition, when plasmid DNAs of cytokines, proven to enhance immune responses, such as IL-2, IL-12, IL-15, IL-21, and GM-CSF, were co-injected with the gp100 plasmid DNA, increased CD8+ T-cell responses against gp100 and improved tumor-free survival were observed in a preclinical melanoma model (178). Clinical trials evaluating the clinical benefit in humans are currently ongoing. Powell and Rosenberg utilized a gp100-derived peptide, modified by substituting methionine for threonine at position 2 for increased HLA-A*0201 binding affinity, and thus elicited enhanced T-cell responses for multiple peptide vaccinations in five HLA-A*0201–positive patients with completely resected melanoma who remained at high risk for tumor recurrence after tumor resection. The initial three patients were vaccinated every three weeks for a total of 16 injections, and the final two patients were vaccinated weekly for 10 weeks followed by a 3-week break between treatment courses. After immunization, the patients developed high frequencies of gp100-specific CD8$^+$ T lymphocytes, which were still functionally tumor-reactive and circulating in the blood at one year follow-up (179). The patients remained free of recurrence at one year after last immunization, and no autoimmune reactivity was observed in the study. Recently, these investigators studied nine patients with metastatic melanoma after vaccination with the modified gp100-derived peptide, followed by ex vivo expansion of the HLA-A*0201–restricted, gp100 peptide-specific T cells, and subsequent adoptive transfer of the expanded T-cell population in combination with high-dose interleukin-2 and the cancer vaccine after chemotherapy-induced lymphodepletion (180). Although the presence of circulating tumor-reactive CD8+ T cells was demonstrated in the blood, no objective clinical response was described in these patients.

Prostate-specific membrane antigen (PSMA), initially thought to be a unique cancer antigen, is a self-antigen that is highly overexpressed on prostate cancer cells, but is also expressed on normal prostate cells, the brain, salivary glands, and biliary tree (181). PSMA is overexpressed on the neovasculature of other solid tumors, such as renal cancer, lung, bladder, pancreatic cancer, and melanoma, but is not found on normal vasculature (182). In a preclinical model, vaccination with xenogeneic PSMA DNA-induced monoclonal antibodies to both mouse and human PSMA provided the basis for evaluating PSMA DNA vaccination in clinical trials (183).

Cell-Based Vaccines

Cell-based vaccine strategies utilizing autologous or allogeneic tumor cells, genetically modified to secrete cytokines for enhanced antigen presentation and improved immune responses, were evaluated in the treatment of solid tumors. A phase 1 trial to assess the safety and feasibility of prostate cancer antigens was performed by Simons et al. (184) In this study, prostate tumor cells were surgically harvested from 11 patients with metastatic prostate cancer. Cells were cultured and complementary DNA (cDNA) encoding GM-CSF was retrovirally transduced into the tumor cells. Sufficient numbers of genetically modified cancer cells were obtained from 8 out of 11 patients. These GM-CSF–modified prostate cancer cells were lethally irradiated and injected intracutaneously up to six times every three weeks. The vaccine was well tolerated, although characterized by local inflammation of the vaccination sites. Biopsies of these infiltrates three days after the injection demonstrated the presence of autologous prostate cancer cells, dendritic cells, macrophages, eosinophils, and lymphocytes. A delayed-type hypersensitivity (DTH) reaction against challenge with irradiated, nontransduced, autologous tumor cells after completion of the vaccination series was newly induced in seven out of

eight vaccinated patients. Biopsies of the DTH sites demonstrated infiltration with T lymphocytes as well as few B lymphocytes. In addition, monoclonal antibody responses against three prostate cancer-derived epitopes (not observed in the prevaccination sera from three of the eight vaccinated patients) was also documented (184). The broader application and a larger phase 2 clinical trial were limited by the impracticability of this approach, including the low yield of prostate cancer cells obtained after cell cultures and the necessity to manufacture the vaccine on an individual basis. A prostate cancer vaccine, termed GVAX, consisting of two allogeneic prostate cancer cell lines genetically modified to secrete GM-CSF, has been subsequently tested in a phase 2 clinical trial in hormone-refractory prostate cancer patients, and a phase 3 trial evaluating the vaccine alone or in combination with docetaxel in this patient cohort has been initiated (185).

The principle of using autologous tumor cells genetically modified to secrete GM-CSF was also explored in metastatic melanoma and metastatic non-small cell lung cancer (NSCLC). Vaccination with irradiated, autologous melanoma cells engineered to secrete GM-CSF, with a replication-defective adenoviral vector encoding human GM-CSF, was performed in 34 patients with metastatic melanoma. Vaccines were injected intradermally or subcutaneously at increasing doses from 1×10^6, 4×10^6, or 1×10^7, depending on overall yield at weekly intervals, until the vaccine supply was exhausted. Side effects were restricted to local skin reactions, and 25 patients could be assessed for DTH reaction. In this study, 17 of 25 patients developed a DTH reaction from autologous, nontransduced melanoma cells, and metastatic lesions that were resected after vaccination showed focal infiltration with T lymphocytes and plasma cells with tumor necrosis in 10 of 16 patients (186,187). A similar strategy was subsequently tested in a phase 1 trial of 35 patients with metastatic NSCLC. This produced DTH reaction to nontransduced autologous NSCLC cells in 18 of 22 assessable patients and improved clinical outcomes in some patients (188). To circumvent the requirement of genetic transduction of individual tumors, a phase 1=2 trial was conducted in which autologous NSCLC cells were admixed with an allogeneic bystander cell line (K562, a human erythroleukemia cell line) and genetically transduced to secrete GM-CSF at a cell ratio of 2:1 for intradermal vaccination. Forty-nine patients were vaccinated at two-week intervals for a total of 3–12 vaccinations, with doses ranging from $5–80 \times 10^6$ autologous NSCLC cells mixed with half the amount of GM-CSF–secreting K562 cells per vaccine (189). Although the GM-CSF secretion was found to be 25-fold higher compared with a previous trial vaccine derived from autologous NSCLC cells modified to secrete

GM-CSF (190), the frequency of vaccine site reactions, tumor response, and time to progression was inferior to the autologous cell vaccines of the previous trial.

PRINCIPLES OF T-CELL–MEDIATED IMMUNE RESPONSE MODIFICATION

In recent years, our knowledge of T-cell–induced lysis of tumor cells and persistence of antigen-specific T cells induced by vaccination has led to the integration of CTLA-4 blockade into clinical trials after vaccination. In addition, the immunoregulatory capacity of T-regulatory cells is currently under investigation. Studies are assessing the effects of selective depletion or infusion of this T-cell subset on enhanced T-cell–mediated tumor effect or amelioration of GVHD, respectively.

Cytotoxic T-Lymphocyte–Associated Antigen (CTLA)-4

T-cell responses are down-regulated by the stimulation of cytotoxic T-lymphocyte–associated antigen (CTLA-4) expressed on the cell surface of activated T lymphocytes. CTLA-4 protein is usually located in intracellular vesicles and increasingly expressed on the surface of T lymphocytes with increased activation of the cells. CTLA-4 expression serves as a counter-regulatory molecule to the activating receptor CD28 on T lymphocytes. The ligands CD80/B7.1 or CD86/B7.2, expressed on antigen-presenting cells, bind to CD28 on the T cells, either inducing their activation or binding to CTLA-4, which prevents overactivation and serves as a negative modulator of T-cell homeostasis (44,45). CTLA-4 activation induces antigen-specific cell death of activated T lymphocytes and prevents proliferation of autoimmune-reactive T cells (191,192). Blockade of CTLA-4 with nonagonistic antibodies to enhance DNA vaccine-mediated T-cell response has been tested in preclinical models (193–195), and the anti-CTLA-4 antibody ipilimumab has been found safe in early clinical trials with promising results, particularly in melanoma and renal cancer (196–198).

T-Regulatory Cells (Tregs)

T-cell tolerance is achieved through negative selection in the thymus of potentially autoreactive T lymphocytes (199). Despite this thymic selection, T cells can escape the process and are found in the peripheral blood of healthy individuals. T-regulatory cells (Tregs), characterized recently by their expression of CD4$^+$CD25$^+$FOXP3$^+$, constitute a T-lymphocyte population that controls pathologic immune responses and is involved in the maintenance of lymphocyte homeostasis.

Several preclinical studies have demonstrated that Tregs prevent autoreactive T-cell responses (200,201), while other studies demonstrated that Tregs can inhibit antigen-specific T-cell responses and T-cell–mediated antitumor effects (46). Ex vivo expansion of these cells for the treatment of autoimmune diseases has been attempted, but these cells have poor in vitro proliferative potential (202,203), and the use of rapamycin, which induces preferential proliferation of Tregs, is currently under investigation (204). In contrast, the depletion of Tregs has been demonstrated to enhance T-cell–mediated antitumor effects in preclinical models (205). In a preclinical melanoma model, Sutmuller et al. combined CTLA-4 blockade with in vivo depletion of Tregs to obtain maximal tumor rejection by tyrosinase-specific T cells after vaccination with B-16-GM-CSF tumor-cell vaccine (206).

The immunoregulatory capacity of Tregs is currently also being investigated for control of GVHD following allogeneic bone marrow transplantation. Several groups have demonstrated that infusion of regulatory T cells can ameliorate GVHD without reducing the graft-versus-leukemia effect in preclinical models (207–209). Clinical trials investigating the potential of regulatory T cells in humans are anticipated.

CONCLUSIONS

Immunotherapies are rapidly evolving and will be increasingly integrated with standard therapies for the treatment of solid tumors and hematologic malignancies. However, the broader application of immunotherapies currently has limitations that need to be resolved. Biologic therapies, such as the production of cancer vaccines or the generation of antigen-specific T lymphocytes, have to be produced under strict manufacturing conditions, currently limiting these approaches to larger centers that provide an institutional environment for these therapeutic trials. Regulatory obstacles for these therapies have to be overcome. The generation of a cancer vaccine or of antigen-specific T lymphocytes includes the incorporation of novel agents needed for the production of the final product. These agents often require prior independent investigational new drug (IND) and Food and Drug Administration (FDA) approval. To facilitate the development of immunotherapies, the pharmaceutical industry must be involved in the production of materials and products that fulfill regulatory FDA criteria. An increased awareness of the implementation and integration of immunotherapies into clinical trials resulted in the first FDA/National Cancer Institute (NCI)–sponsored workshop in February 2007 entitled, "Bringing Therapeutic Cancer Vaccines and Immunotherapy to Licensure."

The workshop, attended by representatives from the FDA, investigators, and industry, discussed strategies to advance the approval process for these therapies.

An additional limitation of immunotherapies, once proven safe and effective, is associated with the time-consuming and labor-intensive process of production. Many cancer vaccines can be produced only on an individual basis, such as the anti-idiotype cancer vaccines, after the idiotype has been determined. The generation of antigen-specific T lymphocytes also has to be performed on an individual basis, targeting the antigen-derived peptide presented by the individuals' HLA type. For this reason, the individuals' HLA alleles and the peptide sequences derived from the antigen presented in these HLA alleles have to be determined prior to generating these peptide-specific T cells. Novel approaches for improving and overcoming some of these limitations are under investigation. Pulsing of antigen-presenting cells with overlapping pentadecapeptides overspanning the entire amino acid sequence of known antigens for the generation of peptide-specific T cells circumvents prior knowledge of the HLA restriction of the peptide derived from the antigen. This strategy may be applied to generate specific T cells for all patients, independently of HLA type (210,211).

In addition, the identification and generation of more potent antigen-presenting cells has improved the cytotoxic potential of antigen-specific T cells and permits the generation of T lymphocytes targeting cancer-derived antigens with low immunogenicity (212,213). The development of artificial antigen-presenting cells consisting of nonimmunogenic mouse fibroblasts transduced to express selected HLA alleles and co-stimulatory molecules, which can be expanded without limit in vitro, may circumvent the necessity to repeatedly generate antigen-presenting cells for each individual, and may provide "off-the-shelf" access to these cells for the generation of antigen-specific T lymphocytes (214,215). Recent studies have demonstrated gene transfer of T-cell receptors, thereby redirecting the specificity of T cells to tumor antigens (216–219). This approach may produce antigen-specific T cells without the necessity of producing antigen-presenting cells.

Monoclonal antibodies are easily obtained and can be administered to all individuals who might benefit from this therapy. Current radioimmunotherapy trials that used β-emitting isotopes, such as ^{131}iodine and ^{90}yttrium, conjugated to anti-CD20, anti-CD33, or anti-CD45 monoclonal antibodies, demonstrated promising results and safe administration. The incorporation of α-emitters, such as ^{213}bismuth and ^{225}acinium, into trials for the treatment of minimal residual disease is currently under investigation and holds great promise because of the short range and high linear energy transfer (220,221).

It is anticipated that immunotherapies will continue to evolve, and as results of clinical trials become available, the benefits and limitations of these therapies will be better defined. Combination immunotherapies, such as the ex vivo expansion of antigen-specific T lymphocytes collected from patients after administration of a cancer vaccine and reinfusion of the expanded cell population and/or the administration of an immune response modifying agent, eg, anti-CTLA-4 antibody, could improve the outcome of these therapies once regulations limiting these approaches have been overcome.

*R*eferences

1. Roberts MM, To LB, Gillis D, et al. Immune reconstitution following peripheral blood stem cell transplantation, autologous bone marrow transplantation and allogeneic bone marrow transplantation. *Bone Marrow Transplant*. 1993;12: 469–475.
2. de Gast GC, Verdonck LF, Middeldorp JM, et al. Recovery of T cell subsets after autologous bone marrow transplantation is mainly due to proliferation of mature T cells in the graft. *Blood*. 1985;66:428–431.
3. Mackall CL, Fleisher TA, Brown MR, et al. Age, thymopoiesis, and CD4+ T-lymphocyte regeneration after intensive chemotherapy. *N Engl J Med*. 1995;332:143–149.
4. Koehne G, Zeller W, Stockschlaeder M, et al. Phenotype of lymphocyte subsets after autologous peripheral blood stem cell transplantation. *Bone Marrow Transplant*. 1997;19:149–156.
5. Pettengell R. Autologous stem cell transplantation in follicular non-Hodgkin's lymphoma. *Bone Marrow Transplant*. 2002;29(Suppl 1):S1–S4.
6. Kewalramani T, Zelenetz AD, Nimer SD, et al. Rituximab and ICE as second-line therapy before autologous stem cell transplantation for relapsed or primary refractory diffuse large B-cell lymphoma. *Blood*. 2004;103:3684–3688.
7. Hamlin PA, Zelenetz AD, Kewalramani T, et al. Age-adjusted International Prognostic Index predicts autologous stem cell transplantation outcome for patients with relapsed or primary refractory diffuse large B-cell lymphoma. *Blood*. 2003;102:1989–1996.
8. Diehl V, Josting A. Hodgkin's disease. *Cancer J*. 2000;6(Suppl 2):S150–S158.
9. Josting A. Autologous transplantation in relapsed and refractory Hodgkin's disease. *Eur J Haematol Suppl*. 2005;66: 141–145.
10. Majhail NS, Weisdorf DJ, Defor TE, et al. Long-term results of autologous stem cell transplantation for primary refractory or relapsed Hodgkin's lymphoma. *Biol Blood Marrow Transplant*. 2006;12:1065–1072.
11. Barlogie B, Shaughnessy J, Tricot G, et al. Treatment of multiple myeloma. *Blood*. 2004;103:20–32.
12. Attal M, Harousseau JL, Facon T, et al. Single versus double autologous stem-cell transplantation for multiple myeloma. *N Engl J Med*. 2003;349:2495–2502.
13. Bruno B, Rotta M, Patriarca F, et al. A comparison of allografting with autografting for newly diagnosed myeloma. *N Engl J Med*. 2007;356:1110–1120.
14. Fefer A, Sullivan KM, Weiden P, et al. Graft versus leukemia effect in man: the relapse rate of acute leukemia is lower after allogeneic than after syngeneic marrow transplantation. *Prog Clin Biol Res*. 1987;244:401–408.
15. Weiden PL, Flournoy N, Thomas ED, et al. Antileukemic effect of graft-versus-host disease in human recipients of allogeneic-marrow grafts. *N Engl J Med*. 1979;300:1068–1073.

16. Kolb HJ, Mittermuller J, Clemm C, et al. Donor leukocyte transfusions for treatment of recurrent chronic myelogenous leukemia in marrow transplant patients. *Blood.* 1990;76:2462–2465.

17. Kolb HJ, Schattenberg A, Goldman JM, et al. Graft-versus-leukemia effect of donor lymphocyte transfusions in marrow grafted patients. *Blood.* 1995;86:2041–2050.

18. Mackinnon S, Papadopoulos EB, Carabasi MH, et al. Adoptive immunotherapy evaluating escalating doses of donor leukocytes for relapse of chronic myeloid leukemia after bone marrow transplantation: separation of graft-versus-leukemia responses from graft-versus-host disease. *Blood.* 1995;86:1261–1268.

19. Drobyski WR, Keever CA, Roth MS, et al. Salvage immunotherapy using donor leukocyte infusions as treatment for relapsed chronic myelogenous leukemia after allogeneic bone marrow transplantation: efficacy and toxicity of a defined T-cell dose. *Blood.* 1993;82:2310–2318.

20. Collins RH, Jr., Shpilberg O, Drobyski WR, et al. Donor leukocyte infusions in 140 patients with relapsed malignancy after allogeneic bone marrow transplantation. *J Clin Oncol.* 1997;15:433–444.

21. Falkenburg JH, Wafelman AR, Joosten P, et al. Complete remission of accelerated phase chronic myeloid leukemia by treatment with leukemia-reactive cytotoxic T lymphocytes. *Blood.* 1999;94:1201–1208.

22. Riddell SR, Watanabe KS, Goodrich JM, et al. Restoration of viral immunity in immunodeficient humans by the adoptive transfer of T cell clones. *Science.* 1992;257:238–241.

23. Heslop HE, Ng CY, Li C, et al. Long-term restoration of immunity against Epstein-Barr virus infection by adoptive transfer of gene-modified virus-specific T lymphocytes. *Nat Med.* 1996;2:551–555.

24. Rooney CM, Smith CA, Ng CY, et al. Infusion of cytotoxic T cells for the prevention and treatment of Epstein-Barr virus-induced lymphoma in allogeneic transplant recipients. *Blood.* 1998;92:1549–1555.

25. Vales-Gomez M, Reyburn HT, Mandelboim M, et al. Kinetics of interaction of HLA-C ligands with natural killer cell inhibitory receptors. *Immunity.* 1998;9:337–344.

26. Farag SS, Fehniger TA, Ruggeri L, et al. Natural killer cell receptors: new biology and insights into the graft-versus-leukemia effect. *Blood.* 2002;100:1935–1947.

27. Aversa F, Terenzi A, Tabilio A, et al. Full haplotype-mismatched hematopoietic stem-cell transplantation: a phase II study in patients with acute leukemia at high risk of relapse. *J Clin Oncol.* 2005;23:3447–3454.

28. Ruggeri L, Capanni M, Urbani E, et al. Effectiveness of donor natural killer cell alloreactivity in mismatched hematopoietic transplants. *Science.* 2002;295:2097–2100.

29. McLaughlin P, Grillo-Lopez AJ, Link BK, et al. Rituximab chimeric anti-CD20 monoclonal antibody therapy for relapsed indolent lymphoma: half of patients respond to a four-dose treatment program. *J Clin Oncol.* 1998;16:2825–2833.

30. Czuczman MS, Grillo-Lopez AJ, White CA, et al. Treatment of patients with low-grade B-cell lymphoma with the combination of chimeric anti-CD20 monoclonal antibody and CHOP chemotherapy. *J Clin Oncol.* 1999;17:268–276.

31. Witzig TE, Gordon LI, Cabanillas F, et al. Randomized controlled trial of yttrium-90-labeled ibritumomab tiuxetan radioimmunotherapy versus rituximab immunotherapy for patients with relapsed or refractory low-grade, follicular, or transformed B-cell non-Hodgkin's lymphoma. *J Clin Oncol.* 2002;20:2453–2463.

32. Press OW, Unger JM, Braziel RM, et al. A phase 2 trial of CHOP chemotherapy followed by tositumomab/iodine I 131 tositumomab for previously untreated follicular non-Hodgkin lymphoma: Southwest Oncology Group Protocol S9911. *Blood.* 2003;102:1606–1612.

33. Zelenetz AD. A clinical and scientific overview of tositumomab and iodine I 131 tositumomab. *Semin Oncol.* 2003;30:22–30.

34. Schwartz MA, Lovett DR, Redner A, et al. Dose-escalation trial of M195 labeled with iodine 131 for cytoreduction and marrow ablation in relapsed or refractory myeloid leukemias. *J Clin Oncol.* 1993;11:294–303.

35. Jurcic JG, Caron PC, Nikula TK, et al. Radiolabeled anti-CD33 monoclonal antibody M195 for myeloid leukemias. *Cancer Res.* 1995;55:5908s–5910s.

36. Jurcic JG, Scheinberg DA. Radionuclides as conditioning before stem cell transplantation. *Curr Opin Hematol.* 1999;6:371–376.

37. Sievers EL, Appelbaum FR, Spielberger RT, et al. Selective ablation of acute myeloid leukemia using antibody-targeted chemotherapy: a phase I study of an anti-CD33 calicheamicin immunoconjugate. *Blood.* 1999;93:3678–3684.

38. Davis TA, Maloney DG, Czerwinski DK, et al. Anti-idiotype antibodies can induce long-term complete remissions in non-Hodgkin's lymphoma without eradicating the malignant clone. *Blood.* 1998;92:1184–1190.

39. Levy R, Miller RA. Therapy of lymphoma directed at idiotypes. *J Natl Cancer Inst Monogr.* 1990;10:61–68.

40. Miller RA, Maloney DG, Warnke R, et al. Treatment of B-cell lymphoma with monoclonal anti-idiotype antibody. *N Engl J Med.* 1982;306:517–522.

41. Akbari O, Panjwani N, Garcia S, et al. DNA vaccination: transfection and activation of dendritic cells as key events for immunity. *J Exp Med.* 1999;189:169–178.

42. O'Hagan DT. Recent advances in vaccine adjuvants for systemic and mucosal administration. *J Pharm Pharmacol.* 1998;50:1–10.

43. Ulmer JB, DeWitt CM, Chastain M, et al. Enhancement of DNA vaccine potency using conventional aluminum adjuvants. *Vaccine.* 1999;18:18–28.

44. Tivol EA, Borriello F, Schweitzer AN, et al. Loss of CTLA-4 leads to massive lymphoproliferation and fatal multiorgan tissue destruction, revealing a critical negative regulatory role of CTLA-4. *Immunity.* 1995;3:541–547.

45. Waterhouse P, Marengere LE, Mittrucker HW, et al. CTLA-4, a negative regulator of T-lymphocyte activation. *Immunol Rev.* 1996;153:183–207.

46. Lanzavecchia A, Sallusto F. Regulation of T cell immunity by dendritic cells. *Cell.* 2001;106:263–266.

47. Gale RP, Champlin RE. How does bone-marrow transplantation cure leukaemia? *Lancet.* 1984;2:28–30.

48. Kolb HJ. Donor leukocyte transfusions for treatment of leukemic relapse after bone marrow transplantation. EBMT Immunology and Chronic Leukemia Working Parties. *Vox Sang.* 1998;74(Suppl 2):321–329.

49. Kolb HJ. Management of relapse after hematopoietic cell transplantation. In: Thomas ED BKG, Forman ST, eds. *Hematopoietic Cell Transplantation.* Blackwell Science Inc; 1999:929–936.

50. Cardoso AA, Schultze JL, Boussiotis VA, et al. Pre-B acute lymphoblastic leukemia cells may induce T-cell anergy to alloantigen. *Blood.* 1996;88:41–48.

51. Stripecke R, Cardoso AA, Pepper KA, et al. Lentiviral vectors for efficient delivery of CD80 and granulocyte-macrophage-colony-stimulating factor in human acute lymphoblastic leukemia and acute myeloid leukemia cells to induce antileukemic immune responses. *Blood.* 2000;96:1317–1326.

52. Choudhury A, Gajewski JL, Liang JC, et al. Use of leukemic dendritic cells for the generation of antileukemic cellular cytotoxicity against Philadelphia chromosome-positive chronic myelogenous leukemia. *Blood.* 1997;89:1133–1142.

53. Smit WM, Rijnbeek M, van Bergen CA, et al. Generation of dendritic cells expressing bcr-abl from CD34-positive chronic myeloid leukemia precursor cells. *Hum Immunol.* 1997;53:216–223.

54. Choudhury BA, Liang JC, Thomas EK, et al. Dendritic cells derived in vitro from acute myelogenous leukemia cells stimulate autologous, antileukemic T-cell responses. *Blood.* 1999;93:780–786.

55. Cignetti A, Bryant E, Allione B, et al. CD34(+) acute myeloid and lymphoid leukemic blasts can be induced to differentiate into dendritic cells. *Blood.* 1999;94:2048–2055.

56. Dunussi-Joannopoulos K, Weinstein HJ, Nickerson PW, et al. Irradiated B7-1 transduced primary acute myelogenous leukemia (AML) cells can be used as therapeutic vaccines in murine AML. *Blood.* 1996;87:2938–2946.

57. Mutis T, Schrama E, Melief CJ, et al. CD80-Transfected acute myeloid leukemia cells induce primary allogeneic T-cell responses directed at patient specific minor histocompatibility antigens and leukemia-associated antigens. *Blood.* 1998;92:1677–1684.

58. Cardoso AA, Seamon MJ, Afonso HM, et al. Ex vivo generation of human anti-pre-B leukemia-specific autologous cytolytic T cells. *Blood.* 1997;90:549–561.

59. Ljungman P, Aschan J, Lewensohn-Fuchs I, et al. Results of different strategies for reducing cytomegalovirus-associated mortality in allogeneic stem cell transplant recipients. *Transplantation.* 1998;66:1330–1334.

60. Boeckh M, Leisenring W, Riddell SR, et al. Late cytomegalovirus disease and mortality in recipients of allogeneic hematopoietic stem cell transplants: importance of viral load and T-cell immunity. *Blood.* 2003;101:407–414.

61. Papadopoulos EB, Ladanyi M, Emanuel D, et al. Infusions of donor leukocytes to treat Epstein-Barr virus-associated lymphoproliferative disorders after allogeneic bone marrow transplantation. *N Engl J Med.* 1994;330:1185–1191.

62. Bonini C, Ferrari G, Verzeletti S, et al. HSV-TK gene transfer into donor lymphocytes for control of allogeneic graft-versus-leukemia. *Science.* 1997;276:1719–1724.

63. Haque T, Wilkie GM, Taylor C, et al. Treatment of Epstein-Barr-virus-positive post-transplantation lymphoproliferative disease with partly HLA-matched allogeneic cytotoxic T cells. *Lancet.* 2002;360:436–442.

64. Rooney CM, Smith CA, Ng CY, et al. Use of gene-modified virus-specific T lymphocytes to control Epstein-Barr-virus-related lymphoproliferation. *Lancet.* 1995;345:9–13.

65. Walter EA, Greenberg PD, Gilbert MJ, et al. Reconstitution of cellular immunity against cytomegalovirus in recipients of allogeneic bone marrow by transfer of T-cell clones from the donor. *N Engl J Med.* 1995;333:1038–1044.

66. Peggs KS, Verfuerth S, Pizzey A, et al. Adoptive cellular therapy for early cytomegalovirus infection after allogeneic stem-cell transplantation with virus-specific T-cell lines. *Lancet.* 2003;362:1375–1377.

67. Einsele H, Roosnek E, Rufer N, et al. Infusion of cytomegalovirus (CMV)-specific T cells for the treatment of CMV infection not responding to antiviral chemotherapy. *Blood.* 2002;99:3916–3922.

68. Call KM, Glaser T, Ito CY, et al. Isolation and characterization of a zinc finger polypeptide gene at the human chromosome 11 Wilms' tumor locus. *Cell.* 1990;60:509–520.

69. Rauscher FJ, 3rd. The WT1 Wilms tumor gene product: a developmentally regulated transcription factor in the kidney that functions as a tumor suppressor. *Faseb J.* 1993;7:896–903.

70. Buckler AJ, Pelletier J, Haber DA, et al. Isolation, characterization, and expression of the murine Wilms' tumor gene (WT1) during kidney development. *Mol Cell Biol.* 1991;11:1707–1712.

71. Park S, Schalling M, Bernard A, et al. The Wilms tumour gene WT1 is expressed in murine mesoderm-derived tissues and mutated in a human mesothelioma. *Nat Genet.* 1993;4:415–420.

72. Gaiger A, Reese V, Disis ML, et al. Immunity to WT1 in the animal model and in patients with acute myeloid leukemia. *Blood.* 2000;96:1480–1489.

73. Miwa H, Beran M, Saunders GF. Expression of the Wilms' tumor gene (WT1) in human leukemias. *Leukemia.* 1992;6:405–409.

74. Tamaki H, Ogawa H, Inoue K, et al. Increased expression of the Wilms tumor gene (WT1) at relapse in acute leukemia. *Blood.* 1996;88:4396–4398.

75. Ohminami H, Yasukawa M, Fujita S. HLA class I-restricted lysis of leukemia cells by a CD8(+) cytotoxic T-lymphocyte clone specific for WT1 peptide. *Blood.* 2000;95:286–293.

76. Oka Y, Elisseeva OA, Tsuboi A, et al. Human cytotoxic T-lymphocyte responses specific for peptides of the wild-type Wilms' tumor gene (WT1) product. *Immunogenetics.* 2000;51:99–107.

77. Gao L, Bellantuono I, Elsasser A, et al. Selective elimination of leukemic CD34(+) progenitor cells by cytotoxic T lymphocytes specific for WT1. *Blood.* 2000;95:2198–2203.

78. Doubrovina ES, Doubrovin MM, Lee S, et al. In vitro stimulation with WT1 peptide-loaded Epstein-Barr virus-positive B cells elicits high frequencies of WT1 peptide-specific T cells with in vitro and in vivo tumoricidal activity. *Clin Cancer Res.* 2004;10:7207–7219.

79. Bories D, Raynal MC, Solomon DH, et al. Down-regulation of a serine protease, myeloblastin, causes growth arrest and differentiation of promyelocytic leukemia cells. *Cell.* 1989;59:959–968.

80. Dengler R, Munstermann U, al-Batran S, et al. Immunocytochemical and flow cytometric detection of proteinase 3 (myeloblastin) in normal and leukaemic myeloid cells. *Br J Haematol.* 1995;89:250–257.

81. Molldrem JJ, Clave E, Jiang YZ, et al. Cytotoxic T lymphocytes specific for a nonpolymorphic proteinase 3 peptide preferentially inhibit chronic myeloid leukemia colony-forming units. *Blood.* 1997;90:2529–2534.

82. Molldrem JJ, Lee PP, Wang C, et al. Evidence that specific T lymphocytes may participate in the elimination of chronic myelogenous leukemia. *Nat Med.* 2000;6:1018–1023.

83. Molldrem JJ, Lee PP, Wang C, et al. A PR1-human leukocyte antigen-A2 tetramer can be used to isolate low-frequency cytotoxic T lymphocytes from healthy donors that selectively lyse chronic myelogenous leukemia. *Cancer Res.* 1999;59:2675–2681.

84. Mailander V, Scheibenbogen C, Thiel E, et al. Complete remission in a patient with recurrent acute myeloid leukemia induced by vaccination with WT1 peptide in the absence of hematological or renal toxicity. *Leukemia.* 2004;18:165–166.

85. Oka Y, Tsuboi A, Taguchi T, et al. Induction of WT1 (Wilms' tumor gene)-specific cytotoxic T lymphocytes by WT1 peptide vaccine and the resultant cancer regression. *Proc Natl Acad Sci USA.* 2004;101:13885–13890.

86. Roopenian D, Choi EY, Brown A. The immunogenomics of minor histocompatibility antigens. *Immunol Rev.* 2002;190:86–94.

87. Korngold B, Sprent J. Lethal graft-versus-host disease after bone marrow transplantation across minor histocompatibility barriers in mice. Prevention by removing mature T cells from marrow. *J Exp Med.* 1978;148:1687–1698.

88. Wallny HJ, Rammensee HG. Identification of classical minor histocompatibility antigen as cell-derived peptide. *Nature.* 1990;343:275–278.

89. Goulmy E. Human minor histocompatibility antigens. *Curr Opin Immunol.* 1996;8:75–81.

90. den Haan JM, Sherman NE, Blokland E, et al. Identification of a graft versus host disease-associated human minor histocompatibility antigen. *Science.* 1995;268:1476–1480.

91. Randolph SS, Gooley TA, Warren EH, et al. Female donors contribute to a selective graft-versus-leukemia effect in male recipients of HLA-matched, related hematopoietic stem cell transplants. *Blood.* 2004;103:347–352.

92. Stern M, Passweg JR, Locasciulli A, et al. Influence of donor/recipient sex matching on outcome of allogeneic hematopoietic stem cell transplantation for aplastic anemia. *Transplantation.* 2006;82:218–226.

93. Goulmy E, Schipper R, Pool J, et al. Mismatches of minor histocompatibility antigens between HLA-identical donors and recipients and the development of graft-versus-host disease after bone marrow transplantation. *N Engl J Med.* 1996;334:281–285.

94. Tseng LH, Lin MT, Hansen JA, et al. Correlation between disparity for the minor histocompatibility antigen HA-1 and the development of acute graft-versus-host disease after allogeneic marrow transplantation. *Blood.* 1999;94:2911–2914.

95. Socie G, Loiseau P, Tamouza R, et al. Both genetic and clinical factors predict the development of graft-versus-host disease after allogeneic hematopoietic stem cell transplantation. *Transplantation.* 2001;72:699–706.

96. Lin MT, Gooley T, Hansen JA, et al. Absence of statistically significant correlation between disparity for the minor histocompatibility antigen-HA-1 and outcome after allogeneic hematopoietic cell transplantation. *Blood.* 2001;98:3172–3173.

97. Pietz BC, Warden MB, DuChateau BK, et al. Multiplex genotyping of human minor histocompatibility antigens. *Hum Immunol.* 2005;66:1174–1182.

98. Wu CJ, Ritz J. Induction of tumor immunity following allogeneic stem cell transplantation. *Adv Immunol.* 2006;90:133–173.

99. van Els CA, D'Amaro J, Pool J, et al. Immunogenetics of human minor histocompatibility antigens: their polymorphism and immunodominance. *Immunogenetics.* 1992;35:161–165.

100. Martin PJ. How much benefit can be expected from matching for minor antigens in allogeneic marrow transplantation? *Bone Marrow Transplant.* 1997;20:97–100.

101. Mutis T, Gillespie G, Schrama E, et al. Tetrameric HLA class I-minor histocompatibility antigen peptide complexes demonstrate minor histocompatibility antigen-specific cytotoxic T lymphocytes in patients with graft-versus-host disease. *Nat Med.* 1999;5:839–842.

102. Dickinson AM, Wang XN, Sviland L, et al. In situ dissection of the graft-versus-host activities of cytotoxic T cells specific for minor histocompatibility antigens. *Nat Med.* 2002;8:410–414.

103. Marijt WA, Heemskerk MH, Kloosterboer FM, et al. Hematopoiesis-restricted minor histocompatibility antigens HA-1- or HA-2-specific T cells can induce complete remissions of relapsed leukemia. *Proc Natl Acad Sci USA.* 2003;100:2742–2747.

104. Kloosterboer FM, van Luxemburg-Heijs SA, van Soest RA, et al. Direct cloning of leukemia-reactive T cells from patients treated with donor lymphocyte infusion shows a relative dominance of hematopoiesis-restricted minor histocompatibility antigen HA-1 and HA-2 specific T cells. *Leukemia.* 2004;18:798–808.

105. Allen RD. The new genetics of bone marrow transplantation. *Genes Immun.* 2000;1:316–320.

106. Trinchieri G. Biology of natural killer cells. *Adv Immunol.* 1989;47:187–376.

107. Foa R, Meloni G, Tosti S, et al. Treatment of residual disease in acute leukemia patients with recombinant interleukin 2 (IL2): clinical and biological findings. *Bone Marrow Transplant.* 1990;6(Suppl 1):98–102.

108. Meloni G, Vignetti M, Pogliani E, et al. Interleukin-2 therapy in relapsed acute myelogenous leukemia. *Cancer J Sci Am.* 1997;3(Suppl 1):S43–S47.

109. Fehniger TA, Cooper MA, Caligiuri MA. Interleukin-2 and interleukin-15: immunotherapy for cancer. *Cytokine Growth Factor Rev.* 2002;13:169–183.

110. Storkus WJ, Alexander J, Payne JA, et al. Reversal of natural killing susceptibility in target cells expressing transfected class I HLA genes. *Proc Natl Acad Sci USA.* 1989;86:2361–2364.

111. Shimizu Y, DeMars R. Demonstration by class I gene transfer that reduced susceptibility of human cells to natural killer cell-mediated lysis is inversely correlated with HLA class I antigen expression. *Eur J Immunol.* 1989;19:447–451.

112. Moretta A, Bottino C, Pende D, et al. Identification of four subsets of human CD3-CD16+ natural killer (NK) cells by the expression of clonally distributed functional surface molecules: correlation between subset assignment of NK clones and ability to mediate specific alloantigen recognition. *J Exp Med.* 1990;172:1589–1598.

113. Ruggeri L, Capanni M, Casucci M, et al. Role of natural killer cell alloreactivity in HLA-mismatched hematopoietic stem cell transplantation. *Blood.* 1999;94:333–339.

114. Giebel S, Locatelli F, Lamparelli T, et al. Survival advantage with KIR ligand incompatibility in hematopoietic stem cell transplantation from unrelated donors. *Blood.* 2003;102:814–819.

115. Hsu KC, Keever-Taylor CA, Wilton A, et al. Improved outcome in HLA-identical sibling hematopoietic stem-cell transplantation for acute myelogenous leukemia predicted by KIR and HLA genotypes. *Blood.* 2005;105:4878–4884.

116. Shilling HG, Young N, Guethlein LA, et al. Genetic control of human NK cell repertoire. *J Immunol.* 2002;169:239–247.

117. Coiffier B, Haioun C, Ketterer N, et al. Rituximab (anti-CD20 monoclonal antibody) for the treatment of patients with relapsing or refractory aggressive lymphoma: a multicenter phase II study. *Blood.* 1998;92:1927–1932.

118. Comoli P, Basso S, Zecca M, et al. Preemptive Therapy of EBV-Related Lymphoproliferative Disease after Pediatric Haploidentical Stem Cell Transplantation. *Am J Transplant.* 2007;7:1648–1655.

119. Savoldo B, Rooney CM, Quiros-Tejeira RE, et al. Cellular immunity to Epstein-Barr virus in liver transplant recipients treated with rituximab for post-transplant lymphoproliferative disease. *Am J Transplant.* 2005;5:566–572.

120. Cutler C, Miklos D, Kim HT, et al. Rituximab for steroid-refractory chronic graft-versus-host disease. *Blood.* 2006;108:756–762.

121. Ratanatharathorn V, Ayash L, Reynolds C, et al. Treatment of chronic graft-versus-host disease with anti-CD20 chimeric monoclonal antibody. *Biol Blood Marrow Transplant.* 2003;9:505–511.

122. Keating M, O'Brien S. High-dose rituximab therapy in chronic lymphocytic leukemia. *Semin Oncol.* 2000;27:86–90.

123. Huhn D, von Schilling C, Wilhelm M, et al. Rituximab therapy of patients with B-cell chronic lymphocytic leukemia. *Blood.* 2001;98:1326–1331.

124. Manshouri T, Do KA, Wang X, et al. Circulating CD20 is detectable in the plasma of patients with chronic lymphocytic leukemia and is of prognostic significance. *Blood.* 2003;101:2507–2513.

125. Keating MJ, Flinn I, Jain V, et al. Therapeutic role of alemtuzumab (Campath-1H) in patients who have failed fludarabine: results of a large international study. *Blood.* 2002;99:3554–3561.

126. Osterborg A, Dyer MJ, Bunjes D, et al. Phase II multicenter study of human CD52 antibody in previously treated chronic lymphocytic leukemia. European Study Group of CAMPATH-1H Treatment in Chronic Lymphocytic Leukemia. *J Clin Oncol.* 1997;15:1567–1574.

127. Rai KR, Freter CE, Mercier RJ, et al. Alemtuzumab in previously treated chronic lymphocytic leukemia patients who also had received fludarabine. *J Clin Oncol.* 2002;20:3891–3897.

128. Bowen AL, Zomas A, Emmett E, et al. Subcutaneous CAMPATH-1H in fludarabine-resistant/relapsed chronic lymphocytic and B-prolymphocytic leukaemia. *Br J Haematol.* 1997;96:617–619.

129. Lundin J, Kimby E, Bjorkholm M, et al. Phase II trial of subcutaneous anti-CD52 monoclonal antibody alemtuzumab (Campath-1H) as first-line treatment for patients with B-cell chronic lymphocytic leukemia (B-CLL). *Blood.* 2002;100:768–773.

130. Stilgenbauer S, Dohner H. Campath-1H-induced complete remission of chronic lymphocytic leukemia despite p53 gene mutation and resistance to chemotherapy. *N Engl J Med.* 2002;347:452–453.

131. Andrews RG, Torok-Storb B, Bernstein ID. Myeloid-associated differentiation antigens on stem cells and their progeny identified by monoclonal antibodies. *Blood.* 1983;62:124–132.

132. Griffin JD, Linch D, Sabbath K, et al. A monoclonal antibody reactive with normal and leukemic human myeloid progenitor cells. *Leuk Res.* 1984;8:521–534.

133. Matutes E, Rodriguez B, Polli N, et al. Characterization of myeloid leukemias with monoclonal antibodies 3C5 and MY9. *Hematol Oncol.* 1985;3:179–186.

134. Radich J, Sievers E. New developments in the treatment of acute myeloid leukemia. *Oncology (Williston Park).* 2000;14:125–131.

135. Ruffner KL, Matthews DC. Current uses of monoclonal antibodies in the treatment of acute leukemia. *Semin Oncol.* 2000;27:531–539.

136. Scheinberg DA, Tanimoto M, McKenzie S, et al. Monoclonal antibody M195: a diagnostic marker for acute myelogenous leukemia. *Leukemia.* 1989;3:440–445.

137. Caron PC, Dumont L, Scheinberg DA. Supersaturating infusional humanized anti-CD33 monoclonal antibody HuM195 in myelogenous leukemia. *Clin Cancer Res.* 1998;4:1421–1428.

138. Feldman E, Kalaycio M, Weiner G, et al. Treatment of relapsed or refractory acute myeloid leukemia with humanized anti-CD33 monoclonal antibody HuM195. *Leukemia.* 2003;17:314–318.

139. Jurcic JG, DeBlasio T, Dumont L, et al. Molecular remission induction with retinoic acid and anti-CD33 monoclonal antibody HuM195 in acute promyelocytic leukemia. *Clin Cancer Res.* 2000;6:372–380.

140. Jurcic JG. Antibody therapy for residual disease in acute myelogenous leukemia. *Crit Rev Oncol Hematol.* 2001;38:37–45.

141. Zein N, Sinha AM, McGahren WJ, et al. Calicheamicin gamma 1I: an antitumor antibiotic that cleaves double-stranded DNA site specifically. *Science.* 1988;240:1198–1201.

142. Larson RA, Sievers EL, Stadtmauer EA, et al. Final report of the efficacy and safety of gemtuzumab ozogamicin (Mylotarg) in patients with CD33-positive acute myeloid leukemia in first recurrence. *Cancer.* 2005;104:1442–1452.

143. Bastie JN, Suzan F, Garcia I, et al. Veno-occlusive disease after an anti-CD33 therapy (gemtuzumab ozogamicin). *Br J Haematol.* 2002;116:924.

144. Rajvanshi P, Shulman HM, Sievers EL, et al. Hepatic sinusoidal obstruction after gemtuzumab ozogamicin (Mylotarg) therapy. *Blood.* 2002;99:2310–2314.

145. Giles FJ, Kantarjian HM, Kornblau SM, et al. Mylotarg (gemtuzumab ozogamicin) therapy is associated with hepatic venoocclusive disease in patients who have not received stem cell transplantation. *Cancer.* 2001;92:406–413.

146. Matthews DC, Appelbaum FR, Eary JF, et al. Phase I study of (131)I-anti-CD45 antibody plus cyclophosphamide and total body irradiation for advanced acute leukemia and myelodysplastic syndrome. *Blood.* 1999;94:1237–1247.

147. Witzig TE, Molina A, Gordon LI, et al. Long-term responses in patients with recurring or refractory B-cell non-Hodgkin lymphoma treated with yttrium 90 ibritumomab tiuxetan. *Cancer.* 2007;109:1804–1810.

148. Gordon LI, Molina A, Witzig T, et al. Durable responses after ibritumomab tiuxetan radioimmunotherapy for CD20+ B-cell lymphoma: long-term follow-up of a phase 1/2 study. *Blood.* 2004;103:4429–4431.

149. Kaminski MS, Zelenetz AD, Press OW, et al. Pivotal study of iodine I 131 tositumomab for chemotherapy-refractory low-grade or transformed low-grade B-cell non-Hodgkin's lymphomas. *J Clin Oncol.* 2001;19:3918–3928.

150. Fisher RI, Kaminski MS, Wahl RL, et al. Tositumomab and iodine-131 tositumomab produces durable complete remissions in a subset of heavily pretreated patients with low-grade and transformed non-Hodgkin's lymphomas. *J Clin Oncol.* 2005;23:7565–7573.

151. Horning SJ, Younes A, Jain V, et al. Efficacy and safety of tositumomab and iodine-131 tositumomab (Bexxar) in B-cell lymphoma, progressive after rituximab. *J Clin Oncol.* 2005;23:712–719.

152. Witzig TE, Flinn IW, Gordon LI, et al. Treatment with ibritumomab tiuxetan radioimmunotherapy in patients with rituximab-refractory follicular non-Hodgkin's lymphoma. *J Clin Oncol.* 2002;20:3262–3269.

153. Press OW, Unger JM, Braziel RM, et al. Phase II trial of CHOP chemotherapy followed by tositumomab/iodine I-131 tositumomab for previously untreated follicular non-Hodgkin's lymphoma: five-year follow-up of Southwest Oncology Group Protocol S9911. *J Clin Oncol.* 2006;24:4143–4149.

154. Gopal AK, Rajendran JG, Gooley TA, et al. High-dose [131I] tositumomab (anti-CD20) radioimmunotherapy and autologous hematopoietic stem-cell transplantation for adults > or = 60 years old with relapsed or refractory B-cell lymphoma. *J Clin Oncol.* 2007;25:1396–1402.

155. Pantelias A, Pagel JM, Hedin N, et al. Comparative biodistributions of pretargeted radioimmunoconjugates targeting CD20, CD22, and DR molecules on human B-cell lymphomas. *Blood.* 2007;109:4980–4987.

156. Condon C, Watkins SC, Celluzzi CM, et al. DNA-based immunization by in vivo transfection of dendritic cells. *Nat Med.* 1996;2:1122–1128.

157. Randolph GJ, Inaba K, Robbiani DF, et al. Differentiation of phagocytic monocytes into lymph node dendritic cells in vivo. *Immunity.* 1999;11:753–761.

158. Kwak LW, Campbell MJ, Czerwinski DK, et al. Induction of immune responses in patients with B-cell lymphoma against the surface-immunoglobulin idiotype expressed by their tumors. *N Engl J Med.* 1992;327:1209–1215.

159. Hsu FJ, Caspar CB, Czerwinski D, et al. Tumor-specific idiotype vaccines in the treatment of patients with B-cell lymphoma—long-term results of a clinical trial. *Blood.* 1997;89:3129–3135.

160. Bendandi M, Gocke CD, Kobrin CB, et al. Complete molecular remissions induced by patient-specific vaccination plus granulocyte-monocyte colony-stimulating factor against lymphoma. *Nat Med.* 1999;5:1171–1177.

161. Neelapu SS, Gause BL, Nikcevich DA, et al. Phase III randomized trial of patient-specific vaccination for previously untreated patients with follicular lymphoma in first complete remission: protocol summary and interim report. *Clin Lymphoma.* 2005;6:61–64.

162. Weng WK, Czerwinski D, Timmerman J, et al. Clinical outcome of lymphoma patients after idiotype vaccination is correlated with humoral immune response and immunoglobulin G Fc receptor genotype. *J Clin Oncol.* 2004;22:4717–4724.

163. Weng WK, Czerwinski D, Levy R. Humoral immune response and immunoglobulin G Fc receptor genotype are associated with better clinical outcome following idiotype vaccination in follicular lymphoma patients regardless of their response to induction chemotherapy. *Blood.* 2007;109:951–953.

164. Gold P, Freedman SO. Demonstration of tumor-specific antigens in human colonic carcinomata by immunological tolerance and absorption techniques. *J Exp Med.* 1965;121:439–462.

165. Lindenmann J. Speculations on idiotypes and homobodies. *Ann Immunol (Paris).* 1973;124:171–184.

166. Jerne NK. Towards a network theory of the immune system. *Ann Immunol (Paris).* 1974;125C:373–389.

167. Foon KA, John WJ, Chakraborty M, et al. Clinical and immune responses in resected colon cancer patients treated with anti-idiotype monoclonal antibody vaccine that mimics the carcinoembryonic antigen. *J Clin Oncol.* 1999;17:2889–2895.

168. Cheung NK, Guo HF, Heller G, et al. Induction of Ab3 and Ab3' antibody was associated with long-term survival after anti-G(D2) antibody therapy of stage 4 neuroblastoma. *Clin Cancer Res.* 2000;6:2653–2660.

169. Foon KA, Lutzky J, Baral RN, et al. Clinical and immune responses in advanced melanoma patients immunized with an anti-idiotype antibody mimicking disialoganglioside GD2. *J Clin Oncol.* 2000;18:376–384.

170. Wagner U, Kohler S, Reinartz S, et al. Immunological consolidation of ovarian carcinoma recurrences with monoclonal anti-idiotype antibody ACA125: immune responses and survival in palliative treatment. See the biology behind: K. A. Foon and M. Bhattacharya-Chatterjee, Are solid tumor anti-idiotype vaccines ready for prime time? *Clin Cancer Res.* 2001;7:1112–1115, 1154–1162.

171. Yao TJ, Meyers M, Livingston PO, et al. Immunization of melanoma patients with BEC2-keyhole limpet hemocyanin plus BCG intradermally followed by intravenous booster immunizations with BEC2 to induce anti-GD3 ganglioside antibodies. *Clin Cancer Res.* 1999;5:77–81.

172. Johnston SA, Tang DC. Gene gun transfection of animal cells and genetic immunization. *Methods Cell Biol.* 1994;43 (Pt A):353–365.

173. Epstein JE, Gorak EJ, Charoenvit Y, et al. Safety, tolerability, and lack of antibody responses after administration of a PfCSP DNA malaria vaccine via needle or needle-free jet injection, and comparison of intramuscular and combination intramuscular/intradermal routes. *Hum Gene Ther.* 2002;13:1551–1560.

174. Houghton AN. Cancer antigens: immune recognition of self and altered self. *J Exp Med.* 1994;180:1–4.

175. Bowne WB, Srinivasan R, Wolchok JD, et al. Coupling and uncoupling of tumor immunity and autoimmunity. *J Exp Med.* 1999;190:1717–1722.

176. Weber LW, Bowne WB, Wolchok JD, et al. Tumor immunity and autoimmunity induced by immunization with homologous DNA. *J Clin Invest.* 1998;102:1258–1264.

177. Hawkins WG, Gold JS, Dyall R, et al. Immunization with DNA coding for gp100 results in CD4 T-cell independent antitumor immunity. *Surgery.* 2000;128:273–280.

178. Ferrone CR, Perales MA, Goldberg SM, et al. Adjuvanticity of plasmid DNA encoding cytokines fused to immunoglobulin Fc domains. *Clin Cancer Res.* 2006;12:5511–5519.

179. Powell DJ, Jr., Rosenberg SA. Phenotypic and functional maturation of tumor antigen-reactive CD8+ T lymphocytes in patients undergoing multiple course peptide vaccination. *J Immunother.* (1997) 2004;27:36–47.

180. Powell DJ, Jr., Dudley ME, Hogan KA, et al. Adoptive transfer of vaccine-induced peripheral blood mononuclear cells to patients with metastatic melanoma following lymphodepletion. *J Immunol.* 2006;177:6527–6539.

181. Silver DA, Pellicer I, Fair WR, et al. Prostate-specific membrane antigen expression in normal and malignant human tissues. *Clin Cancer Res.* 1997;3:81–85.

182. Chang SS, O'Keefe DS, Bacich DJ, et al. Prostate-specific membrane antigen is produced in tumor-associated neovasculature. *Clin Cancer Res.* 1999;5:2674–2681.

183. Gregor PD, Wolchok JD, Turaga V, et al. Induction of autoantibodies to syngeneic prostate-specific membrane antigen by xenogeneic vaccination. *Int J Cancer.* 2005;116:415–421.

184. Simons JW, Mikhak B, Chang JF, et al. Induction of immunity to prostate cancer antigens: results of a clinical trial of vaccination with irradiated autologous prostate tumor cells engineered to secrete granulocyte-macrophage colony-stimulating factor using ex vivo gene transfer. *Cancer Res.* 1999;59:5160–5168.

185. Simons JW, Sacks N. Granulocyte-macrophage colony-stimulating factor-transduced allogeneic cancer cellular immunotherapy: the GVAX vaccine for prostate cancer. *Urol Oncol.* 2006;24:419–424.

186. Soiffer R, Lynch T, Mihm M, et al. Vaccination with irradiated autologous melanoma cells engineered to secrete human granulocyte-macrophage colony-stimulating factor generates potent antitumor immunity in patients with metastatic melanoma. *Proc Natl Acad Sci USA.* 1998;95:13141–13146.

187. Soiffer R, Hodi FS, Haluska F, et al. Vaccination with irradiated, autologous melanoma cells engineered to secrete granulocyte-macrophage colony-stimulating factor by adenoviral-mediated gene transfer augments antitumor immunity in patients with metastatic melanoma. *J Clin Oncol.* 2003;21:3343–3350.

188. Salgia R, Lynch T, Skarin A, et al. Vaccination with irradiated autologous tumor cells engineered to secrete granulocyte-macrophage colony-stimulating factor augments antitumor immunity in some patients with metastatic non-small-cell lung carcinoma. *J Clin Oncol.* 2003;21:624–630.

189. Nemunaitis J, Jahan T, Ross H, et al. Phase 1/2 trial of autologous tumor mixed with an allogeneic GVAX vaccine in advanced-stage non-small-cell lung cancer. *Cancer Gene Ther.* 2006;13:555–562.

190. Nemunaitis J, Sterman D, Jablons D, et al. Granulocyte-macrophage colony-stimulating factor gene-modified autologous tumor vaccines in non-small-cell lung cancer. *J Natl Cancer Inst.* 2004;96:326–331.

191. Greenwald RJ, Oosterwegel MA, van der Woude D, et al. CTLA-4 regulates cell cycle progression during a primary immune response. *Eur J Immunol.* 2002;32:366–373.

192. Gribben JG, Freeman GJ, Boussiotis VA, et al. CTLA4 mediates antigen-specific apoptosis of human T cells. *Proc Natl Acad Sci USA.* 1995;92:811–815.

193. van Elsas A, Hurwitz AA, Allison JP. Combination immunotherapy of B16 melanoma using anti-cytotoxic T lymphocyte-associated antigen 4 (CTLA-4) and granulocyte/macrophage colony-stimulating factor (GM-CSF)-producing vaccines induces rejection of subcutaneous and metastatic tumors accompanied by autoimmune depigmentation. *J Exp Med.* 1999;190:355–366.

194. van Elsas A, Sutmuller RP, Hurwitz AA, et al. Elucidating the autoimmune and antitumor effector mechanisms of a treatment based on cytotoxic T lymphocyte antigen-4 blockade in combination with a B16 melanoma vaccine: comparison of prophylaxis and therapy. *J Exp Med.* 2001;194:481–489.

195. Gregor PD, Wolchok JD, Ferrone CR, et al. CTLA-4 blockade in combination with xenogeneic DNA vaccines enhances T-cell responses, tumor immunity and autoimmunity to self antigens in animal and cellular model systems. *Vaccine.* 2004;22:1700–1708.

196. Peggs KS, Quezada SA, Korman AJ, et al. Principles and use of anti CTLA4 antibody in human cancer immunotherapy. *Curr Opin Immunol.* 2006;18:206–213.

197. Small EJ, Tchekmedyian NS, Rini BI, et al. A pilot trial of CTLA-4 blockade with human anti-CTLA-4 in patients with hormone-refractory prostate cancer. *Clin Cancer Res.* 2007;13:1810–1815.

198. Phan GQ, Yang JC, Sherry RM, et al. Cancer regression and autoimmunity induced by cytotoxic T lymphocyte-associated antigen 4 blockade in patients with metastatic melanoma. *Proc Natl Acad Sci USA.* 2003;100:8372–8377.

199. Van Parijs L, Abbas AK. Homeostasis and self-tolerance in the immune system: turning lymphocytes off. *Science.* 1998;280:243–248.

200. Curotto de Lafaille MA, Lafaille JJ. CD4(+) regulatory T cells in autoimmunity and allergy. *Curr Opin Immunol.* 2002;14:771–778.

201. Jonuleit H, Schmitt E. The regulatory T cell family: distinct subsets and their interrelations. *J Immunol.* 2003;171:6323–6327.

202. Earle KE, Tang Q, Zhou X, et al. In vitro expanded human CD4+CD25+ regulatory T cells suppress effector T cell proliferation. *Clin Immunol.* 2005;115:3–9.

203. Hoffmann P, Eder R, Kunz-Schughart LA, et al. Large-scale in vitro expansion of polyclonal human CD4(+)CD25high regulatory T cells. *Blood.* 2004;104:895–903.

204. Battaglia M, Stabilini A, Roncarolo MG. Rapamycin selectively expands CD4+CD25+FoxP3+ regulatory T cells. *Blood.* 2005;105:4743–4748.

205. Casares N, Arribillaga L, Sarobe P, et al. CD4+/CD25+ regulatory cells inhibit activation of tumor-primed CD4+ T cells with IFN-gamma-dependent antiangiogenic activity, as well as long-lasting tumor immunity elicited by peptide vaccination. *J Immunol.* 2003;171:5931–5939.

206. Sutmuller RP, van Duivenvoorde LM, van Elsas A, et al. Synergism of cytotoxic T lymphocyte-associated antigen 4 blockade and depletion of CD25(+) regulatory T cells in antitumor therapy reveals alternative pathways for suppression of autoreactive cytotoxic T lymphocyte responses. *J Exp Med.* 2001;194:823–832.

207. Jones SC, Murphy GF, Korngold R. Post-hematopoietic cell transplantation control of graft-versus-host disease by donor CD425 T cells to allow an effective graft-versus-leukemia response. *Biol Blood Marrow Transplant.* 2003;9:243–256.

208. Hanash AM, Levy RB. Donor CD4+CD25+ T cells promote engraftment and tolerance following MHC-mismatched hematopoietic cell transplantation. *Blood.* 2005;105:1828–1836.

209. Ermann J, Hoffmann P, Edinger M, et al. Only the CD62L+ subpopulation of CD4+CD25+ regulatory T cells protects from lethal acute GVHD. *Blood.* 2005;105:2220–2226.

210. Kern F, Faulhaber N, Frommel C, et al. Analysis of CD8 T cell reactivity to cytomegalovirus using protein-spanning

pools of overlapping pentadecapeptides. *Eur J Immunol.* 2000;30:1676–1682.

211. Trivedi D, Williams RY, O'Reilly RJ, et al. Generation of CMV-specific T lymphocytes using protein-spanning pools of pp65-derived overlapping pentadecapeptides for adoptive immunotherapy. *Blood.* 2005;105:2793–2801.

212. Ratzinger G, Baggers J, de Cos MA, et al. Mature human Langerhans cells derived from CD34+ hematopoietic progenitors stimulate greater cytolytic T lymphocyte activity in the absence of bioactive IL-12p70, by either single peptide presentation or cross-priming, than do dermal-interstitial or monocyte-derived dendritic cells. *J Immunol.* 2004;173:2780–2791.

213. Young JW, Merad M, Hart DN. Dendritic cells in transplantation and immune-based therapies. *Biol Blood Marrow Transplant.* 2007;13:23–32.

214. Latouche JB, Sadelain M. Induction of human cytotoxic T lymphocytes by artificial antigen-presenting cells. *Nat Biotechnol.* 2000;18:405–409.

215. Papanicolaou GA, Latouche JB, Tan C, et al. Rapid expansion of cytomegalovirus-specific cytotoxic T lymphocytes by arti-ficial antigen-presenting cells expressing a single HLA allele. *Blood.* 2003;102:2498–2505.

216. Brentjens RJ, Latouche JB, Santos E, et al. Eradication of systemic B-cell tumors by genetically targeted human T lymphocytes co-stimulated by CD80 and interleukin-15. *Nat Med.* 2003;9:279–286.

217. Brentjens RJ. Novel Approaches to Immunotherapy for B-cell Malignancies. *Curr Oncol Rep.* 2004;6:339–347.

218. Rossig C, Brenner MK. Chimeric T-cell receptors for the targeting of cancer cells. *Acta Haematol.* 2003;110:154–159.

219. Savoldo B, Rooney CM, Di Stasi A, et al. Epstein Barr virus-specific cytotoxic T lymphocytes expressing the anti-CD30{zeta} artificial chimeric T-cell receptor for immunotherapy of Hodgkin's disease. *Blood.* 2007;110(7):2620–2630.

220. McDevitt MR, Ma D, Lai LT, et al. Tumor therapy with targeted atomic nanogenerators. *Science.* 2001;294:1537–1540.

221. Jurcic JG, Larson SM, Sgouros G, et al. Targeted alpha particle immunotherapy for myeloid leukemia. *Blood.* 2002;100:1233–1239.

Principles of Radiotherapy

4

Yoshiya Yamada

The risk of radiation-induced secondary cancers is a difficult late effect of radiation therapy. Ever since the discovery of x-rays by Conrad Roentgen in 1895, radiation has been closely tied to medical applications, and it has been known to have significant biologic effects from the very beginning of the radiologic era. Antoine-Henri Becquerel, who discovered that uranium compounds emitted radiation in 1896, was the first to record the biological effect of radiation when he inadvertently left a vial of radium in his vest pocket, noting skin erythema two weeks later. This later turned into a skin ulcer, which took several weeks to heal. Pierre Curie repeated the experiment in 1901 by deliberately causing a radiation burn on his forearm. An Austrian surgeon, Leopold Freund, demonstrated in 1896 to the Vienna Medical Society that radiation could cause a hairy mole to disappear (1).

From these beginnings, radiation therapy has evolved into an important modality of treating benign and malignant illness. Radiotherapy has been shown to either contribute to the cure or be the primary curative therapy for cancers that affect every organ system in the body. Improvements in computer and imaging technology have expanded the role of radiotherapy, allowing for the effective noninvasive management of tumors without the morbidity commonly associated with surgical or chemotherapeutic strategies. Radiotherapy may offer curative options for patients who may not be able to tolerate radical surgery. Radiotherapy is not limited by the anatomic or functional constraints of surgical resection, and thus is able to treat cancer in a regional paradigm, such as in the treatment of many lymphomas or spare significant morbidity and functional loss or deformity associated with radical resections. Because radiation effects are typically locoregional, patients can be spared the generalized toxicity associated with cytotoxic chemotherapy. Radiotherapy is not dependent upon the circulatory system to reach the target tissue. Hence, toxicity is limited to the tissues to which radiation is administered, but the benefits of radiation are also limited to the area to which radiation is given. Radiotherapy is also an integral part of combined modality therapy with systemic therapy and/or surgery. Nearly two-thirds of all cancer patients will receive radiation therapy at some point during their illness, and in 2004, nearly 1 million patients were treated with radiotherapy in the United States (2). As the incidence of cancer increases with an increasingly aging population, it is expected that even more patients will benefit from radiotherapy. Currently there are about 3,900 radiation oncologists in the United States.

RADIATION PHYSICS

Radiation therapy can be broadly defined as the use of ionizing radiation for the treatment of neoplasms. The most commonly utilized form of radiation is photon radiation, commonly known as x-rays (artificially produced) or gamma rays (emitted from naturally decaying isotopes). Photons are packets of energy that can interact with the atoms that make up the deoxyribonucleic

KEY POINTS

- Nearly two-thirds of all cancer patients will receive radiation therapy at some point during their illness, and in 2004, nearly 1 million patients were treated with radiotherapy in the United States.
- Improvements in computer and imaging technology have expanded the role of radiotherapy, allowing for the effective noninvasive management of tumors without the morbidity commonly associated with surgical or chemotherapeutic strategies.
- The most commonly utilized form of radiation is photon radiation, commonly known as x-rays (artificially produced) or gamma rays (emitted from naturally decaying isotopes).
- Radiation dose (Gray or Gy) is commonly defined as joules per kilogram (energy per unit mass) where 1 Gy equals 1 joule/kg.
- A technique called intensity modulated radiotherapy (IMRT) has allowed steep dose gradients around tumors, as high as 10% per millimeter.
- As opposed to treating tumors with the radiation source distant from the tumor, brachytherapy (placing radioactive sources inside of tumors) is another way to deliver very high-dose radiation and limit normal tissue doses.
- The effects of radiation therapy on tissues are dependent upon the inherent radiosensitivity of the tissue or organ in question, the dose of radiation given, and the volume of tissue irradiated.
- Radiation effects have been traditionally classified as early or late effects.
- Early effects are generally seen during the course of treatment or within six weeks of radiation therapy.
- Late effects are considered those that appear months to years after radiation, and are more likely in tissues with low proliferative potential, such as connective tissue (fibrosis) or neural tissue (neuropathy).
- Microvascular damage (endothelial thickening to the point that red blood cells are not able to pass through) has thought to play an important role in the late toxicity, causing hypoxic stress and cellular death.

acid (DNA) of a cell, causing disruption of chemical bonds and DNA strand breaks, which ultimately leads to irreparable damage (3). Cells not able to repair this damage may not be able to successfully complete mitosis, resulting in the death of both mother and daughter cells. Many cells will also undergo apoptotic death, when the cell detects DNA damage, without completing mitosis (4).

Radiation dose (Gray or Gy) is commonly defined as joules per kilogram (energy per unit mass) where 1 Gy equals 1 joule/kg (5). Since radiation is ionizing energy, radiotherapy does not induce heat or other manifestations of energy transfer that can be felt by patients. Thus, patients feel no pain during radiation administration. Because radiation effects are stochastic, they may cause similar effects on healthy normal cells. In order to reduce the side effects of radiotherapy, radiation oncologists attempt to concentrate the radiation in tumors and minimize the amount of radiation absorbed by surrounding normal tissues.

THE THERAPEUTIC RATIO

Tumor control probability and normal tissue complication probability is usually dose-dependent. Efforts to minimize radiation dose to normal tissue result in lower normal tissue complication probabilities, while increasing dose to the tumor should increase tumor control probabilities. Hence, a basic mantra of radiation oncology is to increase the gap between toxicity and tumor control probability curves (Fig. 4.1), commonly referred to as the therapeutic ratio.

One strategy to minimize radiation toxicity is to use the appropriate photon energy. Most radiation beams are created in machines that accelerate electrons to very high energies (typically 4–25 megaelectron volts or MV) called linear accelerators or linacs (3). Because of the very high energy of the resultant photons, they tended to penetrate deeper into the body as the energy increases. Thus, by choosing the appropriate beam energy, the radiation oncologist can limit radiation damage to superficial structures in the case of deep-seated tumors, or use lower-energy beams for superficial tumors to limit dose to deeper normal structures.

Another method of improving the therapeutic ratio is to shape radiation fields to match the three-dimensional shape of the target volume, thereby limiting the exposure of normal tissues to high doses of radiation (5). The shape of the radiation beam can also be manipulated by placing using thick lead or cerrobend blocks into the head of the linac to block out radiation except to the tumor. Modern linacs utilize a device known as the multileaf collimator (Fig. 4.2), which has multiple individually motorized leaves of thick tungsten 3–10 mm wide. These leaves can be pushed in or out of the radiation field to approximate the tumor outline and similarly block radiation from

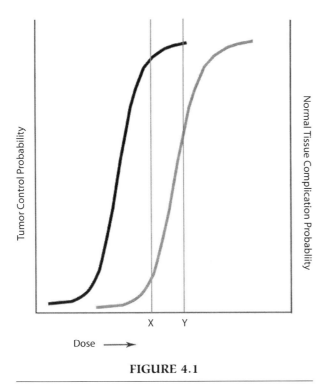

FIGURE 4.1

The therapeutic ratio. The aim of successful treatment is to increase the tumor control probability (black curve) while reducing the treatment complication (gray curve). Increase dose delivered to the tumor will typically increase the probability of cure, but will also increase the likelihood of toxicity. By reducing the amount of radiation given to normal tissues and/or the volume of normal tissue exposed to radiation, toxicity can be reduced (shifting the complication curve to the right of the tumor control curve). Because of the sigmoid nature of these curves, a moderate increase in dose (X to Y) can often result in a much higher probability of complications with only a modest gain in tumor control probability.

areas where it is not necessary or desired. Most tumors are complex shapes, and will present different outlines when viewed from different angles. When multiple beams of shaped radiation fields intersect in the tumor, the result is a cloud of radiation where the high-dose volume is similar to the actual three-dimensional characteristics of the tumor. By conforming the high-dose region to just the tumor, higher doses of radiation can be delivered while the surrounding tissues can be relatively spared of high doses, and thus healthy tissue can be relatively spared the effects of higher doses, limiting the toxicity of treatment and improving the therapeutic ratio.

An important recent innovation has been the use of intensity modulation. By using fast computers, radiation doses can be changed or modulated within different regions of each radiation field. Hence, the radiation not only conforms to the three-dimensional

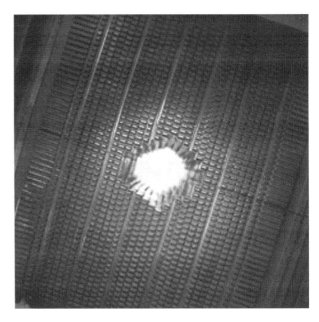

FIGURE 4.2

Multileaf collimator. The multileaf collimator is a device that is made up of many leaves of tungsten, each of which is individually motorized. This allows a computer to control the position of each leaf while the radiation beam is on. By adjusting the position of each leaf and the time spent at that position, the intensity of radiation at any particular part of the radiation field can be manipulated or modulated. When multiple beams of modulated radiation come from different directions and intersect in the target, the cumulative dose that results can be made to closely follow the three-dimensional characters of even complicated target volumes.

outline of the tumor, but can be modulated to reduce dose to areas of the field, which might approach a dose-sensitive normal structure that might be just in front or behind the field, or account for a change in the tumor outline, which may not be appreciable from different angles. This technique, called intensity modulated radiotherapy (IMRT), has allowed steep dose gradients around tumors as high as 10% per millimeter (5). Figure 4.3 illustrates how spinal cord doses are minimized relative to the tumor.

Uncertainty of where the radiation actually goes in relation to the intended target has always been a problem in radiation therapy. In traditional radiation therapy, patients undergo a procedure called simulation to radiographically identify the center of the target. During simulation, either two-dimensional (standard x-rays) or three-dimensional imaging (computed tomography [CT]/magnetic resonance imaging [MRI]/positron emission tomography [PET] or a combination) is utilized to identify the target center in relation to the

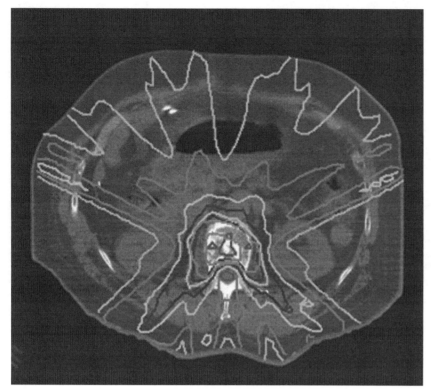

FIGURE 4.3

Radiation treatments are often represented by dose maps, called dose distributions, which depict different levels of dose intensity. The dose distribution shown is an example of a highly conformal radiation treatment plan that delivers 2400 cGy to the target while the spinal cord, which is an important dose-sensitive structure, receives less than 1400 cGy. Because the treatment was delivered using intensity-modulated techniques, the high-dose region of the treatment plan conformed very tightly to the tumor; hence, much less radiation was given to the spinal cord, even though it was only a few millimeters away. This was administered in a single treatment.

patient's anatomy. Small skin marks are made to allow the patient to be triangulated relative to the treatment machine to allow for daily administration of radiation. When patients are treated in this manner, a number of uncertainties must be accounted for. For example, respiration may cause substantial cranial-caudal displacement of a lung tumor during radiation administration. There are day-to-day variations in setting up the patient relative to the treatment machine. There may also be uncertainty regarding the true extent of disease. All of these must be taken into account when planning treatment. Allowances for potential positional errors during multiple radiation treatments (fractions) require that the radiation portals be enlarged beyond the dimensions of the target. Enlarging the margin of radiation around the tumor may result in unacceptably high doses of radiation to normal tissues. Reducing treatment-related uncertainties means less exposure of nearby normal tissues. Positional uncertainties can be reduced by the use of immobilization devices that are designed to minimize positioning errors and patient motion. Most recently, the advent of image-guided techniques, such as cone-beam CT of patients just about to undergo treatment, have greatly increased the accuracy of radiation to within a few millimeters of precision, allowing for even higher biologically effective doses to be delivered without a higher risk of toxicity (6).

Advances in imaging technology have also reduced the uncertainties associated with radiotherapy. When the tumor-bearing volume can be more precisely defined, tissue not needing treatment can be otherwise spared from radiation exposure. MRI and more recently PET imaging have been incorporated into the process of treatment planning to more accurately identify the volume at risk, as well as better visualization of normal tissues to be avoided.

Proton Beams

Charged particles, such as proton beam radiotherapy, are another type of ionizing radiation that is garnering more and more interest. Photons have no mass and therefore no kinetic energy. Charged particles do have mass and kinetic energy, and are subject to the physics of kinetic energy. One very useful aspect unique to charged particles is the Bragg peak effect (Fig. 4.4) in which accelerated particles such as protons deliver their inherent energy within a very narrow depth spectrum in tissue (3). Protons, in effect, have almost no "exit" dose, while photons are attenuated, as they interact with atoms within tissue but are likely to "exit" out of the back of the tumor. The kinetic energy of particle beams also results in higher amounts of energy deposition per linear distance, or linear energy transfer

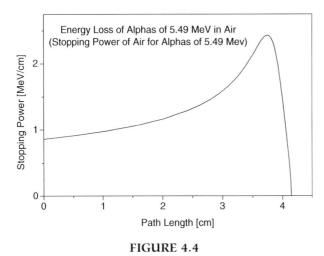

FIGURE 4.4

The Bragg peak effect. Because many charged particles have mass, they also have kinetic energy. Protons are accelerated to very high velocities. As they interact with other atoms, they tend to transfer their inherent energy to the atoms with which they interact. As they lose kinetic energy and slow down, they tend to give up more of their energy to the atoms they "bump into." Hence, towards the end of their trajectory, most of their energy is deposited over a very short distance. This phenomenon is call the Bragg peak effect. There is no "exit dose" after the peak effect. Photons (x-rays) have no mass, and hence have no kinetic energy, and do not demonstrate the Bragg peak effect.

(LET) (4). This depends upon the energy of the beam. For practical purposes, the conversion of proton beam doses to photon beam doses is expressed in Cobalt Gray equivalents by multiplying the proton beam doses by a factor of 1.1. However, other charged particles, such as carbon ions, have a much higher LET than photons and are more likely to inflict damage along the track the particle travels.

Brachytherapy

As opposed to treating tumors with the radiation source distant from the tumor, brachytherapy (placing radioactive sources inside of tumors) is another way to deliver very high-dose radiation and limit normal tissue doses. In brachytherapy, the dose falls off at an inverse to the square of the distance. Thus, the radiation dose quickly falls even a short distance from the implanted source. A commonly used isotope is iodine 125, which emits very weak gamma rays (29 KeV). The dose of radiation absorbed by the tissues immediately surrounding the source (within 1 cm) is very high; hence, if I 125 sources are placed strategically within a tumor, a very high dose can be given without exposing neighboring organs to much radiation (7).

Radiobiology

An understanding of radiobiology (how radiation affects different tissues) can also help improve the therapeutic ratio. The effects of radiation therapy on tissues is dependent upon the inherent radiosensitivity of the tissue or organ in question, the dose of radiation given, and the volume of tissue irradiated (1). The dose per fraction (treatment) is also an important determinant of toxicity. In general, a higher dose per fraction has a greater biologic impact, for both normal tissue as well as tumor. Thus, if larger doses of radiation are administered per fraction, the same probability of tumor control can be achieved with a lower total cumulative dose in comparison with a treatment schedule utilizing a small dose of radiation per fraction, which would require a higher total dose to achieve the same level of tumor control (8). A smaller dose per fraction may be desirable when it is important to spare radiosensitive organs that may be near the target volume or when a large volume of tissue needs to be treated. Since the total time required to deliver the prescribed radiation also has biologic effects, the dose rate, or how quickly radiation is given, is also important (9). This is especially significant in brachytherapy. The total dose prescribed may be reduced when using isotopes with a higher dose rate in comparison with an implant utilizing lower dose rate sources.

Time is thought to be critical because it may affect how well a cell can recover from radiation damage. A cell that has more time to repair damage is less sensitive to radiation effects. Thus, it is often noted that tissues that have a high rate of turnover, such as the bone marrow, are very sensitive to radiation. Time also allows the irradiated tissue to repopulate or replace cells lost to radiation. Because cells in different phases of the cell cycle have different sensitivities to radiation, giving time for cells to randomly distribute themselves to different phases of the cell cycle will ensure that at least some of the cells will be in more sensitive phases when the next fraction of radiation is delivered. Thus, fractionating radiation treatment allows time for reassortment and can make tissues more radiosensitive. Other factors, such as the oxygenation status of the tissue, may also be important. Hypoxic tissues are less sensitive to radiotherapy, and so allowing time to permit reoxygenation to increase the oxygen tension within the tumor is thought to increase the effects of radiation. Thus, most radiation schedules give radiation in multiple treatments or fractions to allow opportunity for normal tissues to repair radiation effects and repopulate. It also allows for reassortment of tumor cells into more radiosensitive phases of the cell cycle and reoxygenation of hypoxic tumors to increase the radiation effect (1).

There is great interest in the use of chemicals to increase the effect of radiation (radiosensitizers, such as many chemotherapeutic agents, which also target DNA) or protect normal tissues from the effects of radiation (radioprotectors such as amifostine) (10). The cell cycle appears to be regulated by a variety of protein kinases, which are under the control of complex signal transduction pathways. These may also be manipulated to increase the sensitivity of tumors to radiation (11).

Although dose is a significant contributor to the effects of radiation on normal tissue, another important factor to consider is the volume of irradiated tissue. In general, when a significant volume of an organ has been irradiated, the risk of radiation effects is higher. Whole-organ irradiation carries a much higher risk of organ failure compared to partial-organ irradiation. Hence, a higher dose or larger volume is more likely to result in radiation toxicity. For example, whole-brain radiation is typically much more morbid than stereotactic radiosurgery, which focuses a high dose of radiation to a very small volume (12).

Radiation effects have been traditionally classified as early or late (13). Early effects are generally seen during the course of treatment or within six weeks of radiation therapy. Early effects are usually manifest in tissues that are quite sensitive to radiation, such as the skin or oral mucosa, which are highly proliferative. Fortunately, most early or acute effects of radiation are temporary. Late effects are considered those that appear months to years after radiation, and are more likely in tissues with low proliferative potential, such as connective tissue (fibrosis) or neural tissue (neuropathy). Although the mechanisms involved are not completely well understood, the late effects of radiotherapy, such as fibrosis, are often irreversible. Often, microvascular damage (endothelial thickening to the point that red blood cells are not able to pass through) has thought to play an important role in late toxicity, causing hypoxic stress and cellular death. Endothelial thickening can take months to years to manifest. Loss of cells due to apoptosis after radiation-induced DNA damage also is likely to play a role. At high doses (>8 Gy) per fraction, there are likely greater effects on the endothelial lining mediated by the ceramide pathway, and could help explain the significantly higher risk of late radiation effects seen with higher doses per fraction (14).

Another difficult late effect of radiation therapy is the risk of radiation-induced secondary cancers. For example, radiation therapy represented the first curative treatment for Hodgkin disease, but requires regional radiation therapy of the lymph nodes. When breast tissue was included in these fields to treat mediastinal lymph nodes, the risk of subsequent breast cancer was found to be more than 10 times greater than in women who had never had such treatment (15 times greater in women who were irradiated between the ages of 20–30) (15). Overall, the risk of second cancers is approximately 2% higher over a patient's lifetime, but exposure to radiation at a younger age or to a large volume of normal tissue carries a higher risk (16).

PATIENT MANAGEMENT AND DECISION MAKING

A radiation oncologist must weigh many factors when approaching treatment of a patient. Radiation effects are dependent upon the inherent radiosensitivity and the volume of irradiated tissue, the dose of radiation delivered, and the dose fraction schedule employed for treatment, and must be considered when weighing the risks and benefits of such therapy. This requires a careful evaluation of the patient, paying particular attention to the potential toxicities of therapy weighed against the probabilities of benefit.

A common approach is to assess both patient factors and tumor factors associated with the case. Patient factors include the patient's ability to tolerate treatment, such as Karnofsky Performance Status (17), organ function, nutrition, or bone marrow reserve. Patient symptoms and signs are considered. The prognosis is also important to assess, and prior treatment must be considered. When evaluating tumor factors, histology, the extent of disease, location of the disease, and adjacent normal structures, as well as potentially involved areas of the body must also be factored in. A tissue diagnosis of a disease for which radiation can potentially be useful is critical.

An important decision point is to assess whether the intent of treatment is palliative or curative. In potentially curable disease, a higher level of toxicity is generally acceptable. However, with advances in systemic therapy, patients with incurable cancers may enjoy longer and longer survivals, and may warrant a more aggressive approach to controlling gross disease. Also, as patients live longer, quality of life is still an important issue. Aggressive treatment may add or detract to a patient's long-term quality of life, depending upon the situation. Hence, it is important for radiation oncologists to assess each patient thoroughly in order to recommend appropriate therapy.

SUMMARY

Cancer treatment is becoming increasingly complicated, and a multidisciplinary approach to treatment is appropriate in many cases. For example, radiation therapy can have adverse effects on wound healing (18), and if the patient is to undergo surgery after radiation,

radiation treatment should be planned in such a way as to minimize the effects on the surgical bed. Chemotherapy can also potentiate the effects of radiation on both normal tissue and tumor (19). Hence, evaluation of a patient from surgical and medical oncology perspectives, as well as radiation oncology, and input from other allied specialties, such as pathology, radiology, neurology, and physiatry, will often produce the most optimal approach.

References

1. Hall EJ, Giaccia, AJ. *Radiobiology for the Radiologist*, 6th ed. Philadelphia: Lippincott Williams & Wilkins; 2006.
2. American Society for Radiation Oncology. Fast Facts About Radiation Therapy; 2007. http://www.astro.org/pressroom/fastfacts/
3. Khan FM. *Physics of Radiation Therapy*, 3rd ed. Philadelphia: Lippincott Williams & Wilkins; 2003.
4. Tannock IH, Richard. *Basic Science of Oncology*. 3rd ed. New York: McGraw-Hill Professional; 1998.
5. Measures ICRU. Report 10b, Physical Aspects of Irradiation. Vol 10b: ICRU; 1964.
6. Yamada Y, Lovelock DM, Yenice KM, et al. Multifractionated image-guided and stereotactic intensity-modulated radiotherapy of paraspinal tumors: a preliminary report. *Int J Radiat Oncol Biol Phys.* 2005;62:53–61.
7. Nag S. *Principles and Practice of Brachytherapy*. Armonk: Futura Publishing Company; 1997.
8. Brenner DJ, Martinez AA, Edmundson GK, et al. Direct evidence that prostate tumors show high sensitivity to fractionation (low alpha/beta ratio), similar to late-responding normal tissue. *Int J Radiat Oncol Biol Phys.* 2002;52:6–13.
9. Fowler JF. The radiobiology of prostate cancer including new aspects of fractionated radiotherapy. *Acta Oncol.* 2005;44:265–276.
10. Brizel D, Overgaard J. Does amifostine have a role in chemoradiation treatment? *Lancet Oncol.* 2003;4:378–381.
11. Weinberg R. *The Biology of Cancer: Garland Science*. New York: Taylor and Francis Group; 2007.
12. Flickinger JC, Kondziolka D, Lunsford LD. Clinical applications of stereotactic radiosurgery. *Cancer Treat Res.* 1998;93:283–297.
13. Thames HD WH, Peters LJ, Fletcher GH. Changes in early and late radiation responses with altered dose fractionation: implications for dose-survival relationships. *Int J Radiat Biol Phys.* 1982;8:219–226.
14. Garcia-Barros M, Paris F, Cordon-Cardo C, et al. Tumor response to radiotherapy regulated by endothelial cell apoptosis. *Science.* 2003;300:1155–1159.
15. Hancock SL, Tucker MA, Hoppe RT. Breast cancer after treatment of Hodgkin's disease. *J Natl Cancer Inst.* 1993;85:25–31.
16. Hall EJ, Wuu CS. Radiation-induced second cancers: the impact of 3D-CRT and IMRT. *Int J Radiat Oncol Biol Phys.* 2003;56:83–88.
17. Karnofsky DA BJ. *The Clinical Evaluation of Chemotherapeutic Agents in Cancer*. New York: Columbia University Press; 1949.
18. Tibbs MK. Wound healing following radiation therapy: a review. *Radiother Oncol.* 1997;42:99–106.
19. Philips TL FK. Quantification of combined radiation therapy and chemotherapy effects on critical normal tissues. *Cancer.* 1976;37:1186–1200.

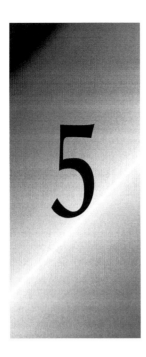

Principles of Neurosurgery in Cancer

Mark H. Bilsky

Metastatic spinal tumors are a major source of morbidity in cancer patients. The overriding goals for treatment are palliative in order to improve or maintain neurological status, provide spinal stability, and achieve local, durable tumor control. The principle treatments for spinal tumors are radiation and/or surgery. Recent advances in surgical and radiation techniques, such as image-guided intensity modulated radiation therapy (IGRT), have made treatment of spine metastases safer and more effective. Additionally, the development of newer chemotherapy, hormonal, and immunotherapy treatments has led to improved systemic control of many types of cancers. All interventions used to treat spinal tumors and their outcomes affect a patient's rehabilitation potential. Rehabilitative medicine plays a large role in achieving meaningful palliation and improved quality of life for patients with spinal tumors. A fundamental understanding of treatment decisions and outcomes will help in the assessment of cancer patients.

PRESENTATION

Spinal tumors typically present with pain (1). Three pain syndromes associated with spinal tumors are biologic, mechanical instability, and radiculopathy. All of these have important treatment implications. The vast majority of patients will present with a history of biologic pain, which is nocturnal or early morning pain that resolves over the course of the day. The pain

generator appears to be a reaction to inflammatory mediators secreted by the tumor. The diurnal variation in endogenous steroid secretion by the adrenal gland is decreased at night causing this flare-up of inflammatory pain. Biologic pain is responsive to exogenous steroids and very often responsive to radiation.

Differentiating biologic pain from mechanical pain is critically important to treating physicians. As opposed to biologic pain, mechanical pain, in broad terms, is movement-related pain and denotes significant lytic bone destruction. These patients often require surgery to stabilize the spine or possibly percutaneous cement augmentation with vertebroplasty or kyphoplasty. Physical therapy will typically not improve mechanical instability pain and may lead to an exacerbation of instability and neurologic progression.

The movement-related pain that denotes instability is dependent on the spinal level involved (1–3,8). Patients with atlantoaxial instability have flexion and extension pain, but also have a component of rotational pain. This is differentiated from the subaxial cervical spine, where flexion and extension pain are predominant with no rotational component. Our experience suggests that thoracic instability is worse in extension. While thoracic instability is relatively rare, it may be seen in patients with burst fractures with extension into a unilateral joint. These patients are very comfortable in kyphosis while leaning forward, but extension of the unstable kyphosis produces unremitting pain. Patients will often give a history of sitting in a reclining chair

KEY POINTS

- The overriding goals for treatment of spinal metastases are palliative in order to improve or maintain neurological status, provide spinal stability, and achieve local, durable tumor control.
- The three pain syndromes associated with spinal tumors are biologic, mechanical instability, and radiculopathy.
- Myelopathy indicates the presence of high-grade spinal cord compression that is treated with radiation for radiosensitive tumors (eg, multiple myeloma, lymphoma) or surgery for radioresistant tumors (non-small cell lung, renal cell, or thyroid carcinoma).
- The NOMS framework is designed to facilitate surgical and radiotherapeutic decision making into readily identifiable components: neurologic (N), oncologic (O), mechanical stability (M), and systemic disease and medical comorbidities (S).
- Spinal stabilization is dependent on instrumentation, with a very small expectation that patients will achieve arthrodesis. The instrumentation should be constructed with biomaterials that are magnetic resonance imaging (MRI)–compatible to facilitate imaging for recurrence.
- Typically, anterior resection and reconstruction are supplemented with posterior instrumentation in order to avoid subsidence of anterior grafts or to avoid losing anterior fixation in patients who have adjacent segment tumor progression.

- Currently, pedicle and lateral mass screw-rod systems are principally used to reconstruct cancer patients. These are placed a minimum of two levels superior and inferior to the level of the decompression.
- Distributing the load with multiple fixation points is more important in tumor reconstruction than saving motion segments, as is typically done for degenerative and trauma surgery.
- In the thoracic and lumbar spine, circumferential decompression and reconstruction is performed using a posterolateral transpedicular approach (PTA). This obviates the need to enter the chest or retroperitoneum, which is often poorly tolerated in the cancer population. This approach has relatively low morbidity and provides stabilization that allows patients to be mobilized early in the postoperative period. If patients are neurologically normal, the expectation is that they will sit in the chair postoperative day 1, walk day 2, stairs day 4, and home days 5 to 7. These patients are not placed in external orthoses.
- The ability to rehabilitate patients immediately after treatment takes on exaggerated significance in the cancer population, because nonambulatory patients are often excluded from further systemic therapy.
- Back or neck strengthening exercises are discouraged in patients who have undergone PTA due to the risk of creating hardware failure in patients with a low expectation of arthrodesis.

for several weeks because they cannot lie recumbent in bed. In the lumbar spine, the most common pattern of instability is mechanical radiculopathy (Fig. 5.1). These patients have searing radicular leg pain on axial load, such as sitting or standing. Radiographically, this is manifest as a burst or compression with extension into the neural foramen. This presentation is a mechanical problem as axial load narrows the neural foramen, resulting in compression of the nerve root. This pain does not typically respond to radiation therapy.

A large number of patients present with ongoing axial load pain resulting from a burst or compression fracture. These patients are not grossly unstable, but may benefit from percutaneous cement augmentation of the vertebral body with procedures such as vertebroplasty or kyphoplasty. The mechanism of pain relief is unclear, but a number of published series have shown significant pain relief in cancer patients (4). Technical limitations restrict the use of these procedures to the

lumbar spine and thoracic spine below the T3 level and in the absence of epidural disease.

The third pain syndrome is radiculopathy, or nerve root pain. The recognition of radiculopathy pain is important, as it denotes that tumor extends into the neural foramen and very often is beginning to compress the spinal cord. Early recognition of radiculopathy that prompts MRI may avoid progression to high-grade spinal cord compression and myelopathy. Additionally, radiculopathy may mimic bone pain or brachial or lumbosacral plexopathy. For example, pain from an L2 radiculopathy and pathologic hip fracture both present with pain radiating to the groin. These can often be distinguished by using provocative tests, such as hip rotation, which elicits hip but not spine pain. However, metastatic disease often involves multiple bones, so spine and hip disease may occur concurrently. For this reason, the workup of pain radiating to the groin includes both hip films and an MRI of the spine. Diagnosis to

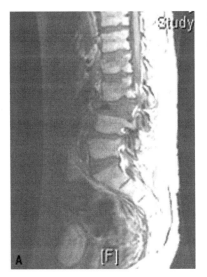 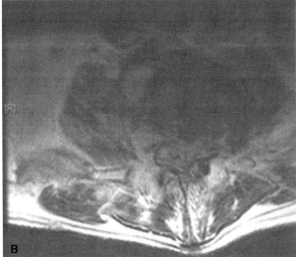

FIGURE 5.1

A. Sagittal T1: weighted image showing L3 burst fracture. B. Axial T2: weighted image showing high grade thecal sac compression.

differentiate the pain generator may include electromyograms (EMGs) and nerve conduction studies.

The development of myelopathy should be treated with some degree of urgency prompting early MRI studies. Myelopathy indicates the presence of high-grade spinal cord compression that is treated with radiation for radiosensitive tumors (eg, multiple myeloma, lymphoma) or surgery for radioresistant tumors (non-small cell lung, renal cell, or thyroid carcinoma).

Early myelopathy is often manifest by involvement of the spinothalamic tracts with loss of pinprick, typically followed by loss of motor function. Dorsal column deficits are often a late finding with resultant loss of proprioception. Bowel and bladder loss are also lost late in the evolution of myelopathy except when tumor involves the conus medullaris at approximately T12-L1 or diffuse sacral replacement, where they may be a very early sign. Spinal cord compression that results in loss of bowel and bladder is most often associated with perineal numbness, which is absent with other causes, such as narcotics or prostate hypertrophy. Early recognition of myelopathy and therapeutic intervention improve the chance for meaningful recovery. This recovery often results in early return of motor function, although sensory modalities will often recover more slowly. Loss of proprioception is particularly difficult as recovery is often suboptimal and makes ambulation extremely difficult, despite normal motor function. Once a patient is paralyzed, meaningful recovery of ambulation and bowel and bladder function are rare (<5%).

DECISION FRAMEWORK: NOMS

The principle decisions in the treatment of spinal disease are radiation therapy or surgery. The NOMS framework is designed to facilitate decision making into readily identifiable components: neurologic (N), oncologic (O), mechanical stability (M), and systemic disease and medical comorbidities (S). The neurologic considerations include the severity of myelopathy, functional radiculopathy, and degree of epidural spinal cord compression. The oncologic consideration is based on tumor histology to establish the radiosensitivity of the tumor. Patients with radiosensitive tumors, such as multiple myeloma and lymphoma, can undergo radiation therapy as first-line therapy. Unfortunately, most tumors are resistant to conventional-dose radiation (eg, 30 Gy in 10 fractions). These tumors include most solid tumors, such as renal cell, lung, and colon carcinoma. For patients with tumor in the bone or dural impingement without spinal cord compression, stereotactic radiosurgery (SRS) can be used to effectively control tumors. Currently, SRS is being delivered at 24 Gy single fraction, with 95% local tumor control at a median follow-up of 16 months (9). This is significantly better than the 20% response rates seen using conventional external beam radiation in radioresistant tumors (5). Surgery in this population as initial therapy is based on data from the study published by Patchell et al. (6) comparing surgery and radiotherapy (RT) to RT alone in patients with solid, ie, radioresistant, tumors. Patients undergoing surgery and RT had significantly better outcomes with regard to maintenance and recovery of ambulation and survival. SRS is not a viable option in patients with high-grade spinal cord compression because the high dose is above spinal cord tolerance and would result in radiation-induced myelopathy. However, SRS is an effective postsurgical adjuvant for radioresistant tumors.

Mechanical instability is a second indication for operation. A number of principles have evolved for reconstruction of spinal tumors that may be somewhat different from those used for degenerative, trauma, or scoliosis surgery. Spinal stabilization is dependent on instrumentation, with a very small expectation that patients will achieve arthrodesis. The instrumentation should be constructed with biomaterials that are MRI-compatible to facilitate imaging for recurrence. Stainless steel is difficult to image using MRI and should be avoided in tumor patients. Anterior reconstruction is performed using a number of constructs, including polymethyl methacrylate (PMMA), titanium or polyetheretherketone (PEEK) carbon fiber cages, or allo- or autograft bone.

Typically, anterior resection and reconstruction are supplemented with posterior instrumentation in order to avoid subsidence of anterior grafts or to avoid losing anterior fixation in patients who have adjacent segment tumor progression. Currently, pedicle and lateral mass screw-rod systems are principally used to reconstruct cancer patients. These are placed a minimum of two levels superior and inferior to the level of the decompression. Distributing the load with multiple fixation points is more important in tumor reconstruction than saving motion segments, as is typically done for degenerative and trauma surgery. In the thoracic and lumbar spine, circumferential decompression and reconstruction is performed using a posterolateral transpedicular approach (PTA) (Fig. 5.2). This obviates the need to enter the chest or retroperitoneum, which is often poorly tolerated in the cancer population. This approach has relatively low morbidity and provides stabilization that allows patients to be mobilized very early in the postoperative period. If patients are neurologically normal, the expectation is that they will sit in the chair postoperative day 1, walk day 2, stairs day 4, and home days 5 to 7. These patients are not placed in external orthoses.

Finally, decision making is heavily dependent on what the patient can tolerate from a systemic cancer standpoint and the significance of medical comorbidities. Given the palliative nature of the surgery, with the overriding goal of improving quality of life, an assessment of the ability to tolerate radiation, surgery, or both is essential. Preoperative oncology assessment includes complete spinal axis imaging and extent of disease workup using either computed tomography (CT) of the chest, pelvis, and abdomen as well as bone scan or positron emission tomography (PET) scan. Medical workup may include Doppler ultrasound of the lower extremities and cardiology and pulmonary clearance. The ability to rehabilitate patients immediately after treatment takes on exaggerated significance in the cancer population because nonambulatory patients are often excluded from further systemic therapy.

REHABILITATIVE MEDICINE

The impact of rehabilitative medicine to optimize outcomes in spine oncology patients cannot be overstated. Early mobilization is essential for these patients. The majority of patients continue physical therapy following discharge to improve stamina and to improve gait if there are issues. We discourage back or neck strengthening exercises due to the risk of creating hardware failure in patients with a low expectation of arthrodesis. Early ambulation typically requires a walker, but the expectation at six weeks is that they will be independent. While physical therapists typically work with patients several days per week, physiatrists may only see patients on a weekly or biweekly basis unless ongoing pain or functional issues require closer attention. Careful assessment by the rehabilitation team is often instrumental in identifying changes in a patient's condition. A change in the patient's baseline pain may be a harbinger of recurrent disease or instrumentation failure. This pain prompts repeat plain radiographs and/or a repeat MRI of the spine.

Physiatrists have introduced therapeutic modalities that have significantly improved postradiation and surgical outcomes. Perhaps the most significant is the Botox injections for paraspinal muscle spasm (7). This agent has been remarkably useful in treating postradiation fibrosis, functional spasm, and postoperative muscle spasm, particularly in the cervical and thoracic spine to treat trapezius pain.

CONCLUSION

The treatment of spinal metastases is palliative and designed to improve a patient's quality of life. The NOMS decision framework helps delineate important decisions regarding treatment with radiation therapy and/or surgery. Currently, surgery is reserved for patients with high-grade spinal cord compression resulting from RT-resistant tumors and gross spinal

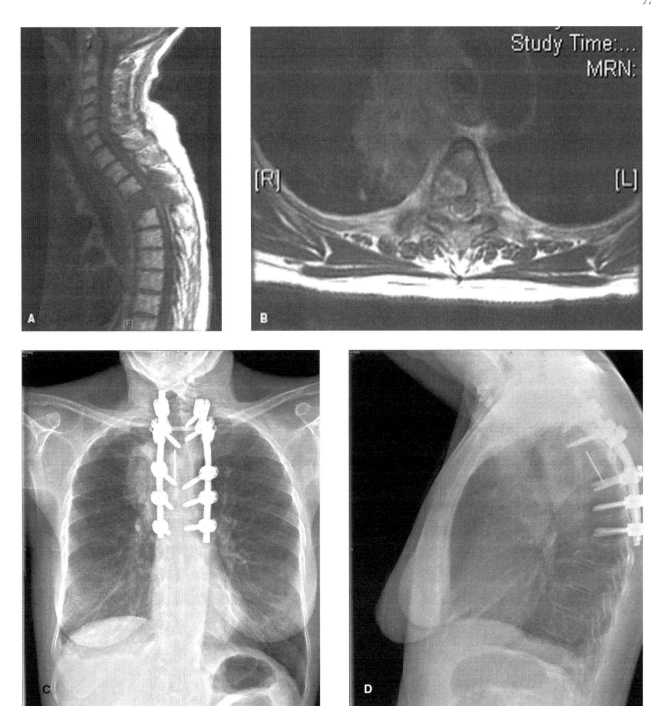

FIGURE 5.2

A. Sagittal T1-weighted image showing T4 burst fracture with circumferential bone disease. B. Axial T2-weighted image showing minimal epidural compression with circumferential bone disease and a large right-sided paraspinal mass. C. Post-operative AP radiograph. D. Post-operative lateral radiograph.

instability. Conventional external beam radiation is used for patients with radiosensitive tumors and radiosurgery for patients with RT-resistant tumors without spinal cord compression or as a postoperative adjuvant. Regardless of radiation or surgery, the goals of pain relief, restoration of neurologic function, and ambulation are essential to treatment in this patient population. Rehabilitative medicine plays an enormous role in meaningful palliation.

References

1. Bilsky M, Smith M. Surgical approach to epidural spinal cord compression. *Hematol Oncol Clin North Am.* 2006;20:1307–1317.
2. Bilsky MH, Boakye M, Collignon F, Kraus D, Boland P. Operative management of metastatic and malignant primary subaxial cervical tumors. *J Neurosurg Spine.* 2005;2:256–264.
3. Bilsky MH, Shannon FJ, Sheppard S, Prabhu V, Boland PJ. Diagnosis and management of a metastatic tumor in the atlantoaxial spine. *Spine.* 2002;27:1062–1069.
4. Hentschel SJ, Burton AW, Fourney DR, Rhines LD, Mendel E. Percutaneous vertebroplasty and kyphoplasty performed at a cancer center: refuting proposed contraindications. *J Neurosurg Spine.* 2005;2:436–440.
5. Maranzano E, Latini P. Effectiveness of radiation therapy without surgery in metastatic spinal cord compression: final results from a prospective trial. *Int J Radiat Oncol Biol Phys.* 1995;32:959–967.
6. Patchell RA, Tibbs PA, Walsh JW, et al. A randomized trial of surgery in the treatment of single metastases to the brain. *N Engl J Med.* 1990;322:494–500.
7. Stubblefield MD, Levine A, Custodio CM, Fitzpatrick T. The role of botulinum toxin type A in the radiation fibrosis syndrome: a preliminary report. *Arch Phys Med Rehabil.* 2008;89:417–421.
8. Wang JC, Boland P, Mitra N, et al. Single-stage posterolateral transpedicular approach for resection of epidural metastatic spine tumors involving the vertebral body with circumferential reconstruction: results in 140 patients. Invited submission from the Joint Section Meeting on Disorders of the Spine and Peripheral Nerves, March 2004. *J Neurosurg Spine.* 2004;1:287–298.
9. Yamada Y, Bilsky MH, Lovelock DM, et al. High-dose, single-fraction image-guided intensity-modulated radiotherapy for metastatic spinal lesions. *Int J Radiat Oncol Biol Phys.* 2008;71(2):484–490.

Principles of Orthopedic Surgery in Cancer

Carol D. Morris
Corey Rothrock

The musculoskeletal manifestations of cancer are far-reaching. Both benign and malignant tumors of bone can occur at any age and in any of the 206 bones in the human body. Soft tissue tumors follow a similar pattern, presenting in both pediatric and adult patients virtually anywhere in the body. The surgical management of bone and soft tissue tumors largely depends on the origin of the tumor. Both bone and soft tissue sarcomas are largely treated with curative intent in the form of limb salvage surgery or amputation. Secondary tumors of bone, or metastatic disease, are usually treated with palliative intent, which most often requires stabilization of the bone without removing the entire tumor. While tumors may metastasize to soft tissue, this pattern of spread is far less common. The role of the orthopedic oncologist is often twofold: (1) to eradicate cancer in muscle and bones and (2) rebuild the resulting defects in a functionally acceptable manner. This chapter will review the surgical principles of treating both primary and secondary musculoskeletal malignancies in the extremities.

GENERAL PRINCIPLES

Diagnosis and Staging

A thoughtful and methodical strategy for the diagnosis of bone and soft tissue tumors cannot be overemphasized. Because primary bone and soft tissue malignancies are relatively rare, they are diagnostically challenging, and a delay in diagnosis is not uncommon. An accurate diagnosis is based on a combination of clinical, imaging, and histological data.

Always start with a thorough history and physical exam. Most patients with malignant bone tumors present with pain. "Night pain," defined as pain that awakes one from sleep, is a classic complaint among patients with bone tumors and should always be investigated. Functional pain refers to pain with ambulation or certain activities, and can be indicative of an impending fracture. Most patients with functional pain should be placed on a restricted weight-bearing status. Pathologic fractures through primary bone sarcomas carry devastating consequences, often requiring immediate amputation of the affected limb to control tumor spread. In contrast, the majority of soft tissue sarcomas are painless unless nerve or bone involvement is present. Often, patients report a history of trauma that has brought attention to the affected area.

A patient's medical history can be contributory. In patients with a known diagnosis of cancer, bone pain must always be investigated to rule out metastatic disease. Certain clinical syndromes such as neurofibromatosis or Paget disease, are associated with sarcomas (1). Patients that have undergone radiation for other conditions are at risk of developing secondary sarcomas (2). Up to 10% of primary bone tumors will present pathologic fractures.

On physical examination, primary bone tumors are often associated with a painful mass. Other important aspects of the exam include altered gait, decreased

KEY POINTS

- Both bone and soft tissue sarcomas are largely treated with curative intent in the form of limb salvage surgery or amputation.
- Secondary tumors of bone, or metastatic disease, are usually treated with palliative intent, which most often requires stabilization of the bone without removing the entire tumor.
- The role of the orthopedic oncologist is often two-fold: (1) to eradicate cancer in muscle and bones, and (2) to rebuild the resulting defects in a functionally acceptable manner.
- Most patients with malignant bone tumors present with pain.
- "Night pain" is defined as pain that awakes one from sleep. This is a classic complaint among patients with bone tumors and should always be investigated.
- Functional pain refers to pain with ambulation or certain activities and can be indicative of an impending fracture. Most patients with functional pain should be placed on a restricted weight-bearing status.
- The majority of soft tissue sarcomas are painless unless nerve or bone involvement is present.

- There are four types of oncologic excisions: intralesional, marginal, wide, and radical.
- Approximately 90% of all extremity sarcomas can be successfully removed without amputation.
- Limb salvage surgery requires that oncologic outcome is not compromised and the resultant limb has reasonable functional capacity.
- The main reason to perform amputation in the oncology setting is the inability to achieve negative tumor margins at the time of definitive surgery.
- The most common indication for rotationplasty is a child with considerable remaining growth as endoprosthetic reconstruction in very skeletally immature patients will require multiple revisions for lengthening and failures.
- A pathologic fracture is a fracture that has occurred through diseased bone.
- An impending fracture is one that is likely to occur with normal physiologic loading (turning in bed, ambulation, etc).
- As a general rule, lower extremity fractures should be surgically fixed if the patient's life expectancy is at least six weeks. Upper extremity fractures are usually not fixed if the life expectancy is less than three months.

range of motion of the adjacent joint, joint effusions, regional lymphadenopathy, overlying skin changes, and neurovascular status. When metastatic disease is suspected, the physical exam should also focus on the suspected primary site (thyroid, breast, etc.). For soft tissue tumors, the mass is evaluated for its size, mobility, and firmness in addition to more discreet findings, such as a Tinel sign, bruits, or transillumination. Large (>5 cm) and deep soft tissue masses should be considered malignant until proven otherwise (Fig. 6.1).

All bone tumors require an x-ray. In fact, despite advances in imaging modalities, the plane x-ray remains the most telling diagnostic study (Fig. 6.2). When a primary bone sarcoma is suspected, magnetic resonance imaging (MRI) of the entire bone, computed tomography (CT) scan of the chest, and whole-body bone scan are necessary for complete staging. For soft tissue tumors, MRI is the most revealing imaging modality, as it allows for excellent definition of the mass, including characteristic signal patterns and the relation of the mass to adjacent neurovascular structures (Fig. 6.3). In addition, soft tissue sarcomas (STS) are staged with CT of the chest, and more recently, positron emission tomography (PET) scans are being incorporated into staging protocols, though the role of PET scan has yet to be fully validated. For metastatic bone disease in which the primary cancer has already been identified,

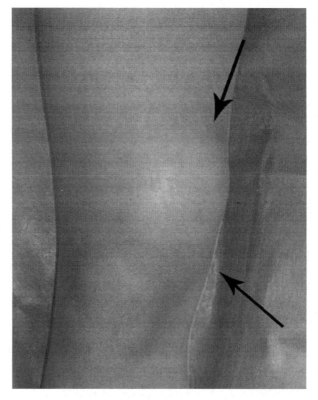

FIGURE 6.1

Clinical picture of a distal mesial thigh soft tissue mass.

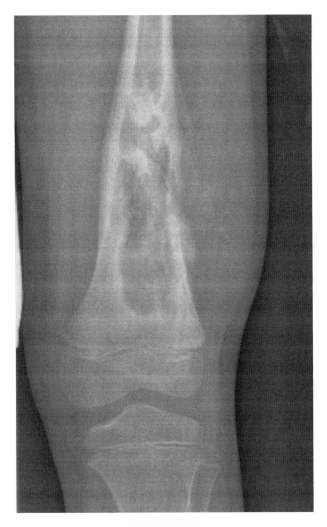

FIGURE 6.2

Classic x-ray appearance of an osteogenic sarcoma of the distal femur of a skeletally immature patient showing a permeative lesion with a wide zone of transition, cortical destruction with soft tissue extension, and periosteal elevation.

imaging is directed at the bone of interest to guide treatment. If the primary cancer is unknown, CT scan of the chest/abdomen/pelvis is performed to elucidate the primary cancer, as well as bone scan to identify other bony sites of disease.

Biopsy

The biopsy is an important part of the staging process. The purpose of the biopsy is to obtain tissue for pathologic analysis in order to make a diagnosis. Often referred to as the first step of a successful limb salvage operation, the biopsy must be done carefully so as not to adversely affect the outcome. It is preferentially performed by a surgeon with experience in

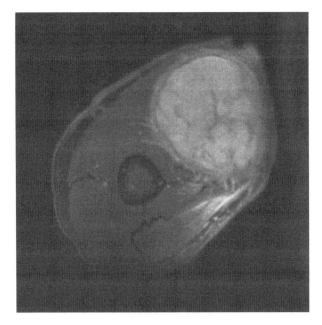

FIGURE 6.3

Typical MRI appearance of a high-grade soft tissue sarcoma in the upper extremity demonstrating a large heterogeneous mass.

musculoskeletal oncology who will ultimately perform the definitive procedure. There are several types of biopsies: fine needle aspirates (FNA), core needle, open incisional, and open excisional (Fig. 6.4). The type of biopsy performed depends on a host of factors, including the size and location of the mass and the experience of the interpreting pathologist.

Needle biopsies are advantageous in that they can be performed in the office or by an interventional radiologist, are minimally invasive, and when done properly, are associated with minimal tissue contamination. Obviously, needle biopsy is associated with a small tissue sample, which can be problematic if special stains or studies are required to make an accurate diagnosis. In an open incisional biopsy, a generous tissue sample is obtained by surgically incising into the tumor. Open biopsies require considerable expertise, as several technical points must be considered: orientation along the limb salvage incision or directly adjacent to it, meticulous hemostasis, and avoidance of extra compartmental and neurovascular contamination. Any tissue exposed at the time of biopsy is theoretically contaminated and must be excised at the time of definitive surgery. A poorly performed open biopsy can have devastating consequences and is associated with more complex tumor resections, including unnecessary amputation (3,4). Open bone biopsies can create stress risers in the bone, which in turn, can result in pathologic fractures. Splinting and protected weight

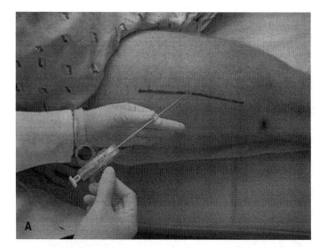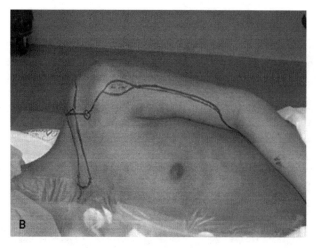

FIGURE 6.4

A: Needle biopsy of a thigh mass performed with a Tru-cut core needle. Note that the limb salvage incision is drawn out first. B: Open biopsy of the proximal humerus. The biopsy tract is incorporated into the definitive limb salvage incision.

bearing are often required following open bone biopsy to avoid such a complication. Excisional biopsy implies that the entire tumor is removed at the time of biopsy. Excisional biopsy is usually reserved for benign tumors, small malignant tumors (<3 cm), or situations in which incisional biopsy would cause considerable contamination. The decision to perform an excisional biopsy must be weighed carefully, as the potential associated complications when performed inadequately or unnecessarily are significant (Fig. 6.5).

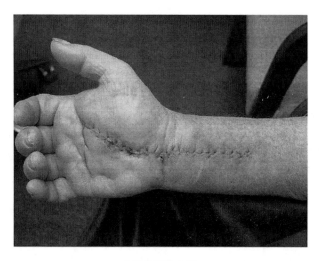

FIGURE 6.5

An open excisional biopsy was performed for a presumed benign tumor of the wrist, which turned out to be a sarcoma. The median nerve was isolated at the time of surgery. The area of contamination is quite large, making conversion to limb salvage difficult.

Oncologic Excisions

There are four types of oncologic excisions: intralesional, marginal, wide, and radical (5). The names of the excisions refer to the surgical margin by which the tumor is removed. In intralesional surgery, the surgeon enters the tumor, leaving microscopic and sometimes gross tumor behind. Intralesional excisions are usually reserved for benign bone tumors such as cyst. In selected instances, low-grade sarcomas, such as low-grade chondrosarcoma, can be treated with a combination of intralesional surgery and an effective adjuvant, such as liquid nitrogen (6). In marginal excisions, the tumor is excised through the "reactive" zone around the tumor or around the pseudocapsule of the tumor. This reactive zone is inflammatory in nature and theoretically contains tumor cells. Marginal excisions are typically performed for benign soft tissue masses such as lipoma. Most malignant tumors should be removed with wide or radical margins. A wide excision completely removes the tumor en bloc with a cuff of normal tissue around the tumor (Fig. 6.6A,B). The vast majority of bone and soft tissue sarcomas are removed by wide excision. Radical resections remove tumors en bloc by resecting the entire compartment: the entire bone or the entire muscle compartment from the origin to the insertion. Radical resections may be performed if "skip" lesions are present, but rarely need to be performed. Due to advances in superior imaging techniques as well as effective adjuvant treatments, such as chemotherapy and radiation, tumors can be excised with fairly narrow margins. Decreasing the amount of normal tissue that needs to be removed around the tumor improves functional outcomes without compromising oncologic results.

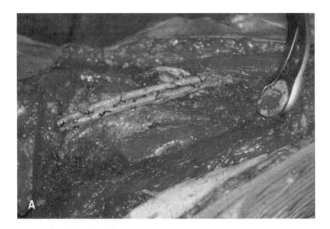

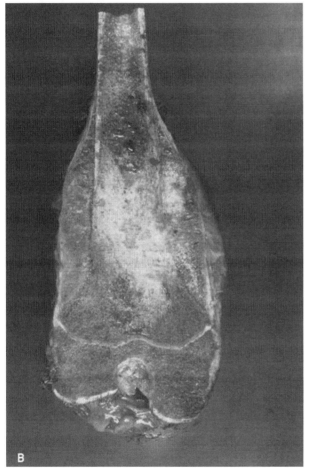

FIGURE 6.6

A: The resultant defect in the thigh following wide excision of a distal femur sarcoma. B: The gross pathology specimen of a distal femur sarcoma removed with wide margins.

SURGICAL MANAGEMENT OF PRIMARY BONE AND SOFT TISSUE SARCOMAS

Limb Salvage Surgery

Surgery is the cornerstone of treatment for bone and soft tissue sarcomas. Approximately 90% of all extremity sarcomas can be successfully removed without amputation. During the late 1970s and the 1980s, limb salvage surgery for sarcomas began to gain popularity. This was due to a variety of factors, including advances in imaging, effective adjuvant treatments, and advances in reconstruction. Several investigations have reported equivalent survival in patients undergoing limb salvage versus amputation (7,8). Limb salvage surgery requires that oncologic outcome is not compromised and the resultant limb has reasonable functional capacity. There are many variables to consider when deciding if an individual is an appropriate candidate for limb salvage surgery, such as vocational demands of the patient, response to neoadjuvant treatment, remaining skeletal growth in children, and cultural expectations.

Once a tumor has been removed, the resultant defect must be reconstructed. Soft tissue tumors may require soft tissue reconstructions, such as tendon transfers, nerve grafts, or flap coverage. In addition to soft tissue defects, bone tumors require reconstruction of the removed bone and often adjacent joint. Orthopedic oncologists typically utilize four reconstruction options in limb salvage surgery for bones: allografts, autografts, metallic prostheses, or allograft-prosthetic composites.

Allografts

Human bone allografts have been used for decades as a biologic solution for skeletal defects. They offer several advantages over synthetic implants, including attachments for host ligaments and muscle and the potential to serve as long-term solutions since the graft continues to incorporate with the host bone over time. Disadvantages of allografts include possible disease transmission, fractures, and nonunions at the host bone interface. Allografts can be used to reconstruct virtually any bone or joint. Clearly, certain anatomic sites have a more successful track record than others.

The American Association of Tissue Banks (AATB), in conjunction with the Food and Drug Administration (FDA), regulates the procurement, testing, and distribution of human allografts (9). Grafts are typically obtained though AATB-approved tissue banks. Once a decision has been made to use a structural allograft, the surgeon contacts a tissue bank to obtain a properly sized allograft that matches the dimensions of the patient's bone and possesses the desired soft tissue. Some medical centers have internal bone banks.

Osteoarticular allografts are large segments of bone with a cryopreserved articular surface (Fig. 6.7A). They can be used to reconstruct very large defects, with the adjacent joint most commonly around the knee and shoulder. Once the tumor is removed, the allograft is cut and sculpted to fit the defect. The allograft is then secured to the host bone using orthopedic hardware

(Fig. 6.7B). The surrounding ligaments and tendons are then attached to the allograft (Fig 6.7C). For example, in the knee, the anterior cruciate ligament (ACL), posterior cruciate ligament (PCL), collateral ligaments, and capsule would all be reapproximated giving rise to stable knee joint. With time, the allograft incorporates with the host bone creating a stable, durable limb (Fig. 6.7D). Allografts can also be used in an intercalary fashion (Fig. 6.8) as well as for partial defects of long bones (Fig. 6.9).

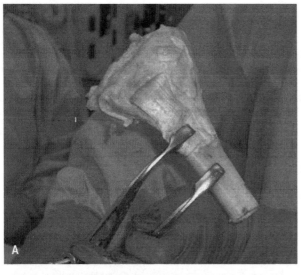

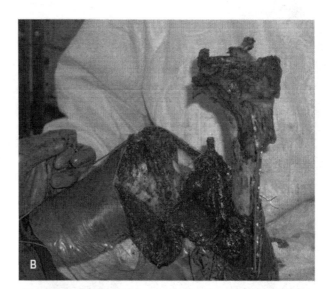

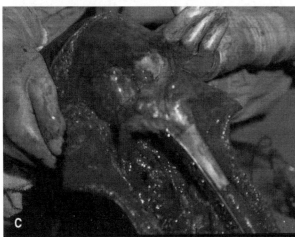

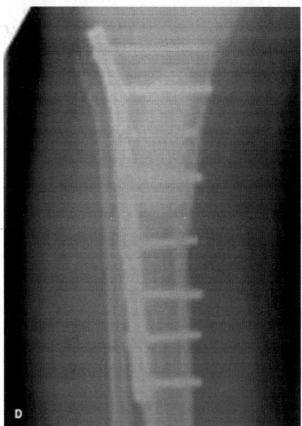

A: A proximal tibial osteoarticular allograft. B: The allograft is secure to the native tibia using a metallic plate and screws. C: The articular surface is reduced and the important soft tissue structures (ACL, PCL, collateral ligaments, patellar tendon) are repaired. D: X-ray appearance of a healed proximal tibial osteoarticular allograft.

FIGURE 6.7

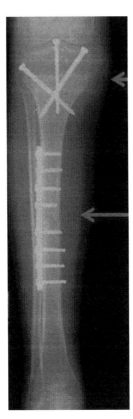

X-ray appearance of a healed intercalary allograft of the tibia. The arrows indicate the osteotomy sites proximally and distally. The patient's articular surface was preserved.

FIGURE 6.8

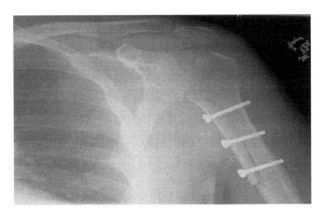

FIGURE 6.9

X-ray appearance of a hemicortical allograft used to reconstitute a partial defect on the medial proximal humerus.

The success of the allograft reconstruction is dependent on a variety of factors, but most importantly the ability to obtain union of the graft-host bone junction. Adequate internal fixation, external splints, and protected weight bearing all serve to enhance union rates, which are approximately 80% in most large series (10–12).

Postoperatively, patients with allografts can mobilize fairly quickly. Almost all allograft reconstructions require an extended period of protected weight bearing until there is evidence of union at the allograft-host bone junction, as demonstrated on imaging. Progressive weight bearing is allowed relative to the amount of healing observed. When intra-articular soft tissue reconstructions are performed, as with osteoarticular allografts, the joint is typically immobilized for several weeks.

Metallic Prostheses

Megaprostheses are most commonly used to reconstruct large-segment bone defects. Historically, implants were fabricated on a custom basis for each patient. Currently, modular systems offering virtually limitless sizing options are widely available. Noncustom metallic implants are available for all commonly reconstructed anatomic sites: shoulder, elbow, hip, and knee (Fig. 6.10). Even smaller joints, such as the wrist and ankle, have "off -the-shelf" implant options.

Large megaprostheses are instantly durable, a quality that can be desirable in patients being treated for malignancies, since it can be difficult to maneuver assistive devices while undergoing chemotherapy or recovering from thoracotomy. In addition, modular systems give the operating surgeon great latitude during the reconstructive phase of the surgery. For example, if the proximal femur is found to be compromised by tumor or lack of bone quality following distal femoral resection, the entire femur can be replaced from hip to knee with minimal effort.

The major disadvantage of metallic prostheses is that they will all eventually fail when the patient is fortunate enough to be cured of disease. With increasing survival rates for most bone sarcomas, prosthetic revision has become increasingly common. Great research and development have gone into improving prosthetic designs. The weakest link in an endoprosthesis is where the metal stem attaches to bone. Currently, most stems are secured with cement or a press-fit technique that relies on bony in-growth of the stem. Both septic and aseptic loosening account for the vast majority of prosthetic failures (Fig. 6.11). Newer designs attempt to circumvent the problem of aseptic loosening.

Postoperatively, most patients with metallic prosthetic reconstructions can mobilize immediately. Exceptions might be reconstructions in which free flap or skin graft is required for wound closure. In general, cemented prostheses allow for immediate full weight bearing. Press-fit prostheses usually require a period of partial weight bearing, though this is highly dependent on surgeon preference and anatomic location. Joint mobilization is typically initiated when the surrounding soft tissue demonstrates adequate healing. Situations requiring soft tissue reconstruction will likely require longer periods of joint immobilization.

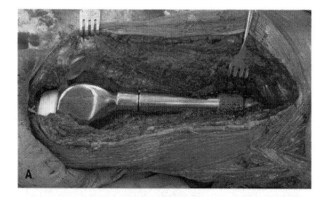

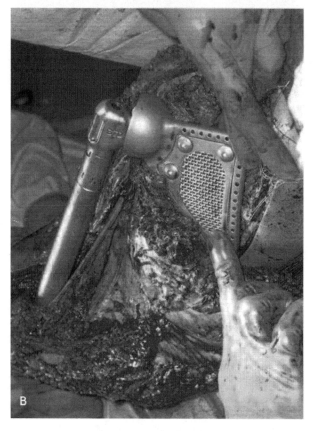

FIGURE 6.10

A: Intraoperative appearance of a distal femur replacement. B: Intraoperative appearance of a total scapula and proximal humerus replacement.

Allograft-Prosthetic Composites

Allograft-prosthetic composites (APCs) are the best of both worlds: the immediate structural integrity of a metallic prosthesis combined with the superior biologic soft tissue attachments of allografts. They have become an increasingly popular reconstruction method (13,14). Alloprosthetic composites are most commonly employed in the proximal tibia and proximal humerus. In the proximal tibia, the allograft provides for secure

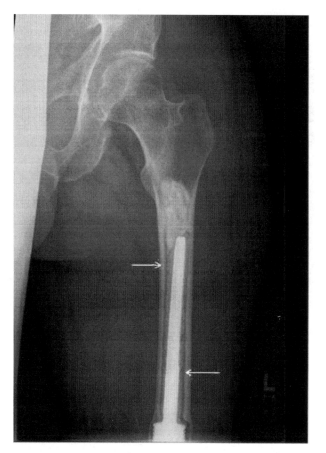

FIGURE 6.11

Aseptic loosening of a distal femoral prosthesis. The cement mantle is fractured and there is a lucency between the cement and the bone (arrows).

attachment of the patellar tendon, reconstituting an intact and sturdy extensor mechanism (15). In the proximal humerus, the rotator cuff tendons and capsule are attached to the remaining soft tissue on the allograft. This allows for a stable and hopefully functional joint. In addition, alloprosthetic composites have been used in the proximal femur to take advantage of the gluteus medius attachment to prevent a Trendelenburg gait.

Regardless of the location, the surgical method is similar. The articular surface of the allograft is cut off and the stem of the implant placed in the allograft. The implant can be skewered through the bone (Fig. 6.12A) or simply into the allograft alone. The implant is typically cemented into the allograft, as bony in-growth is not expected. The skewered stem is then placed in the host bone by either press-fit or cemented techniques. Depending on the stability of the construct, the graft and host bone may or may not require additional fixation (Fig. 6.12B). The soft tissues, including tendon, ligaments, and capsule, are then reconstructed with heavy suture.

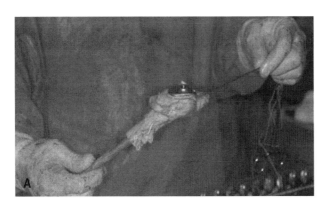

FIGURE 6.12

A: A proximal humerus alloprosthetic composite. A long-stemmed humerus component is skewered through the allograft. Sutures have been placed through soft tissue attachments on the allograft. B: X-ray appearance of a proximal humerus alloprosthetic composite. The construct was secured to the patient's bone with additional internal fixation, facilitating complete healing of the allograft and host bone junction.

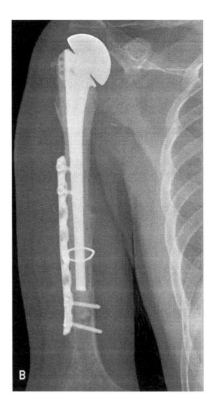

Alloprostheses offer many advantages. The soft tissue advantages are obvious, as the tendon and muscle attachments are functionally superior to those attached to metal. In addition, bone stock is reconstituted, allowing for greater revision options in the future. Also, the exact size matching of the allograft is not as crucial, since the articular surface is replaced with metal. The main disadvantage of APC reconstruction is the lengthy operative time required compared to other techniques, which may theoretically lead to increased rates of infection (16).

Postoperatively, protected weight bearing is required to allow the allograft host bone junction to heal. In addition, the joint must be immobilized for an extended period to allow the soft tissue reconstruction to heal.

Autografts

Autografts are typically used to reconstruct intercalary defects. Tumors located in the diaphysis of the humerus and tibia are ideal for this reconstruction option. The most common autograft donor sites are the fibula and iliac crest. To enhance healing, often their corresponding vascular pedicle is transposed and reconnected by a microvascular anastomosis. Obviously, these types of procedures require a multidisciplinary team. The union rates of vascularized bone grafts are high, making them an attractive alternative (17). If the anastomosis

is patent long-term, the graft tends to hypertrophy with time, assuming the diameter and strength of the replaced bone.

Autograft reconstructions usually require the longest period of protected weight bearing compared to other reconstruction options. Because the initial size mismatch between the autograft and the host bone (Fig. 6.13), extended periods (often greater than one year) of protected weight bearing and brace immobilization must be implemented to avoid fracture.

Special Considerations in Limb Salvage Surgery

CHILDREN. Skeletally immature patients are a particularly challenging group to reconstruct, as children require extremely durable constructs that allow for adjustments in longitudinal growth. The knee, the most common site for primary bone tumors, possesses the two most important growth plates to lower-extremity longitudinal growth. The distal femoral growth plate contributes approximately 1 cm a year, whereas the proximal tibia contributes approximately 0.6 cm a year. Obviously, obliterating these growth plates in a young child will lead to a considerable (and usually unacceptable) leg length discrepancy by skeletal maturity. In general, reconstruction strategies aim to (1) preserve growth plates when possible, (2) utilize

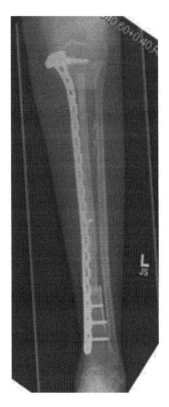

FIGURE 6.13

A vascularized fibular autograft used to reconstruct an intercalary segment of the contralateral tibia following wide excision of a chondrosarcoma.

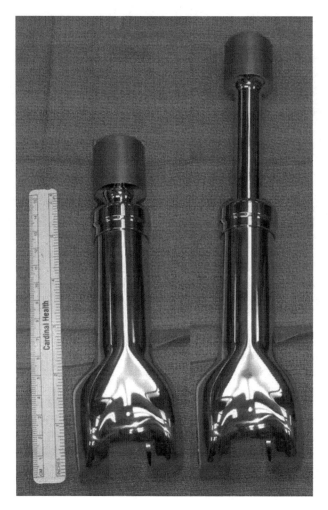

FIGURE 6.14

An expandable distal femoral prosthesis.

extensible metallic prostheses, or (3) expand the
remaining bone by a technique called bone transport.
For example, a nine-year-old boy with a distal femoral
osteogenic sarcoma has approximately 11 cm of
growth remaining in the knee region, assuming he
will grow until the age of 16. The complexity of the
surgical management of this child is considerable. No
doubt, above-knee amputation or rotationplasty will
provide the most simple, most predictable, and least
restrictive option. Limb salvage options might include
using an extensible metallic prosthesis (Fig. 6.14) or
an osteoarticular allograft. While these options seem
attractive, they have considerable limitations, such as
limited athletic activity to prolong the longevity of
the implant, numerous future surgical procedures for
lengthening and implant failure, and a lifetime risk of
implant infection. Certainly, newer prosthetic designs
with noninvasive expansion mechanisms attempt to
address some of the current limitations.

PELVIS. Pelvic reconstruction following tumor
excision probably represents the most complicated and
technically difficult of orthopedic oncologic procedures.

Patients often experience postoperative complications
and require lengthy periods of immobilization. When
the acetabulum can be spared, often, reconstruction can
be avoided. When the acetabulum must be sacrificed,
"hip replacement" is required. Reconstructions can
be accomplished with metallic implants, allografts,
and allograft-prosthetic composites (Figs. 6.15 and
6.16). Joint instability is a major problem following
acetabular reconstruction. Usually, the majority, and
in some cases all, of the surrounding muscles have
been transected or sacrificed, leading to both static
and dynamic instability with minimal active control
of the extremity. The disability is magnified if portions
of the sciatic or femoral nerve are sacrificed or injured.
In cases of severe instability, a hip orthosis may be
required until adequate scarring of the surrounding
soft tissue has been achieved. Patients status-post pelvic
reconstruction require several months of rehabilitation
to maximize their functional capacity.

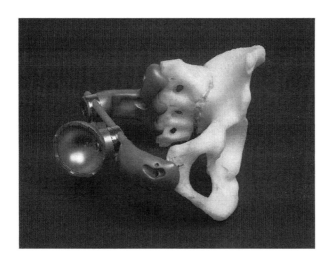

FIGURE 6.15

A custom metal pelvis prosthesis.

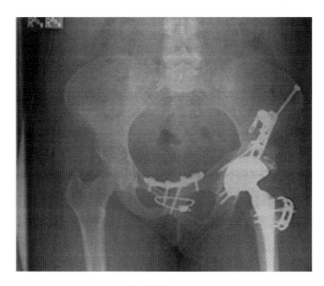

FIGURE 6.16

An x-ray of a pelvis allograft into which a bipolar hip prosthesis has been placed.

Complications Following Limb Salvage Surgery

Unfortunately, complications following limb salvage surgery are plentiful. Approximately 10%–15% of all megaprostheses and/or allografts will become infected during a patient's lifetime. Infection is a particularly difficult problem to manage, requiring removal of the involved prosthesis, placement of an antibiotic-impregnated spacer, a lengthy period of intravenous antibiotics, followed by replacement of a new prosthesis. Cases in which the infection cannot be cleared or there is inadequate surrounding soft tissue, amputation may be required. Implant loosening or breakage

is also common and almost guaranteed given enough time (Fig. 6.17). The more active the patient, the more quickly and more likely implant failure will occur. Prosthetic designs and biologic supplements are actively pursued areas of research aimed to prolong implant survival. Joint instability secondary to force mismatch from muscle or nerve resection can be problematic, leading to dislocation (Fig. 6.18). Solutions such as revision to a constrained implant or prolonged immobilization will usually solve this problem.

Amputation

Only 10% of patients with primary bone and soft tissue sarcomas will require amputation for local tumor control. The main reason to perform amputation in the oncology setting is the inability to achieve negative tumor margins at the time of definitive surgery. This commonly occurs in cases of neglected tumors (Fig. 6.19) Other indications include recurrent disease, fracture, considerable remaining growth in a young child, superior function compared to limb salvage,

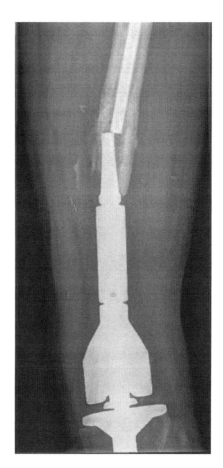

FIGURE 6.17

An x-ray of a broken cemented femoral stem.

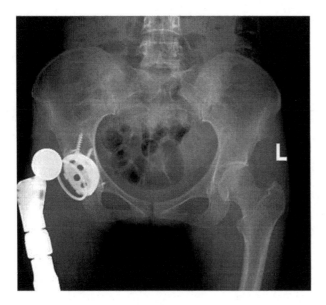

FIGURE 6.18

An unstable right hip following wide excision and reconstruction of the proximal femur and surrounding soft tissue.

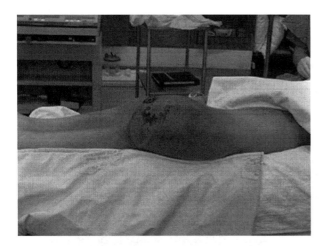

FIGURE 6.19

A very large osteogenic sarcoma of the distal femur with overlying skin compromise.

and infected reconstructions. Tumors of the foot are often treated with below-knee amputation, not because of surgical margins, but rather because of superior function.

Levels of lower-extremity amputation and upper-extremity amputation are shown in Figs. 6.20 and 6.21, respectively. The level of amputation in tumor surgery is entirely directed by the location of the tumor. In general, the higher the level of amputation, the greater the energy expenditure above baseline.

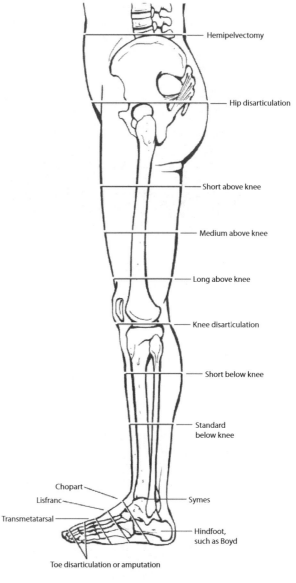

FIGURE 6.20

Amputation levels in the lower extremity.

There are many advantages to amputation in cancer surgery. In certain tumors that are unaffected by adjuvants such as chemotherapy or radiation, amputation allows for the most complete removal of tumor. Local recurrence rates are lower with amputation. Usually, additional surgical procedures are not required following amputation compared to those needed for complications of limb salvage surgery. Finally, both upper- and lower-extremity prosthetic designs have enjoyed tremendous advancement in past decade with excellent function and cosmesis.

There are also disadvantages of amputation compared to limb salvage. Most amputees experience phantom sensation and some experience phantom pain.

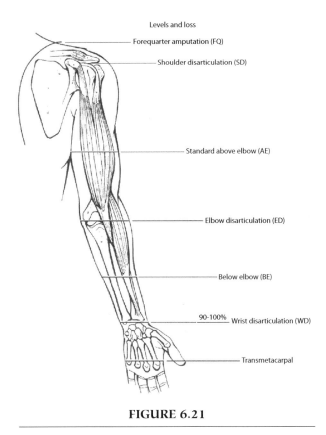

Levels and loss
— Forequarter amputation (FQ)
— Shoulder disarticulation (SD)
— Standard above elbow (AE)
— Elbow disarticulation (ED)
— Below elbow (BE)
90-100% — Wrist disarticulation (WD)
— Transmetacarpal

FIGURE 6.21

Amputation levels in the upper extremity.

Phantom pain can be particularly debilitating and usually requires prolonged pharmacologic intervention. Painful neuromas can occur at the stump of a transected nerve and can cause problems with weight bearing. Proprioception is compromised following amputation, leading to initial difficulties with gait training. Children with considerable remaining growth can get bony overgrowth at the terminal end of the bone, requiring surgical revision.

Lower-Extremity Amputations

Below-knee amputation (BKA) is typically performed for tumors of the foot, ankle, or distal tibia. The ideal length of residual tibia is 12–17 cm distal to the medial joint line (Fig. 6.22). BK amputees expend approximately 40% more kcal/min than nonamputees to maintain a normal gait and ambulate about 35% slower. Whereas a BKA performed for vascular compromise tends to use a large posterior flap, a BKA in cancer surgery utilizes a "fish-mouth" type incision for maximal tumor margins.

Above-knee amputation (AKA) is performed for unresectable tumors of the proximal tibia, distal femur, and popliteal fossa. AKA amputees expend 89% more kcal/min than nonamputees and walk 43% slower.

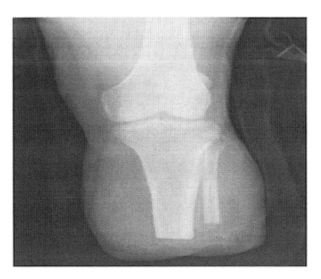

FIGURE 6.22

An x-ray of a below-knee amputation. The fibula is usually transected more proximally than the tibia.

A "fish-mouth" incision is usually used, with an effort to make the anterior flap slightly larger than the posterior flap such that the distal incision is more posterior. Muscle balance is an important technical consideration. If amputation is performed proximal to the adductor tendon insertion, an adductor myodesis should be performed to balance the hip abductor proximally. Also, when the quadriceps myodesis is performed, the hip should be in full extension to avoid overtightening, leading to a hip flexion contracture.

In selected patients, both BKA and AKA are ideal for immediate prosthetic fitting following the definitive surgery. When the surgeon has closed the wound, a sterile dressing is applied. A prosthetist then applies an immediate postoperative prosthesis (IPOP) under the same anesthesia (Fig. 6.23). This temporary prosthesis is not meant to be used for weight bearing. The sensation and cosmetic appearance of an immediate artificial limb is thought to decrease the frequency and severity of phantom pain as well as assist in emotional acceptance. The IPOP typically comes off within a week after surgery once the swelling decreases. In patients with delayed healing secondary to radiation or chemotherapy, immediate prosthetic fitting can cause wound complications and is contraindicated (Fig. 6.24).

Hemipelvectomy is performed for tumors of the hip and pelvis. The resection can include the entire inominate bone (Fig. 6.25) or just portions of it. Hemipelvectomy is often preferred to limb salvage for pelvic tumors, as the associated complications are fewer. Wound complications following hemipelvectomy can be considerable, with rates greater than

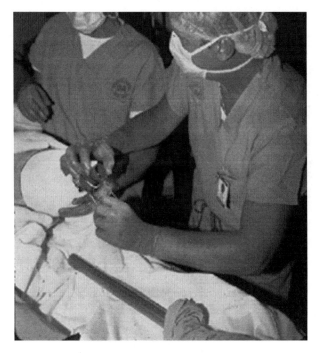

FIGURE 6.23

Following above-knee amputation, prosthetists place an immediate postoperative prosthesis (IPOP) while the patient is still under anesthesia.

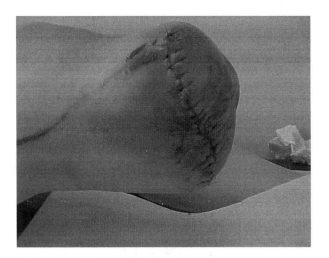

FIGURE 6.24

Wound breakdown following IPOP placement in a patient-post below-knee amputation. The patient had previously undergone radiation to the limb.

50% in some series. Most patients who undergo hemipelvectomy do not ultimately use a prosthesis for ambulation.

Postoperatively, all patients that undergo amputation, regardless of level, are monitored for wound complications and phantom pain. These patients

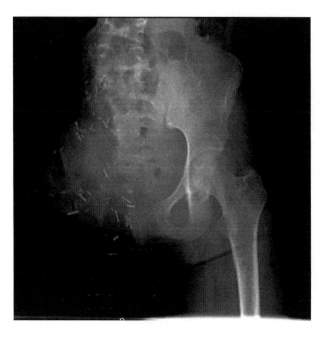

FIGURE 6.25

An x-ray following external hemipelvectomy.

benefit greatly from early evaluation by rehabilitation or physiatry departments. Issues of standing balance and shaping of the residual limb are best addressed as early as possible. For hemipelvectomy patients in which the ischium has been removed, sitting balance needs to be addressed. The timing of prosthetic fitting and weight bearing is ultimately determined by the operating surgeon and is largely based on wound status.

Upper-Extremity Amputations

Upper-extremity amputations are far less common than lower-extremity amputations. Below-elbow amputations are quite functional. Successful prosthetic rehabilitation can be achieved in the majority of patients. Forearm strength and rotation are proportional to the maintained length. Even very short residual below-elbow limbs are preferable to through-elbow or above-elbow amputation. Maintenance of the biceps insertion is important. For above-elbow amputations, at least 5 cm of remaining humerus is required for prosthetic fitting. For proximal tumors, shoulder disarticulation is preferable to forequarter amputation when possible. The scapula provides cosmetic symmetry and is important for wearing clothes.

Rotationplasty

Rotationplasty is an innovative way to manage tumors around the knee that would otherwise require above-knee amputation. Originally described in the 1930s for limbs affected by tuberculosis, rotationplasty was performed for malignant tumors about the knee starting in the 1970s (18,19). The procedure involves removing the entire knee in continuity, with both the distal femur and proximal tibia en bloc, with all of the surrounding soft tissue except the popliteal artery and vein and the tibial and peroneal nerves. The distal portion of the extremity is then rotated 180 degrees, and the bones and soft tissues are reapproximated (Fig. 6.26). The resulting limb is functionally a below-knee amputation (Fig. 6.27A,B). Variations on the theme have been described around the hip and even in the upper extremity (20,21).

The most common indication for rotationplasty is a child with considerable remaining growth, as endoprosthetic reconstruction in skeletally immature patients will require multiple revisions for lengthening and failures. In addition, rotationplasty might be desirable for individuals with high physical demands. Other indications include compromised soft tissue around the knee, pathologic fractures, failed limb salvage procedures, and local recurrence. Compared to above-knee amputation, rotationplasty is void of phantom pain, demonstrates normal proprioception, and provides durable weight bearing without painful neuromas. The obvious disadvantage is the cosmetic appearance. While the procedure is still performed frequently in Europe, the advent of extensible endoprostheses has lead to decreased enthusiasm among parents who desire a more normal-appearing extremity for their child.

Postoperatively, patients are not permitted to bear weight through the extremity until the osteosynthesis

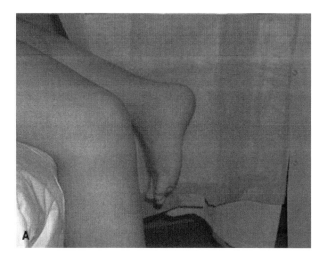

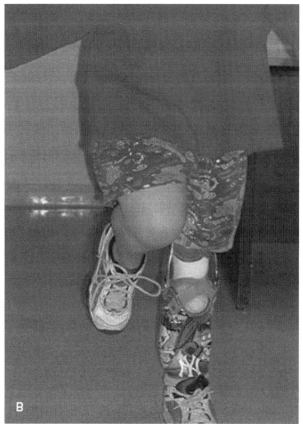

FIGURE 6.27

A: A clinical picture of a young boy post rotationplasty for a malignant tumor of the knee. Note that the heel is at the level of the contralateral knee. B: He has excellent physical coordination following prosthetic fitting of the rotated limb with a modified BKA prosthesis.

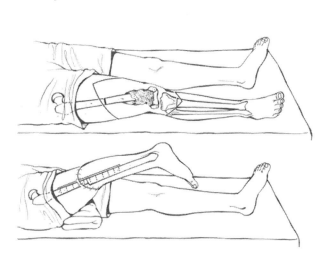

FIGURE 6.26

A schematic representation of a rotationplasty.

site between the distal femur and proximal tibia has fully healed. Ankle range of motion and strengthening is initially restricted as well to allow tendon and muscle connections to heal.

SURGICAL MANAGEMENT OF SKELETAL METASTASES

The management of patients with skeletal metastases represents one of the most challenging aspects of orthopedic oncology. These patients are typically quite ill and in considerable pain. Bone pain from metastatic disease has a tremendous impact on the patient's quality of life. The role of the orthopedic oncologist is largely to maximize the patient's quality of life by treating impending and pathologic fractures for the purposes of pain control and to restore and maintain function and mobility. In certain instances of isolated bone metastases, cure, or at the very least lengthy disease-free intervals, may be achieved with surgical excision (22).

A pathologic fracture is a fracture that has occurred through diseased bone (Fig. 6.28). An impending fracture is one that is likely to occur with normal physiologic loading (turning in bed, ambulation, etc.) (Fig. 6.29). Today, numerous nonsurgical interventions are available to treat impending fractures or lesions at risk of evolving into impending fractures, including radiation, bisphosphonates, and a host of minimally invasive ablative techniques.

When is surgery indicated for pathologic bone lesions? Various investigations have attempted to quantify the risk of fracture depending on imaging and clinical characteristics (23–25). None of these scoring systems has the ability to accurately predict fracture risk. The decision to proceed with surgical fixation is largely dependent on a combination of imaging characteristics, pain, functional deficits, anatomic location

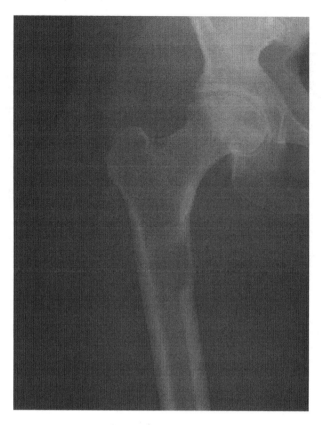

FIGURE 6.29

An impending pathological fracture of the femur through metastatic breast cancer.

of the lesion, and remaining life expectancy. As a rule, lower-extremity fractures should be surgically fixed if the patient's life expectancy is at least six weeks, whereas upper-extremity fractures are usually not fixed if the life expectancy is less than three months. Of course, many factors come into play when making such decisions.

When the decision is made to proceed with surgery, a few basic goals must be achieved:

1. The reconstruction must permit immediate weight bearing.
2. The reconstruction should last the patient's lifetime.
3. "One bone, one operation," meaning the entire bone and any other concerning lesions within the bone must be addressed at the time of surgery.

While these goals seem simple and intuitive, they can be difficult to achieve. New systemic biologic agents are changing the patterns of metastatic disease and the associated survival times. What was once thought to be an adequate fixation technique may not last long

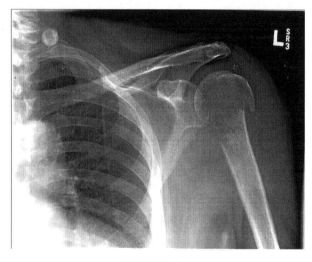

FIGURE 6.28

A pathologic proximal humerus fracture through metastatic renal cancer.

enough (Fig. 6.30). In general, the ends of long bones are treated with prosthetic replacements. This is especially true around the hip. Usually, oncologic prostheses are need as they possess varying stem lengths to splint the entire bone (Fig. 6.31). Diaphyseal lesions can be treated with standard intramedullary nails (Fig. 6.32). When possible, the metastasis should be excised. This potentially extends the longevity of the reconstruction, retarding local tumor progression. The remaining cavitary defect should be filled with cement, as it provides increased strength and prevents tumor reaccumulation. Even thermal and physical adjuvants, such as liquid nitrogen, can be used to supplement the surgery to halt local bone destruction (Fig. 6.33). An important aspect of the preoperative evaluation is considering other bones that may be at risk of fracture. For example, if a patient has a pathologic hip fracture, the upper extremities should be assessed for impending fracture, as the weight bearing will temporarily be transferred to the upper extremities during recovery.

Postoperative Care

Most patients will benefit from postoperative radiation to again prevent tumor progression and prevent loss of

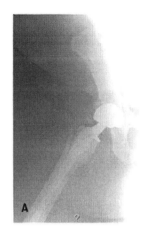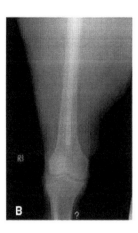

FIGURE 6.31

A long-stemmed cemented hemiarthroplasty of the hip. The shaft splints the entire bone prophylactically, addressing micrometastases in the remaining femur.

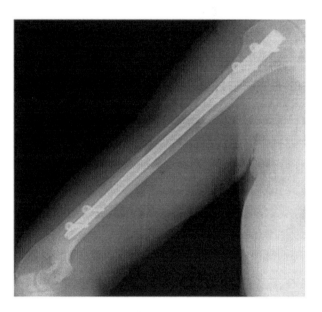

FIGURE 6.32

An intramedullary nail fixation of an impending humeral shaft fracture.

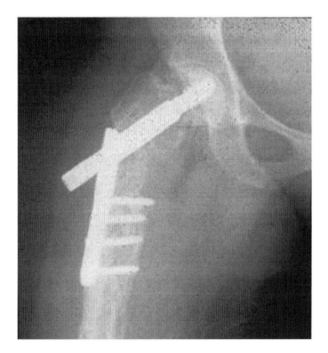

FIGURE 6.30

Failed internal fixation of a proximal femur fracture through metastatic thyroid cancer. The patient outlived the durability of the reconstruction. Revision to an endoprosthesis was performed.

fixation (26). All patients should be mobilized immediately. Standard precautions should be observed for joint replacement to prevent dislocation, but otherwise there should be no weight-bearing restrictions. Postoperative complications are unfortunately common owing to the overall medical status of these patients. Infection and deep venous thrombosis are usually treated prophylactically. Aggressive pulmonary toilet is encouraged. Nutritional supplementation may be beneficial.

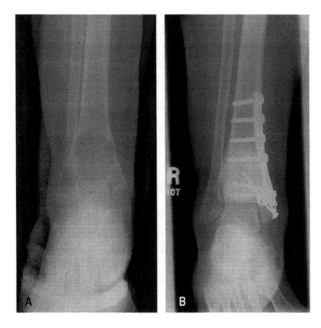

FIGURE 6.33

A pathological fracture (A) of the distal tibia through a plasma cell neoplasm. The lesion was treated with curettage, liquid nitrogen, cement, and internal fixation (B). The cement permitted immediate structural integrity, allowing full weight bearing.

*R*eferences

1. Mankin HJ, Hornicek FJ. Paget's sarcoma: a historical and outcome review. *Clin Orthop Relat Res.* 2005;438:97–102.
2. Brady MS, Gaynor JJ, Brennan MF. Radiation-associated sarcoma of bone and soft tissue. *Arch Surg.* 1992;127:1379–1385.
3. Mankin HJ, Lange TA, Spanier SS. The hazards of biopsy in patients with malignant primary bone and soft-tissue tumors. *J Bone Joint Surg Am.* 1982;64:1121–1127.
4. Mankin HJ, Mankin CJ, Simon MA. The hazards of the biopsy, revisited. Members of the Musculoskeletal Tumor Society. *J Bone Joint Surg Am.* 1996;78:656–663.
5. Enneking WF, Spanier SS, Goodman MA. A system for the surgical staging of musculoskeletal sarcoma. *Clin Orthop Relat Res.* 1980;153:106–120.
6. Marco RA, Gitelis S, Brebach GT, Healey JH. Cartilage tumors: evaluation and treatment. *J Am Acad Orthop Surg.* 2000;8:292–304.
7. Rougraff BT, Simon MA, Kneisl JS, Greenberg DB, Mankin HJ. Limb salvage compared with amputation for osteosarcoma of the distal end of the femur. A long-term oncological, functional, and quality-of-life study. *J Bone Joint Surg Am.* 1994;76:649–656.
8. Williard WC, Hajdu SI, Casper ES, Brennan MF. Comparison of amputation with limb-sparing operations for adult soft tissue sarcoma of the extremity. *Ann Surg.* 1992;215:269–275.
9. Accessed at http://www.aatb.org/.
10. Muscolo DL, Ayerza MA, Aponte-Tinao LA. Massive allograft use in orthopedic oncology. *Orthop Clin North Am.* 2006;37:65–74.
11. Hornicek FJ, Gebhardt MC, Tomford WW, et al. Factors affecting nonunion of the allograft-host junction. *Clin Orthop Relat Res.* 2001;382:87–98.
12. Mankin HJ, Gebhardt MC, Jennings LC, Springfield DS, Tomford WW. Long-term results of allograft replacement in the management of bone tumors. *Clin Orthop Relat Res.* 1996;324:86–97.
13. Gitelis S, Piasecki P. Allograft prosthetic composite arthroplasty for osteosarcoma and other aggressive bone tumors. *Clin Orthop Relat Res.* 1991;270:197–201.
14. Harris AI, Gitelis S, Sheinkop MB, Rosenberg AG, Piasecki P. Allograft prosthetic composite reconstruction for limb salvage and severe deficiency of bone at the knee or hip. *Semin Arthroplasty.* 1994;5:85–94.
15. Donati D, Colangeli M, Colangeli S, Di Bella C, Mercuri M. Allograft-prosthetic composite in the proximal tibia after bone tumor resection. *Clin Orthop Relat Res.* 2008;466:459–465.
16. Zehr RJ, Enneking WF, Scarborough MT. Allograft-prosthesis composite versus megaprosthesis in proximal femoral reconstruction. *Clin Orthop Relat Res.* 1996;322:207–223.
17. Pollock R, Stalley P, Lee K, Pennington D. Free vascularized fibula grafts in limb-salvage surgery. *J Reconstr Microsurg.* 2005;21:79–84.
18. Merkel KD, Gebhardt M, Springfield DS. Rotationplasty as a reconstructive operation after tumor resection. *Clin Orthop Relat Res.* 1991;270:231–236.
19. de Bari A, Krajbich JI, Langer F, Hamilton EL, Hubbard S. Modified Van Nes rotationplasty for osteosarcoma of the proximal tibia in children. *J Bone Joint Surg Br.* 1990;72:1065–1069.
20. Winkelmann WW. Hip rotationplasty for malignant tumors of the proximal part of the femur. *J Bone Joint Surg Am.* 1986;68:362–369.
21. Athanasian EA, Healey JH. Resection replantation of the arm for sarcoma: an alternative to amputation. *Clin Orthop Relat Res.* 2002:204–208.
22. Althausen P, Althausen A, Jennings LC, Mankin HJ. Prognostic factors and surgical treatment of osseous metastases secondary to renal cell carcinoma. *Cancer.* 1997;80:1103–1109.
23. Snell W, Beals RK. Femoral metastases and fractures from breast cancer. *Surg Gynecol Obstet.* 1964;119:22–24.
24. Harrington KD. New trends in the management of lower extremity metastases. *Clin Orthop Relat Res.* 1982;169:53–61.
25. Mirels H. Metastatic disease in long bones. A proposed scoring system for diagnosing impending pathologic fractures. *Clin Orthop Relat Res.* 1989;249:256–264.
26. Townsend PW, Smalley SR, Cozad SC, Rosenthal HG, Hassanein RE. Role of postoperative radiation therapy after stabilization of fractures caused by metastatic disease. *Int J Radiat Oncol Biol Phys.* 1995;31:43–49.

Principles of Breast Surgery in Cancer

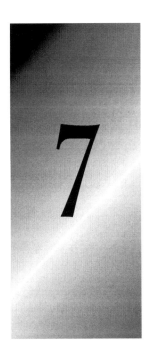

Sarah A. McLaughlin
Tari A. King

While the earliest recorded descriptions of breast surgery date back to the ancient Egyptians, modern breast surgery practice is considered to have begun in the late 1890s with the work of Dr. William S. Halsted. In the 100 years since, the art of breast surgery has been a process in evolution, searching for a balance between what is the oncologically safest procedure and what is the least deforming one.

To date, the role of systemic chemotherapy and antiestrogen hormonal therapies has become increasingly important, but breast cancer remains largely a surgical disease. Surgery offers the best chance for a cure. This chapter covers the basic principles of breast surgery. Although some historical data is included, it focuses on the current concepts of screening, preoperative diagnosis by needle biopsy, surgical options for the breast, and sentinel lymph node (SLN) biopsy for axillary staging.

ANATOMY

The adult breast lies between the second and sixth ribs vertically and between the sternal edge medially and the midaxillary line laterally. The rounded breast has a lateral projection into the axilla, known as the axillary tail of Spence. The breast rests on the pectoralis major muscle and is separated from it by the retromammary space. This space represents a distinct plane between the investing fascia of the breast tissue and the pectoralis

major fascia, and is identified by a thin layer of loose areolar tissue through which small vessels and lymphatic channels pass. When a mastectomy is performed, the breast tissue is removed, incorporating the retromammary space and the pectoralis major fascia.

The glandular breast consists of segments of ducts (lobes) that are arranged radially and extend outward and posteriorly from the nipple-areolar complex. Each duct undergoes a complex system of branching, ultimately ending in the terminal ductal-lobular units (TDLU). The lobules are the milk-forming glands of the lactating breast; the ducts are the channels. It is in the TDLUs that most breast cancers arise (1).

The blood supply to the breast is primarily through superficial arteries branching from the internal thoracic (mammary) artery or the lateral mammary artery from the lateral thoracic artery. The venous drainage follows the arterial patterns, and these veins ultimately drain into either the internal thoracic or the axillary vein. The innervation of the breast is supplied via the anterior and lateral cutaneous branches of the second to sixth intercostal nerves.

The thoracic wall is comprised of 12 thoracic vertebrae, 12 ribs, costal cartilages, and sternum and associated muscles. Table 7.1 lists the muscles of the thoracic wall. The most common muscular variations seen in breast surgery include the finding of a rectus sternalis muscle or the finding of a Langer axillary arch. The rectus sternalis can be found in nearly 8% of patients and represents an extension of muscular

KEY POINTS

- The role of systemic chemotherapy and antiestrogen hormonal therapies has become increasingly important, but breast cancer remains largely a surgical disease.
- When a suspicious abnormality in the breast is palpated or identified by imaging, a biopsy should be obtained for tissue diagnosis.
- In 1894, William Halsted popularized the removal of the breast, pectoralis muscles, and axillary lymph nodes in levels 1, 2, and 3. This procedure was known as the radical mastectomy (RM) or Halsted mastectomy.
- In 1948, Patey and Dyson proposed leaving the pectoralis muscles and named the removal of only the breast and axillary contents the modified radical mastectomy (MRM).
- With more than 25 years of follow-up, it is well accepted that there is no survival difference between RM and MRM.
- Today, the treatment options for patients with early-stage (T1 or T2) breast cancer are total mastectomy (TM) or breast-conservation therapy (BCT).
- BCT involves excision of the tumor and a small portion of surrounding normal breast parenchyma to achieve negative surgical margins and whole-breast adjuvant radiation therapy.
- TM involves removal of the skin, nipple and areolar complex, and breast tissue, including the pectoralis major fascia.
- Sentinel lymph node mapping and biopsy has replaced axillary node dissection as the standard of care for staging the axilla in clinically node-negative patients.
- Intraoperative evaluation of the sentinel lymph node allows for immediate axillary lymph node dissection in cases with identifiable metastatic disease.
- Although sentinel lymph node (SLN) biopsy is considered less invasive than axillary lymph node dissection (ALND), lymphedema may still occur in roughly 3%–7% of patients undergoing an SLN biopsy as compared with 15%–20% of patients undergoing ALND.

and aponeurotic fibers from the rectus abdominus that run medial to the pectoralis major and parallel to the sternum. The sternalis is of anatomic interest only. Langer axillary arch is found in 3%–6% of patients and is a band of latissimus dorsi muscle fibers crossing the axilla superficially and inserting into the pectoralis major muscle medially. Langer arch can cause compression of the axillary artery or vein, or confusion during axillary dissection, but once identified, can be divided without risk.

The pectoralis minor muscle is enveloped in the clavipectoral fascia. It is by opening this fascia along the lateral border of this muscle that the axilla is entered. The axilla contains the axillary vessels and their branches, the brachial plexus, and lymph nodes. The borders of the axilla are listed in Table 7.2. The long thoracic, thoracodorsal, medial pectoral (located lateral to the pectoralis minor muscle), and intercostal brachial nerves are routinely identified during an axillary dissection. While the long thoracic nerve is always preserved

TABLE 7.1
Muscles of the Thoracic Wall and Axilla

MUSCLE	ACTION	NERVE
Pectoralis major	Flexion, adduction, medial rotation of arm	Medial and lateral pectoral
Pectoralis minor	Draws scapula down and forward	Medial pectoral
Subclavius	Draws shoulder down and forward	Long thoracic
Serratus anterior	Rotation of scapula; draws scapula forward	Long thoracic
Subscapularis	Medial rotation of arm	Upper and lower sub scapular
Teres major	Adduction, extension, medial rotation of arm	Lower subscapular
Latissimus dorsi	Adduction, extension, medial rotation of arm; draws shoulder down and backward	Thoracodorsal

TABLE 7.2	
Axillary Boundaries	
BOUNDARIES	**STRUCTURES**
Anterior	Pectoralis major, pectoralis minor, clavipectoral fascia
Posterior	Subscapularis, teres major, latissimus dorsi
Medial	Serratus anterior, 1st–4th ribs, intercostal muscles
Lateral	Humerus, coracobrachialis, biceps muscles

(to avoid a "winged scapula"), the thoracodorsal and medial pectoral nerves are generally preserved, but can be sacrificed in cases of advanced disease when the nerves are encased in tumor. The intercostal brachial nerves run from medial to lateral through the axilla and supply sensation to the medial and posterior upper arm. Although these nerves can be saved, one or two are frequently sacrificed to allow better visualization and access to the subscapular nodes. As a result, patients may complain of varying degrees of regional patchy numbness in the medial and posterior upper arm, some of which may improve in time.

The lymph nodes in the axilla are divided into three levels. Level 1 is located lateral to the border of the pectoralis minor muscle and includes the external mammary, axillary, and scapular nodes. Level 2 is found deep in the pectoralis minor muscle and includes some central and subclavicular nodes. Level 3 is medial to the medial border of the pectoralis minor muscle and extends to Halsted ligament and the costoclavicular ligament of the first rib. This level includes the infraclavicular nodes and, rarely, a supraclavicular node. Interpectoral (Rotter) nodes are found between the pectoralis major and pectoralis minor muscles. While the exact number of axillary nodes is unknown and varies between patients, it is generally accepted that a complete axillary lymph node dissection (ALND) removes approximately 15–20 lymph nodes.

RISK ASSESSMENT, SCREENING, AND DIAGNOSIS

Breast cancer is the most common cancer in women and is second to lung cancer as the most common cause of cancer-related death in women. In 2006, the American Cancer Society (ACS) estimated that nearly 212,920 women would be diagnosed with the disease (2). According to National Cancer Institute (NCI)

Surveillance Epidemiology and End Results (SEER) databases, one in eight women will develop breast cancer in her lifetime. Furthermore, breast-related symptoms, benign or malignant, are one of the most common reasons women seek medical care. For these reasons, an informed discussion regarding patient risk factors and appropriate screening tools should be undertaken with each patient.

It is important to distinguish women who may be at higher-than-normal risk for developing breast cancer. Many factors influence the development of breast cancer, most of which cannot be modified. These include older patient age, a family history of one or more first- or second-degree relatives with breast cancer, and a personal history of biopsy-proven atypical hyperplasia or lobular carcinoma in situ (LCIS). In addition, a history of mantle radiation can significantly increase a woman's risk of developing breast cancer over the next 10–15 years of her life. Modifiable risk factors include the use of postmenopausal hormone replacement therapy (HRT), which can increase one's risk of developing breast cancer by 30%, and possibly parity, with most data suggesting that a multiparous woman is at less risk of developing breast cancer than a nulliparous woman. The most commonly used risk assessment tool is the gail model, which can estimate a woman's overall risk of developing breast cancer over the next five years of her life and over her lifetime as a whole (3). However, this model is limited in patients with a strong family history.

The purpose of breast cancer screening is to facilitate early diagnosis and to decrease breast cancer mortality. The classic triad for routine breast cancer screening includes monthly breast self-exams, annual clinical breast exams, and annual mammography. Beginning at age 25, breast self-exams should be performed at approximately the same time each month or following the completion of menses, as this is the point when the breasts are the least tender. A breast self-exam is best performed while in the shower or while lying down with the ipsilateral arm above the head. An annual clinical breast exam can be performed by an internist, gynecologist, or surgeon. This exam should be a multipositional breast exam and include an evaluation of the axillary and supraclavicular lymph nodes.

The ACS and the NCI recommend annual mammography for all women 40 years and older. Women with a family history of a first-degree relative with breast cancer should begin annual mammography 10 years prior to the age of their relative's diagnosis of breast cancer or age 40, whichever comes first. Mammography is the ideal imaging modality to identify and evaluate both masses and calcifications. The sensitivity of mammography for breast cancer detection ranges between 70% and 85%, while its specificity exceeds 95% (4–6). A complete mammographic examination includes two views of each breast: a mediolateral oblique (MLO) view and a craniocaudal (CC) view. If an abnormality is seen, further images are obtained of the area in question using compression or magnification views.

Mammographic accuracy is limited in younger women and in women with dense breasts. Therefore, adjuncts to the routine screening mammogram include breast ultrasound and, in selected patients, magnetic resonance imaging (MRI) of the breast. Ultrasound can be used as a screening tool or for targeted assessment. Ultrasound cannot replace a screening mammogram because it cannot identify calcifications, which may be the earliest radiologic sign of carcinoma in situ, and because its interpretation is highly operator-dependent. If a mass is identified on mammogram or by palpation, ultrasound can help determine if it is solid or cystic and if its borders are regular or irregular. Malignant masses tend to be irregular, hypoechoic, and "taller than wide."

Data are accumulating to support MRI screening as an adjunct to screening mammography in certain high-risk populations. Currently, the only high-risk population that may derive a benefit from a screening MRI in addition to an annual mammogram is patients with a genetic predisposition to breast cancer, such as that conferred by a mutation in the BRCA 1 or 2 genes (7). The ACS has recently developed guidelines to standardize the recommendations for the use of MRI screening in addition to mammography (8) and plans to develop similar guidelines standardizing MRI techniques. While the sensitivity of MRI for detecting a breast cancer ranges from 86%–100%, the specificity is broad, ranging from 37%–97% (9), resulting in many false-positive biopsies. As a result, this limits its use as a screening modality.

When a suspicious abnormality in the breast is palpated or identified by imaging, a biopsy should be obtained for tissue diagnosis. Biopsy can be performed by direct palpation in a doctor's office, under image guidance, or in the operating room. A fine-needle aspiration (FNA) can be performed of a palpable mass by making several passes with a 22- or 25-gauge needle. The resulting specimen is then ejected onto a glass slide and smeared onto a second slide. The slides are placed into a 95% ethanol solution for fixation and transport to a cytopathologist. An FNA specimen will typically allow for determination between a benign or malignant mass. A core needle biopsy (CNB) employs a large-bore 14-gauge cutting needle that is passed through the mass or image abnormality and retrieves large cores of tissue. This process can be performed by palpation or with mammographic (stereotactic), ultrasound, or MRI

guidance. Vacuum assistance can be added as well to obtain larger volumes of tissue. After CNB, a titanium clip is commonly placed to mark the biopsy area. CNB is the preferred method of diagnosis, as it provides a tissue sample for definitive diagnosis and appropriate surgical planning prior to the operation. In addition to providing a diagnosis, tissue cores can be used to determine the estrogen (ER) or progesterone (PR) receptor, or *HER2/neu* status, of the cancer.

If a CNB cannot be completed, or if the results of the CNB are considered discordant from the image findings, an open surgical biopsy may be needed. Discordance suggests that radiologic images and pathologic diagnosis do not correlate, or that while the images suggest a malignant process, the biopsy pathology is benign. Surgical biopsy of nonpalpable lesions requires needle wire localization placed under stereotactic, sonographic, or MRI guidance. A specimen radiograph is then obtained in the operating room, documenting retrieval of the abnormality.

PATHOLOGY AND STAGING

It is generally believed that most breast cancers arise in the terminal duct-lobular units (TDLU). Breast cancers are then classified as being either in situ or invasive lesions. In situ cancers, specifically ductal carcinoma in situ (DCIS), develop from the epithelial cells lining the lactiferous ducts. Clusters of these cells are separated by orderly, distinct spaces, but all are confined within the basement membrane and surrounded by normal myoepithelial cells (Fig. 7.1). Because DCIS has not penetrated the basement membrane, it lacks the ability to metastasize. Invasive cancers also begin within the TDLU, but characteristically lack any uniform architecture. These tumors grow haphazardly without respect for the basement membrane boundaries, and thus infiltrate into the surrounding stroma (Fig. 7.1). Because invasive cancers extend outside of the TDLU, they have the potential to metastasize to regional lymph nodes or distant sites.

Lobular carcinoma in situ (LCIS) is an abnormal proliferative process arising from the epithelial cells lining the terminal lobules. LCIS cells have bland nuclei that expand and fill the acini of the lobules, but maintain the cross-sectional integrity of the lobular unit. Although LCIS retains the word "carcinoma" in its name, LCIS is not a cancer; instead, it is a multicentric marker of risk. The risk that a woman with LCIS will develop breast cancer is approximately 8- to 10-fold higher than the average woman, or about 25%–30% over her lifetime (Table 7.3). In women who develop cancer after a diagnosis of LCIS, more than 50% of the cancers will be of ductal origin. Classically, LCIS

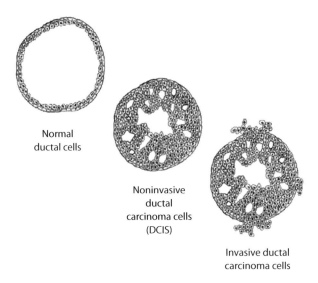

Normal
ductal cells

Noninvasive
ductal
carcinoma cells
(DCIS)

Invasive ductal
carcinoma cells

FIGURE 7.1

Pictorial illustration of normal breast duct, a duct filled with duct carcinoma in situ (*Note*: all cells are confined within the basement membrane of the duct), and invasive ductal carcinoma. Note that the cells have penetrated the basement membrane of the duct and are infiltrating into the surrounding stroma.

TABLE 7.3
Cancer Risk and Borderline Lesions

HISTOLOGY	RELATIVE RISK	ABSOLUTE RISK
Normal	1.0	10%
Hyperplasia, no atypia	~1.0	10%
ADH or ALH	~5.0	10%–20%
LCIS	~10.0	25%–30%

Abbreviations: ADH, atypical ductal hyperplasia; ALH, atypical lobular hyperplasia; LCIS, lobular carcinoma in situ.

Note: Relative risk is a *ratio of incidences* or (CA incidence with factor x)/ (CA incidence without factor x). Absolute risk is a percentage or the proportion of a defined population who develop cancer.

and carcinoma in situ. In all likelihood, atypical hyperplasias are part of a spectrum of lesions that may have the potential to progress to carcinoma in situ. The challenge of distinguishing a severely atypical hyperplasia from an early DCIS is well known to pathologists. The risk that a woman with an atypical hyperplasia will develop breast cancer is about four to five times the average woman's risk (Table 7.3). However, if the woman has both atypical hyperplasia and a significant family history of breast cancer, her risk may be nine times higher than that of the average woman. If ADH or ALH is found at CNB, a surgical excision of that area is recommended to rule out an associated malignant lesion. The incidence of breast cancer at excisional biopsy is inversely related to the size of the core needle used for biopsy. For example, when ADH is diagnosed by 14-gauge CNB, cancer is found in the surgical specimen in 50% of patients; however, when ADH is diagnosed by 11-gauge CNB, cancer is found in the surgical specimen in 20% of patients (10). Furthermore, if ADH is diagnosed by a vacuum-assisted CNB, cancer is found in the surgical specimen in 10%–15% of patients. Of all patients who are upstaged from ADH to cancer after surgical excision, 75% will have DCIS and the remaining 25% will have invasive disease.

DCIS is the earliest form of breast cancer and accounted for 61,980 cases of breast cancer in 2006 (2). Over the last 20 years, there has been a dramatic rise in the incidence of DCIS, primarily due to the implementation of routine mammographic screening and the increasing capability of imaging to detect small lesions.

DCIS begins in the terminal ducts and is confined within them. As DCIS cells multiply, they are pushed centrally within the duct and away from their blood supply, causing cell death and calcification. These pleomorphic calcifications may be the first mammographic signs of DCIS. It is believed that most cases of DCIS will progress to invasive ductal cancer if they are left untreated.

Four subtypes of DCIS exist and are categorized according to their architectural structure: solid, micropapillary, cribriform, and comedo. In many published series, the comedo form predominates over the other three noncomedo forms. Comedo necrosis is characterized by its high nuclear grade, increased mitotic activity, and central necrosis.

Regardless of pathologic subtype, all forms of DCIS require surgical excision with negative margins for optimal treatment. While lumpectomy, with or without radiation therapy or mastectomy, may be appropriate, the ultimate treatment will depend on the amount of DCIS present, the patient's age and breast size, the ability to achieve negative margins, and the type of DCIS found. Lymph nodes are not routinely

lacks mammographic findings. Therefore, the finding of LCIS at biopsy is often incidental and, although controversial, a CNB diagnosis of LCIS should generally be surgically excised to rule out an associated malignant lesion. If LCIS is the only finding at excision, however, negative margins are not required because LCIS is a marker of risk and not a cancer.

Atypical ductal hyperplasia (ADH) and atypical lobular hyperplasia (ALH) represent borderline proliferative processes that histologically lie somewhere between the usual type of hyperplasia without atypia evaluated unless the DCIS presents as a mass (with a higher likelihood of microinvasion), or if a mastectomy is planned. In the TNM staging system, DCIS is categorized as a stage 0 breast cancer.

Invasive mammary cancer accounts for approximately 80% of all breast cancers. Invasive cancer is broadly divided into two categories based on their growth patterns: ductal or lobular. Ductal cancers tend to grow as a coherent mass and appear clinically as a palpable mass or mammographically as a mass, architectural distortion, or group of calcifications. Lobular cancers tend to permeate the breast in a single file, referred to as "Indian file" nature, making them harder to detect both clinically and mammographically. Invasive ductal cancer (IDC) is the most common type of breast cancer, accounting for 50%–70% of cases, followed by invasive lobular cancer (ILC) which represents 10%–15% of all invasive cancers. Less common variants of invasive ductal cancer include tubular, mucinous, papillary, medullary, and metaplastic carcinoma. While the first three are generally considered less aggressive due to their typically good prognostic features, like low nuclear grade and low mitotic index, medullary and metaplastic cancers tend to have poor prognostic features and are, therefore, considered more aggressive. Other, rarer tumors of the breast include squamous carcinoma, both benign and malignant phyllodes tumors, primary breast sarcoma or lymphoma, and metastases to the breast (most commonly from the contralateral breast, leukemia, lymphoma, lung, thyroid, cervix, ovary, and kidney).

The prognosis of invasive breast cancer is determined by the size of the tumor, histologic and nuclear grade, the presence of lymphovascular invasion, the number of nodal metastases, the hormone receptor status (ER or PR), and *HER2/neu* stains.

Inflammatory breast cancer (IBC) carries a poor prognosis and accounts for roughly 1%–6% of all invasive breast cancers. The incidence of IBC is highest among African Americans (10.1%), followed by Caucasians (6.2%), and then by other ethnic groups (5.1%) (11). IBC is a clinical diagnosis that implies the simultaneous development of inflammatory changes in the skin of the breast and the development of an aggressive tumor within the breast. The classic diagnosis as defined by Haagensen in 1971 includes diffuse erythema and edema of the skin, peau d'orange, tenderness, warmth, induration, and diffuse tumor within the breast (12). If IBC is suspected, a skin biopsy may confirm dermal lymphatic invasion by tumor emboli. However, a negative biopsy does not rule out the diagnosis of IBC. Patients with IBC generally present with a history of worsening erythema and skin changes, despite being treated with antibiotics for mastitis or cellulitis of the breast. IBC is regarded as stage IIIC breast cancer. Optimal therapy includes neoadjuvant chemotherapy, followed by a modified radical mastectomy incorporating all involved skin, and postmastectomy chest-wall radiation. Overall five-year survival for IBC is approximately 40%.

Male breast cancer (MBC) accounts for less than 1% of all breast cancers and less than 0.5% of all cancers occurring in men. Male breasts lack lobules; therefore, nearly all male breast cancers are of ductal origin, and more than 80% are invasive. Most MBCs present as a palpable, retroareolar mass and are best treated with a mastectomy. Since routine screening is not performed for MBC, most MBCs present at a later stage than female breast cancer. However, MBC carries the same prognosis, stage for stage, as female breast cancer.

BREAST SURGERY

Historically, the first major advance in breast cancer surgery was described by William Halsted in 1894. Halsted theorized that breast cancer was a local-regional disease that spread in an orderly, centripetal fashion. In his manuscripts, he popularized the removal of the breast, pectoralis muscles, and axillary lymph nodes in levels 1, 2, and 3. This procedure was known as the radical mastectomy (RM) or Halsted mastectomy, and revolutionized the way 19th century surgeons approached breast cancer surgery. Following RM, Halsted documented a local recurrence rate of 6% at three years, which was significantly lower than the 70% shown by his 19th century colleagues (13); however, the operation was severely disfiguring. In 1948, Patey and Dyson proposed leaving the pectoralis muscles and named the removal of only the breast and axillary contents the "modified radical mastectomy" (MRM). With more than 25 years of follow-up, it is well accepted that there is no survival difference between RM and MRM (14).

In the 1970s, Bernard Fisher proposed an alternate theory, hypothesizing that breast cancer was, in fact, a systemic disease and that variations in local-regional therapy were unlikely to affect overall survival. He popularized breast conservation surgery (BCT), which was ultimately studied in a prospective, randomized fashion in thousands of women by The National Surgical Adjuvant Breast and Bowel Project (NSABP), NCI, and the Milan trialists groups. These groups compared MRM, lumpectomy alone, and lumpectomy plus radiation in a variety of study designs. Although local recurrences were higher in those patients having lumpectomy without radiation (approximately 4% per year vs 1% per year), there was no difference in overall or distant disease-free survival at 20 years follow-up between the groups (15).

Today, the treatment options for patients with early stage (T1 or T2) breast cancer are TM or breast-conservation surgery with adjuvant radiation therapy. Both options include an evaluation of the axillary lymph nodes. Approximately 80% of patients are eligible for BCT. Relative and absolute contraindications to BCT are listed in Table 7.4. BCT involves excision of the tumor and a small portion of surrounding normal breast parenchyma. Incisions are made along the lines of skin tension, and in general incision placement should be planned to facilitate subsequent excision if mastectomy is required. Unless the cancer is palpable, needle localization using mammographic (stereotactic), ultrasound (US), or MRI guidance is required to assist in surgical excision. Frequently, a specimen radiograph is performed to document retrieval of the cancer and the biopsy site marker. Surgical clips may be left to denote the extent of the excisional cavity to aid in radiation treatment planning. Successful BCT mandates achieving negative surgical margins, although the definition of a negative surgical margin continues to be a matter of debate. In all NSABP conservation trials, no tumor at the inked margin was considered negative. However, other studies report negative margins ranging from 1–3 mm. Regardless of definition, patients who are properly selected for BCT and have their cancer entirely removed have acceptable local recurrence rates, generally less than 10% at five years, when compared with patients who have undergone a mastectomy for similar sized early-stage breast cancer.

TM involves removal of the skin, nipple and areolar complex, and breast tissue, including the pectoralis major fascia. Many patients with early-stage breast cancer who have a TM (either by choice or out of necessity) are candidates for immediate breast reconstruction. When immediate reconstruction is chosen, a smaller ellipse or oval of skin is removed, incorporating the nipple and areolar complex. This procedure is called a skin-sparing mastectomy. By taking less skin, the breast retains its natural skin envelope and inframammary fold, which ultimately helps re-create a more natural and cosmetically acceptable reconstructed breast. Breast reconstruction can be performed with implant-based techniques or with tissue-transfer techniques, depending on the patient's body habitus and desired reconstructive outcomes.

All patients with an invasive cancer should undergo a pathologic evaluation of the axillary lymph nodes to allow for appropriate staging and treatment. Until the late 1990s, the standard of care was for each patient to undergo an axillary lymph node dissection (ALND) in addition to BCT or mastectomy. In 1997, Giuliano introduced the concept of the axillary sentinel lymph node (SLN) biopsy for patients with breast cancer and provided histopathologic validation of this hypothesis (16). This theory is based on the idea that the lymphatic drainage within the breast is uniform and constant, and that the breast drains in an orderly fashion to a "sentinel" node within the axilla. The SLN biopsy procedure entails the use of an intradermal injection of a radiolabeled isotope (technecium sulfur colloid) and a vital blue dye. Isotope can be injected intradermally or intraparenchymally with equal chances of success. Blue dye is injected intraparenchymally or into the subareolar plexus (Fig. 7.2). Any node that is found to be "hot" with the use of a gamma probe, or visualized as "blue," is considered a sentinel lymph node (17). In the Memorial Sloan-Kettering Cancer Center experience, the median number of SLNs removed per axilla is three. Intraoperative evaluation of the SLN, either by frozen section or by touch prep analysis, allows for immediate ALND in cases with identifiable metastatic

TABLE 7.4	
Absolute and Relative Contraindications to BCT	
ABSOLUTE	**RELATIVE**
Multicentric cancer	Poor cosmetic outcome
Inflammatory breast cancer	Tumor > 5 cm
Inability to receive radiation therapy[a]	

[a]May include history of previous irradiation to the breast, history of collagen vascular disease, or limited access to care.

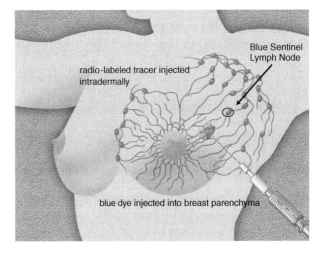

FIGURE 7.2

Pictorial illustration of the sentinel lymph node (SLN) mapping technique. Radiolabeled isotope is injected intradermally, and blue dye is injected intraparenchymally. The SLN is then identified in the axillary nodal basin as a hot and/or blue lymph node.

disease. If tumor is found, an immediate ALND can be performed. Subsequent routine pathologic analysis, with or without enhanced evaluation, including immunohistochemistry, is performed on all SLNs. If nodal metastases are identified, the standard of care at this time is delayed ALND.

The accuracy of SLN biopsy has been validated in multiple centers and with a variety of techniques—isotope or blue dye alone, intradermal or intraparenchymal injection, and injection of tracers over the tumor or into the subareolar plexus. Despite differing techniques, the accuracy of SLN biopsy has been demonstrated to be 97% and has been validated with "backup" ALND in 69 studies involving more than 8,000 women. Equally as important, the false-negative rate of SLN biopsy across these series has remained acceptable at 7% (18). The risk of axillary recurrence after negative SLN biopsy appears to be small and is reported at levels less than 1%; however, follow-up is limited at only two years (19). Longer follow-up is needed to compare the risk of local recurrence after SLN biopsy with the known risk of axillary recurrence after a full ALND, which is approximately 0%–2%, with follow-up ranging from 72 to 180 months (2,20,21).

Although SLN biopsy is considered less invasive than ALND, lymphedema may still occur in roughly 3%–7% of patients undergoing an SLN biopsy as compared with 15%–20% of patients undergoing ALND. There is also a small risk of isosulfan blue dye allergy, presenting most commonly as hives, in 1% of patients, but this has been reported to include anaphylaxis in less than 0.5% of patients. Additional morbidities of SLN biopsy include paresthesias in up to 7% of patients and decreased range of motion of the shoulder or arm in 3%–5% of patients. Longer follow-up of patients having SLN biopsy is ongoing, but the practice of SLN biopsy is considered the standard of care for staging the axilla in women with invasive breast cancer.

In patients with pure DCIS, an SLN biopsy is generally not indicated, as pure DCIS does not have metastatic potential. However, in less than 10% of cases, DCIS can present as a mass. In patients with DCIS presenting as a mass and diagnosed by CNB, SLN biopsy may be performed at the time of lumpectomy, as these cases have a much higher likelihood of harboring microinvasive disease, which carries the risk of nodal metastases in 5% of cases (22). Alternatively, patients can undergo excision of the DCIS alone for definitive diagnosis and return to the operating room (OR) for SLN biopsy should invasive disease be identified. In patients with DCIS who choose mastectomy or who have contraindications to BCT and must have a mastectomy, SLN biopsy should be strongly considered at the time of mastectomy because SLN mapping cannot be performed after mastectomy. If a patient were diagnosed with a focus of invasive breast cancer, a traditional ALND would be the only option for axillary staging.

RADIATION THERAPY

Currently, radiation to the entire breast, known as whole-breast irradiation, is the standard of care following BCT. Radiation therapy is generally given after chemotherapy if this is also indicated. Radiation treatments can be administered to the breast with the patient lying supine or prone, depending on the original tumor location and the patient's body habitus. A total of 5000 Gy are given over six weeks. The first 25 treatments incorporate the entire breast, while the last 5 may or may not be given as a "boost" just to the tumor bed. At this time, a multicenter randomized trial (NSABP-39) is ongoing to determine the effectiveness of partial-breast radiation techniques compared with whole-breast irradiation.

Some patients require postmastectomy radiation treatments to the chest wall, with or without radiation to the regional lymph nodes. This is generally recommended in patients with locally advanced breast cancers, tumors larger than 5 cm, inflammatory breast cancer, and in patients with four or more positive lymph nodes. Radiation treatment to the axilla is rarely added, but may be used after complete axillary dissection in patients with more than 10 positive nodes. The combination of both ALND and radiation treatment to the axilla can greatly increase the risk of lymphedema, with reported rates of more than 50%.

References

1. Wellings SR, Jensen HM, Marcum RG. An atlas of subgross pathology of the human breast with special reference to possible precancerous lesions. J Natl Cancer Inst. 1975;55(2):231–273.
2. Louis-Sylvestre C, Clough K, Asselain B, et al. Axillary treatment in conservative management of operable breast cancer: dissection or radiotherapy? Results of a randomized study with 15 years of follow-up. J Clin Oncol. 2004;22(1):97–101.
3. Gail MH, Brinton LA, Byar DP, et al. Projecting individualized probabilities of developing breast cancer for white females who are being examined annually. J Natl Cancer Inst. 1989;81(24):1879–1886.
4. Poplack SP, Tosteson AN, Grove MR, Wells WA, Carney PA. Mammography in 53,803 women from the New Hampshire mammography network. Radiology. 2000;217(3):832–840.
5. Banks E, Reeves G, Beral V, et al. Influence of personal characteristics of individual women on sensitivity and specificity of mammography in the Million Women Study: cohort study. BMJ. 2004;329(7464):477.
6. Smith-Bindman R, Chu P, Miglioretti DL, et al. Physician predictors of mammographic accuracy. J Natl Cancer Inst. 2005;97(5):358–367.

7. Kuhl CK, Schrading S, Leutner CC, et al. Mammography, breast ultrasound, and magnetic resonance imaging for surveillance of women at high familial risk for breast cancer. *J Clin Oncol*. 2005;23(33):8469–8476.

8. Saslow D, Boetes C, Burke W, et al. American cancer society guidelines for breast screening with MRI as an adjunct to mammography. *CA Cancer J Clin*. 2007;57(2):75–89.

9. Morris EA, Schwartz LH, Dershaw DD, van Zee KJ, Abramson AF, Liberman L. MR imaging of the breast in patients with occult primary breast carcinoma. *Radiology*. 1997;205(2):437–440.

10. Liberman L, Cohen MA, Dershaw DD, Abramson AF, Hann LE, Rosen PP. Atypical ductal hyperplasia diagnosed at stereotaxic core biopsy of breast lesions: an indication for surgical biopsy. *AJR Am J Roentgenol*. 1995;164(5):1111–1113.

11. Levine PH, Steinhorn SC, Ries LG, Aron JL. Inflammatory breast cancer: the experience of the surveillance, epidemiology, and end results (SEER) program. *J Natl Cancer Inst*. 1985;74(2):291–297.

12. Haagensen C. *Diseases of the Breast*, 2nd ed. Philadelphia: Saunders; 1971.

13. Halstead W. The results of radical operations for the cure of carcinoma of the breast. *Ann Surg*. 1907;(46):1–19.

14. Fisher B, Jeong JH, Anderson S, Bryant J, Fisher ER, Wolmark N. Twenty-five-year follow-up of a randomized trial comparing radical mastectomy, total mastectomy, and total mastectomy followed by irradiation. *N Engl J Med*. 2002;347(8):567–575.

15. Fisher B, Anderson S, Bryant J, et al. Twenty-year follow-up of a randomized trial comparing total mastectomy, lumpectomy, and lumpectomy plus irradiation for the treatment of invasive breast cancer. *N Engl J Med*. 2002;347(16):1233–1241.

16. Turner RR, Ollila DW, Krasne DL, Giuliano AE. Histopathologic validation of the sentinel lymph node hypothesis for breast carcinoma. *Ann Surg*. 1997;226(3):271–276; discussion 6–8.

17. Cody HS, 3rd, Borgen PI. State-of-the-art approaches to sentinel node biopsy for breast cancer: study design, patient selection, technique, and quality control at Memorial Sloan-Kettering Cancer Center. *Surg Oncol*. 1999;8(2):85–91.

18. Kim T, Giuliano AE, Lyman GH. Lymphatic mapping and sentinel lymph node biopsy in early-stage breast carcinoma: a metaanalysis. *Cancer*. 2006;106(1):4–16.

19. Naik AM, Fey J, Gemignani M, et al. The risk of axillary relapse after sentinel lymph node biopsy for breast cancer is comparable with that of axillary lymph node dissection: a follow-up study of 4008 procedures. *Ann Surg*. 2004;240(3):462–468; discussion 8–71.

20. Recht A, Pierce SM, Abner A, et al. Regional nodal failure after conservative surgery and radiotherapy for early-stage breast carcinoma. *J Clin Oncol*. 1991;9(6):988–996.

21. Veronesi U, Salvadori B, Luini A, et al. Conservative treatment of early breast cancer. Long-term results of 1232 cases treated with quadrantectomy, axillary dissection, and radiotherapy. *Ann Surg*. 1990;211(3):250–259.

22. Klauber-DeMore N, Tan LK, Liberman L, et al. Sentinel lymph node biopsy: is it indicated in patients with high-risk ductal carcinoma-in-situ and ductal carcinoma-in-situ with microinvasion? *Ann Surg Oncol*. 2000;7(9):636–642.

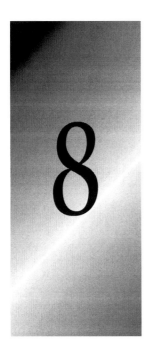

Principles of Breast Reconstruction in Cancer

Joseph J. Disa
Colleen M. McCarthy

Women who elect to undergo mastectomy for the treatment or prophylaxis of breast cancer may consider breast reconstruction in an attempt to improve their outward appearance, their sense of femininity, and ultimately, their self-esteem. For these women, the preservation of a normal breast form through breast reconstruction has been shown to have a positive effect on their psychological well-being.

RECONSTRUCTIVE OPTIONS

Contemporary techniques provide numerous options for postmastectomy reconstruction. These options include single-stage reconstruction with a standard or adjustable implant, tissue expansion followed by placement of a permanent implant, combined autologous tissue/implant reconstruction, or autogenous tissue reconstruction alone.

Procedure selection is based on a range of patient variables, including availability of local, regional, and distant donor tissues; size and shape of the desired breast(s); surgical risk; and most importantly, patient preference. Although autogenous tissue reconstruction is generally thought to produce the most natural-looking and feeling breast(s), the relative magnitude of these procedures is great. Many women will instead opt for a prosthetic reconstruction, choosing a less invasive operative procedure with a faster recovery time. Individualized selection of a reconstructive technique for each patient will be a predominant factor in achieving a reconstructive success.

TIMING OF RECONSTRUCTION

Immediate postmastectomy reconstruction is currently considered the standard of care in breast reconstruction. Numerous studies have demonstrated that reconstruction performed concurrently with mastectomy is an oncologically safe option for women with breast cancer (1). Immediate reconstruction is assumed to be advantageous when compared with delayed procedures based on improved cost-effectiveness and reduced inconvenience for the patient. Moreover, studies have shown that women who undergo immediate reconstruction have less psychological distress about the loss of a breast and have a better overall quality of life (2).

Technically, reconstruction is facilitated in the immediate setting because of the pliability of the native skin envelope and the delineation of the natural infra-mammary fold. The increasing use of postoperative radiotherapy for earlier staged breast cancers has, however, challenged this thinking. Adjuvant radiotherapy

KEY POINTS

- Women who elect to undergo mastectomy for the treatment or prophylaxis of breast cancer may consider breast reconstruction in an attempt to improve their outward appearance, their sense of femininity, and ultimately, their self-esteem.
- Breast reconstruction options include single-stage reconstruction with a standard or adjustable implant, tissue expansion followed by placement of a permanent implant, combined autologous tissue/implant reconstruction, or autogenous tissue reconstruction alone.
- Reconstruction performed concurrently with mastectomy is an oncologically safe option for women with breast cancer.
- Women who undergo immediate reconstruction have less psychological distress about the loss of a breast and have a better overall quality of life.
- Prosthetic reconstruction techniques include single-stage implant reconstruction with either a standard or adjustable permanent prosthesis, two-stage tissue expander/implant reconstruction, and combined implant/autogenous tissue reconstruction.

- To date, there is no definitive evidence linking breast implants to cancer, immunologic diseases, neurologic problems, or other systemic diseases.
- Reconstructive techniques using the lower abdominal donor site include the pedicled transverse rectus abdominis myocutaneous (TRAM) flap, the free TRAM flap, the free muscle-sparing TRAM, the deep inferior epigastric perforator (DIEP) flap, and the superficial inferior epigastric artery (SIEA) flap.
- There is some data to suggest that muscle- and fascia-sparing techniques, such as the use of DIEP flaps, result in measurably better postoperative truncal strength. Interestingly, however, muscle-sparing techniques do not appear to decrease the risk of abdominal bulging or hernia formation.
- Because surgical scars fade and tissue firmness subsides with time, the results of autologous breast reconstruction tend to improve as the patient ages rather than deteriorate, as with prosthetic reconstruction.

has been shown to increase the risk of postoperative complications (3,4). Based on the data, whether or not to perform immediate reconstruction for patients in whom radiation therapy is planned remains controversial. Similarly, for those who may be unwilling to decide about reconstruction while adjusting to their cancer diagnosis, delayed breast reconstruction may be an option.

IMPLANT-BASED RECONSTRUCTION

Techniques

Prosthetic reconstruction techniques include single-stage implant reconstruction with either a standard or an adjustable permanent prosthesis, two-stage tissue expander/implant reconstruction, and combined autogenous tissue/implant reconstruction.

Single-Stage Implant Reconstruction

Immediate single-stage breast reconstruction with a standard implant is best suited to the occasional patient with adequate skin at the mastectomy site and small, nonptotic breasts. Selection criteria for single-stage,

adjustable implant reconstruction is similar; yet, it is the preferred technique when the ability to adjust the volume of the device postoperatively is desired. In small-breasted women where the skin deficiency is minimal, the implant can be partially filled at the time of reconstruction and gradually inflated to the desired volume postoperatively.

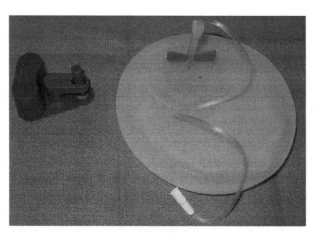

FIGURE 8.1

Textured surface, integrated valve, biodimensional-shaped tissue expander with a Magnasite fill port-locating device.

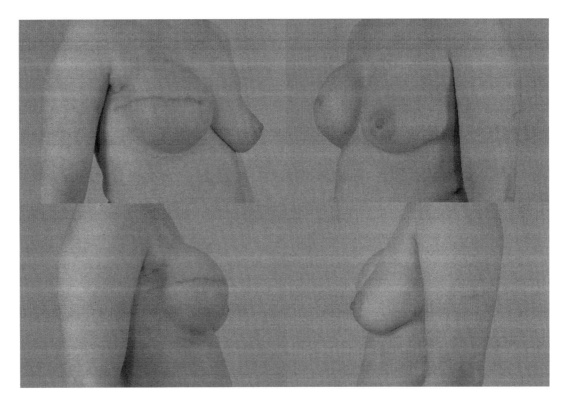

FIGURE 8.2

Unilateral right breast reconstruction with tissue expander. The expander is intentionally overfilled to maximize projection and inferior-pole skin.

Two-Stage Tissue Expander/Implant Reconstruction

While satisfactory results can be obtained with single-stage reconstruction, in the vast majority of patients, a far more reliable approach involves two-stage expander/implant reconstruction. Tissue expansion is used when there is insufficient tissue after mastectomy to create the desired size and shape of a breast in a single stage.

A tissue expander is placed under the skin and muscles of the chest wall at the primary procedure (Fig. 8.1). Postoperatively, tissue expansion is performed over a period of weeks or months, the soft tissues stretched until the desired breast volume is achieved (Fig. 8.2). Exchange of the temporary expander for a permanent implant occurs at a subsequent operation. A capsulotomy is often performed at this second stage. By releasing the surrounding scar capsule, breast projection and breast ptosis are increased. Similarly, precise positioning of the inframammary fold can be addressed (Fig. 8.3).

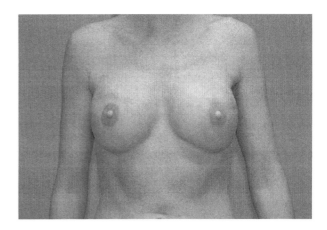

FIGURE 8.3

Bilateral breast reconstruction with silicone gel implants after nipple areola reconstruction.

Combined Autogenous Tissue/ Implant Reconstruction

Nearly every patient who undergoes a mastectomy is a candidate for some form of implant-based reconstruction. Implant reconstruction alone is contraindicated, however, in the presence of an inadequate skin envelope. A large skin excision at the time of mastectomy, due to previous biopsies or locally advanced disease, may preclude primary coverage of a prosthetic device. Similarly, previous chest wall irradiation and/or postmastectomy radiotherapy are considered by many a relative contraindication for implant-based breast reconstruction (5,6).

In patients with thin, contracted, or previously irradiated skin, the ipsilateral latissimus dorsi myocutaneous flap can provide additional skin, soft tissue, and muscle, obviating the need for or facilitating the process of tissue expansion. The skin island is designed under the bra line or along the lateral margin of the muscle, and the flap is tunneled anteriorly into the mastectomy defect. Although the latissimus dorsi myocutaneous flap is extremely reliable, the tissue bulk is usually inadequate. Thus, a permanent implant is often placed beneath the flap to provide adequate volume.

The latissimus dorsi flap is advantageous in that it can provide additional vascularized skin and muscle to the breast mound in a single operative procedure. Its disadvantages include the creation of new chest scars, a back donor scar, and the fact that the transfer of autogenous tissue does not, in this setting, eliminate the need for an implant.

Implant Selection

Currently, both saline and silicone gel implants are available for use in breast reconstruction. While the stigma surrounding the use of silicone-filled implants still exists, issues of silicone safety have been carefully investigated (7). To date, there is no definitive evidence linking breast implants to cancer, immunologic diseases, neurologic problems, or other systemic diseases. The use of silicone gel implants generally allows for a softer, more natural-appearing breast. Alternatively, the use of saline-filled implants allows for minor volume adjustments to be made at the time of implant placement. And while saline-filled implants may offer the greatest piece of mind for some patients in terms of safety, implant palpability and rippling is more likely.

Complications

Prosthetic breast reconstruction is a relatively simple technique that is generally well tolerated. Complications are generally centered on the breast, with minimal systemic health implications and minimal overall patient morbidity. Thus, implant reconstruction can often be performed on patients who might not be suitable candidates for the more complex surgical procedure required for breast reconstruction with autogenous tissue.

Perioperative complications, including hematoma, seroma, infection, skin flap necrosis, and implant exposure/extrusion, can occur. Late complications include implant deflation or rupture and capsular contracture. Capsular contracture occurs when the scar tissue or capsule that normally forms around the implant tightens and squeezes the implant. While capsular contracture occurs to some extent around all implants, in some, the degree of contracture will increase in severity over time (8). A pathologic capsular contracture or implant malfunction may require revisional surgery years following completion of reconstruction.

Advantages and Disadvantages

Implant reconstruction has the distinct advantage of combining a lesser operative procedure with the capability of achieving excellent results. The use of tissue expansion provides donor tissue with similar qualities of skin texture, color, and sensation compared to the contralateral breast. Donor-site morbidity is eliminated with use of a prosthetic device; by using the patient's mastectomy incision to place the prosthesis, no new scars are introduced.

Although implant techniques are technically easier than autologous reconstruction, with shorter hospitalization and a quicker recovery, they can provide additional reconstructive challenges. Patients who undergo tissue expander/implant breast reconstruction will experience varying degrees of discomfort and chest wall asymmetry during the expansion phase. In addition, patients must make more frequent office visits for percutaneous expansion. The breast mound achieved with implant reconstruction is generally more rounded, less ptotic, and will often require a contralateral matching procedure in order to achieve symmetry.

AUTOGENOUS TISSUE RECONSTRUCTION

Techniques

Numerous options exist for autogenous tissue reconstruction. Reconstructive techniques using the lower abdominal donor site include the pedicled transverse rectus abdominis myocutaneous (TRAM) flap, the free TRAM flap, the free muscle-sparing TRAM, the deep inferior epigastric perforator (DIEP) flap, and the superficial inferior epigastric artery (SIEA) flap. The TRAM or related flap is the most frequently used method for autogenous breast reconstruction. TRAM and TRAM-related flaps are designed so that the skin islands are oriented transversely across the lower abdomen and the resulting "abdominoplastylike scar" is camouflaged. Other autogenous tissue alternatives include the latissimus dorsi flap, gluteal flaps, the Rubens fat pad flap, and perforator flaps from the gluteal and lateral thigh donor sites.

Pedicled TRAM Flap Reconstruction

The blood supply of the pedicled TRAM flap is derived from the superior epigastric artery. The rectus muscle serves as the vascular carrier for a large ellipse of lower abdominal skin and fat. After harvest of the flap, a subcutaneous tunnel from the abdominal donor site to the mastectomy defect is created in order to accommodate the flap. The abdominal donor site is closed by reapproximating the anterior rectus sheath and by advancing the remaining superior skin edge of the donor site as a modified abdominoplasty. The ipsilateral, the contralateral, or bilateral rectus muscles may be used. The muscle-sparing TRAM flap, which is limited to the portion of muscle that encompasses the lateral and medial rows of perforating vessels, is a modification of the TRAM flap, which theoretically minimizes violation of the abdominal wall and the risk of donor-site morbidity. The muscle-sparing TRAM can be performed either as a pedicled flap or free tissue transfer.

Free TRAM Flap Reconstruction

The microvascular, or free, TRAM flap is based upon the more dominant inferior epigastric vascular pedicle, which permits transfer of larger volumes of tissue with a minimal risk of fat necrosis. Similarly, because the blood supply to a free TRAM is more robust, the procedure can be used with a greater degree of safety in patients with risk factors such as tobacco use, diabetes, and obesity. Microvascular anastomoses are generally performed to the thoracodorsal or internal mammary vessels. Insetting of the free tissue transfer is facilitated because the flap is not tethered by a pedicle. In addition, the potential abdominal contour deformity arising from the bulk of the transposed pedicled flap is eliminated (Figs. 8.4 and 8.5).

DIEP Flap Reconstruction

The DIEP flap is a further refinement of the conventional muscle-sparing free TRAM flap. The overlying skin and subcutaneous tissues are perfused by transmuscular perforators originating from the deep inferior epigastric artery. When a perforating vessel is found, it is dissected away from the surrounding muscle and traced to its origin from the vascular pedicle. Because no muscle is harvested, donor-site morbidity is theoretically minimized (9,10). Harvest of the DIEP flap can be a tedious dissection, however, which can prolong surgical time. In addition, flap vascularity may be less than that of free TRAM flap because of the small size and number of the perforating vessels in some patients. A higher risk of venous insufficiency, partial flap loss, and fat necrosis compared with free TRAM flaps has been reported (11) (Fig. 8.6).

SIEA Flap Reconstruction

The SIEA flap can be used in breast reconstruction, with an aesthetic outcome similar to that of TRAM and DIEP flaps. The SIEA flap allows for transfer of a moderate volume of lower abdominal tissue based on

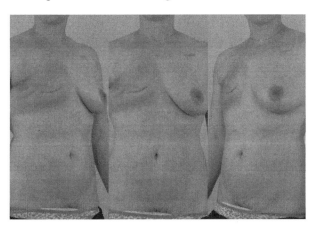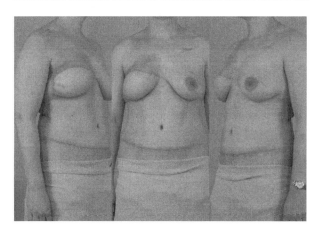

FIGURE 8.4

A: Right modified radical mastectomy and postoperative irradiation. Note radiation-induced skin changes on right chest wall. B: Delayed right breast reconstruction with a free TRAM flap. Photo taken prior to planned nipple areolar reconstruction.

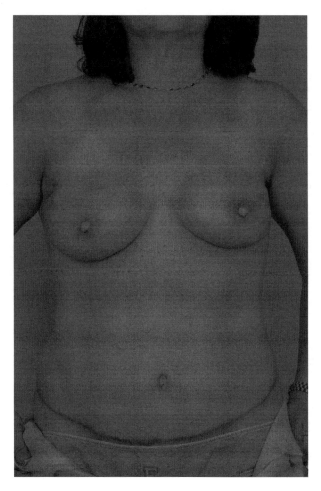

FIGURE 8.5

Bilateral free TRAM flap reconstruction was performed immediately following bilateral skin-sparing mastectomies. Bilateral nipple areolae reconstruction has been completed.

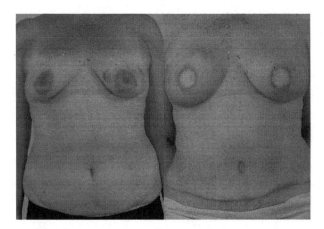

FIGURE 8.6

Bilateral free DIEP flap reconstruction following bilateral skin-sparing mastectomies, preoperative (left) and postoperative (right).

the superficial inferior epigastric artery. Based solely on the superficial system, the flap can be elevated off the anterior rectus sheath without excision or incision of the rectus abdominis muscle. Abdominal donor-site morbidity is theoretically eliminated. Because of the absence or inadequacy of the superficial epigastric vessels in up to 70% of patients, however, the use of the flap is limited (12).

Further Options in Autologous Tissue Reconstruction

A patient desiring a TRAM or related flap must have adequate tissues in the lower abdomen to be considered a candidate. Additionally, a patient's lifestyle must allow for the potential diminution of truncal strength. One of the primary reasons for use of an alternate flap includes inadequate abdominal fat in a patient with a slender body habitus. In addition, high-risk abdominal scars may predispose to flap necrosis and/or wound healing problems at the abdominal donor site. In a situation where a patient is an inappropriate TRAM flap candidate, yet still desires an autogenous reconstruction, alternate flap options include the Rubens fat pad flap, gluteal myocutaneous flaps, and perforator flaps from the gluteal and lateral thigh donor sites. These free flaps are much less commonly employed and have distinct disadvantages when compared with flaps from the abdominal donor site.

Complications

Autogenous reconstruction is more complex than implant-based reconstruction and requires a much lengthier, more invasive surgical procedure. Postmastectomy reconstruction with a TRAM or related flap generally requires a five-to-seven-day hospitalization and a four-to-six-week convalesce. Because of the magnitude of the procedure, complications do occur. Fortunately, major complications are uncommon.

Use of the free TRAM flap decreases the rate of complications compared to pedicled TRAM flaps. The incidence of both fat necrosis and partial flap loss is close to 5% in most series, as compared to 15%–20% in pedicled flaps (13,14). The rate of total flap loss is 1%–2% in most series and is comparable to those published for the pedicled TRAM flap (15). Smoking, chest wall irradiation, significant abdominal scarring, and obesity are associated with an increased complication rate (11).

There is some data to suggest that muscle- and fascia-sparing techniques, such as the use of DIEP flaps, result in measurably better postoperative truncal strength (9,10). Postoperative abdominal hernia, or more commonly, abdominal wall laxity remains a persistent issue for some patients choosing TRAM reconstruction. Interestingly, muscle-sparing techniques do not appear to decrease the risk of abdominal bulging or hernia formation (16).

Alterations in shape and size of the reconstructed breast are sometimes required, and donor site adjustments do exist. Common secondary adjustments include liposuction of the flap for improved contour, abdominal scar revision and hernia repair, and fat necrosis excision.

Advantages and Disadvantages

Breast reconstruction with autologous tissue can generally achieve more durable, natural-appearing results than reconstruction based on prosthetic implants alone. The breast mound reconstructed with autologous tissue is closer in consistency to the native breast. Because surgical scars fade and tissue firmness subsides with time, the results of autologous breast reconstruction tend to improve as the patient ages rather than deteriorate, as with prosthetic reconstruction. Complete restoration of the breast mound in a single stage is possible in most patients.

Permanent dependency on prosthesis can also lead to long-term complications, such as implant leak or deflation, often occurring many years after an otherwise successful reconstruction. Autogenous tissue reconstructions, therefore, may be especially appropriate for younger patients, who might be expected to live longer and be particularly susceptible to the longer-term problems of prosthetic reconstructions.

ADJUVANT THERAPY AND BREAST RECONSTRUCTION

Earlier breast cancers are being increasingly treated with adjuvant chemotherapy and radiotherapy in an attempt to increase survival. Chemotherapy does not increase the risk of postoperative complications. Previous reports have also demonstrated that patients who undergo immediate breast reconstruction are not predisposed to delays in administration of adjuvant chemotherapy compared with patients undergo mastectomy alone (17–19). The possible implications of adjuvant radiotherapy on the timing of breast reconstruction are, however, both profound and controversial.

Not only is tissue expansion difficult in the previously irradiated tissues, but the risks of infection, expander exposure, and subsequent extrusion are increased. Recent reports have demonstrated that patients who received postoperative radiotherapy had a significantly higher incidence of capsular contracture than controls. For these reasons, it is generally agreed

that autologous breast reconstruction is preferable in patients who have a history of previous chest wall irradiation and/or will require adjuvant postmastectomy radiotherapy.

Unfortunately, even though autologous tissue alone is preferred in this setting, autologous reconstructions may also be adversely affected by postmastectomy radiation. Contracture of the breast skin, development of palpable fat necrosis, and atrophy of the flap resulting in distortion of the reconstructed breast are described (20).

The increasing use of postmastectomy radiation and chemotherapy in patients with early-stage breast cancer necessitates increased communication between the medical oncologist, radiation oncologist, breast surgeon, and plastic surgeon during treatment planning. Paramount to a successful outcome is a frank discussion between the plastic surgeon and the patient about the potential risks of adjuvant radiotherapy on immediate reconstruction versus the additional surgery required for delayed reconstruction. There is no single "standard of care" in the setting of adjuvant radiotherapy, and each case must be individualized.

CONCLUSIONS

Breast reconstruction following mastectomy has been shown to have a positive impact on patients' physical and mental quality of life. Autologous tissue reconstruction has been advocated over implant-based reconstruction by some because of the potential for superior aesthetic results. In addition, the permanency of results and elimination of dependency on a permanent prosthesis are advantageous. Prosthetic reconstruction, however, has the capability of producing excellent results in the properly selected patient. Implant reconstruction is a less invasive surgical technique that is generally well tolerated.

The overriding goal of reconstructive breast surgery is to satisfy the patient with respect to her own self-image and expectations for the aesthetic result. Individualized selection of a reconstructive technique for each patient will be the predominant factor in achieving a reconstructive success.

References

1. Sandelin K, Billgren AM, Wickman M. Management, morbidity, and oncologic aspects in 100 consecutive patients with immediate breast reconstruction. *Ann Surg Oncol.* 1998;5:159–165.
2. Al Ghazal SK, Sully L, Fallowfield L, Blamey RW. The psychological impact of immediate rather than delayed breast reconstruction. *Eur J Surg Oncol.* 2000;26:17–19.

3. Spear SL, Onyewu C. Staged breast reconstruction with saline-filled implants in the irradiated breast: recent trends and therapeutic implications. *Plast Reconstr Surg.* 2000;105:930–942.

4. Cordeiro PG, Pusic AL, Disa JJ, McCormick B, VanZee K. Irradiation after immediate tissue expander/implant breast reconstruction: outcomes, complications, aesthetic results, and satisfaction among 156 patients. *Plast Reconstr Surg.* 2004;113:877–881.

5. Krueger EA, Wilkins EG, Strawderman M, et al. Complications and patient satisfaction following expander/implant breast reconstruction with and without radiotherapy. *Int J Radiat Oncol Biol Phys.* 2001;49:713–721.

6. Evans GR, Schusterman MA, Kroll SS, et al. Reconstruction and the radiated breast: is there a role for implants? *Plast Reconstr Surg.* 1995;96:1111–1115.

7. Hulka BS, Kerkvliet NL, Tugwell P. Experience of a scientific panel formed to advise the federal judiciary on silicone breast implants. *NEJM.* 2000;342:812–815.

8. Clough KB. Prospective evaluation of late cosmetic results following breast reconstruction: II. TRAM flap reconstruction. *Plast Reconstr Surg.* 2001;107:1710–1716.

9. Blondeel N, Vanderstraeten GG, Monstrey SJ, et al. The donor site morbidity of free DIEP flaps and free TRAM flaps for breast reconstruction. *Br J Plast Surg.* 1997;50:322–330.

10. Futter CM, Webster MH, Hagen S, Mitchell SL. A retrospective comparison of abdominal muscle strength following breast reconstruction with a free TRAM or DIEP flap. *Br J Plas Surg.* 2000;53:578–583.

11. Kroll SS. Fat necrosis in free transverse rectus abdominis myocutaneous and deep inferior epigastric perforator flaps. *Plast Reconstr Surg.* 2000;106:576–583.

12. Chevray PM. Breast reconstruction with superficial inferior epigastric artery flaps: a prospective comparison with TRAM and DIEP flaps. *Plast Reconstr Surg.* 2004;114:1077–1083.

13. Watterson PA, Bostwick J, III, Hester TR, Jr., Bried JT, Taylor GI. TRAM flap anatomy correlated with a 10-year clinical experience with 556 patients. *Plast Reconstr Surg.* 1995;95:1185–1194.

14. Kroll SS, Netscher DT. Complications of TRAM flap breast reconstruction in obese patients. *Plast Reconstr Surg.* 1989;84:886–892.

15. Serletti JM, Moran SL. Free versus the pedicled TRAM flap: a cost comparison and outcome analysis. *Plast Reconstr Surg.* 1997;100:1418–1424.

16. Nahabedian MY, Dooley W, Singh N, Manson PN. Contour abnormalities of the abdomen after breast reconstruction with abdominal flaps: the role of muscle preservation. *Plast Reconstr Surg.* 2002;109:91–101.

17. Nahabedian. Infectious complications following breast reconstruction with expanders and implants. *Plast Reconstr Surg.* 2003;112:467–476.

18. Vandeweyer E, Deraemaecker R, Nogaret JM, Hertens D. Immediate breast reconstruction with implants and adjuvant chemotherapy: a good option? *Acta Chir Belg.* 2003;103:98–101.

19. Wilson CR, Brown IM, Weiller-Mithoff E, George WD, Doughty JC. Immediate breast reconstruction does not lead to a delay in the delivery of adjuvant chemotherapy. *Eur J Surg Oncol.* 2004;30:624–627.

20. Tran NV, Evans GR, Kroll SS, et al. Postoperative adjuvant irradiation: effects on transverse rectus abdominis muscle flap breast reconstruction. *Plast Reconstr Surg.* 2000;106:313–317.

Principles of Spine Imaging in Cancer

9

Eric Lis
Christopher Mazzone

Cancer patients with symptoms referable to the spine present a unique imaging challenge. Metastatic disease can involve any portions of the spine. Most commonly, the epidural space is involved. Intradural disease, either leptomeningeal or intramedullary (spinal cord) metastasis, is less common. In addition, several complications of cancer therapy can affect the spine, sometimes mimicking metastatic disease. Problems that are often unique to cancer patients may be superimposed on more mundane and common processes that can involve any nonmalignant spine, particularly degenerative disease.

Metastatic disease to the spine is quite common, complicating the course of 5%–10% of cancer patients (1). As determined by autopsy, about 5% of patients that succumb to cancer exhibit spinal cord or cauda equina compression (2). The osseous spine is involved in about 30%–70% of patients with metastatic cancer (3). Overall, the spine is the most common site of bone metastasis, followed by the bony pelvis and femurs (4,5). The incidence of intradural metastasis (leptomeningeal and intramedullary) is much less than of epidural metastasis, accounting for fewer than 5% of metastatic disease to the spine (6).

The goal of this chapter is to impart an understanding of fundamental spine imaging anatomy to the clinician as well as to advance their knowledge of the most common lesions involving the spine in cancer patients. The choice of optimal imaging modalities for evaluation of such lesions will be discussed. Lesions that occur directly or indirectly from cancer treatment and may mimic metastatic disease will be reviewed. The diagnosis and treatment of spine metastasis and related processes in the cancer patient require a multidisciplinary approach and, with the proper use of imaging, will lead to earlier diagnosis, better management options, and ultimately improved neurological, functional, and potentially oncologic outcomes.

BASIC IMAGING ANATOMY AND TERMINOLOGY

The spine is best divided up into three anatomic spaces. The first and largest space is the epidural (extradural) space. The epidural space surrounds the thecal sac-dural sac and is everything outside of the thecal sac. Metastatic tumors that typically involve the epidural space usually arise within the osseous spine vertebrae. These are the typical vertebral-body metastases that expand into the epidural space and encroach upon the spinal canal and its contents. Less commonly, tumors such as leukemia and lymphoma can involve the epidural space without primary involvement of the osseous spine.

Intradural tumors can be broken down into two basic groups: intradural extramedullary and intramedullary lesions. Intradural extramedullary metastasis, more commonly referred to as leptomeningeal disease, is tumor that secondarily involves the leptomeninges and the subarachnoid (cerebrospinal fluid [CSF]) space. Occasionally, these lesions can be large enough to

KEY POINTS

- Metastatic disease can involve any portions of the spine, with the epidural space most commonly involved.
- Intradural tumors can be broken down into two basic groups: intradural extramedullary and intramedullary lesions. Intradural extramedullary metastasis, more commonly referred to as leptomeningeal disease, is tumor that secondarily involves the leptomeninges and the subarachnoid (cerebrospinal fluid [CSF]) space.
- The most common imaging modalities that are readily available to cancer patients with symptoms referable to the spine are plain films, computed

tomography (CT), magnetic resonance imaging (MRI), and CT-myelography.
- MRI is the modality of choice for imaging of the spine in cancer patients.
- Although MRI has largely replaced CT myelography, it is still commonly performed on patients who have a contraindication to MRI or who have had prior spine reconstruction with instrumentation that results in artifact, making an MRI study nondiagnostic.
- It is important to remember that when the imaging is inconsistent with the clinical findings, a discussion and review of the imaging with the radiologist or neuroradiologist is indicated.

extrinsically deform or compress the spinal cord and are potentially confused with epidural disease. Least common is the intramedullary metastasis, which is a lesion arising within the substance of the spinal cord.

One of the best ways to understand the radiographic anatomy of the spine is with a postmyelogram computed tomography (CT) scan (Fig. 9.1A, C, and E). The thecal sac CSF space is opacified by contrast and is easily identified. The spinal cord is seen centrally, with the nerve route of the cauda equina also easily

identified. To review previously mentioned concepts, the epidural space would be everything outside of the opacified thecal sac. This space is predominately occupied by the vertebrae, but also includes epidural fat, ligaments, and vascular plexuses. Working inward, the next space is the intradural extramedullary space. This is everything between the spinal cord and the dura, and is, for practical purposes, the contrast-opacified CSF space. Typically, metastatic disease that involves the meninges of the spine would appear as filling defects

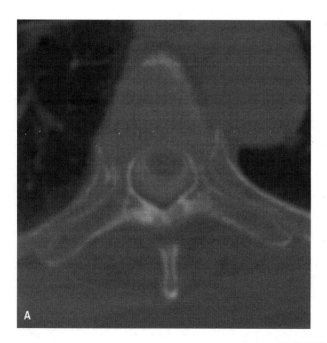 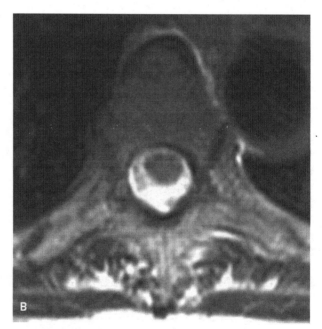

FIGURE 9.1 A–E

A: Axial postmyelogram CT through the mid-thoracic spine. B: Matching axial T2 weighted MRI.

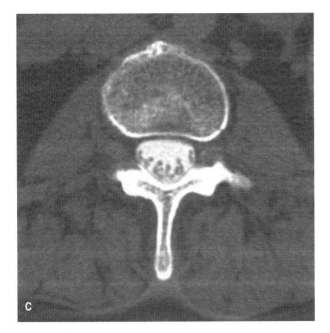

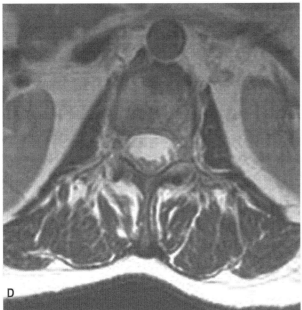

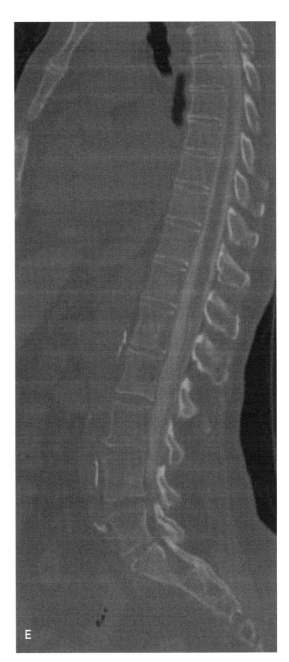

FIGURE 9.1 A–E (Continued)

Basic compartments of the spine. C: Postmyelogram axial CT through the cauda equina. D: Matching axial T2 weighted MRI. E: Postmyelogram CT reformatted in the sagittal plane. The postmyelogram images (A, C, E) show opacification of the subarachnoid space (intradural extramedullary), which is the space where leptomeningeal metastases are seen. The spinal cord (intramedullary) is outlined by the CSF. Similarly, the nerve roots of the cauda equina are well demonstrated (C, D). In simple terms, the epidural space is everything outside of the opacified thecal-CSF space, most of which is made up of bone vertebrae, fat, and ligaments.

or nodules along the surface of the cauda equina or spinal cord. The intradural intramedullary compartment is the spinal cord itself and is outlined by the opacified thecal sac. This basic understanding of spinal anatomy is easily applicable to magnetic resonance imaging (MRI).

DIAGNOSTIC SPINE IMAGING

The most common imaging modalities that are readily available to cancer patients with symptoms referable to the spine are plain films, CT, MRI, and CT-myelography. Adjunctive modalities, such as bone scans, positron emission tomography (PET) scans, and spinal angiography, are beyond the scope of this chapter.

Spine MRI

MRI is currently the most sensitive and specific imaging modality in evaluating spine tumors and, as such, is the modality of choice for imaging of the spine in cancer patients. Contraindications to MRI generally include the presence of any metallic material susceptible to magnetic fields. This includes a cardiac pacemaker, implanted cardiac defibrillator, cochlear implant, carotid artery vascular clamp, neurostimulator, insulin or infusion pump, implanted drug infusion device, bone growth/fusion stimulator, and certain aneurysm clips.

Adequate imaging of the entire spine can easily be performed with any of the commercially available MRI units. Thorough MR imaging of the spine usually requires both T1 and T2 weighted images obtained in the sagittal plane with selected axial images through regions of interest (7,8). Typically, the entire spine can be imaged in an hour or less by using a large field of view that essentially divides the spine into upper and lower halves, with slight overlap of the lower thoracic spine to ensure complete coverage (Fig. 9.2). Ideally, the part of the spine that is clinically symptomatic should be imaged first in case the patient is unable to complete the study. Axial images are prescribed as needed.

T1 weighted images provide anatomic definition, marrow detail, and a generally good overview of the spinal column. CSF is hypointense (dark), and fat is hyperintense (bright). Typically, most bone metastases are hypointense on T1 weighted sequences relative to the marrow, which is often slightly hyperintense secondary to its fat content in adults (Fig. 9.3). Fast spin echo (FSE) T2 weighted sequences have essentially replaced standard T2 weighted sequences secondary to a significant decrease in imaging time. CSF is hyperintense on T2 weighted images, with FSE T2 images providing excellent definition of both the spinal cord and CSF spaces. However, bone metastases are often less conspicuous on FSE T2 images, as fat is somewhat hyperintense. This can be compensated for by using the short tau inversion recovery (STIR) technique, which is essentially a fat-suppressed T2 image that makes many tumors appear hyperintense to adjacent

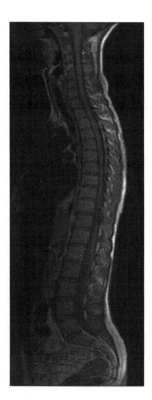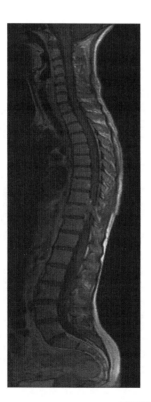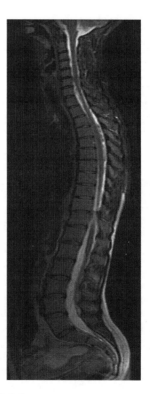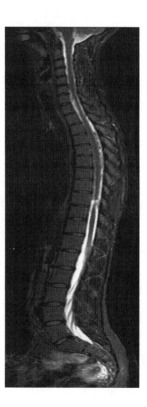

FIGURE 9.2

Normal MRI survey of the total spine in the sagittal plane. The images are merged from upper and lower spine studies and do not align perfectly. Left to right: Sagittal T1, matching postcontrast T1, FSE T2, and T2 STIR (D). Notice the hyperintense dorsal epidural fat, especially in the lumbar spine, as well as the hyperintense subcutaneous fat, both of which are suppressed on the T2 STIR images. Notice that the enhancement is limited to vascular structure, particularly the ventral epidural venous plexus.

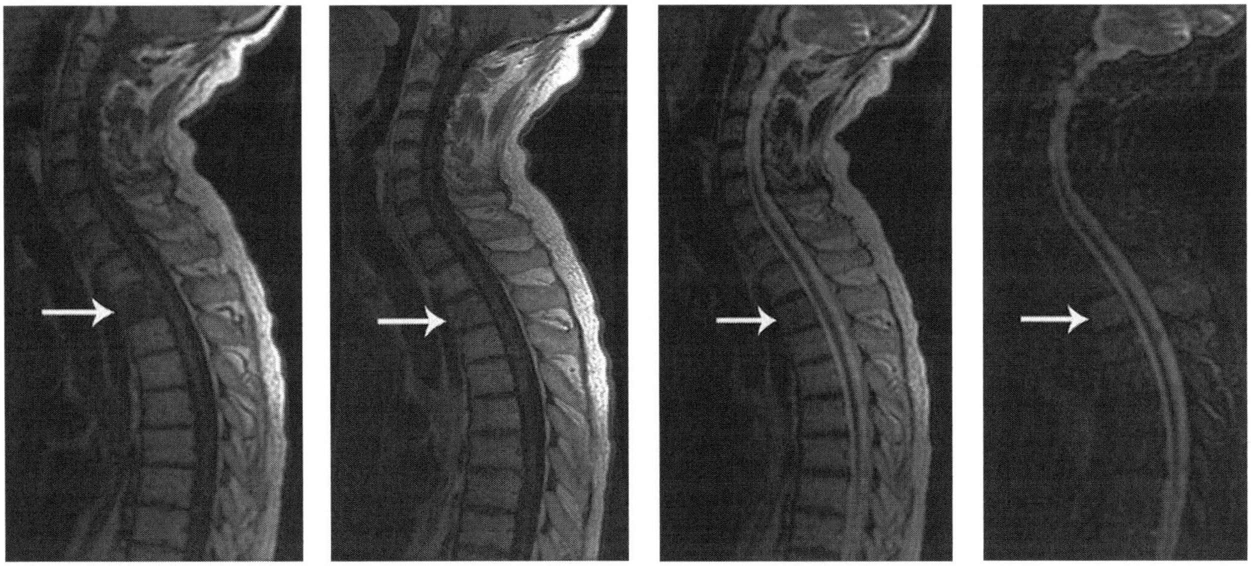

FIGURE 9.3

Typical MRI appearance of a T3 metastasis (arrow) in a patient with esophageal cancer. Left to right: Sagittal T1 with matching contrast-enhanced T1, T2, and T2 STIR images.

marrow and is also sensitive in identifying marrow edema. Most vertebral metastases are usually hypointense on T1 weighted images and hyperintense on T2 weighted images and also hyperintense, though generally more conspicuous, on T2 STIR images (Fig. 9.4). Sclerotic metastases are commonly hypointense on all pulse sequences (Fig. 9.5).

Other pulse sequences that are less common but are occasionally added to spine studies in certain situations include gradient echo (GRE) sequences, which are often useful in identifying blood products, or diffusion weighted images (DWI), which can play a role in spinal cord ischemia and the identification of bacterial abscesses. Some advanced MRI pulse sequences that are commonly utilized in brain imaging, such as DWI, perfusion imaging, and spectroscopy, are now being looked at on an investigational basis to evaluate neoplastic disease in the spine; however, they are generally limited by technical challenges. Ultra-fast sequences, such as half number of excitations (NEX) single-shot (SS) FSE T2 sequences, are useful when patient motion degrades standard images. This type of pulse sequence is able to image the lower or upper half of the spine in the sagittal or axial plane in less than 15 seconds. It comes at the cost of lesion conspicuity, but usually provides enough information to exclude any problem requiring immediate intervention (Fig. 9.6).

The use of gadolinium-based contrast agents are particularly useful in the identification of leptomeningeal disease or intramedullary spinal cord tumors, both of which typically enhance, as do most osseous metastatic and epidural disease. Gadolinium may also be useful in the evaluation of the postoperative spine to differentiate scar from tumor and for the evaluation of infection abscess. Enhancement of the nerve roots of the cauda equina may sometimes be seen with the administration of gadolinium in patients with acute inflammatory demyelinating polyradiculoneuropathy (AIDP) and chronic idiopathic demyelinating polyradiculoneuropathy (CIDP).

Spine Plain Films

Plain films of the spine are readily available but generally a poor screening for metastatic disease. About 30%–50% bone destruction is needed before a lytic lesion can be identified on a radiograph. Vertebral compression fractures are easily identified, though the degree of canal compromise can be difficult to determine (Fig. 9.7). Plain films can be obtained while weight bearing, possibly identifying deformities or malalignments that would be otherwise undetected in supine non-weight bearing positions required for CT and MRI. In the postoperative patient, plain films are most useful in assessing the alignment of the spine and the structural integrity of the reconstruction hardware (Fig. 9.8).

Spine CT

Over the last decade, the introduction of multidetector helical CT scanners has greatly improved the use

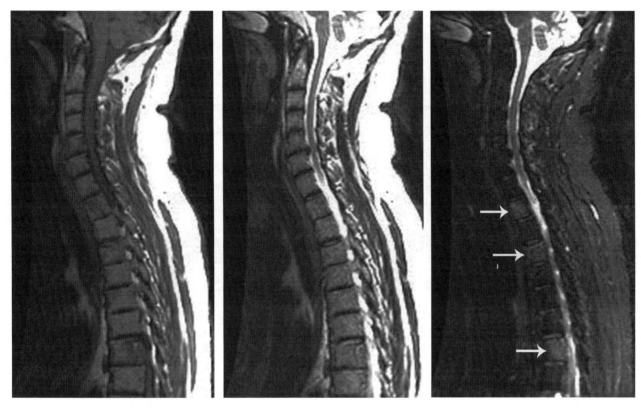

FIGURE 9.4

A patient with melanoma and multiple spine metastases. Left to right: Sagittal T1, FSE T2, and T2 STIR MRI showing multiple spine metastases. Notice that the metastases (arrows) are much more conspicuous on the T2 STIR image, especially when compared to the standard FSE T2 image.

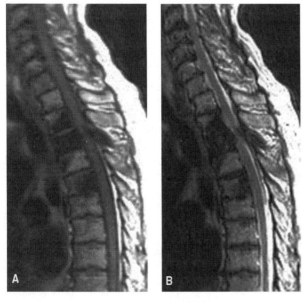

FIGURE 9.5

Sagittal T1 (A) and matching FSE T2 (B) MRI in a patient with metastatic prostate cancer and sclerotic metastasis that remain hypointense on both the T1 and T2 weighted sequences.

of CT as a spine imaging modality. Axial images can be quickly acquired through the entire spine in a matter of minutes and reconstructed in even thinner slice thicknesses for sagittal and coronal reformations. An unenhanced CT scan is not sensitive for the identification of epidural soft tissue tumor, especially when compared to MRI, but is extremely good at demonstrating lytic or sclerotic bony changes and cortical destruction (Fig. 9.9). Contrast will improve epidural soft tissue conspicuity, but is limited in identifying leptomeningeal and intramedullary tumor. Similarly, CT is not very good at identifying marrow infiltration without bony changes.

CT Myelography

Before MRI, myelography and then CT myelography was the diagnostic study of choice for the evaluation of the spine in regard to nerve root or spinal cord compression. The descriptive epidural, intradural, and intramedullary compartments were essentially brought to the forefront with myelography.

Myelography, when combined with a postmyelogram CT scan, is very sensitive in the detection

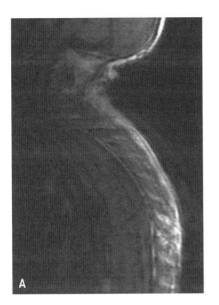 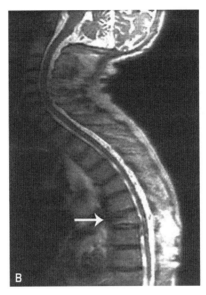 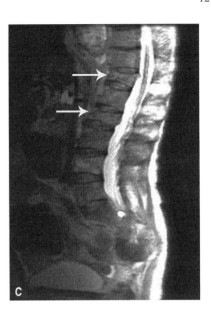

FIGURE 9.6

A patient with multiple myeloma with acute back pain. Sagittal T1 weighted MRI (A) is essentially nondiagnostic secondary to motion. Sagittal SS FSE T2 MRI of the upper and lower halves of the spine (B, C) demonstrates multiple partial collapse deformities (arrows) without cord compression.

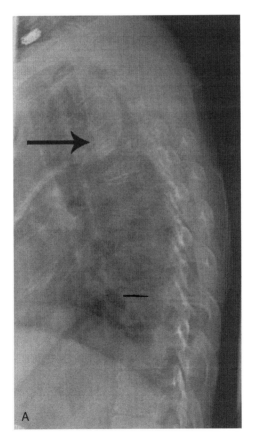 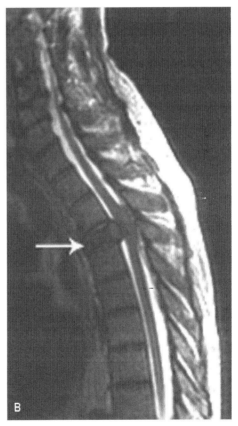

FIGURE 9.7

A: A lateral plain film of the thoracic spine in a patient with bladder cancer showing a T4 collapse deformity but essentially giving no information about the degree of canal compromise or the condition of the spinal cord. B: Sagittal T2 weighted MRI in the same patient showing spinal cord compression.

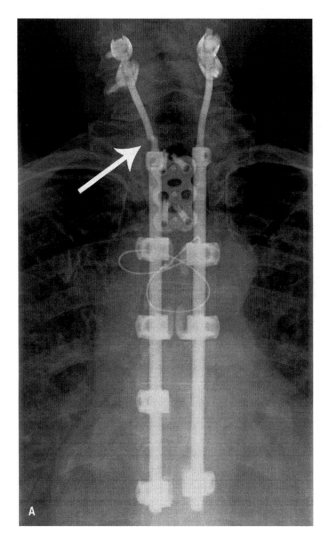 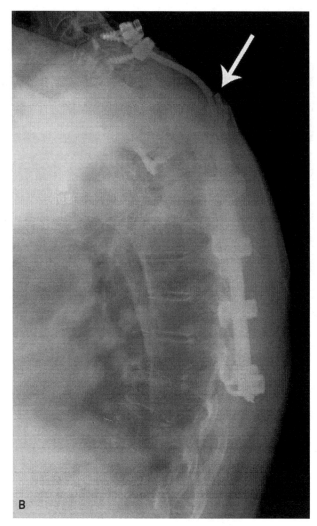

FIGURE 9.8

AP and lateral plain films (A,B) in a patient with multiple myeloma showing a broken posterior stabilization rod. Such a defect would not be detectable on MRI or CT.

of epidural tumor and spinal cord compression. A myelogram consists of infusing a small amount of nonionic water-soluble contrast into the subarachnoid space via a lumbar puncture or, less commonly, a cervical C1-2 puncture (Fig. 9.10E). The intrathecal contrast is then advanced in a controlled fashion throughout the spinal column with fluoroscopic spot images obtained. Attention is given to regions of the spine where the flow of intrathecal contrast is either held up or "blocked," usually secondary to epidural tumor in cancer patients. A myelogram is usually followed by a CT scan of the spine, which adds much detail and anatomic definition. A small amount CSF is also obtained at the time of the procedure, which can sent for analysis. The presence of neoplastic cells on cytopathologic evaluation is indicative of leptomeningeal disease. Myelography is generally safe, though

it is an invasive procedure that can have side effects, including neurological decompensation in patients with high-grade blocks.

Although MRI has largely replaced CT myelography, it is still commonly performed on patients that have a contraindication to MRI or who have had prior spine reconstruction with instrumentation that results in artifact, making an MRI study nondiagnostic.

PUTTING THE IMAGING TOGETHER

Before proceeding to the specifics of the most common disease processes that involve the spine and cancer patients, it is worthwhile to discuss a patient with one typical spine lesion imaged with the previously

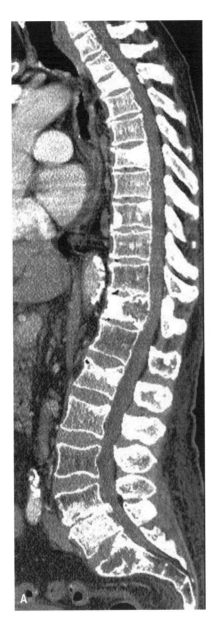
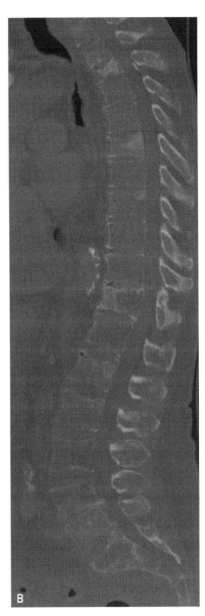

FIGURE 9.9

Reformatted contrast-enhanced CT scan in the sagittal plane in soft-tissue windows (A) and in bone windows (B) showing multiple lytic and sclerotic metastases, as well as several partial collapse deformities in this patient with an unknown primary.

discussed modalities. This will illustrate the clinical value and differences of each modality. The patient is a 61-year-old female with a history of breast cancer who presents to her oncologist with worsening back pain (Fig. 9.11).

EPIDURAL TUMOR

The epidural space is the most common compartment of the spine to be involved by metastatic disease, with the majority of epidural lesions arising from the verte-

brae. Back pain is the most common presenting symptom of metastatic epidural disease. Early and accurate diagnosis is of tremendous importance, as the treatments offered and the functional outcomes depend on the neurologic, oncologic, medical, and spinal stability status of the patient at the time of presentation.

At the Memorial Sloan-Kettering Cancer Center, spinal canal compromise is sometimes graded on MRI axial images using a standard scale: 0 to 3 (Fig. 9.12) (9). Grade 0 is vertebral body or posterior element disease with possibly early epidural involvement but

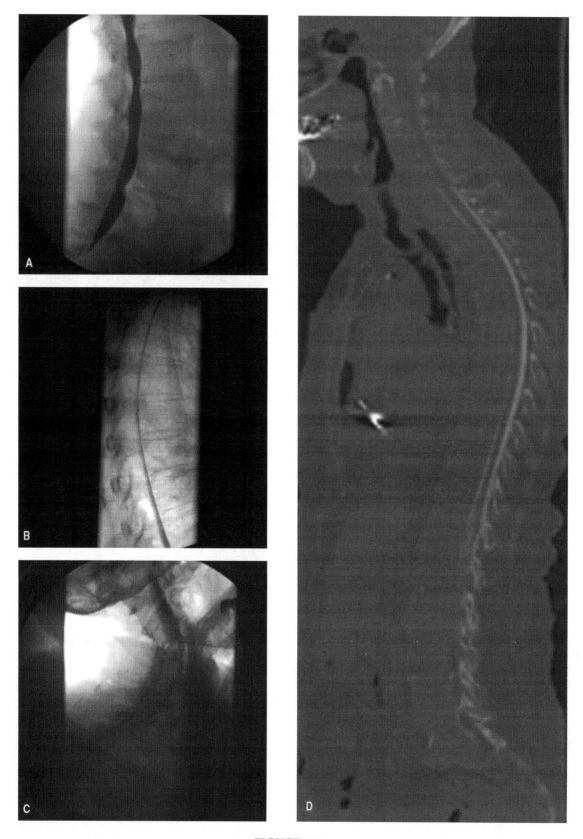

FIGURE 9.10

A–C: Lateral spot films obtained during a myelogram showing free passage of the intrathecal contrast throughout the spinal canal. D: A postmyelogram CT scan reformatted in the sagittal plane.

no mass upon the thecal sac. Essentially, there is no significant canal compromise. Grade 1 is when epidural disease results in partial effacement of the thecal sac but without spinal cord deformity or compression. Grade 1 disease usually is described as causing mild to moderate spinal canal compromise. Grade 2 epidural disease also partially obliterates the thecal sac, but without frank spinal cord compression. Grade 3 disease is complete obliteration of the thecal sac with spinal cord compression. Multiple examples of epidural disease are illustrated and discussed in Figures 9.13–9.19.

Leptomeningeal Metastases, Spinal Cord Metastasis, and Lesions Adjacent to the Spine.

When a patient presents with new or progressive spine symptoms but no epidural disease or non-neoplastic (ie, degenerative) causes are identified to explain their symptoms, a close inspection of the CSF spaces and spinal cord is indicated (Figs. 9.20–9.22). Also, it is usually worth evaluating areas adjacent to the spine (ie, paraspinally) when nothing centrally fits the patient's presentation.

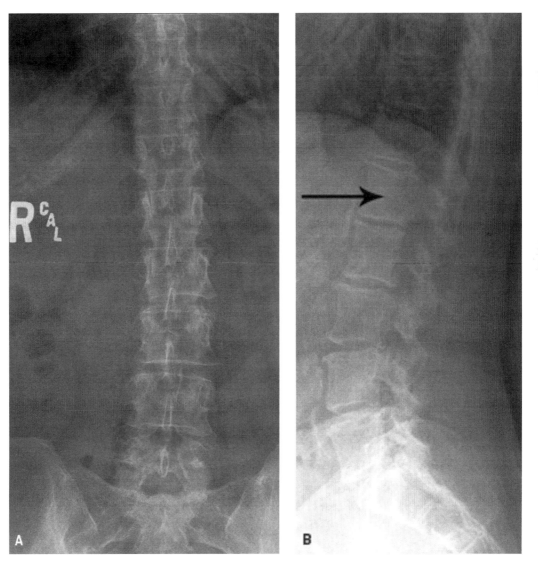

FIGURE 9.11 A–J

The patient is a 61-year-old female with a history of breast cancer with worsening back pain. AP and lateral plain films (A,B) of the lumbar spine show subtle lucency (arrow) along the posterior aspect of the L1 vertebral body.   (*Continued*)

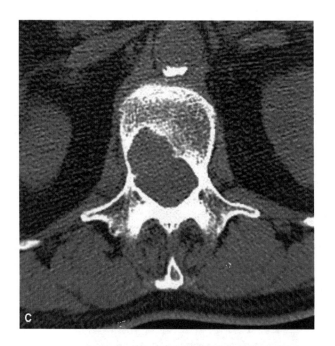

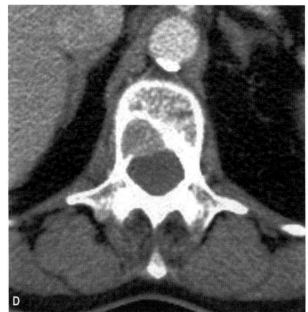

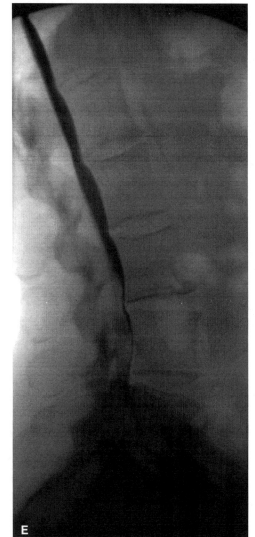

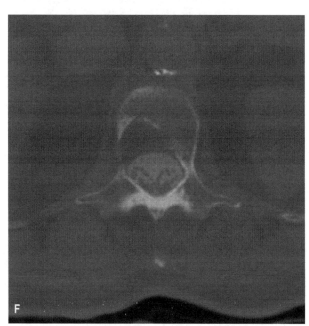

FIGURE 9.11 A–J (Continued)

A nonconstrast axial CT scan (C) through L1 shows a lytic metastasis with destruction of the posterior vertebral body cortex. Any significant epidural component cannot be determined by this image. A contrast-enhanced axial CT image (D) demonstrates enhancement of the metastasis with little epidural involvement and no significant canal compromise. A lateral plain film from a myelogram (E) shows free flow of the intrathecal contrast by L1 with an axial postmyelogram CT (F) through L1 showing the lesion that is without significant canal compromise. Notice the normal nerve roots of the cauda equina. The same lesion is seen in the sagittal plane on a noncontrast T1 and T2 STIR MRI (G, H) in the axial plane on T1 and T2 weighted images (I, J).

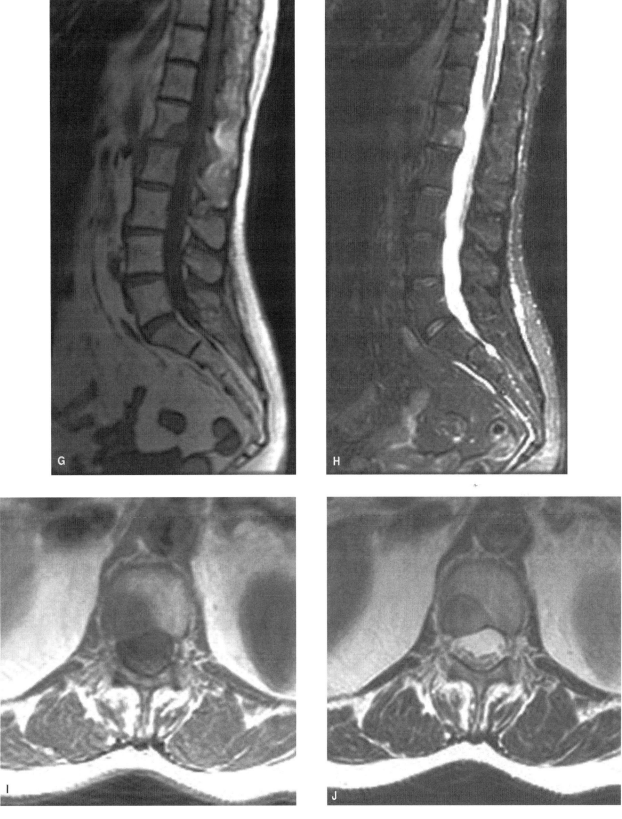

FIGURE 9.11 A–J (*Continued*)

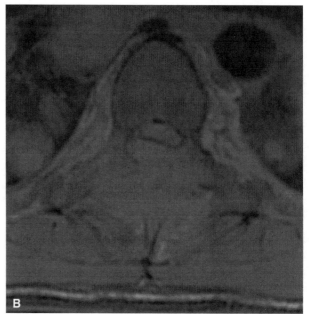

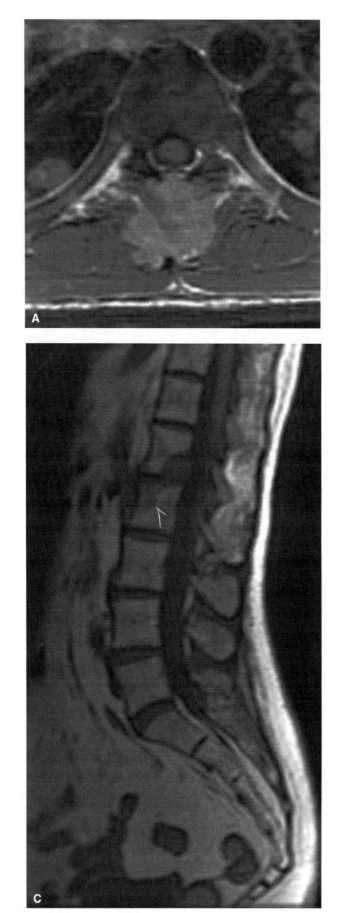

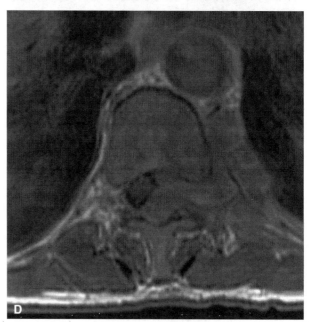

FIGURE 9.12

Grading epidural disease. A: Grade 0 as seen on a contrast-enhanced axial T1 weighted MRI showing an expansile metastasis extending just into the dorsal epidural space-fat but without any mass effect in the thecal sac. B: Grade 1 canal compromise as demonstrated by this postcontrast axial T1 weighted image showing left lateral epidural tumor causing mild to moderate canal compromise but without spinal cord compression. C: Postcontrast axial T1 weighted image depicts Grade 2 canal compromise by left lateral and left dorsal epidural tumor causing moderate canal compromise with spinal cord displacement and impingement but without frank spinal cord compression. D: Grade 3 canal compromise, as seen on this postcontrast axial T1 weighted image, where dorsal epidural tumor results in high-grade canal compromise and marked spinal cord compression.

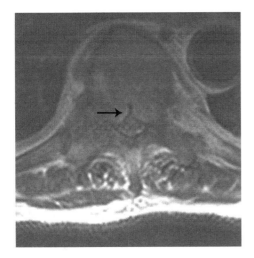

FIGURE 9.13

Axial T2 weighted MRI through the mid-thoracic spine showing biventral epidural tumor. Notice the posterior longitudinal ligament that contains the tumor and demonstrates an inverted V configuration secondary to its strong attachment to the mid-posterior vertebrae.

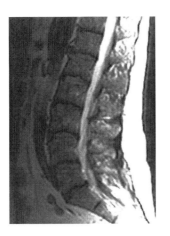 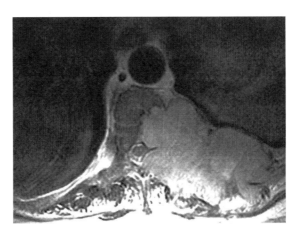 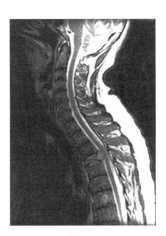

FIGURE 9.14

Tandem lesions. A patient with melanoma presented with worsening left-sided low back pain. Sagittal T2 weighted and axial T2 weighted (A, B) MRI show a left-side chest wall mass with vertebral and epidural involvement. A completion sagittal T2 MRI through the upper spine (C) shows a pathological collapse of T4 with cord compression that was relatively clinically silent but more critical. This is to emphasize the importance of imaging the entire spine in cancer patients.

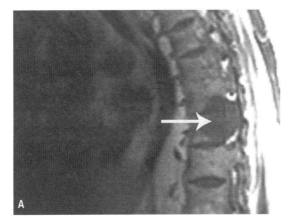 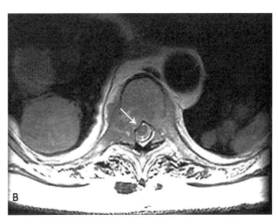

FIGURE 9.15

Metastatic leiomyosarcoma with right posterior chest wall pain that radiates anteriorly. A: Sagittal T1 weighted MRI demonstrates an expansile metastasis (arrow) encroaching upon the adjacent neural foramina. B: Axial T2 image showing epidural involvement with mild spinal canal compromise (arrow). Multiple pulmonary metastases are also visible.

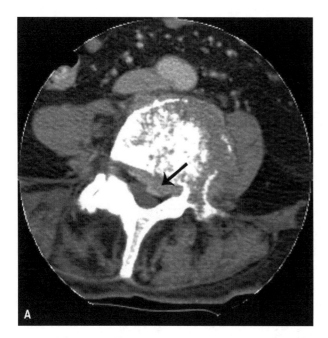

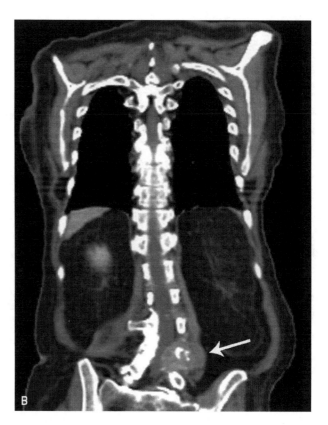

A patient with bladder cancer that has a worsening left L4 radiculopathy. A contrast-enhanced CT image through L4 (A) with coronal reformations (B) showing expansile metastatic disease involving L4, resulting in moderate canal compromise and involvement of the adjacent left-sided neural foramina.

FIGURE 9.16

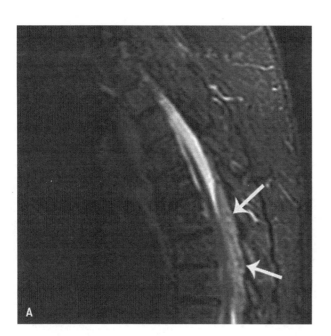

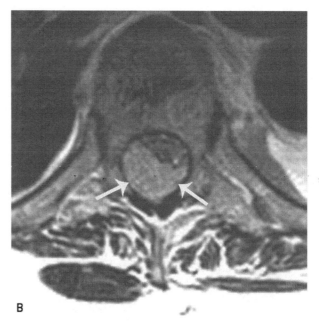

FIGURE 9.17

A patient presenting with back pain and weakness found to have lymphoma. A: Sagittal T2 STIR and B: axial T2 MRI demonstrate a thoracic dorsal epidural mass (arrows) causing high-grade spinal canal compromise and spinal cord compression. Notice that there is no obvious involvement of the vertebrae, a finding not uncommon with some of the hematologic malignancies, such as lymphoma.

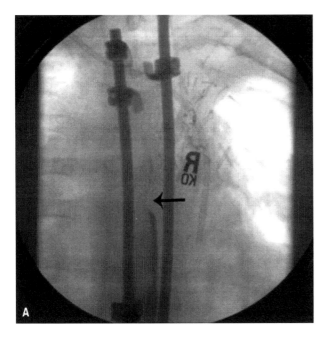

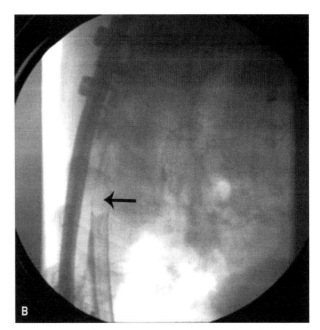

This patient has had multiple thoracic decompressive spine surgeries for recurrent sarcoma. Instrumentation degraded the MRI, so a myelogram was performed to evaluate for epidural disease. Spot images from a myelogram in the frontal and lateral projections (A, B) show epidural compression (arrows) of the thecal sac with a small amount of contrast sneaking past the region of spinal canal compromise. A postmyelogram CT scan (C) reformatted in the coronal plane showing a large paraspinal mass (arrows) with epidural extension into the spinal canal with spinal cord compression.

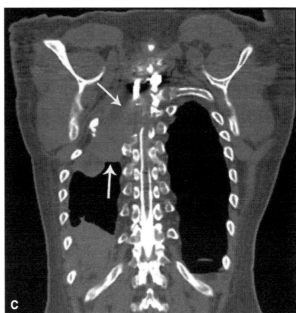

FIGURE 9.18

Lesions Mimicking Metastatic Disease

Cancer patients may present with spinal symptoms or imaging that is indeterminate for metastatic disease but which reflects direct or indirect sequelae of treatment. Spinal infections may occur in the immunocompro-mised patient, and secondary malignancies may occur because of prior radiation treatment. Nonmalignant osteoporotic type fractures of the spine are particularly common and may cause severe back pain (Figs. 9.23–9.31).

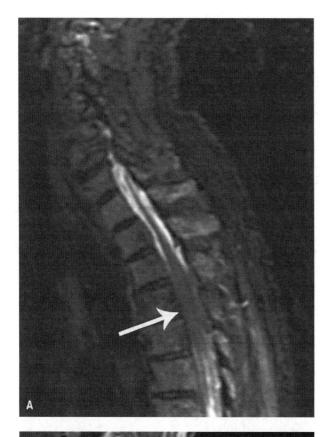

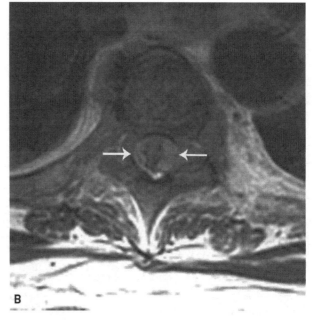

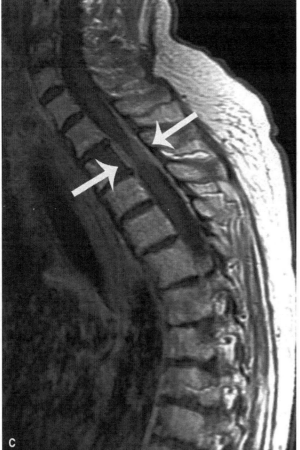

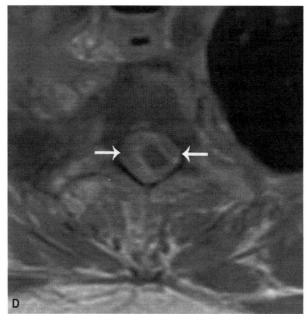

FIGURE 9.19

Sagittal T2 STIR MRI (A) revealing somewhat indistinct thoracic spinal cord. Axial T2 image (B) through this region showing bilateral lateral epidural tumor with cord compression (arrows). MRI from a different patient with lung cancer demonstrating circumferential epidural tumor with spinal cord compression (arrows) on postcontrast (C) sagittal and (D) axial T1 weighted images.

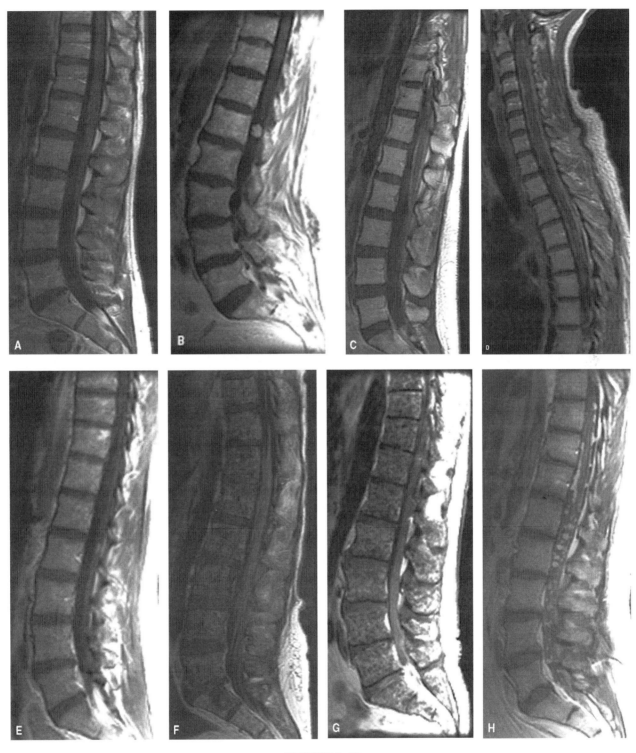

FIGURE 9.20

The variable appearance of leptomeningeal disease on MRI. This is a series of postcontrast sagittal T1 weighted MRIs of the spine in patients with documented leptomeningeal disease. A: Normal, no suspicious enhancement identified. B: Focal nodular enhancement. C, D: Plaquelike and nodular coating of the spinal cord. E: Scattered segmental plaques of enhancement. F: Confluent enhancing plaques of tumor extending along the cauda equina. G: Confluent-enhancing disease nearly filling the lumbar thecal sac. H: Extensive nodular leptomeningeal disease.

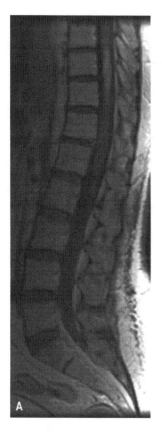
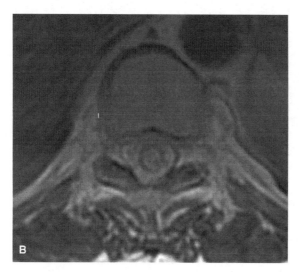
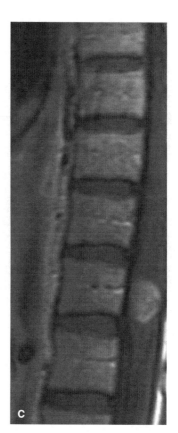

FIGURE 9.21

A patient with metastatic breast cancer and urinary incontinence. Contrast-enhanced sagittal T1 weighted MRI (A) showing a lower thoracic spinal cord metastasis. Axial T2 weighted image (B) showing the lesion within the spinal cord. A second patient with breast cancer and a metastasis to the conus as seen on a postcontrast sagittal T1 MRI (C).

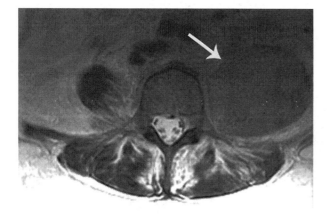

FIGURE 9.22

Lymphoma with left leg weakness. The MRI of the spine was essentially negative. A left psoas mass was identified and likely accounts for the symptoms.

CONCLUSION

MRI is generally the procedure of choice and the first imaging modality used to evaluate patients with symptoms referable to the spine. Exceptions include the presence of a contraindication to MRI, the suspicion of spinal stabilization hardware failure, or the presence of suspected tumor in an area where imaging is degraded, such as around hardware. Other imaging modalities can play a complementary role. It is important to remember that when the imaging is inconsistent with the clinical findings, a discussion and review of the imaging with the radiologist or neuroradiologist is indicated. Such collaboration can often lead to the elucidation of a subtle finding that will affect patient treatment and potential outcome.

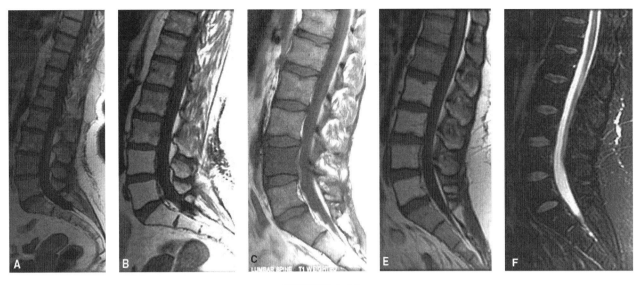

FIGURE 9.23

Radiation change. A: Sagittal T1 weighted MRI of the lumbosacral spine. B: The same patient three months after radiation to the pelvis showing the typical fatty change of the marrow, L4, L5, and the sacrum that now demonstrates homogenous hyperintensity on this T1 weighted image. The margins of the radiation port are usually well defined, as in this case. C: A second patient with L4 lymphoma as seen on this sagittal T1 weighted image. D: A postradiation sagittal T1 weighted image shows well demarcated radiation change-fatty change in the lumbar spine in addition to resolution of the L4 lesion and with homogenous suppression on the fat-suppressed T2 STIR image (E).

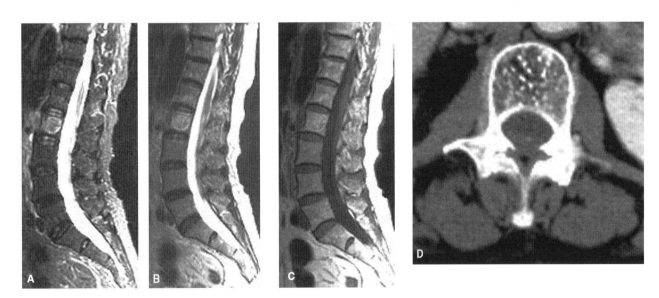

FIGURE 9.24

Hemangioma of bone. These benign lesions are common and should not be confused with metastatic disease. The patient has a history of lung cancer and focal bone scan activity in L2. Sagittal T2 STIR (A) and T2 weighted MRI (B) of the lumbar spine showing a focal hyperintense lesion in L2. A matching T1 weighted image (C) shows the lesion to be slightly hyperintense to isointense to adjacent marrow. An axial CT image through L2 (D) shows a coarsened trabecular pattern consistent with a hemangioma.

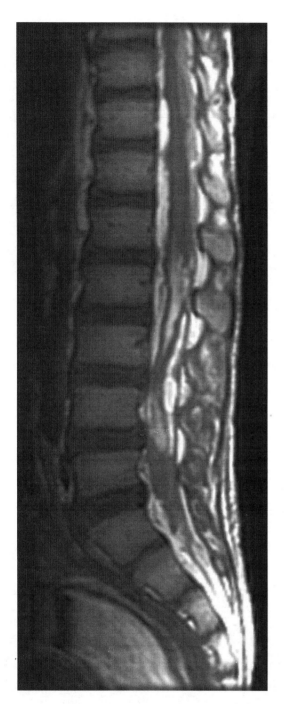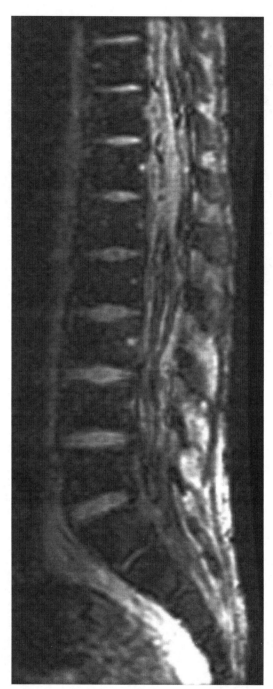

FIGURE 9.25

The patient has leukemia and developed lower-extremity weakness shortly after a lumbar puncture and intrathecal chemotherapy. Sagittal T1 weighted image (A) of the lumbar spine shows irregular hyperintensity in and about the thecal sac. A matching sagittal GRE image (B) shows regions of decreased signal supportive of hemorrhage.

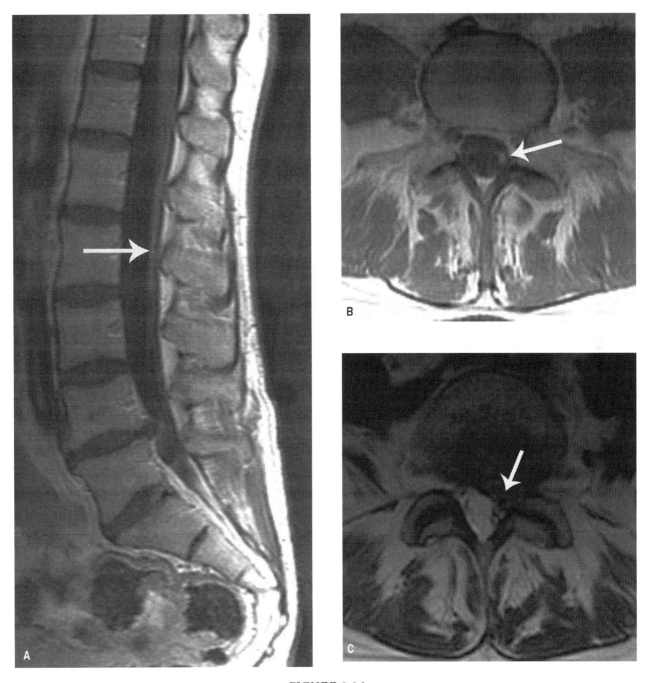

FIGURE 9.26

The patient has a history of lymphoma and developed an L5 radiculopathy. Postcontrast sagittal (A) and axial T1 weighted MRI (B) through the lumbar spine show segmental enhancement of the left L5 nerve root (arrows). This was determined to be reactive and secondary to impingement by a large left L4-5 disc herniation, as seen on an axial T2 weighted image (C, arrow), and not to represent leptomeningeal disease.

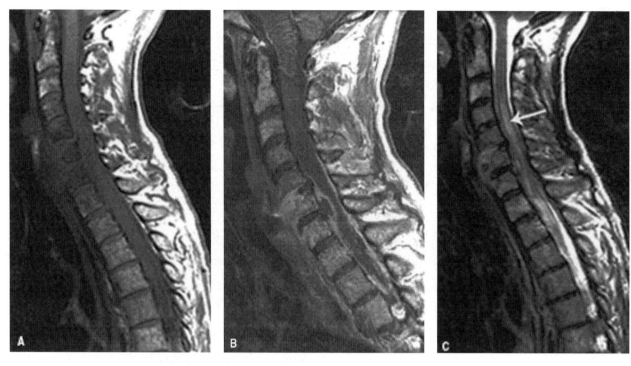

FIGURE 9.27

A patient with recurrent head and neck cancer that developed weakness and neck pain. Sagittal T1 weighted MRI (A) of the cervical spine followed by a contrast-enhanced sagittal T1 weighted image(B) and a matching sagittal T2 weighted image (C) showing discitis/osteomyelitis with C5-6 and C6-7 epidural abscesses. Note the spinal cord edema (arrow) on the T2 weighted images.

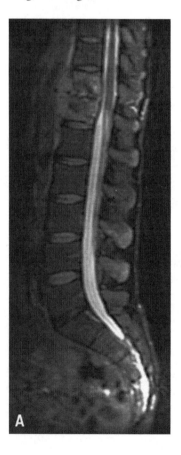

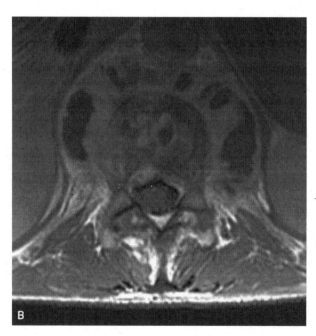

FIGURE 9.28

A patient with a remote history of lymphoma developed back pain and was thought to have a recurrence. Sagittal T2 STIR (A) demonstrates increased marrow signal in T11 and T12 with paraspinal soft tissue. Axial contrast-enhanced T1 weighted image (B) shows paraspinal disease with cystic change. CT-guided biopsy confirmed tuberculosis.

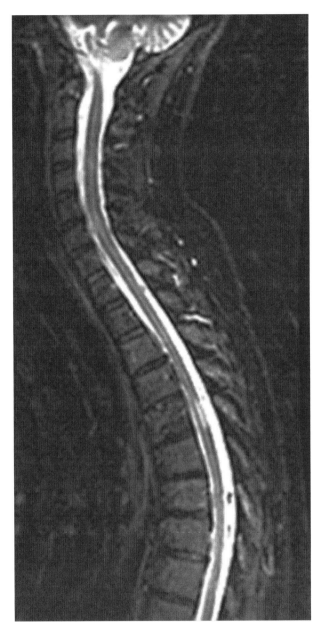

FIGURE 9.29

The patient is status-post bone marrow transplant for leukemia. Sagittal T2 STIR image of the spinal cord demonstrates
nonspecific signal changes in the spinal cord. Subsequent
biopsy revealed likely nonspecific demyelination.

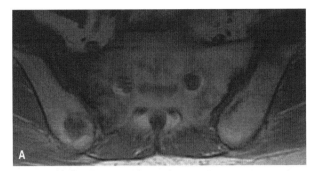

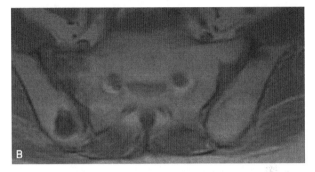

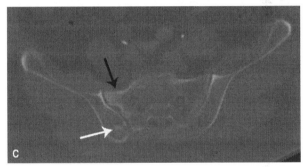

FIGURE 9.30

Osteoporotic fractures. Fractures of the spine, including
the sacrum, commonly occur secondary to therapy-related
or senile bone loss in cancer patients. A: A patient with a
history of colon cancer presents with low back pain. An
axial T1 weighted MRI demonstrates marrow changes in the
right sacral ala. CT-guided biopsy was negative for tumor.
Follow-up (B) axial T1 weighted MRI shows improvement
with an axial CT image (C) showing patchy sclerosis (black
arrow) most compatible with a healing stress fracture. Incidentally identified is a bone island in the right posterior iliac
bone (white arrow).

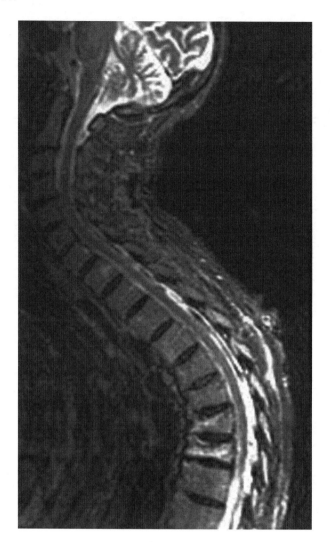
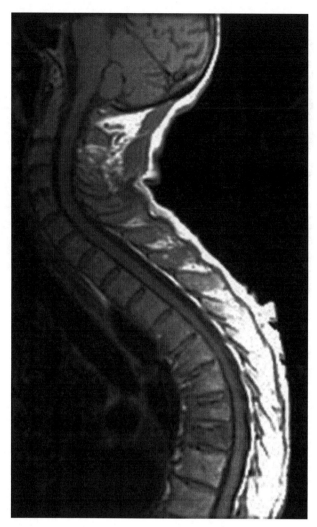

FIGURE 9.31

Typical-appearing osteoporotic fractures of the thoracic spine in a patient with a history of lung cancer. Sagittal T2 STIR (A) and sagittal T1 weighted MRI (B). Biopsy at the time of kyphoplasty was negative for tumor.

References

1. Bach F, Larsen BH, et al. Metastatic spinal cord compression: occurrence, symptoms, clinical presentations and prognosis in 398 patients with spinal cord compression. *Acta Neurochir.* 1990;170:37–43.
2. Barron KD, Hirano A, et al. Experiences with metastatic neoplasms involving the spinal cord. *Neurology.* 1959;8:91–106.
3. Fornasier V, Horne J. Metastases to the vertebral column. *Cancer.* 1975;36:590–594.
4. Galasko C. The anatomy and pathways of skeletal metastases. In: Weiss L, Gilbert H, eds. *Bone Metastasis.* Boston: GK Hall & Co; 1981:49–63.
5. Harrington K. Metastatic diseases of the spine. In: Harrington K, ed. *Orthopaedic Management of Metastatic Bone Disease.* St. Louis: CV Mosby; 1988:309–383.
6. Costigan D, Winkelman M. Intramedullary spinal cord metastasis. A clinicopathological study of 13 cases. *J Neurosurg.* 1985;62:227–233.
7. Algra PR, Bloem JL, et al. Detection of vertebral metastases: comparison between MR imaging and bone scintigraphy. *Radiographics.* 1991;11:219–232.
8. Riggieri PM. Pulse sequences in lumbar spine imaging. *Magn Reson Imaging Clin N Am.* 1999;7:425–437.
9. Bilsky M, Smith M. Surgical approach to epidural spinal cord compression. *Hematol Oncol Clin North Am.* 2006;20(6):1307–1317.

Principles of Plexus Imaging in Cancer

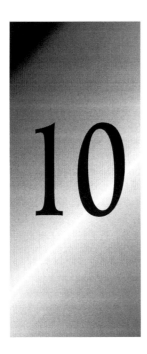

Jon Lewis
George Krol

Involvement of plexus in a patient with cancer may be due to a tumor arising directly from neural components, direct (contiguous) metastatic spread from adjacent organs, or compression by adjacent tumor masses (eg, enlarged nodes). Most common iatrogenically induced causes include sequelae or complications of surgical intervention or radiation therapy (RT). Clinical presentation in all these conditions is frequently similar, thus a common term "plexopathy" is used. Symptoms include pain, paresthesias, focal weakness, autonomic symptoms, sensory deficits, and muscle atrophy (1,2). Although history may suggest possible cause, physical examination is of limited value in evaluation of plexopathy. Conventional radiologic methods (plain radiographs) are usually negative, although may be helpful in advanced disease. Both computed tomography (CT) and magnetic resonance imaging (MRI) have been utilized all along, but in recent years, MRI has emerged as a leading method of imaging of plexus regions. Technical improvements (neurography) made it possible to visualize individual nerves directly (3–6). A reliable method of visualization of diseased nerve/plexus seems more difficult to find. As new techniques are introduced, improving resolution and depicting more detail and chemical composition of tissue, there arises a need for more thorough knowledge of utilization of imaging in normal and diseased state. This chapter will discuss the role of conventional and new modalities in the assessment of plexus disease, including indications, current techniques, advantages and pitfalls, and selection of methods of choice.

NORMAL ANATOMY OF PLEXUSES

Plexus is defined as a network of connections of nerve roots, giving rise to further interconnecting or terminal branches. As ventral (motor) and dorsal (sensory) roots leave the spinal cord, they soon unite within the spinal canal to form a spinal nerve. After exiting neural foramina, they form a network of interconnections (plexus), from ventral roots, trunks, and cords to individual nerves. Although there are many such stations in the body, the three main plexuses are cervical, brachial, and lumbosacral. Plexopathy may result when any of these segments of the plexus becomes involved. Since it may not be possible to visualize directly the abnormality within the nerve, one may have to rely on altered adjacent tissue to make a diagnosis. Thus, the knowledge of normal configuration, adjacent tissue characteristics, and spatial relationships of plexus components in reference to bony landmarks, vascular structures, and muscles is very important in detection of abnormality and interpretation of plexus disease.

Cervical and Brachial Plexus

The cervical plexus lies on the ventral surface of the medial scalene and levator scapulae muscles. It is formed by ventral rami of the cervical nerves C1 through C4. Each ramus at C2, C3, and C4 levels divides into two branches, superior and inferior. These, in turn, unite in the following way: superior branch of C2 with C1, inferior branch of C2 with superior branch of C3, inferior

KEY POINTS

- Involvement of plexus in a patient with cancer may be due to a tumor arising directly from neural components, direct (contiguous) metastatic spread from adjacent organs, or compression by adjacent tumor masses (eg, enlarged nodes).
- Magnetic resonance imaging (MRI), with and without contrast, has emerged as a leading method of imaging of plexus regions.
- Development of picture archiving and communication system (PACS) revolutionized the way the studies are viewed and interpreted by radiologists. Perhaps the best example is a cine mode option, which creates three-dimensional perception, allowing for better understanding of extent and configuration of lesions and their relation to adjacent normal structures, particularly vessels.
- The main advantages of MRI over computed tomography (CT) are ability of multiplanar scan-

ning without change of patient's position, superior resolution, and tissue characterization.
- Primary plexus neoplasms, including schwannomas, perineuriomas, neurofibromas, and malignant peripheral nerve sheath tumors (MPNST), are usually present as well-defined, rounded, or oval masses orientated along the longitudinal axis of the nerve.
- Plexus may be compressed or infiltrated by an extrinsic neoplasm, arising from adjacent structures, with breast, neck, lung, and lymph node malignancies being most common offenders for brachial region and pelvic tumors for lumbosacral plexus.
- MRI in radiation-induced fibrosis (RIF) may reveal thickening and indistinct outline of plexus components, without identifiable focal mass.

branch of C3 with superior branch of C4, and inferior branch of C4 joins C5 to become part of the brachial plexus. Terminal cutaneous, muscular, and communicating branches supply skin and muscles in occipital area, upper neck, supraclavicular, upper pectoral region, and diaphragm.

The brachial plexus is formed by ventral rami of spinal nerves exiting through the neural foramina of the cervical spine at C5 to T1 levels (dorsal rami innervate posterior paravertebral muscles). Inconsistent contributions may arise from C4 and T2 segments. As the spinal nerves leave the foramina between vertebral artery anteriorly and facet joint posteriorly, they soon create the first station of connections between anterior and middle scalene muscles: C5 and C6 nerves unite to form superior trunk, C7 becomes middle trunk, and C8 and T1 form inferior trunk. Subclavian artery proceeds with the brachial plexus components within the triangle anteriorly to the trunks and subclavian vein courses in front of anterior scalene muscle. The trunks divide just laterally to the lateral margin of scalene muscles into three anterior and three posterior divisions. Pectoralis major and serratus anterior muscles constitute anterior and posterior boundaries, respectively. Anterior divisions of superior and middle trunks join to form lateral cord; anterior division of inferior trunk becomes medial cord, and posterior divisions of all three trunks unite to form posterior cord. The medial cord, which receives fibers from inferior C8 to T1 trunk, gives off the ulnar nerve. The lateral cord, containing contributions from superior and middle trunks (C5–C7) becomes the

largest nerve of the upper extremity, the median nerve. The posterior cord contains fibers from all three trunks (C5–T1); its main pathway is the radial nerve. Other terminal branches include suprascapular, musculocutaneous, axillary, thoracodorsal, medial cutaneous, and long thoracic nerves (Figs. 10.1 and 10.2), (7,8).

Lumbosacral Plexus

The lumbosacral plexus is formed by ventral rami of the lumbar and sacral nerves, T12–S4. Lumbar part is formed by roots from T12—L4, and sacral component by L4–S4 roots. These divide into anterior and posterior divisions, which give rise to anterior and posterior branches, respectively. Anterior branches of the lumbar plexus include (in craniocaudal direction): iliohypogastric, ilioinguinal, genitofemoral, and obturator nerves; the same of sacral plexus are tibial component of sciatic nerve, posterior femoral cutaneous, and pudendal nerves. Posterior branches of lumbar plexus include lateral femoral cutaneous and femoral nerves, and those of sacral plexus are: peroneal component of sciatic nerve, superior and inferior gluteal, and piriformis nerves. The roots of lumbar plexus lie on the ventral surface of the posterior abdominal wall, proceeding in diagonal fashion anterolaterally, between fibers of psoas and iliacus muscles. The largest femoral nerve continues behind the inguinal ligament, supplying anterior and medial aspects of the thigh. The sacral plexus proceeds laterally along the posterior wall of the pelvis, where it lies between iliac vessels anterolaterally and piriform

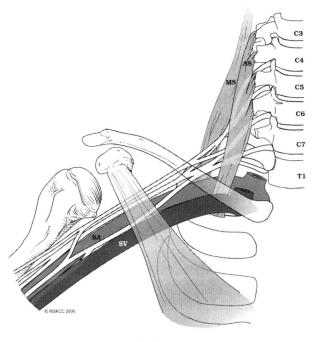

FIGURE 10.1

Brachial plexus proceeds laterally towards axillary fossa through the scalene triangle (bordered by anterior scalene [AS] and middle scalene [MS] muscles anteroposteriorly and first rib inferiorly), where it is located posteriorly to subclavian artery. Subclavian vein travels anteriorly to the anterior scalene muscle. SC—subclavian artery; SV—subclavian vein.

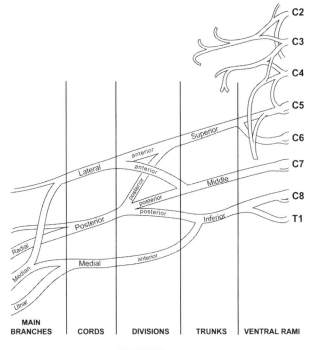

FIGURE 10.2

Schematic representation of cervical and brachial plexus network. Cervical plexus (C1–C4): Ventral rami C2, C3, and C4 divide, giving off superior and inferior branch at each level. Superior branch of C2 and C1 ramus unite to form ansa cervicalis. Adjacent inferior and superior branches of C2, C3, and C4 merge and give off lesser occipital, greater auricular, transverse cervical, supraclavicular, and phrenic nerves (unmarked). Brachial plexus (C5–T1): Superior, middle, and inferior trunks are formed by ventral rami of C5/C6, C7, and C8/T1, respectively. Each trunk divides into anterior and posterior divisions. Anterior divisions of superior and middle trunks form lateral cord; anterior division of inferior trunk becomes medial cord, and posterior divisions of all three trunks unite to form posterior cord. Major nerves of the arm—median, ulnar, and radial—receive contributions predominantly from lateral, medial, and posterior cords, respectively.

muscle posteromedially (Fig. 10.3). Terminal branches innervate pelvic organs, and the sciatic nerve, the largest nerve of the body, proceeds through the greater sciatic notch to supply regions of posterior thigh and below the knee (5).

RADIOGRAPHIC METHODS OF IMAGING

Evaluation of plexus with conventional radiography is difficult and yields little information (9). However, it may be used in preliminary evaluation of plexopathy, mainly to exclude major abnormality, such as bone destruction, fracture, lung infiltration, or ligamentous calcifications. Potential of computed tomography in detection of plexus disease has been realized by early investigators (10–15). Introduced in recent years, a new technique of multichannel scanning allows for uninterrupted data acquisition during continuous tube rotation and table advance (16). Further anatomical detail and tissue characteristics have been provided by MRI. Special sequences have been developed for selective imaging of nerve tissue (neurography). Sonography

and positron emission tomography (PET) scanning also have been reported to provide valuable contributions (17–19). Development of picture archiving and communication system (PACS) revolutionized the way the studies are viewed and interpreted by radiologists. Perhaps the best example is a cine mode option, which enables three-dimensional perception, allowing for better understanding of extent and configuration of lesions and their relation to adjacent normal structures, particularly vessels. However, despite valuable contributions from these imaging methods, the assessment of plexus regions frequently presents a challenging problem for a clinician as well as a radiologist.

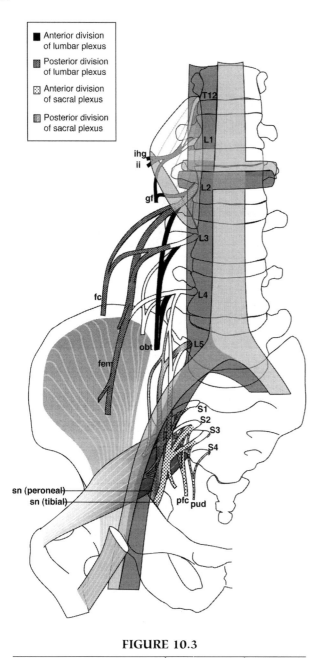

FIGURE 10.3

Simplified coronal diagram of lumbosacral plexus depicted on a background of psoas, iliacus, and piriformis muscles. Anatomy of the lumbosacral plexus is much less intricate and more variable than that of brachial plexus. Anterior and posterior divisions unite and/or divide to form terminal branches (the trunks and cords are not distinguished). Anterior divisions of lumbar plexus unite to form iliohypogastric (ihg), ilioinguinal (ii), genitofemoral (gf), and obturator (obt) branches, whereas posterior divisions give rise to femoral cutaneous (fc) and femoral (fem) nerves. Of sacral plexus, anterior divisions divide to give rise to tibial component of sciatic nerve (sn), posterior femoral cutaneous (pfc), and pudendal nerves (pud), while posterior divisions give off peroneal component of sciatic nerve (sn), part of femoral cutaneous, gluteal, and piriformis nerves.

Technique

Because of its small size, the cervical plexus is rarely evaluated radiographically as a separate entity. Rather, it is included as a part of head, cervical spine, or neck examinations. Cervical plexus extends from C1 down to C4, thus scanning from skull base down to C5, utilizing small field of view (FOV) (25 cm), is sufficient. The anatomical brachial plexus extends approximately from C5 down to T2 vertebral levels. Adequate coverage of the plexus is provided by scanning the region from C4 to T3. However, we extend lower range with larger FOV down to T6 to include peripheral components within axillary fossas. Contiguous 4–5-mm spaced axial sections are obtained perpendicular to the table top. Coned-down view of the area in question may be added to the study. The elements of normal plexus are small and are depicted as nodular or linear areas of soft tissue density. They are difficult to identify and may not be outlined at all (20), particularly on inferior quality examination. Contrast injection is recommended (9), not only for identification of normal vascular structures and differentiation from lymph nodes, but also for more complete information on the enhancement pattern of the lesion. For this purpose, an intravenous injection in dynamic mode is preferred, using initial bolus of 50 cc, followed by contiguous infusion at the rate of 1 cc/second to a total of 100 cc of nonionic contrast (Omnipaque 300 or equivalent). The infusion should be administered on the site opposite to suspected pathology, since high concentration of intravenous contrast may produce streaking artifacts, obscuring detail (20).

Adequate coverage of the lumbosacral plexus includes axial sections from T12 down to the tip of the coccyx to visualize greater sciatic notches (GSN). Axial images with 4–5-mm slice thickness and FOV large enough to include both sacroiliac joints are usually sufficient. Intravenous contrast administration (100 cc of Omnipaque 300 or equivalent in dynamic mode or bolus injection) is recommended unless contraindicated. An intraoral contrast (Gastrografin, given two hours in advance) may be beneficial in assessment of plexus pathology, mainly to delineate distal urinary tract and colon, respectively.

MR Technique

The main advantages of MRI over CT are ability of multiplanar scanning without change of patient's position, superior resolution, and tissue characterization (21,22). Adequate anatomical coverage of the plexus must be assured. Thus, for brachial plexus, axial sections from levels of C3 down to T6 coronal sections, including glenohumeral joints and sagittal sections to cover both axillary fossas, should be obtained. For lumbosacral plexus, the coverage in axial plane needs to extend from T12 to coccyx. Sections of 5-mm thickeness/0.25 gap are obtained in axial, sagittal, and coronal planes. We prefer scanning in direct axial, sagittal, and coronal planes (23), although oblique scanning planes have been advocated for brachial (24) and sacral plexus (25) to optimize visualization of plexus components and sciatic nerve. T1, fast spin echo T2, and short tau inversion recovery (STIR) (fat suppression) should be obtained. Use of phased-array coils is recommended for greater resolution of detail (26,27). Intravenous contrast (Magnevist or equivalent) is utilized routinely in a dose of 0.1 mmol/kg of body weight.

Visualization of Normal Plexus Components on CT and MRI

Conventional (noncontrast) CT offers rather poor definition of structures within the subarachnoid sac (spinal cord, roots of cauda equina). Nerve roots exiting laterally through foramina are more consistently seen, particularly in lumbar spine and sacrum, because of larger size and more abundant epidural fat. They are depicted as punctate or linear structures of muscle density, contrasting against the adjacent darker fat within the foramen or vicinity (Fig. 10.4). Trunks and cords of the brachial plexus are usually blended with muscle fibers and major vessels more distally. With abundant fat tissue, individual nerve components may be visible as discrete, linear areas of soft tissue density, proceeding posteriorly along the subclavian artery (Fig. 10.5). Those of the lumbar plexus enter paraspinal musculature (psoas) and are difficult to identify with certainty. Femoral and obturator nerves may be visible, contrasted against the intrapelvic/intra-abdominal fat. The largest sciatic nerve (Fig. 10.6) is more consistently identified in the lateral aspect of GSN posteriorly to the ischial spine.

MRI depicts the plexus components with much greater accuracy (19,22,28), still improved when phased-array coils are used (27,29). Conventional T1 weighted sequences are routinely utilized for anatomic detail. Although individual nerves down to 2 mm in

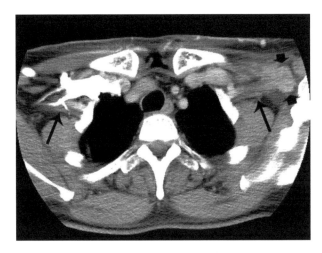

FIGURE 10.5

Axial CT image through thoracic inlet. Fibers of brachial plexus proceed posteriorly to vascular bundle (arrows). A lobulated mass (arrowheads) is visible more laterally on the left, representing recurrent metastatic breast cancer.

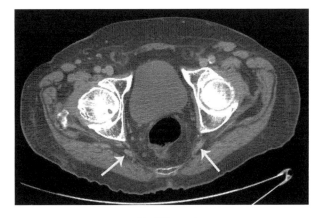

FIGURE 10.6

Axial CT section through the greater sciatic notch (GSN). Sciatic nerves (arrows) are visualized in the lateral aspect of GSN posteriorly to the ischial spine.

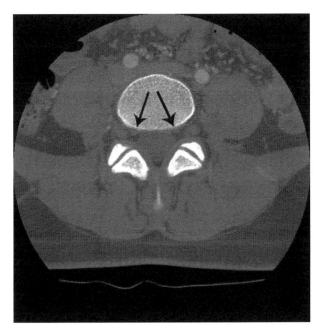

FIGURE 10.4

Axial CT section through inferior plate of L4. Nerve roots are clearly seen bilaterally (arrows) contrasting against a low-density background of fat tissue.

diameter can be seen (27), much of the success depends upon relaxation properties of adjacent tissues. Thus, even a smaller branch surrounded by fat or fluid (cerebrospinal fluid [CSF]) can be seen clearly, while a larger neural trunk encompassed by infiltrative process will blend with the abnormal tissue and may not be recognized at all. T2 weighted sequences (fast spin echo [FSE]) provide best detail of normal nerve when contrast interphase of fluid (CSF) or abnormal tissue (eg, edema) is present.

Thus, spinal nerves within the canal are demonstrated in good detail on T1 and T2 sequences because they contrast against fat (epidural) and fluid (CSF), respectively. Special sequences have been designed to create "myelographic effect," depicting the cord and roots within the thecal sac throughout the spine (30). Fat suppression sequences (STIR being most commonly used) null fat signal, thus rendering background fat tissue darker and nerve more clearly visible (31,32). The option can be applied to both T1 and T2 weighted sequences, and is most valuable in conjunction with contrast enhancement.

The normal neural components of plexus can be identified with various success on a good-quality MRI. Nerve roots within the foramina and immediate vicinity are routinely seen. As they descend with the muscle fibers, trunks and cords of the brachial plexus can be identified on axial images, proceeding between anterior and middle scalene group laterally to exit through the scalene triangle. Extended segments of the plexus may be demonstrated on one well-placed axial and/or coronal T1 weighted anatomic image (Fig. 10.7). Sagittal sections through and laterally to the scalene triangle outline the individual divisions as punctate areas of soft tissue intensity within the fat background, with subclavian artery and vein anteriorly (Fig. 10.8). Similarly, the lumbar and sacral roots within the subarachnoid space and neural foramina are seen in detail, while interconnecting network within the psoas complex is more difficult to identify. On axial sections, femoral nerve may be visualized as a single trunk proceeding anterolaterally along the ventral aspect of posterior abdominal wall. The greater sciatic nerve within the notch is more consistently seen, either as a single oval structure or as a cluster of several smaller individual nerves (Fig. 10.9), (6,22).

Abnormal Nerve

When involved by a disease, nerve tissue may exhibit swelling, focal or diffuse infiltration, edema, cyst formation, or necrosis. In the early stage, when there is no enlargement of peripheral nerve(s), these changes may not be appreciated on imaging modalities, but become more apparent as the process progresses. On

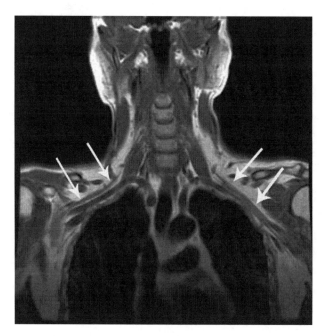

FIGURE 10.7

MRI of the brachial plexus. Long segments of plexus fibers (arrows) are demonstrated on coronal T1 weighted image.

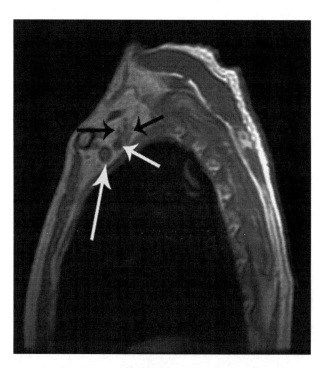

FIGURE 10.8

Sagittal T1 weighted image through the axillary fossa on the same patient as in Figure 10.7. Brachial plexus components (black arrows) depicted as nodular, somewhat irregular, soft tissue densities posteriorly to the artery (short white arrow) and vein (long white arrow), which are the rounded lower-intensity structures anteriorly.

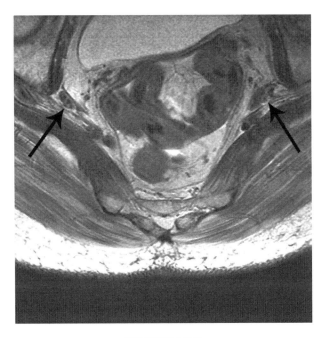

FIGURE 10.9

Sciatic nerves (arrows) depicted on axial T1 weighted MR image through the pelvic region as a conglomerate of individual fibers.

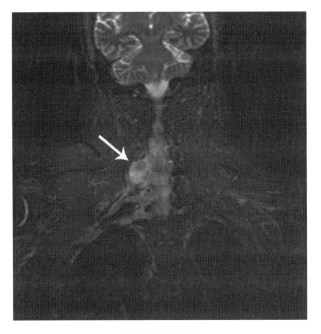

FIGURE 10.11

Coronal STIR MRI noncontrast sequence enhances visualization of the tumor tissue (arrow and bright areas on the right side).

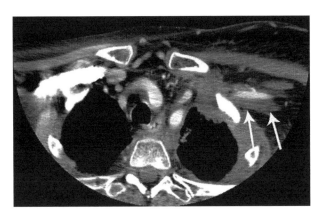

FIGURE 10.10

Recurrent breast cancer. Axial CT image demonstrates general thickening of the neurovascular bundle (arrows).

CT, abnormal nerve or plexus may appear locally or diffusely enlarged, or become indistinguishable from adjacent structures because of infiltrative process or fibrosis. In brachial plexus, this may be manifested as general thickening of neurovascular bundle (Fig. 10.10). Greater tissue discrimination allows MRI to assess the character and extent of disease more precisely. T1 weighted images may show segmental or diffuse enlargement, and increased T2 intensity may be seen within the nerve in case of involvement by infiltrative process or edema. The extent of the abnormal T2 signal may be demonstrated to the better advantage on fat suppression (STIR) sequences (Fig. 10.11). Contiguity (or disruption) of the nerve, increased diameter, change of course or contour (compression), altered intrinsic intensity, or enhancement within involved or compressed segment of the nerve may be observed. Neurography, utilizing combination of T1, T2, STIR, short inversion recovery (IR) sequences, and phased-array surface coils depict these changes with greater accuracy (4,33–35). In a study of 15 patients with neuropathic leg pain and negative or inconclusive conventional MRI conducted by Moore et al. (36), it proved definitely superior, revealing abnormality accounting for clinical findings in all cases.

An interesting phenomenon of increased T2 intensity within normal nerve(s), mimicking a diseased tissue, was reported by Chappell et al. (37) They observed raising intensity within the peripheral nerve as the orientation of longitudinal axis of the nerve approached 55 degrees to main magnetic field Bo. As the brachial plexus is usually scanned close to this "magic angle," T2 hyperintensity within the nerve or plexus should thus be interpreted with caution to avoid false-positive reading. Administration of contrast is essential in proper evaluation of extent of disease. Generally, enhancement of intraspinal or peripheral nerve after administration of conventional dose of gadolinium-based contrast is considered pathological.

Imaging Method of Choice

As x-rays yielded limited information on plexus involvement, early reports praised the ability of CT to demonstrate anatomic detail of normal and diseased plexus and its advantages over conventional radiography (10,14). As early as 1988, Benzel et al. considered CT a method of choice in evaluation of location and extent of nerve sheath tumors of sciatic nerve and sacral plexus, important in determination of resectability of these lesions. Hirakata et al. (15) found CT to be helpful in assessment of patients with Pancoast tumor. They reported obliteration of fat plane between scalene muscles on CT to be an indication of brachial plexus involvement. Addition of sagittal, coronal, and oblique reformatted images improved visualization of brachial plexus and helped to diagnose tumor recurrence (38). Soon after introduction of MRI, and as early as 1987, Castagno and Shuman (39) anticipated that new modality may have substantial clinical utility in evaluating patients with suspected brachial plexus tumor. The advantages of MRI over CT in assessment of plexus were reported in comparative studies by several investigators (40–42). In evaluation of 64 patients with brachial plexopathy of diverse cause by Bilbey et al. (43), the sensitivity of MRI was 63%, specificity 100%, and accuracy 77%. In subgroup of patients with trauma and neoplasm, these were even higher (81%, 100%, and 88%, respectively). Better anatomic definition provided by MRI was considered to improve patient care in the study by Collins et al. (44) In the study of patients with plexopathy following the treatment of breast cancer, Qayyum et al. (45) reported high reliability of MRI, with specificity of 95%, positive predictive value of 96%, and negative predictive value of 95%. MRI without and with contrast enhancement is also a method of choice in evaluating a patient with plexopathy at Memorial Sloan-Kettering Cancer Center.

PRIMARY PLEXUS NEOPLASMS

Primary tumors of peripheral nerve (plexus) are rare, constituting approximately 1% of all cancers. According to World Health Organization (WHO) classification proposed in 2000, four groups are distinguished: (1) schwannomas; (2) perineuriomas; (3) neurofibromas, and (4) malignant peripheral nerve sheath tumors (MPNST). Neurofibromas and schwannomas are most prevalent. On MRI, these tumors usually present as well-defined rounded or oval masses orientated along the longitudinal axis of the nerve (Fig. 10.12). Larger size or plexiform appearance favors neurofibroma, particularly in patients with neurofibromatosis (Fig. 10.13). Both are iso- or slightly hyperintense on T1 and hyperin-

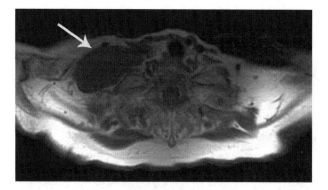

FIGURE 10.12

Brachial plexus schwannoma, depicted on axial T1 weighted MR image. Fusiform mass (arrows) is orientated along the longitudinal axis of the plexus.

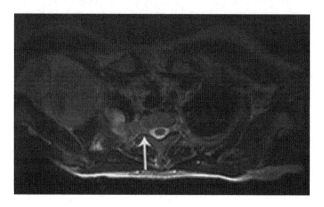

FIGURE 10.13

Patient with neurofibroma. Large mass is demonstrated in axillary fossa, involving brachial plexus and extending into the neural foramen (arrow).

tense on T2 weighted sequences, showing homogenous or inhomogeneous enhancement. Marked T2 hyperintensity may be seen in some patients (46–50). Capsule can be identified in approximately 70% of schwannomas and 30% of neurofibromas (45). A "target sign," consisting of central low-intensity area within the lesion on T2 weighted sequence, was found to be much more frequent in neurofibromas (51,52). On a CT, low density (in reference to the muscle) was a common feature of plexus tumors, and contrast enhancement varied from moderate to marked, as reported by Verstraete (53). MPNSTs are rare, arising either as spontaneous mutation or within preexisting neurofibroma, usually as a transformation to spindle cell sarcoma (54). It may be difficult to distinguish these tumors from their benign counterpart. Larger size, internal heterogeneity, poor definition of peripheral border, invasion of fat planes, and adjacent edema favor malignant variant

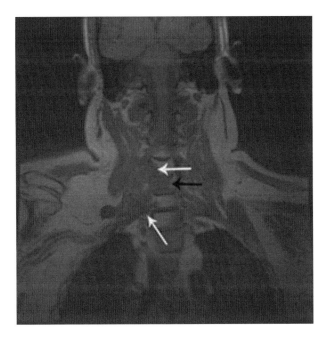

FIGURE 10.14

Malignant PNST, coronal T1 weighted MRI (the same patient as in Figure 10.11). The tumor (white arrows) is poorly defined and infiltrates adjacent cervical vertebrae (black arrow).

(Fig. 10.14) (55–58). Extremely rarely, other malignancies (eg, lymphoma) can arise from the nerve proper (59). There are no pathognomonic radiographic features that could be totally attributed to a particular group; thus, thorough knowledge of clinical information, such as age, gender, duration of symptoms, history of von Recklinghausen disease, etc., is helpful while interpreting the imaging studies.

EXTRINSIC PLEXUS TUMORS

Plexus may be compressed or infiltrated by an extrinsic neoplasm, arising from adjacent structures, with breast, neck, lung, and lymph node malignancies being most common offenders for brachial region and pelvic tumors for lumbosacral plexus (Fig. 10.15). Clinically, pain is a prominent feature of residual or recurrent tumor (1). Although local extent of the lesion may be depicted adequately by CT, infiltration of the plexus is difficult to diagnose, except for advanced disease with gross infiltration of the plexus region. In a study of 14 patients with Pancoast tumor (15), obliteration of fat planes between scalene muscles on CT was found to be suggestive of plexus involvement. The potential of MRI in evaluation of extent of thoracic malignancies and brachial plexus involvement was realized as early as 1989 (40). In the study of chest wall tumors by

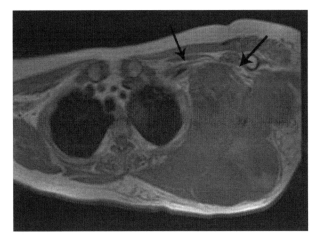

FIGURE 10.15

Axial CT section through thoracic inlet of patient with advanced osteogenic sarcoma of the scapula. Neurovascular elements (arrows) are compressed and displaced anteriorly.

Fortier (60), MRI clearly delineated the margins and revealed evidence of muscle, vascular, or bone invasion. T1 and T2 signal characteristics were nonspecific (apart for lipomas), not allowing for confident distinction of benign from malignant process. Qayyum (45) considered MRI to be a reliable and accurate tool in evaluation of brachial plexopathy due to tumor, reporting sensitivity, and positive predictive value of 96% and specificity and negative predictive value of 95%. Currently, MRI without and with contrast remains a method of choice for the assessment of local tumor extent and plexus involvement. PET scan is considered useful in evaluation of patients with plexopathy, mainly by excluding recurrent tumor (17,18).

RADIATION INJURY

Plexopathy is a recognized complication of radiation therapy, occurring most commonly in brachial plexus (Kori, 1981), following regional treatment of breast, lung, or neck cancers. Clinical presentation of radiation-induced fibrosis (RIF) is that of protracted course, with low-grade pain, as opposed to recurrent tumor, which is progressing more rapidly, with pain being a dominant symptom. Three forms are recognized: acute ischemic, transient, and delayed (radiation fibrosis), the latter being most common (61–63). Radiation-induced fibrosis occurs usually within the first few years after completion of treatment, although latent periods as long as 22 years have been reported (64,65). It is dose-dependent, more likely to occur above 6000 cGy and with larger fraction size. Younger patients and those

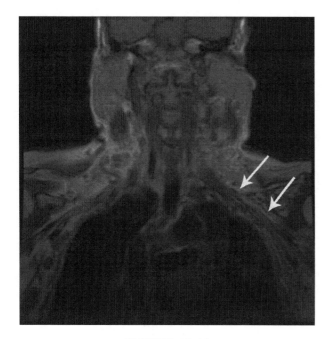

FIGURE 10.16

Patient with breast cancer and suspected postradiation left brachial plexopathy. MRI reveals matting and thickening of the left neurovascular bundle (arrows) without recognizable soft tissue mass, consistent with clinical diagnosis of RIF.

receiving cytotoxic therapy are more vulnerable (1,66). Changes are confined to the radiation port, with clearly demarcated margin from nonirradiated tissue. The main role of imaging is to distinguish this chronic iatrogenic process from a recurrent tumor, which generally carries unfavorable prognosis. CT may demonstrate poor definition of neurovascular bundle and increased density of regional fat without recognizable soft tissue mass (67), and MRI may reveal thickening and indistinct outline of plexus components, again without identifiable focal mass (Fig. 10.16). There is no uniform agreement as to signal intensity patterns and contrast enhancement of RIF. While some investigators reported low intensity of both on T1 and T2 weighted sequences (68), others described variable signal changes (69–71). Parascalene and interscalene T2 hyperintensity was reported by Bowen (72), and the degree of T2 hyperintensity was found to correspond with severity of fibrosis by Hoeller (71). Positive contrast enhancement was reported by most investigators, even in delayed cases (69).

SUMMARY

Clinical assessment of plexus involvement by primary neoplasm, metastases, or conditions related to treatment is limited, and imaging studies (CT, MRI) are routinely requested to further characterize the nature and extent of the process. With its many advantages

over CT, MRI, without and with contrast, is presently considered an imaging method of choice in evaluation of plexus disease. Utilizing high-resolution devices, we are now able to visualize individual nerves (MR neurography). However, there are still many limitations of MRI technique, such as inhomogenous fat suppression or vascular flow artifacts, making the interpretation difficult. Although abnormal signal or enhancement within the individual nerve can be depicted, the process cannot be further characterized (eg, benign or malignant). Recently introduced into clinical practice, higher field strength (3T) MRI may offer superior resolution and improved option for functional imaging. As the state of the art approach at present, it includes thorough clinical examination, followed by high-resolution phase-array MRI without and with contrast. Dynamic CT should be reserved for patients unable to have MRI and instances when additional information on bone detail or vascular anatomy is also needed. PET scan plays a complementary role to MRI in assessment of neoplastic involvement.

References

1. Kori SH, Foley KM, et al. Brachial plexus lesions in patients with cancer: 100 cases. *Neurology.* 1981;31(1):45–50.
2. Jaeckle KA. Neurological manifestations of neoplastic and radiation-induced plexopathies. *Semin Neurol.* 2004;24(4):385–393.
3. Filler AG, Howe FA, et al. Magnetic resonance neurography. *Lancet.* 1993;341(8846):659–661.
4. Filler AG, Kliot M, et al. Application of magnetic resonance neurography in the evaluation of patients with peripheral nerve pathology. *J Neurosurg.* 1996;85(2):299–309.
5. Aagaard BD, Maravilla KR, et al. MR neurography. MR imaging of peripheral nerves. *Magn Reson Imaging Clin N Am.* 1998;6(1):179–194.
6. Freund W, Brinkmann A, et al. MR neurography with multiplanar reconstruction of 3D MRI datasets: an anatomical study and clinical applications. *Neuroradiology.* 2007.
7. Clemente DC. The peripheral nervous system. In: *Gray's Anatomy, Thirtieth American Edition.* Philadelphia: Lea & Febiger Publishers; 1985:1149–1282.
8. Castillo M. Imaging the anatomy of the brachial plexus: review and self-assessment module. *AJR Am J Roentgenol.* 2005;185(6 Suppl):S196–S204.
9. Posniak HV, Olson MC, et al. MR imaging of the brachial plexus. *AJR Am J Roentgenol.* 1993;161(2):373–379.
10. Benzel EC, Morris DM, et al. Nerve sheath tumors of the sciatic nerve and sacral plexus. *J Surg Oncol.* 1988;39(1):8–16.
11. Cooke J, Cooke D, et al. The anatomy and pathology of the brachial plexus as demonstrated by computed tomography. *Clin Radiol.* 1988;39(6):595–601.
12. Dietemann JL, Sick H, et al. Anatomy and computed tomography of the normal lumbosacral plexus. *Neuroradiology.* 1987;29(1):58–68.
13. Gebarski KS, Glazer GM, et al. Brachial plexus: anatomic, radiologic, and pathologic correlation using computed tomography. *J Comput Assist Tomogr.* 1982;6(6):1058–1063.
14. Gebarski KS, Gebarski SS, et al. The lumbosacral plexus: anatomic-radiologic-pathologic correlation using CT. *Radiographics.* 1986;6(3):401–425.
15. Hirakata K, Nakata H, et al. Computed tomography of Pancoast tumor. *Rinsho Hoshasen.* 1989;34(1):79–84.

16. Rydberg J, Liang Y, et al. Fundamentals of multichannel CT. *Semin Musculoskelet Radiol.* 2004;8(2):137–146.

17. Graif M, Martinoli C, et al. Sonographic evaluation of brachial plexus pathology. *Eur Radiol.* 2004;14(2):193–200.

18. Hathaway PB, Mankoff DA, et al. Value of combined FDG PET and MR imaging in the evaluation of suspected recurrent local-regional breast cancer: preliminary experience. *Radiology.* 1999;210(3):807–814.

19. Ahmad A, Barrington S, et al. Use of positron emission tomography in evaluation of brachial plexopathy in breast cancer patients. *Br J Cancer.* 1999;79(3–4):478–482.

20. Krol G, Strong E. Computed tomography of head and neck malignancies. *Clin Plast Surg.* 1986;13(3):475–491.

21. Carriero A, Ciccotosto C, et al. Magnetic resonance imaging of the brachial plexus. Anatomy. *Radiol Med (Torino).* 1991;81(1–2):73–77.

22. Gierada DS, Erickson SJ, et al. MR imaging of the sacral plexus: normal findings. *AJR Am J Roentgenol.* 1993;160(5):1059–1065.

23. Blake LC, Robertson WD, et al. Sacral plexus: optimal imaging planes for MR assessment. *Radiology.* 1996;199(3):767–772.

24. Panasci DJ, Holliday RA, et al. Advanced imaging techniques of the brachial plexus. *Hand Clin.* 1995;11(4):545–553.

25. Almanza MY, Poon-Chue A, et al. Dual oblique MR method for imaging the sciatic nerve. *J Comput Assist Tomogr.* 1999;23(1):138–140.

26. Kichari JR, Hussain SM, et al. MR imaging of the brachial plexus: current imaging sequences, normal findings, and findings in a spectrum of focal lesions with MR-pathologic correlation. *Curr Probl Diagn Radiol.* 2003;32(2):88–101.

27. Maravilla KR, Bowen BC. Imaging of the peripheral nervous system: evaluation of peripheral neuropathy and plexopathy. *AJNR Am J Neuroradiol.* 1998;19(6):1011–1023.

28. Blair DN, Rapoport S, et al. Normal brachial plexus: MR imaging. *Radiology.* 1987;165(3):763–767.

29. Bowen BC, Pattany PM, et al. The brachial plexus: normal anatomy, pathology, and MR imaging. *Neuroimaging Clin N Am.* 2004;14(1):59–85, vii–viii.

30. Gasparotti R, Ferraresi S, et al. Three-dimensional MR myelography of traumatic injuries of the brachial plexus. *AJNR Am J Neuroradiol.* 1997;18(9):1733–1742.

31. Tien RD, Hesselink JR, et al. Improved detection and delineation of head and neck lesions with fat suppression spin-echo MR imaging. *AJNR Am J Neuroradiol.* 1991;12(1):19–24.

32. Howe FA, Filler AG, et al. Magnetic resonance neurography. *Magn Reson Med.* 1992;28(2):328–338.

33. Dailey AT, Tsuruda JS, et al. Magnetic resonance neurography for cervical radiculopathy: a preliminary report. *Neurosurgery.* 1996;38(3):488–492, discussion 492.

34. Erdem CZ, Erdem LO, et al. High resolution MR neurography in patients with cervical radiculopathy. *Tani Girisim Radyol.* 2004;10(1):14–19.

35. Lewis AM, Layzer R, et al. Magnetic resonance neurography in extraspinal sciatica. *Arch Neurol.* 2006;63(10):1469–1472.

36. Moore KR, Tsuruda JS, et al. The value of MR neurography for evaluating extraspinal neuropathic leg pain: a pictorial essay. *AJNR Am J Neuroradiol.* 2001;22(4):786–794.

37. Chappell KE, Robson MD, et al. Magic angle effects in MR neurography. *AJNR Am J Neuroradiol.* 2004;25(3):431–440.

38. Fishman EK, Campbell JN, et al. Multiplanar CT evaluation of brachial plexopathy in breast cancer. *J Comput Assist Tomogr.* 1991;15(5):790–795.

39. Castagno AA, Shuman WP. MR imaging in clinically suspected brachial plexus tumor. *AJR Am J Roentgenol.* 1987;149(6):1219–1222.

40. Rapoport S, Blair DN, et al. Brachial plexus: correlation of MR imaging with CT and pathologic findings. *Radiology.* 1988;167(1):161–165.

41. Thyagarajan D, Cascino T, et al. Magnetic resonance imaging in brachial plexopathy of cancer. *Neurology.* 1995;45 (3 Pt 1):421–427.

42. Taylor BV, Kimmel DW, et al. Magnetic resonance imaging in cancer-related lumbosacral plexopathy. *Mayo Clin Proc.* 1997;72(9):823–829.

43. Bilbey JH, Lamond RG, et al. MR imaging of disorders of the brachial plexus. *J Magn Reson Imaging.* 1994;4(1):13–18.

44. Collins JD, Shaver ML, et al. Compromising abnormalities of the brachial plexus as displayed by magnetic resonance imaging. *Clin Anat.* 1995;8(1):1–16.

45. Qayyum A, MacVicar AD, et al. Symptomatic brachial plexopathy following treatment for breast cancer: utility of MR imaging with surface-coil techniques. *Radiology.* 2000;214(3):837–842.

46. Baba Y, Ohkubo K, et al. MR imaging appearances of schwannoma: correlation with pathological findings. *Nippon Igaku Hoshasen Gakkai Zasshi.* 1997;57(8):499–504.

47. Cerofolini E, Landi A, et al. MR of benign peripheral nerve sheath tumors. *J Comput Assist Tomogr.* 1991;15(4):593–597.

48. Soderlund V, Goranson H, et al. MR imaging of benign peripheral nerve sheath tumors. *Acta Radiol.* 1994;35(3):282–286.

49. Saifuddin A. Imaging tumours of the brachial plexus. *Skeletal Radiol.* 2003;32(7):375–387.

50. Hayasaka K, Tanaka Y, et al. MR findings in primary retroperitoneal schwannoma. *Acta Radiol.* 1999;40(1):78–82.

51. Bhargava R, Parham DM, et al. MR imaging differentiation of benign and malignant peripheral nerve sheath tumors: use of the target sign. *Pediatr Radiol.* 1997;27(2):124–129.

52. Burk DL, Jr., Brunberg JA, et al. Spinal and paraspinal neurofibromatosis: surface coil MR imaging at 1.5 T1. *Radiology.* 1987;162(3):797–801.

53. Verstraete KL, Achten E, et al. Nerve sheath tumors: evaluation with CT and MR imaging. *J Belge Radiol.* 1992;75(4):311–320.

54. Antonescu C, Woodruff J. (2006). Primary tumors of cranial, spinal and peripheral nerves. In: McLendon RE, Rosenblum MK, Bigner DD, eds. *Russell and Rubinstein's Pathology of Tumors of the Nervous System,* 7th ed. Hodder Arnold Publisher; 2006:787–835.

55. Levine E, Huntrakoon M, et al. Malignant nerve-sheath neoplasms in neurofibromatosis: distinction from benign tumors by using imaging techniques. *AJR Am J Roentgenol.* 1987;149(5):1059–1064.

56. Fuchs B, Spinner RJ, et al. Malignant peripheral nerve sheath tumors: an update. *J Surg Orthop Adv.* 2005;14(4):168–174.

57. Geniets C, Vanhoenacker FM, et al. Imaging features of peripheral neurogenic tumors. *Jbr-Btr.* 2006;89(4):216–219.

58. Amoretti N, Grimaud A, et al. Peripheral neurogenic tumors: is the use of different types of imaging diagnostically useful? *Clin Imaging.* 2006;30(3):201–205.

59. Descamps MJ, Barrett L, et al. Primary sciatic nerve lymphoma: a case report and review of the literature. *J Neurol Neurosurg Psychiatry.* 2006;77(9):1087–1089.

60. Fortier M, Mayo JR, Swensen SJ, Munk PL, Vellet DA, Muller NL. MR imaging of chest wall lesions. *Radiographics.* 1994;14(3):597–606.

61. Gerard JM, Franck N, Moussa Z, Hildebrand J. Acute ischemic brachial plexus neuropathy following radiation therapy. *Neurology.* March 1989;39(3):450–451.

62. Salner AL, Botnick LE, et al. Reversible brachial plexopathy following primary radiation therapy for breast cancer. *Cancer Treat Rep.* 1981;65(9–10):797–802.

63. Maruyama Y, Mylrea MM, Logothetis J. Neuropathy following irradiation. An unusual late complication of radiotherapy. *Am J Roentgenol Ther Nucl Med.* September 1967;101(1):216–219.

64. Fathers E, Thrush D, et al. Radiation-induced brachial plexopathy in women treated for carcinoma of the breast. *Clin Rehabil.* 2002;16(2):160–165.

65. Nich C, Bonnin P, et al. An uncommon form of delayed radioinduced brachial plexopathy. *Chir Main.* 2005;24(1):48–51.

66. Olsen NK, Pfeiffer P, Johannsen L, Schroder H, Rose C. Radiation-induced brachial plexopathy: neurological follow-up in

161 recurrence free breast cancer patients. *Int J Radiat Biol Phys.* April 30, 1993;26(1):43–49.

67. Cascino TL, Kori S, et al. CT of the brachial plexus in patients with cancer. *Neurology.* 1983;33(12):1553–1557.

68. Wittenberg KH, Adkins MC. MR imaging of nontraumatic brachial plexopathies: frequency and spectrum of findings. *Radiographics.* 2000;20(4):1023–1032.

69. Wouter van Es H, Engelen AM, et al. Radiation-induced brachial plexopathy: MR imaging. *Skeletal Radiol.* 1997;26(5):284–288.

70. Dao TH, Rahmouni A, et al. Tumor recurrence versus fibrosis in the irradiated breast: differentiation with dynamic gadolinium-enhanced MR imaging. *Radiology.* 1993;187(3):751–755.

71. Hoeller U, Bonacker M, et al. Radiation-induced plexopathy and fibrosis. Is magnetic resonance imaging the adequate diagnostic tool? *Strahlenther Onkol.* 2004;180(10):650–654.

72. Bowen BC, Verma A, et al. Radiation-induced brachial plexopathy: MR and clinical findings. *AJNR Am J Neuroradiol.* 1996;17(10):1932–1936.

73. Garant M, Remy H, et al. Aggressive fibromatosis of the neck: MR findings. *AJNR Am J Neuroradiol.* 1997;18(8):1429–1431.

74. Gierada DS, Erickson SJ. MR imaging of the sacral plexus: abnormal findings. *AJR Am J Roentgenol.* 1993;160(5):1067–1071.

Cancer Statistics

Melissa M. Center
Ahmedin Jemal

Cancer is a complex constellation of hundreds of diseases (1) whose occurrence varies strikingly according to age, sex, race/ethnicity, socioeconomic status, geographic location, and time. Close examination of these variations has provided strong evidence that much of cancer is caused by environmental factors and is potentially avoidable (2). Monitoring time trends in cancer occurrence is also important to assess the effectiveness of cancer prevention and control efforts in the overall population and in subgroups that may be at higher risk. This chapter describes cancer occurrence patterns in the United States for all cancers combined and for seven select cancer sites, which together account for 58% of the total new cases in the United States (3).

DATA SOURCES

In the United States, the Surveillance, Epidemiology, and End Results (SEER) program has been collecting cancer incidence data in nine population-based cancer registries since 1975. These registries, which provide information on temporal trends, cover approximately 10% of the U.S. population. Subsequent expansions of the SEER program provide coverage of approximately 26% of the U.S. population (http://www.seer.cancer .gov) (4). The Centers for Disease Control and Prevention's National Program of Cancer Registries (NPCR) was established in 1994 to improve existing non-SEER

population-based cancer registries and to establish new statewide cancer registries (http://www.cdc.gov/cancer/ npcr). Through the NPCR and SEER programs, cancer data are collected in almost all parts of the United States, although data quality varies across registries.

Mortality data have been collected for most of the United States since 1930, based on information from death certificates. The underlying cause of death is classified according to the most current International Statistical Classification of Diseases (ICD). Beginning with the 1999 mortality data, underlying causes of death are classified according to ICD-10 coding and selection rules, replacing ICD-9, which was used from 1979–1998 (5). The ICD-10 codes for malignant cancer are C00-C97 (6). Mortality data are available from the National Center for Health Statistics (http://www.cdc. gov/nchs/nvss.htm).

MEASUREMENTS OF CANCER OCCURRENCE

Incidence and Mortality

Incidence and mortality rates are two frequently used measures of cancer occurrence. These indices quantify the number of new cancer cases or deaths, respectively, in a specified population over a defined time period. They are commonly expressed as counts per

KEY POINTS

- Cancer is a complex constellation of hundreds of diseases whose occurrence varies strikingly according to age, sex, race/ethnicity, socioeconomic status, geographic location, and time.
- In the United States, the Surveillance, Epidemiology, and End Results (SEER) program has been collecting cancer incidence data in nine population-based cancer registries since 1975.
- Mortality data have been collected for most of the United States since 1930, based on information from death certificates.
- Incidence is the number of new cancer cases or deaths, respectively, in a specified population over a defined time period and is commonly expressed as counts per 100,000 people per year.
- Prevalence measures the proportion of people living with cancer at a certain point in time.
- The relative survival rate for a specific disease reflects the proportion of people alive at a specified period after diagnosis, usually five years, compared

- to that of a population of equivalent age, sex, and race without the disease.
- The risk of developing cancer is affected by age, race, sex, socioeconomic status, geographic location, and calendar year.
- It is estimated that 1,444,920 new cancer cases and 559,650 new deaths due to cancer will occur in the United States in 2007.
- The probability of developing invasive cancer over a lifetime is about 45% for men and 38% for women.
- Survival rates for all cancers combined have increased significantly, from 50% during the period 1975–1977 to 66% during 1996–2003.
- The three most commonly diagnosed cancers in the United States in 2007 will be prostate, lung and bronchus, and colon and rectum in men and breast, lung and bronchus, and colon and rectum in females.
- Lung cancer accounts for the most cancer-related deaths in both men and women.

100,000 people per year and are age-standardized to allow comparisons across populations of varying age structure.

Prevalence

Prevalence measures the proportion of people living with cancer at a certain point in time. In principle, the number of prevalent cases includes newly diagnosed cases, those who are undergoing treatment, and people who are in remission. It is influenced by both the incidence rate of the cancers of interest and by survival or cure rates. In practice, estimates of the number of prevalent cases in the United States represent the total number of cancer cases diagnosed in a specified duration. Therefore, they cannot distinguish precisely between people who have been cured and those with active disease. There were 10.7 million people with a history of cancer (Table 11.1) in the United States in January 2004.

The Probability of Developing or Dying from Cancer

The probability that an individual will develop or die from cancer by a certain age is another measure used

to describe average risk in the general population. The probability, usually expressed as a percentage, can also be expressed as one person in X persons. These estimates are based on the average experience of the general population and may over- or underestimate individual risk because of family history or individual risk factors. The probability of developing cancer or dying of cancer are calculated using Probability of Developing Cancer Software (DevCan) developed by the National Cancer Institute (http://www.srab.cancer.gov/devcan/).

Estimated New Cancer Cases and Deaths

Each year, the American Cancer Society estimates the total number of new cancer cases and deaths that will occur in the nation and in each state in the current year. These estimates are of interest because actual mortality statistics do not become available for approximately three years. The American Cancer Society projections are more readily understood by the public than are projections of cancer rates, and are frequently cited by cancer control planners and researchers (7). The estimates are produced by modeling historic information on the observed number of cancer cases and deaths in past years and modeling trends over time (8,9).

TABLE 11.1

Estimated Number of Prevalent Cases of Selected Cancers, by Sex; United States, 2004

	MALE NO.	%	FEMALE NO.	%	TOTAL NO.	%
All sites	4,848,429	100	5,913,785	100	10,762,214	100
Breast	12,270	0.3	2,407,943	40.7	2,420,213	22.5
Cervix uteri		0.0	250,726	4.2	250,726	2.3
Colon and rectum	521,676	10.8	554,659	9.4	1,076,335	10.0
Esophagus	18,763	0.4	6,022	0.1	24,785	0.2
Kidney and renal pelvis	141,899	2.9	98,367	1.7	240,266	2.2
Liver and intrahepatic bile duct	12,411	0.3	7,018	0.1	19,429	0.2
Lung and bronchus	174,880	3.6	183,248	3.1	358,128	3.3
Melanoma	333,330	6.9	356,691	6.0	690,021	6.4
Pancreas	13,423	0.3	15,024	0.3	28,447	0.3
Prostate	2,024,489	41.8		0.0	2,024,489	18.8

Source: Surveillance, Epidemiology, and End Results Program, 1975–2004, Division of Cancer Control and Population Sciences, National Cancer Institute, 2007.

Survival Rate

The relative survival rate for a specific disease reflects the proportion of people alive at a specified period after diagnosis, usually five years, compared to that of a population of equivalent age, sex, and race without the disease. It adjusts for normal life expectancy (events such as deaths from heart disease, accidents, and diseases of old age).

DEMOGRAPHIC AND GEOGRAPHIC FACTORS

As mentioned, the risk of developing cancer is affected by age, race, sex, socioeconomic status, geographic location, and calendar year.

Age

Age profoundly affects the risk of being diagnosed with cancer. For most cancers, the incidence rates increase with age because of cumulative exposures to carcinogenic agents such as tobacco, infectious organisms, chemicals, and internal factors, such as inherited mutations, hormones, and immune conditions. Figure 11.1 (left panel) depicts the age-related increase in the incidence rate from all cancer combined in men

and women. The incidence rate for age 0–4 years is twice that for ages 5–9 and 10–14 due to cancers such as acute lymphocytic leukemia, neuroblastoma, and retinoblastoma that have higher incidence rates among young children. The decrease in cancer incidence rates after age 84 may largely reflect underdiagnosis. The median age at diagnosis for most cancer sites is 60 or above. Cancers with median ages of diagnosis under 50 include cancers of the testis, bones and joints, thyroid, and cervix and Hodgkin disease.

Sex

Cancer affects both men and women, unless it is sex-specific. However, the incidence rates of most types of cancer are higher in men than in women (Table 11.2). The most extreme example is cancer of the larynx, for which the incidence rate is nearly five times as high in males as in females. The few exceptions in which cancers that affect both sexes are more common in women than men include breast, thyroid, and gallbladder (Table 11.2). Although overall cancer rates are lower in women than in men, the overall prevalence of cancer is higher in women. Of the 10.7 million prevalent cancer cases in 2004, 4.8 million were men, while 5.9 million were women (Table 11.1). This may reflect the high survival rates of women with early-stage breast cancers and the greater longevity of women than men.

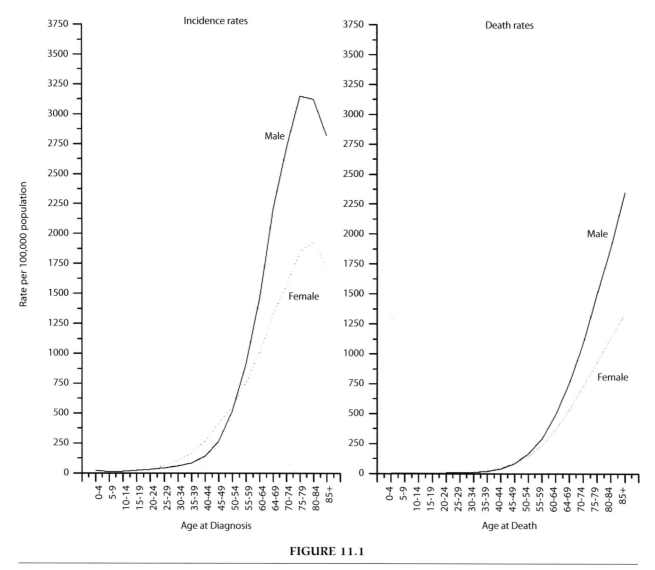

FIGURE 11.1

Age- and sex-specific incidence and death rates from all cancers combined, United States, 2004. Incidence rates from Surveillance, Epidemiology, and End Results (SEER) program statistics database for 1973–2004. Death rates from National Center for Health Statistics, Centers for Disease Control and Prevention.

Race

Cancer rates vary widely across racial and ethnic groups, and as Table 11.3 shows, blacks generally have higher cancer rates compared to whites. Cancer incidence and death rates are 16% and 27% higher, respectively, in black men than in white men. Similarly, cancer death rates are nearly 15% higher in black women than white women, despite lower incidence. While other racial ethnic groups, such as Asian American/Pacific Islanders, have lower incidence and mortality for all sites combined compared to whites and blacks, their rates of certain cancers (stomach, liver and intrahepatic bile duct, cervix) are generally higher. This is thought to reflect greater exposure to specific infectious agents (in the case of stomach and liver cancers), lower use of screening (for cervical cancer), and higher consumption of preserved rather than fresh foods (for stomach cancer) (10).

Socioeconomic Status

Socioeconomic status (SES) is inversely correlated with death rates from cancer and many other causes because it is strongly associated with high-risk factors, such as smoking, drinking, lack of health insurance, access to care, and low screening rates (11–13). A study by Albano et al. found an inverse relationship between level of education and death rates from all cancers combined for African American and white men and for white women. Much of the variation in mortality

TABLE 11.2
*Average Annual Age-Standardized Cancer Incidence Rates^a in Men Compared to Women,
2000–2004, United States*

	MALE RATE	FEMALE RATE	RATE RATIO MALE VS. FEMALE
All sites	555.82	411.32	1.35
Oral cavity and pharynx	15.63	6.12	2.55
Esophagus	7.86	2.01	3.91
Stomach	11.43	5.58	2.05
Small intestine	2.17	1.49	1.46
Colon and rectum	60.76	44.57	1.36
Anus, anal canal, and anorectum	1.30	1.62	0.80
Liver and intrahepatic bile duct	9.51	3.39	2.81
Gallbladder	0.82	1.46	0.56
Pancreas	12.88	10.10	1.28
Larynx	6.64	1.37	4.85
Lung and bronchus	81.19	52.31	1.55
Bones and joints	1.04	0.78	1.33
Soft tissue, including heart	3.69	2.62	1.41
Melanoma of the skin	23.64	14.94	1.58
Breast	1.15	127.85	0.01
Urinary bladder	37.32	9.37	3.98
Kidney and renal pelvis	17.76	8.85	2.01
Eye and orbit	1.00	0.66	1.52
Brain and other nervous system	7.65	5.42	1.41
Thyroid	4.35	12.48	0.35
Hodgkin lymphoma	3.03	2.40	1.26
Non-Hodgkin lymphoma	23.21	16.25	1.43
Myeloma	6.96	4.54	1.53
Leukemia	15.99	9.51	1.68

^{a}Rates are per 100,000 and age-adjusted to the 2000 U.S. standard population.

occurred between those with 12 or fewer years of education compared to those with additional schooling. The mortality rate ratio for all cancers combined in less educated persons compared to more educated persons was 1.43 for African American women, 1.76 for non-Hispanic white women, 2.24 for non-Hispanic white men, and 2.38 for African American men (14). In contrast, higher SES is positively associated with the incidence of some screening-related cancers. For example, the incidence of prostate cancer is higher in high and middle SES groups than in the poor, simply because of greater detection (12).

Geographic Location

Variability in cancer occurrence by place, together with surveillance data on cancer trends, has stimulated important hypotheses about the etiology and potential preventability of many cancers (2,15). High-risk areas for specific cancers may or may not be well characterized by official administrative boundaries, such as county, state, or national borders. For example, in the United States, the area with the highest death rates from cervical cancer spans much of Appalachia (16), where women historically lacked access to regular Pap testing or treatment. This observation motivated the

TABLE 11.3

Age-Standardized Incidence and Death Rates[a] for Selected Cancer Sites by Race and Ethnicity, United States, 2000–2004

	WHITE	AFRICAN AMERICAN	ASIAN/PACIFIC ISLANDER	AMERICAN INDIAN/ ALASKA NATIVE	HISPANIC- LATINO[b]
Incidence					
All sites					
Males	556.7	663.7	359.9	236.3	421.7
Females	423.9	396.9	285.8	203.3	314.5
Breast (female)	132.5	118.3	89.0	51.0	89.4
Colon and rectum					
Males	60.4	72.6	49.7	29.1	47.6
Females	44.0	55.0	35.3	26.9	33.0
Esophagus					
Males	8.0	10.4	4.2	4.9	5.4
Females	1.9	3.2	1.2	1	1.2
Lung and bronchus					
Males	81.0	110.6	55.1	40.3	45.0
Females	54.6	53.7	27.7	27.6	25.3
Liver and bile duct					
Males	7.9	12.7	21.3	10.3	14.4
Females	2.9	3.8	7.9	4.4	5.7
Pancreas					
Males	12.8	16.2	10	7	11
Females	9.9	13.9	8.3	6.8	10
Prostate	161.4	255.5	96.5	52.5	140.6
MORTALITY					
All sites					
Males	234.7	321.8	141.7	187.9	162.2
Females	161.4	189.3	96.7	141.2	106.7
Breast (female)	25.0	33.8	12.6	16.1	16.1
Colon and rectum					
Males	22.9	32.7	15.0	20.6	17.0
Females	15.9	22.9	10.3	14.3	11.1
Esophagus					
Males	7.7	10.2	3.1	6.7	4.2
Females	1.7	3.0	0.8	1.5	1.0
Lung and bronchus					
Males	72.6	95.8	38.3	49.6	36.0
Females	42.1	39.8	18.5	32.7	16.1
Liver and bile duct					
Males	6.5	10.0	15.5	10.7	10.8
Females	2.8	3.9	6.7	6.7	5.0
Pancreas					
Males	12.0	15.5	7.9	7.6	9.1
Females	9.0	12.4	6.9	7.3	7.5
Prostate	25.6	62.3	11.3	21.5	21.2

[a]Per 100,000, age-adjusted to 2000 U.S. standard population.
[b]Mortality rates for American Indian/Alaska Native are based on the CHSDA (Contract Health Service Delivery Area) counties.
[c]Hispanic-Latinos are not mutually exclusive from whites, blacks, Asian/Pacific Islanders, and American Indian/Alaska Natives.

Source: Reis LAG, Harkins D, Krapcho M, et al., eds. SEER Cancer Statistics Review, 1975–2004, National Cancer Institute, based on November 2006 SEER data submission, posted to the SEER Web site, 2007.

U.S. Congress to create the National Breast and Cervical Cancer Early Detection Program (NBCCEDP) to improve access to breast and cervical cancer screening and diagnostic services for low-income women (17).

Temporal Trends

Changes in cancer incidence over time may result from changes in the prevalence of risk factors and/or changes in detection practices due to the introduction or increased use of screening/diagnostic techniques. Furthermore, incidence trends can be affected by reporting delay and changes in disease classification. Trends in mortality rates may also be affected by most of the previously mentioned factors, with the exception of delay in reporting and artifacts of screening, in addition to improvements in cancer treatments over time.

CANCER OCCURRENCE PATTERNS FOR ALL CANCERS COMBINED

All cancers combined include all malignant cases, except nonmelanoma skin cancers. It is estimated that 1,444,920 new cancer cases and 559,650 new deaths due to cancer will occur in the United States in 2007 (18). The probability of developing invasive cancer over a lifetime is about 45% for men and 38% for women (Table 11.4). Age-standardized incidence rates for all cancers combined are 26% higher in men than in women (Table 11.2) and 16% higher in black men than white men (Table 11.3). Survival rates for all cancers combined have increased significantly, from 50% during the period 1975–1977 to 66% during 1996–2003 (Table 11.5).

The interpretation of temporal trends for all cancers combined is complex because cancer is a constellation of more than 100 diseases, each of which is affected by several factors, including risk factors, screening, diagnosis, and treatment. However, the overall cancer trend is substantially influenced by trends of the major cancer sites. The increase in the incidence rate for all cancers combined among men from 1975–1988 (Fig. 11.2) reflects the rise in lung cancer from smoking and the diagnosis of prostate cancer from transurethral resection (19,20). In contrast, the sharp increase and subsequent decrease in the incidence of all cancers combined from 1988–1992 is driven by trends in prostate cancer incidence (Fig. 11.3, left panel) and reflect the introduction of prostate-specific antigen (PSA) testing, followed by the saturation and leveling off of PSA testing (21). The overall increase in incidence rates among women (Fig. 11.2), although slower during the most recent time period, predominantly reflects trends in lung and breast cancer incidence, which in turn, result from the increased consumption of cigarettes in women

born in the 1930s (19) and the increased utilization of mammography along with the increased prevalence of reproductive risk factors (22), respectively. Female breast cancer incidence rates are declining since 2000, likely due to reduction in use of mammography and hormone replacement therapy (23,24).

Among men, the long-term trend in overall cancer death rates (Fig. 11.2) is largely determined by trends in tobacco-related cancers, particularly lung cancer (19). Between 1930 and 1990, lung cancer death rates (per 100,000) rose from 4.3 to 90.4, representing a 21-fold increase (4). Thereafter, lung cancer death rates decreased to 70.3 per 100,000 in 2004 (4). These trends reflect historical smoking patterns. Cigarette consumption peaked during the mid-20th century and gradually decreased following the Surgeon General's report in 1964 (25). In addition to lung cancer, cigarette smoking has been linked to multiple other cancer types, including oral cavity, pharynx, larynx, esophagus, stomach, pancreas, urinary bladder, kidney, liver, cervix, and myeloid leukemia (26).

Improved treatments, increased screening, and changes in dietary habits may have also contributed to the reduction in death rates from all cancers combined since the early 1990s (27). Colorectal and prostate cancers are among the sites for which trends are shown in Figure 11.4 that may be affected by a combination of improved treatment and/or screening.

Among women, the overall cancer death rate decreased from the 1930s through early 1970s, increased until the early 1990s, and decreased thereafter (Fig. 11.2). The long-term decline before the 1970s reflects decreases in deaths from cancer of the stomach, cervix-uterus, and colon and rectum. The dramatic decrease in stomach cancer mortality, which has occurred in most industrialized countries, is thought to result from improvements in food preservation and reduced prevalence of *Helicobacter pylori* infection (28). Among women, the historic decreases in mortality from stomach and cervix-uterus cancers were offset by the increases in lung cancer mortality after 1960 (19). Decreases in the overall cancer death rates since the early 1990s reflect reduction in death rates from colorectal and breast cancers due to improved treatment and increased screening rates and plateauing of trends in lung cancer mortality rates (Fig. 11.4, right panel).

CANCER OCCURRENCE PATTERNS FOR SELECT SITES

The three most commonly diagnosed cancers in the United States in 2007 will be prostate, lung and bronchus, and colon and rectum in men and breast, lung and

TABLE 11.4

Probability of (Percentage) Developing Invasive Cancers Over Specified Age Intervals,
by Sex, United States[a]

	BIRTH TO 39 (%)	40 TO 59 (%)	60 TO 69 (%)	70 AND OLDER (%)	BIRTH TO DEATH (%)
All sites[b]					
Male	1.42 (1 in 70)	8.58 (1 in 12)	16.25 (1 in 6)	38.96 (1 in 3)	44.94 (1 in 2)
Female	2.04 (1 in 49)	8.97 (1 in 11)	10.36 (1 in 10)	26.31 (1 in 4)	37.52 (1 in 3)
Bladder[c]					
Male	0.02 (1 in 4477)	0.41 (1 in 244)	0.96 (1 in 104)	3.50 (1 in 29)	3.70 (1 in 27)
Female	0.01 (1 in 9462)	0.13 (1 in 790)	0.26 (1 in 384)	0.99 (1 in 101)	1.17 (1 in 85)
Breast					
Female	0.48 (1 in 210)	3.86 (1 in 26)	3.51 (1 in 28)	6.59 (1 in 15)	12.28 (1 in 8)
Colon and rectum					
Male	0.08 (1 in 1329)	0.92 (1 in 109)	1.60 (1 in 63)	4.78 (1 in 21)	5.65 (1 in 18)
Female	0.07 (1 in 1394)	0.72 (1 in 138)	1.12 (1 in 89)	4.30 (1 in 23)	5.23 (1 in 19)
Leukemia					
Male	0.16 (1 in 624)	0.21 (1 in 468)	0.35 (1 in 288)	1.18 (1 in 85)	1.50 (1 in 67)
Female	0.12 (1 in 837)	0.14 (1 in 705)	0.20 (1 in 496)	0.76 (1 in 131)	1.06 (1 in 95)
Lung and bronchus					
Male	0.03 (1 in 3357)	1.03 (1 in 97)	2.52 (1 in 40)	6.74 (1 in 15)	7.91 (1 in 13)
Female	0.03 (1 in 2964)	0.82 (1 in 121)	1.81 (1 in 55)	4.61 (1 in 22)	6.18 (1 in 16)
Melanoma of the skin					
Male	0.13 (1 in 784)	0.53 (1 in 190)	0.57 (1 in 175)	1.40 (1 in 72)	2.10 (1 in 48)
Female	0.21 (1 in 471)	0.42 (1 in 236)	0.29 (1 in 348)	0.64 (1 in 156)	1.40 (1 in 71)
Non-Hodgkin lymphoma					
Male	0.13 (1 in 760)	0.45 (1 in 222)	0.57 (1 in 174)	1.61 (1 in 62)	2.19 (1 in 46)
Female	0.08 (1 in 1212)	0.32 (1 in 312)	0.45 (1 in 221)	1.33 (1 in 75)	1.87 (1 in 53)
Prostate					
Male	0.01 (1 in 10553)	2.54 (1 in 39)	6.83 (1 in 15)	13.36 (1 in 7)	16.72 (1 in 6)
Uterine cervix	0.16 (1 in 638)	0.28 (1 in 359)	0.13 (1 in 750)	0.19 (1 in 523)	0.70 (1 in 142)
Uterine corpus	0.06 (1 in 1569)	0.71 (1 in 142)	0.79 (1 in 126)	1.23 (1 in 81)	2.45 (1 in 41)

TABLE 11.5

Changes in Five-Year Relative Survival Rates[a] (%), by Race and Year of Diagnosis in the United States from 1975–2003

Site	ALL RACES			WHITE			AFRICAN AMERICAN		
	1975–1977	1996–2003	Dif.	1975–1977	1996–2003	Dif.	1975–1977	1996–2003	Dif.
All cancers	50	66	16[b]	51	67	16[b]	40	57	17[b]
Brain	24	35	11[b]	23	34	11[b]	27	37	11[b]
Breast (female)	75	89	14[b]	76	90	14[b]	62	78	16[b]
Colon	51	65	14[b]	52	66	14[b]	46	55	9[b]
Esophagus	5	16	11[b]	6	18	12[b]	3	11	8[b]
Hodgkin disease	74	86	13[b]	74	87	13[b]	71	81	10[b]
Kidney	51	66	15[b]	51	66	15[b]	50	66	16[b]
Larynx	67	64	-3[b]	67	66	-1	59	50	-9
Leukemia	35	50	15[b]	36	51	15[b]	34	40	7
Liver and bile duct	4	11	7[b]	4	10	6[b]	2	8	6[b]
Lung and bronchus	13	16	3[b]	13	16	3[b]	12	13	1[b]
Melanoma of the skin	82	92	10[b]	82	92	10[b]	60	77	17
Multiple myeloma	26	34	8[b]	25	34	9[b]	31	32	1
Non-Hodgkin lymphoma	48	64	16[b]	48	65	17[b]	49	56	7
Oral cavity and pharynx	53	60	7[b]	55	62	7[b]	36	41	5
Ovary[c]	37	45	8[b]	37	45	8[b]	43	38	-5
Pancreas	2	5	3[b]	3	5	2[b]	2	5	3[b]
Prostate	69	99	30[b]	70	99	29[b]	61	95	34[b]
Rectum	49	66	17[b]	49	66	17[b]	45	58	13[b]
Stomach	16	24	8[b]	15	22	7[b]	16	24	8[b]
Testis	83	96	13[b]	83	96	13[b]	82	88	6
Thyroid	93	97	4[b]	93	97	4[b]	91	94	3
Urinary bladder	74	81	7[b]	75	81	7[b]	51	65	14[b]
Uterine cervix	70	73	3[b]	71	74	3[b]	65	66	1
Uterine corpus	88	84	-4[b]	89	86	-3[b]	61	61	0

[a]Survival rates are adjusted for normal life expectancy and are based in cases diagnosed from 1975–1977 to 1996–2003 and followed through 2004.
[b]The difference in rates between 1975–1977 and 1996–2003 is statistically significant ($p < 0.05$).
[c]Recent changes in classification of ovarian cancer, namely excluding borderline tumors, have affected 1996–2003 survival rates.

Note: "All sites" excludes basal and squamous cell skin cancers and in situ carcinomas except urinary bladder.

Source: Surveillance, Epidemiology, and End Results Program, 1973–2004, Division of Cancer Control and Population Sciences, National Cancer Institute, 2007.

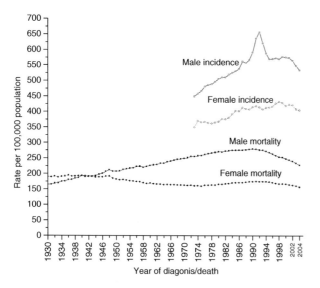

FIGURE 11.2

Trends in all cancers combined incidence and mortality rates, United States, 1930–2004. Incidence rates from Surveillance, Epidemiology, and End Results (SEER) program (http://www.seer.cancer.gov) SEER*Stat Database, 1973–2004. National Cancer Institute, 2007. Death rates from National Center for Health Statistics, Centers for Disease Control and Prevention, 2007.

bronchus, and colon and rectum in females (Fig. 11.5). These cancers account for more than 50% of the new cases in males and in females. Lung and bronchus cancer is the leading cause of cancer death in men and in women, followed by prostate cancer in men, breast cancer in women, and colorectal cancer in men and in women. For both sexes combined, colorectal cancer is the second leading cause of cancer death. The remainder of this section will focus on these four most common cancer sites, as well as three additional cancer sites (liver, esophagus, and pancreas) that are unique with respect to their risk factors, varying histologic types, and low survival rates. These cancers collectively account for 58% of the total new cases in the United States.

Lung and Bronchus Cancer

An estimated 213,380 new cases of lung and bronchus cancer are expected in 2007, accounting for about 15% of cancer diagnoses (18). Overall, men have higher rates of lung and bronchus cancer compared to women and blacks have the highest rates among racial/ethnic groups (Tables 11.2 and 11.3). Lung cancer accounts for the most cancer-related deaths in both men and women. An estimated 160,390 lung cancer deaths, accounting for about 29% of all cancer deaths, are expected to occur

in 2007 (18). The probability of developing invasive lung and bronchus cancer over a lifetime is 7.9% for men and 6.2% for women (Table 11.4).

The incidence rate of lung and bronchus cancer is declining significantly in men, from a high of 102.0 per 100,000 in 1984 to 72.6 per 100,000 in 2004 (4) (Fig. 11.3, left panel). In women, the rate is approaching a plateau after a long period of increase (Fig. 11.3, right panel). Lung cancer death rates have continued to decline significantly in men from 1991–2004 by about 1.9% per year (Fig. 11.4, left panel). Since 1987, more women have died each year from lung cancer than from breast cancer, although female lung cancer death rates are approaching a plateau after continuously increasing for several decades (27) (Fig. 11.4, right panel). These trends in lung cancer mortality reflect the patterns in smoking rates over the past 30 years. Cigarette smoking is by far the most important risk factor for lung cancer. Risk increases with quantity of cigarette consumption and years of smoking duration. Other risk factors include secondhand smoke, occupational or environmental exposures to radon and asbestos (particularly among smokers), certain metals (chromium, cadmium, arsenic), some organic chemicals, radiation, air pollution, and tuberculosis. Genetic susceptibility plays a contributing role in the development of lung cancer, especially in those who develop the disease at a younger age (18).

The five-year survival rate for all stages of lung cancer has slightly increased from 13% in 1975–1977 to 16% in 1996–2003 (Table 11.5), largely due to improvements in surgical techniques and combined therapies. The survival rate is 49% for cases detected when the disease is still localized; however, only 16% of lung cancers are diagnosed at this early stage (4).

Breast Cancer

Breast cancer is the most frequently diagnosed cancer in women, and an estimated 178,480 new cases of invasive breast cancer are expected to occur among women in the United States during 2007 (Fig. 11.5). Breast cancer occurs at higher rates among white women compared to other races/ethnicities, and incidence rates are substantially higher for women aged 50 and older (22). Breast cancer ranks second among cancer deaths in women, and an estimated 40,460 breast cancer deaths are expected among women in 2007 (18). Racial disparities in breast cancer death rates are observed, with black women having a 26% higher death rate than white women (Table 11.3). The higher death rate among black women, despite the lower incidence rate, is due to both later stage at diagnosis and poorer stage-specific survival (22).

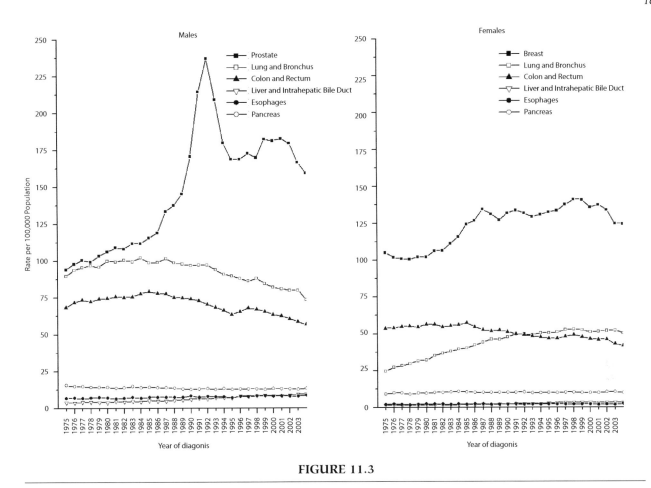

FIGURE 11.3

Annual age-adjusted cancer incidence rates among males and females for selected cancer sites, United States, 1975–2004. Rates are age-adjusted to the 2000 U.S. standard population and adjusted for delays in reporting. Incidence rates from Surveillance, Epidemiology, and End Results (SEER) program (http://www.seer.cancer.gov) SEER*Stat Database, 1973–2004. National Cancer Institute, 2007.

Breast cancer incidence rates increased rapidly among women from 1980–1987, a period when there was increasing uptake of mammography by a growing proportion of U.S. women, and then continued to increase at a slower rate through 1999. After continuously increasing for more than two decades, female breast cancer incidence rates decreased slightly and leveled off from 2001–2004 (Fig. 11.3, right panel). This may reflect the saturation of mammography utilization and reduction in the use of hormone replacement therapy (29). Death rates from breast cancer have steadily decreased in women since 1990 (Fig. 11.4, right panel), with larger decreases in women younger than 50 (a decrease of 3.3% per year) than in those 50 years and older (2.0% per year) (4). The substantial decreases in female breast cancer mortality are thought to reflect early detection (30) and improvements in treatment (31).

Aside from being female, age is the most important factor affecting breast cancer risk. Risk is also increased by inherited genetic mutations in the BRCA1 and BRCA2 genes, a personal or family history of breast cancer, high breast tissue density, biopsy-confirmed hyperplasia (especially atypical hyperplasia), and high-dose radiation to the chest as a result of medical procedures. Reproductive factors that increase risk include a long menstrual history, never having children or delayed childbearing (32), and recent use of oral contraceptives. Some potentially modifiable factors that increase risk include being overweight or obese after menopause, use of postmenopausal hormone therapy (especially combined estrogen and progestin therapy), physical inactivity, and consumption of one or more alcoholic beverages per day (22).

The five-year relative survival rate for all stages of breast cancer has increased from 75% in 1975–1977

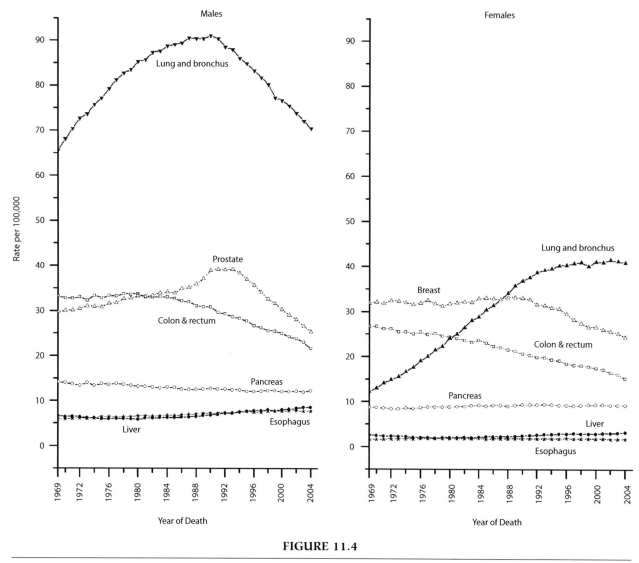

FIGURE 11.4

Trends in annual age-adjusted cancer death rates among males and females for selected cancer types, United States, 1969–2004. Death rates from National Center for Health Statistics, Centers for Disease Control and Prevention, 2007.

to 89% in 1996–2003 (Table 11.5). The five-year relative survival rate for localized breast cancer is 98%, while the rate for cancer that has spread regionally is 84% and that for distant spread is only 27% (4). Mammography can detect breast cancer at an early state, when treatment may be more effective. Numerous studies have shown that early detection saves lives and increases treatment options.

Prostate Cancer

An estimated 218,890 new cases of prostate cancer will occur in the United States during 2007 (Fig. 11.5) (18). Prostate cancer is the most frequently diagnosed cancer

in men. For reasons that remain unclear, incidence rates are significantly higher in black men than in white men (Table 11.3). More than 65% of all prostate cancer cases are diagnosed in men 65 years and older. With an estimated 27,050 deaths in 2007 (18), prostate cancer is a leading cause of cancer death in men.

Incidence rates of prostate cancer have changed substantially over the last 20 years: rapidly increasing from 1988–1992, declining sharply from 1992–1995, and increasing modestly since 1995 (Fig. 11.3, left panel). These trends, in large part, reflect increased prostate cancer screening with the PSA blood test (33). Moderate incidence increases in the last decade are most likely attributable to widespread PSA screening

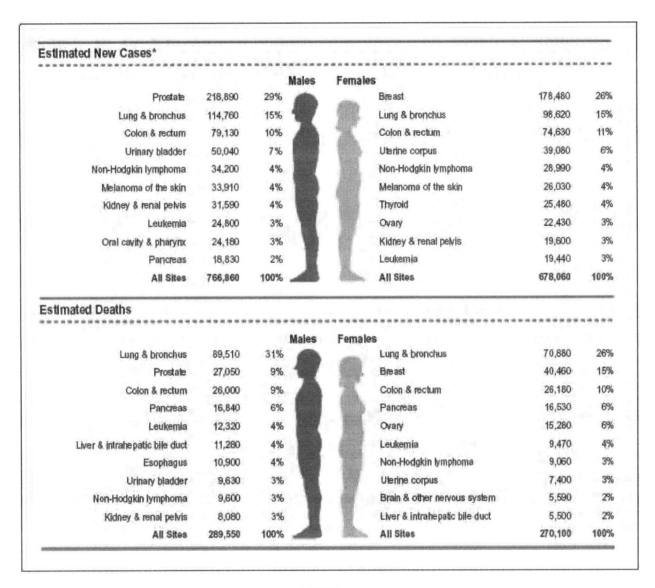

Estimated New Cases*

		Males	Females		
Prostate	218,890	29%	Breast	178,480	26%
Lung & bronchus	114,760	15%	Lung & bronchus	98,620	15%
Colon & rectum	79,130	10%	Colon & rectum	74,630	11%
Urinary bladder	50,040	7%	Uterine corpus	39,080	6%
Non-Hodgkin lymphoma	34,200	4%	Non-Hodgkin lymphoma	28,990	4%
Melanoma of the skin	33,910	4%	Melanoma of the skin	26,030	4%
Kidney & renal pelvis	31,590	4%	Thyroid	25,480	4%
Leukemia	24,800	3%	Ovary	22,430	3%
Oral cavity & pharynx	24,180	3%	Kidney & renal pelvis	19,600	3%
Pancreas	18,830	2%	Leukemia	19,440	3%
All Sites	**766,860**	**100%**	**All Sites**	**678,060**	**100%**

Estimated Deaths

		Males	Females		
Lung & bronchus	89,510	31%	Lung & bronchus	70,880	26%
Prostate	27,050	9%	Breast	40,460	15%
Colon & rectum	26,000	9%	Colon & rectum	26,180	10%
Pancreas	16,840	6%	Pancreas	16,530	6%
Leukemia	12,320	4%	Ovary	15,280	6%
Liver & intrahepatic bile duct	11,280	4%	Leukemia	9,470	4%
Esophagus	10,900	4%	Non-Hodgkin lymphoma	9,060	3%
Urinary bladder	9,630	3%	Uterine corpus	7,400	3%
Non-Hodgkin lymphoma	9,600	3%	Brain & other nervous system	5,590	2%
Kidney & renal pelvis	8,080	3%	Liver & intrahepatic bile duct	5,500	2%
All Sites	**289,550**	**100%**	**All Sites**	**270,100**	**100%**

FIGURE 11.5

Ten leading cancer types for the estimated new cancer cases and deaths, by sex, United States, 2007. Excludes basal and squamous cell skin cancer and in situ carcinomas except urinary bladder. Percentage may not total 100%. (Data from Cancer Facts and Figures, 2007. American Cancer Society.)

among men younger than 65. Prostate cancer incidence rates have leveled off in men 65 and older. Although death rates have been declining among white and African American men since the early 1990s, rates in African American men remain more than twice as high as those in white men (Table 11.3).

The only well-established risk factors for prostate cancer are age, ethnicity, and family history of the disease. Recent genetic studies suggest that strong familial predisposition may be responsible for 5%–10% of prostate cancers. International studies suggest that a diet high in saturated fat may also be

a risk factor (28,34). There is some evidence that the risk of dying from prostate cancer may increase with obesity (35).

More than 90% of all prostate cancers are discovered in the local and regional stages, and the five-year relative survival rate for patients whose tumors are diagnosed at these stages approaches 100% (4). The five-year survival rate for all stages combined has increased from 69% in 1975–1977 to 99% in 1996–2003 (Table 11.5). The dramatic improvements in prostate cancer survival are partly attributable to earlier diagnosis and improvements in treatment.

Colon and Rectum Cancer

An estimated 112,340 cases of colon and 41,420 cases of rectal cancer are expected to occur in 2007 (18). Colorectal cancer is the third most common cancer in both men and women, and it is estimated that in 2004, 1,076,335 persons were living with the disease, representing 10% of all prevalent cancer cases (Table 11.1). Males have a higher incidence of colorectal cancer compared to females (Table 11.2), and more than 90% of cases are diagnosed in individuals 50 and older. Black males and females have higher incidence rates of colorectal cancer compared to whites and all other racial/ethnic groups (Table 11.3). An estimated 52,180 deaths from colon and rectum cancer are expected to occur in 2007, accounting for about 10% of all cancer deaths (18).

Colorectal cancer incidence rates have been decreasing since 1985 for both sexes (Fig. 11.3). The more rapid decrease in the most recent time period (2.5% per year from 1998–2004 (4) partly reflects an increase in screening, which can detect and remove precancerous colorectal polyps (36,37), before they progress to cancer. Colorectal cancer mortality rates have continued to decline in both men and women over the past two decades (Fig. 11.4) because of detection and removal of precancerous polyps (36,37), earlier diagnosis, and improved treatment and supportive care. The risk of colorectal cancer increases with age and is also increased by certain inherited genetic mutations, a personal or family history of colorectal cancer and/or polyps, or a personal history of chronic inflammatory bowel disease. Several modifiable factors are associated with increased risk of colorectal cancer. Among these are obesity, physical inactivity, heavy alcohol consumption, a diet high in red or processed meat, and inadequate intake of fruits and vegetables (18). Beginning at age 50, men and women who are at average risk for developing colorectal cancer should begin screening.

When colorectal cancers are diagnosed at an early, localized stage, the five-year survival is 90%; however, only 39% of colorectal cancers are diagnosed at this stage, mostly due to low rates of screening. After the cancer has spread regionally to involve adjacent organs or lymph nodes, the five-year survival drops to 68%. For persons with distant metastases, five-year survival is 10% (4).

Liver Cancer

In 2007, it is estimated that there will be 19,160 new cases of liver cancer in the United States, accounting for approximately 1.3% of new cancer cases (18). The incidence of liver cancer is substantially greater among men than women. From 2000–2004, the incidence rate for liver cancer was 9.5 per 100,000 among males, while only 3.4 per 100,000 among females (Table 11.2). Incidence also varies by race and ethnicity, with Asian Americans, particularly those of Vietnamese and Korean ethnicities, experiencing the highest rates (10). Liver cancer incidence is highly correlated with age. The incidence peaks among individuals 75–79 years of age and is rare among those less than 50 years of age (Fig. 11.6). Approximately 16,780 deaths due to liver cancer are estimated to occur in 2007, representing 3% of all cancer deaths (18).

About 83% of liver cancers are hepatocellular carcinomas (HCC) affecting hepatocytes, the predominant type of cell in the liver. Worldwide, the major causes of liver cancer are chronic infection with hepatitis B virus (HBV) and hepatitis C virus (HCV). In developing countries, 37% of liver cancers are attributable to HBV, 25% to HCV, 10% to infection of the intrahepatic bile ducts by liver flukes, and 9% to other causes. In developed countries, 14% of liver cancers are attributable to HBV, 14% to HCV, and 71% to other causes, such as alcohol-related cirrhosis and possibly hepatitis from obesity (38). Data for North America

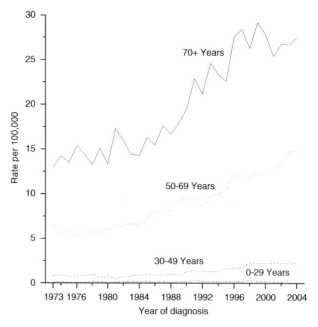

FIGURE 11.6

Age-specific liver cancer incidence, United States, 1973–2004. Incidence rates from Surveillance, Epidemiology, and End Results (SEER) program (http://www.seer.cancer.gov) SEER*Stat Database, 1973–2004. National Cancer Institute, 2007.

indicate that 6.2% of liver cancers are attributed to chronic infection with HBV, 23% are due to chronic infection with HCV, and a substantial portion of the remainder are due to alcohol-related cirrhosis (39). The majority of liver cancers occur in Eastern Asia and sub-Saharan Africa (40). The United States is considered a low rate area for liver cancer; however, the incidence in the United States has been steadily increasing, from 2.9 per 100,000 in 1984 to 6.1 per 100,000 in 2004 (41). Reasons for the increase in incidence are not entirely clear, but may be related to increased prevalence of HCV infection (42).

Survival rates for liver cancer are universally poor, and a five-year survival rate of only 11% was observed during the period 1996–2003 in the United States (Table 11.5). Because survival is so low, prevention mechanisms for the major causes of liver cancer are vitally important. A vaccine that protects against HBV has been available since 1982, and state laws mandating hepatitis B vaccination for middle school children have contributed to achieving high coverage rates among adolescents (43). Although progress in vaccination among adolescents has been made, hepatitis B infections among men over age 19 and women 40 and older have been rising since 1999. Increasing efforts to vaccinate high-risk individuals, including those with multiple sex partners, men who have sex with men, and injection drug users, are recommended to counteract this trend (44). There is no vaccine available for HCV. Universal precautions should be used among health care workers to prevent infection, and The Centers for Disease Control and Prevention (CDC) recommends that routine HCV testing be offered to individuals at high risk for infection.

Esophageal Cancer

It is estimated that 15,560 new cases and 13,940 new deaths due to esophageal cancer will occur in the United States in 2007 (18). Incidence rates for esophageal cancer rise with age and are very low among children and young adults. Males have higher rates of esophageal cancer compared to females, with the male to female ratio (3.91) nearly reaching four-fold (Table 11.2). Cancers of the esophagus typically have two distinct histologic types, squamous cell carcinoma and adenocarcinoma, that display remarkable racial and ethnic differences. Rates of esophageal adenocarcinoma are higher among whites than blacks, while the inverse is true for squamous cell carcinoma. Squamous cell carcinoma occurs in the upper third of the esophagus and is caused mainly by tobacco and alcohol consumption. Adenocarcinoma generally occurs in the lower third of the esophagus and has risk factors that include obesity, gastroesophageal reflux disease (GERD), and Barrett esophagus, which is a premalignant condition involving chronic inflammation and dysplasia (45).

Trends in esophageal cancer have changed dramatically in recent years. The incidence of esophageal cancer has been rising in men and is stable in women (Fig. 11.3). Historically, squamous cell carcinoma has been the most common histologic type; however, its incidence has been decreasing since 1975, first among whites, followed by blacks. In contrast, adenocarcinoma, which used to be relatively rare throughout the world, has risen steeply among white males in the United States while remaining relatively stable among black males (Fig. 11.7) (46). Reasons for the sharp increase in esophageal adenocarcinoma among white men but not among black men are not fully understood; however, a higher prevalence of *Helicobacter pylori* infection in blacks, which may be protective against adenocarcinoma of the esophagus (47), has been suggested to be a factor (48). The increase in adenocarcinoma of the esophagus may also be related to the increase in obesity and GERD in the United States. As smoking is a primary cause of squamous cell carcinoma, the decrease in smoking rates in the United States most likely have contributed to the decrease in this type of esophageal cancer.

Survival from esophageal cancer is low, and survival rates do not differ by histologic type (45). In the United States, the five-year survival rate was 16% during the period 1996–2003. This was a significant improvement from the five-year survival rate of 5% from 1975–1977 (Table 11.5).

Pancreatic Cancer

An estimated 37,170 new cases and 33,370 new deaths due to pancreatic cancer are expected to occur in the United States in 2007 (18). Pancreatic cancer rates are slightly higher in men than in women, with a male-to-female ratio of 1.28 (Table 11.2). Age is an important predictor for pancreatic cancer, as both its incidence and mortality increase with age in a linear fashion. The median age of diagnosis is 72, and the majority of cases occur between ages 65 and 79 (49). In general, pancreatic cancer incidence rates are higher among blacks compared to whites in the United States (Table 11.3).

For both sexes combined, incidence rates increased slightly (by 0.5% per year) from 1993–2004 (4). The death rate from pancreatic cancer has continued to decline since the 1970s in men, while it has leveled off in women after increasing from 1975–1984. Tobacco smoking increases the risk of pancreatic cancer, and incidence rates are more than twice as high for cigarette

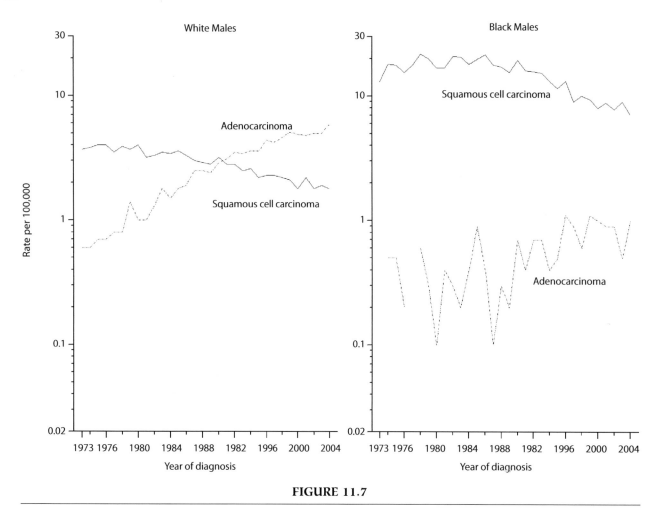

FIGURE 11.7

Age-adjusted incidence rates of esophageal cancer among males by race and histologic type, United States, 1973–2004. Incidence rates from Surveillance, Epidemiology, and End Results (SEER) program (http://www.seer.cancer.gov) SEER*Stat Database, 1973–2004. National Cancer Institute, 2007.

smokers than for nonsmokers. Risk also appears to increase with obesity, chronic pancreatitis, diabetes, and cirrhosis. Surgery, radiation therapy, and chemotherapy are treatment options that may extend survival and/or relieve symptoms in many patients, but seldom produce a cure.

Pancreatic cancer is highly lethal, and survival rates are among the lowest of any cancer. For all stages combined, the five-year survival rate is about 5% (Table 11.5). Even for those people diagnosed with local disease, the five-year survival rate is only 20% (4). Only about 7% of pancreatic cancers are diagnosed at the localized stage, whereas 52% are diagnosed at the distant stage (4). There is no screening test for early detection of pancreatic cancer, and early stages of the disease are usually asymptomatic. Difficulties in early detection, lack of effective treatments, and extremely low survival rates make cancer of the pancreas a serious medical and public health problem.

References

1. Extramural Committee to Assess Measures of Progress Against Cancer. Measurement of progress against cancer. *J Natl Cancer Inst.* 1990;82:825–835.
2. Doll R, Peto R. The causes of cancer: quantitative estimates of avoidable risks of cancer in the United States today. *J Natl Cancer Inst.* 1981;66:1191–1308.
3. Jemal A, Siegel R, Ward E, Murray T, Xu J, Thun MJ. Cancer statistics, 2007. *CA Cancer J Clin.* 2007;57:43–66.
4. Ries LAG, Melbert D, Krapcho M, et al., eds. *SEER Cancer Statistics Review, 1975-2004.* Bethesda, MD: National Cancer Institute, National Cancer Institute; 2007.
5. Anderson RN, Minino AM, Hoyert DL, Rosenberg HM. Comparability of cause of death between ICD-9 and ICD-10: preliminary estimates. *Natl Vital Stat Rep.* 2001;49:1–32.
6. World Health Organization. *International Statistical Classification of Diseases and Related Health Problems.* Geneva: WHO; 1992.
7. Thun MJ, Calle EE, Rodriguez C, Wingo PA. Epidemiological research at the American Cancer Society. *Cancer Epidemiol Biomarkers Prev.* 2000;9:861–868.

8. Tiwari RC, Ghosh K, Jemal A, et al. Derivation and validation of a new method of predicting U.S. and state-level cancer mortality counts for the current calendar year. *CA Cancer J Clin.* 2004;54:8–29.

9. Wingo PA, Landis S, Parker S. Using cancer registry and vital statistics to estimate the number of new cases cancer cases and deaths in the US for the upcoming year. *Journal of Registry Management.* 1998;25:43–51.

10. McCracken M, Olsen M, Chen MS, Jr., et al. Cancer incidence, mortality, and associated risk factors among asian americans of chinese, filipino, vietnamese, korean, and Japanese ethnicities. *CA Cancer J Clin.* 2007;57:190–205.

11. Ward E, Jemal A, Cokkinides V, et al. Cancer disparities by race/ethnicity and socioeconomic status. *CA Cancer J Clin.* 2004;54:78–93.

12. Singh GK, Miller BA, Hankey BF, Edwards BK, eds. *Area Socioeconomic Variations in U.S. Cancer Incidence, Mortality, and Survival, 1975–1999.* Bethesda, MD: National Cancer Institute, National Cancer Institute; 2003.

13. Howard G, Anderson RT, Russell G, Howard VJ, Burke GL. Race, socioeconomic status, and cause-specific mortality. *Ann Epidemiol.* 2000;10:214–223.

14. Albano J, Ward E, Jemal ARA, et al. Cancer mortality by education and Race in the United States *J Natl Cancer Inst.* 2007; 99:1364–1384.

15. Doll R. Epidemiological evidence of the effects of behaviour and the environment on the risk of human cancer. *Recent Results Cancer Res.* 1998;154:3–21.

16. Devesa SS, Grauman DJ, Blot WJ, Pennello GA, Hoover RN, Fraumeni JFJ. *Atlas of Cancer Mortality in the United States 1950–94.* Bethesda: National Institute of Health; 1999.

17. Centers for Disease Control and Prevention (2003), Available at: http://www.cdc.gov/cancer/nbccedp/about.htm.

18. American Cancer Society. *Cancer Facts & Figures 2007.* Atlanta, GA: American Cancer Society; 2007.

19. Thun MJ, Henley SJ, Calle EE. Tobacco use and cancer: an epidemiologic perspective for geneticists. *Oncogene.* 2002;21:7307–7325.

20. Potosky AL, Kessler L, Gridley G, Brown CC, Horm JW. Rise in prostatic cancer incidence associated with increased use of transurethral resection. *J Natl Cancer Inst.* 1990;82: 1624–1628.

21. Potosky AL, Miller BA, Albertsen PC, Kramer BS. The role of increasing detection in the rising incidence of prostate cancer. *JAMA.* 1995;273:548–552.

22. Smigal C, Jemal A, Ward E, et al. Trends in breast cancer by race and ethnicity: update 2006. *CA Cancer J Clin.* 2006;56:168–183.

23. Jemal A, Ward E, Thun MJ. Recent trends in breast cancer incidence rates by age and tumor characteristics among U.S. women. *Breast Cancer Res.* 2007;9:R28.

24. Ravdin PM, Cronin KA, Howlader N, et al. The decrease in breast-cancer incidence in 2003 in the United States. *N Engl J Med.* 2007;356:1670–1674.

25. U.S. Public Health Service. *Smoking and Health. Report of the Advisory Committee to the Surgeon General of the Public Health Service.* Washington, DC: US Department of Health, Education, and Welfare, Public Health Service, Center for Disease Control; 1964.

26. US Department of Health and Human Services. *A Surgeon General's Report on the Health Consequences of Smoking.* Atlanta: US Department of Health and Human Services, Centers for Disease Control and Prevention, Office of Smoking and Health; 2004.

27. Howe HL, Wu X, Ries LA, et al. Annual report to the nation on the status of cancer, 1975–2003, featuring cancer among U.S. Hispanic/Latino populations. *Cancer.* 2006;107:1711–1142.

28. Parkin DM. The global health burden of infection-associated cancers in the year 2002. *Int J Cancer.* 2006;118: 3030–3044.

29. Jemal A, Clegg LX, Ward E, et al. Annual report to the nation on the status of cancer, 1975–2001, with a special feature regarding survival. *Cancer.* 2004;101:3–27.

30. Swan J, Breen N, Coates RJ, Rimer BK, Lee NC. Progress in cancer screening practices in the United States: results from the 2000 National Health Interview Survey. *Cancer.* 2003;97: 1528–1540.

31. Mariotto A, Feuer EJ, Harlan LC, Wun LM, Johnson KA, Abrams J. Trends in use of adjuvant multi-agent chemotherapy and tamoxifen for breast cancer in the United States: 1975–1999. *J Natl Cancer Inst.* 2002;94:1626–1634.

32. Chu K, Tarone R, Kessler L, et al. Recent trends in U.S. breast cancer incidence, survival, and mortality rates. *J Natl Cancer Inst.* 1996;88:1571–1579.

33. Hankey BF, Feuer EJ, Clegg LX, et al. Cancer surveillance series: interpreting trends in prostate cancer—part I: evidence of the effects of screening in recent prostate cancer incidence, mortality, and survival rates. *J Natl Cancer Inst.* 1999;91: 1017–1024.

34. Platz E, Giovannucci E. Prostate cancer. In: Schottenfeld D, Jr. Fraumeni JF, Jr. eds. *Cancer Epidemiology and Prevention Third Edition.* New York: Oxford University Press; 2006; 1128–1150.

35. Gong Z, Agalliu I, Lin DW, Stanford JL, Kristal AR. Obesity is associated with increased risks of prostate cancer metastasis and death after initial cancer diagnosis in middle-aged men. *Cancer.* 2007;109:1192–1202.

36. Mandel JS, Bond JH, Church TR, et al. (1993) Reducing mortality from colorectal cancer by screening for fecal occult blood. Minnesota Colon Cancer Control Study. *N Engl J Med.* 1993;328:1365–1371.

37. Mandel JS, Church TR, Ederer F, Bond JH. Colorectal cancer mortality: effectiveness of biennial screening for fecal occult blood. *J Natl Cancer Inst.* 1999;91:434–437.

38. American Cancer Society. *Cancer Facts & Figures 2005.* Atlanta, GA: American Cancer Society; 2005.

39. Pisani P, Parkin DM, Munoz N, Ferlay J. Cancer and infection: estimates of the attributable fraction in 1990. *Cancer Epidemiol Biomarkers Prev.* 1997;6:387–400.

40. Parkin DM, Bray FI, Devesa SS. Cancer burden in the year 2000. The global picture. *Eur J Cancer.* 2001;37(Suppl 8): S4–S66.

41. Reis L, Melbert D, Krapcho M, et al. *SEER Cancer Statistics Review, 1975–2004.* Bethesda, MD: National Cancer Institute; 2007.

42. El-Serag HB, Davila JA, Petersen NJ, McGlynn KA. The continuing increase in the incidence of hepatocellular carcinoma in the United States: an update. *Ann Intern Med.* 2003;139:817–823.

43. Centers for Disease Cancer and Prevention (CDC). Hepatitis B vaccination—United States, 1982–2002. *MMWR Morb Mortal Wkly Rep.* 2002;51:549–552.

44. Centers for Disease Cancer and Prevention (CDC). Incidence of acute hepatitis B—United States, 1990–2002. *MMWR Morb Mortal Wkly Rep.* 2004;52:1252–1254.

45. Blot W, McLaughlin J, Fraumeni J, Jr. Esophageal cancer. In: Schottenfeld D, Fraumeni JF, Jr. eds. *Cancer Epidemiology and Prevention Third Edition.* New York: Oxford University Press; 2006; 647–706.

46. Ward EM, Thun MJ, Hannan LM, Jemal A. Interpreting cancer trends. *Ann N Y Acad Sci.* 2006;1076:29–53.

47. Ye W, Held M, Lagergren J, et al. Helicobacter pylori infection and gastric atrophy: risk of adenocarcinoma and squamous-cell carcinoma of the esophagus and adenocarcinoma of the gastric cardia. *J Natl Cancer Inst.* 2004;96:388–396.

48. Graham DY, Malaty HM, Evans DG, Evans DJ, Jr., Klein PD, Adam E. Epidemiology of Helicobacter pylori in an asymptomatic population in the United States. Effect of age, race, and socioeconomic status. *Gastroenterology.* 1991;100: 1495–1501.

49. Anderson K, Mack T, Silverman D. Cancer of the pancreas. In: Schottenfeld D, Fraumeni JF, Jr. eds. *Cancer Epidemiology and Prevention Third Edition.* New York: Oxford University Press; 2006;721–762.

II

INTRODUCTION TO EVALUATION AND TREATMENT OF MALIGNANCY

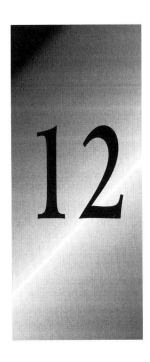

Evaluation and Treatment of Breast Cancer

Heather L. McArthur
Clifford A. Hudis

Breast cancer is the most common potentially life-threatening cancer among women in the United States, with more than 200,000 new cases and more than 40,000 breast cancer-related deaths anticipated in 2008 (1). The most well-defined risk factors for breast cancer include increasing age, prolonged endogenous or exogenous estrogen exposure, and family history. Significant estrogen exposure histories include nulliparity, early menarche, late menopause, obesity, oral contraceptive use, and hormone replacement therapy. Although as many as 20% of women with a new breast cancer diagnosis cite a positive family history, inherited genetic mutations that predispose to breast cancer are rare. For example, only 5%–10% of all breast cancers are attributable to inheritance of a breast cancer susceptibility gene (1,2). However, for those women who do inherit a gene mutation, the lifetime risk of developing breast cancer can be significant. For example, in a meta-analysis of 10 studies evaluating cancer risk among known BRCA1 and BRCA2 mutation carriers, the cumulative lifetime breast cancer risk was 57% in the BRCA1 cohort and 49% in the BRCA2 cohort (3). Other risk factors for developing breast cancer include a prior history of ductal carcinoma in situ (DCIS), lobular carcinoma in situ (LCIS), atypical ductal hyperplasia (ADH), a prior history of invasive breast cancer, and prior radiotherapy to the chest. Associations with environmental factors including smoking, alcohol consumption, and diet have also been established. Despite these risk factors and associations,

however, the etiology of most breast cancer diagnoses is unknown. The difficulty in identifying the majority of women who are at risk of developing breast cancer, combined with the significant burden of disease in the population, has resulted in the widespread adoption of breast cancer screening programs as a public health measure.

Annual mammography, in combination with annual clinical breast examination, is recommended for all women aged 40 years or older who are considered at average risk of developing breast cancer. Screening may be indicated earlier and more frequently for women at higher risk. When an abnormality is detected on screening, breast cancer diagnosis and management typically require a multidisciplinary approach that incorporates some combination of radiology, surgery, pathology, medical oncology, radiation oncology, and/or care by specialists in rehabilitation. This chapter provides an overview of the principles of breast cancer diagnosis and treatment.

DIAGNOSIS

Mammography

In the United States, the adoption of national screening programs accounts for a significant proportion of the improved breast cancer-specific mortality rates observed over the last three decades (4,5). The National Cancer Institute, American Cancer Society,

KEY POINTS

- Breast cancer is the most common potentially life-threatening cancer among women in the United States, with more than 200,000 new cases and more than 40,000 breast cancer-related deaths in 2008.
- The most well-defined risk factors for breast cancer include increasing age, prolonged endogenous or exogenous estrogen exposure, and family history.
- Annual mammography in combination with annual clinical breast examination are recommended for all women aged 40 or older who are considered at average risk of developing breast cancer.
- Patients with a suspicious abnormality on breast imaging and/or a clinically palpable mass should undergo a core needle biopsy to confirm the diagnosis and to facilitate appropriate surgical planning.
- For patients with evidence of breast cancer on core biopsy, definitive surgery is warranted.
- Malignant cells that are confined strictly to the breast ducts (ductal carcinoma in situ, DCIS) or lobules (lobular carcinoma in situ, LCIS), and there-

fore do not have metastatic potential, are designated as carcinoma in situ.
- A diagnosis of early-stage breast cancer denotes disease that is limited to the breast and/or axilla.
- Systemic chemotherapy is an integral component of the adjuvant treatment strategy for many women with early-stage breast cancer.
- Because of the significant risk of locoregional recurrence in the ipsilateral breast and/or axilla after breast conserving surgery, radiotherapy to the conserved breast is indicated. Radiotherapy to the axilla is also indicated when four or more lymph nodes are involved. The role of radiotherapy when one to three axillary lymph nodes are involved is uncertain.
- Metastatic breast cancer (MBC) is associated with a median survival of two to three years. Because MBC is generally incurable, the goals of therapy are to improve quality of life and ideally, improve survival.

American College of Radiology, American Medical Association, and American College of Obstetrics and Gynecology recommend breast cancer screening with routine mammography in conjunction with annual clinical breast examination for all women aged 40 years or older who are at average risk of developing breast cancer. Earlier screening, more frequent breast imaging, and/or adjunctive imaging may be indicated for women at increased risk. Furthermore, women with a strong family history or genetic predisposition may be considered for risk-reducing procedures. To facilitate individual risk estimations, the National Cancer Institute developed a computerized risk assessment tool that synthesizes information on age, race, age at menarche, age of first birth or nulliparity, number of first degree relatives with breast cancer, number of previous benign breast biopsies, and atypical hyperplasia in a previous biopsy into five–year and lifetime invasive breast cancer risk projections (www.cancer.gov/bcrisktool). Appropriate screening regimens may be planned accordingly.

It is important to note that although most breast cancer diagnoses are made as a result of abnormal screening mammograms (6), not all mammography findings represent cancer. If an abnormality is detected on a screening study, a variety of mammography techniques may be employed to better characterize suspi-

cious lesions. These may include magnification views, spot compression views, and variations in angle views. Digital mammography, which has demonstrated superior diagnostic accuracy compared with traditional film techniques for young women, pre- or peri-menopausal women, and women with heterogenous breasts, is also increasingly utilized (Fig. 12.1) (7).

Mammography findings are summarized into diagnostic assessment categories using the American College of Radiology (ACR) Breast Imaging Reporting and Data System (BI-RADS) (www.acr.org). This system was developed in 1993 in order to standardize breast imaging terminology, communication, and reporting in clinical practice and in research. The BI-RADS system not only provides diagnostic and prognostic information, but also incorporates management recommendations (Table 12.1).

Ultrasound

Ultrasound imaging of the breast is sometimes employed as an adjunct to mammography. This imaging modality is frequently used to further characterize palpable or radiographically detectable masses (ie, by distinguishing between solid and cystic masses) and to guide interventional procedures. Ultrasound imaging is not routinely incorporated into the diagnostic paradigm, but has been demonstrated to improve diagnostic specificity by correctly downgrading the diagnosis, particularly among women with a palpable breast mass or an abnormal screening mammogram (8–10).

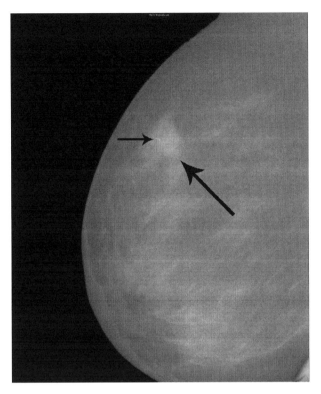

FIGURE 12.1

Digital mammogram obtained following an ultrasound guided biopsy and fine needle aspiration of a poorly differentiated invasive ductal carcinoma (large arrow). Note the clip placed at the biopsy site to facilitate surgical resection (small arrow).

Magnetic Resonance Imaging (MRI)

Almost all invasive breast cancers are visualized on gadolinium contrast-enhanced magnetic resonance imaging (MRI) (Fig. 12.2). Breast MRI has historically been associated with high sensitivity but variable specificity in detecting breast cancer among women are symptomatic, or those who are at high risk but are asymptomatic. In 2007, The American Cancer Society published guidelines for the use of breast cancer screening, suggesting MRI as an adjunct to mammography (11). Breast MRI was recommended for women with a greater than or equal to 20%–25% lifetime risk of developing breast cancer, including women with a known BRCA1 or BRCA2 mutation, a strong family history of breast or ovarian cancer, or a prior history of radiation therapy to the chest for the treatment of lymphoma. Outside of these indications, the role of MRI in breast cancer screening and management remains an ongoing area of investigation.

BREAST BIOPSY

Patients with a suspicious abnormality on breast imaging and/or a clinically palpable mass should undergo a core needle biopsy to confirm the diagnosis and to facilitate appropriate surgical planning. Fine needle aspiration (FNA) of suspicious breast lesions is typically less desirable than core biopsy because of the difficulty in distinguishing noninvasive (in situ) disease from invasive disease, the high incidence of false negative results, and the significant potential for yielding samples that are nondiagnostic. However, because identification of breast cancer that has spread to the axilla may have important clinical implications, FNA may be indicated for evaluation of suspicious axillary masses. Axillary involvement confirmed by FNA is typically managed

TABLE 12.1
Breast Imaging Reporting and Data System (BI-RADS) Mammographic Assessment Categories

ASSESSMENT CATEGORY	RECOMMENDATION	PROBABILITY OF MALIGNANCY
1. Negative	Routine follow-up	0%
2. Benign	Routine follow-up	0%
3. Probably benign	Short interval follow-up	<2%
4. Suspicious	Consider biopsy	2%–95%
5. Highly suggestive of malignancy	Appropriate management	≥95%
6. Incomplete	Further imaging evaluation	Not applicable

Source: Reprinted with permission of the American College of Radiology. No other representation of this material is authorized without expressed, written permission from the American College of Radiology.

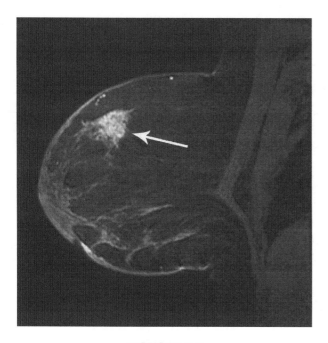

FIGURE 12.2

Breast MRI of the same poorly differentiated invasive ductal carcinoma illustrated on digital mammography in Figure 12.1.

with a complete axillary lymph node dissection, rather than sentinel lymph node biopsy alone, and may have implications for decisions regarding preoperative or neoadjuvant, chemotherapy.

Many centers have adopted stereotactic core needle biopsy techniques that utilize a specialized computer-guided imaging system or ultrasound guided core biopsy to investigate suspicious breast masses. Ultrasound guided biopsy is generally well tolerated and has the advantages of direct visualization of the target lesion and a relatively short study duration. Stereotactic methods are often reserved for patients with microcalcifications whose lesions are not well visualized on ultrasound, or for patients with deep masses close to the chest wall, where the biopsy needle can be inserted safely in parallel to the chest wall. Clips may also be inserted at the time of breast biopsy. Clips can provide radiographic correlation of the biopsied lesion, which may prove particularly important if the lesion is small and could be entirely removed by the biopsy procedure. Clips can also be useful in guiding further surgical interventions, or in following response to therapy for women with locally advanced disease undergoing neoadjuvant chemotherapy.

If breast cancer is identified on core biopsy, assays for hormone receptor status and HER2 status are typically performed on the biopsy specimen (see below). This practice may expedite decisions regarding post-

operative or adjuvant chemotherapy. However, given that breast cancers represent a heterogenous population of cells, and the potential for a false negative result is significant, these assays should be repeated on the excised surgical specimens if the assay results from the core biopsy specimens are reported as negative.

SURGERY

Breast: For patients with evidence of breast cancer on core biopsy, definitive surgery is warranted. Surgery may entail a lumpectomy (or breast conserving approach) or total mastectomy. Breast conserving surgery in combination with adjuvant radiotherapy to the breast is associated with an increased risk of local recurrence when compared to mastectomy, but there is no difference in overall survival (12).

Axilla: Historically, the standard approach to evaluation and management of the axilla was complete axillary dissection. However, surgical management of the axilla may now involve sentinel lymph node biopsy (SLNB), a technique that involves the injection of radioactive colloid or blue dye into the breast to identify the lymph nodes that first receive drainage from the tumor. If lymph node involvement is detected on SLNB, further surgery is typically warranted. The principles of breast surgery, perioperative imaging, and reconstruction are reviewed in detail elsewhere.

DUCTAL CARCINOMA *IN SITU* (DCIS)

Malignant cells that are confined strictly to the breast ducts (DCIS) or lobules (lobular carcinoma in situ, LCIS) are designated as carcinoma in situ (Fig. 12.3). Because there is no evidence of invasion into the surrounding stroma, these cells do not have the capacity for metastasis, a feature that distinguishes in situ from invasive disease. LCIS is not believed to be a direct precursor of invasive disease, but is considered a harbinger of increased risk (13–15). DCIS, however, is an established precursor of invasive disease, although the frequency of progression from untreated DCIS to invasive disease is uncertain. DCIS is treated with definitive local therapy comprised of mastectomy or breast conserving surgery with or without postoperative or adjuvant radiotherapy. If there is no evidence of invasive disease on the excised specimen, then evaluation of the axilla is generally not performed. Five years of additional treatment with tamoxifen, a selective estrogen receptor modulator, may be considered; however, the results of randomized trials have not been consistent (16,17). Furthermore, the potential benefits must be weighed against the risk for thromboembolic events

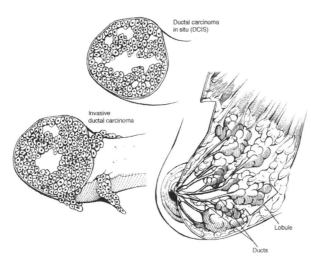

FIGURE 12.3

Ductal carcinoma in situ (DCIS) is an established precursor of invasive disease and is often treated with mastectomy or breast-conserving surgery with or without postoperative or adjuvant radiotherapy.

and the development of new uterine cancers associated with tamoxifen therapy.

STAGING FOR INVASIVE BREAST CANCER

The stage, or burden, of invasive disease at diagnosis is typically divided into either early-stage, locally advanced, or metastatic categories. However, a formal clinical and pathological staging system, developed by the American Joint Committee on Cancer (AJCC), is frequently used (18). In general, AJCC stages I and II are considered early; stage III, locally advanced; and stage IV, metastatic. These formal and informal staging categories endeavor to group together patients with a similar prognosis and may be used to guide further investigations. For example, women with small, node-negative, early-stage disease are at a low risk of distant spread. Consequently, the yield of further imaging studies is extremely low in this population. Women with large, bulky, node-positive disease, however, are at significant risk of distant spread and should therefore be considered for further evaluation at diagnosis to exclude established metastatic disease. The National Comprehensive Cancer Network currently recommends the following staging investigations for patients with early-stage (T1-2, N0-1) breast cancer: history and physical examination, complete blood count (CBC), liver function tests, chest imaging, and diagnostic mammogram (www.nccn.org/professionals/physician_gls).

Additional investigations with bone scan and abdominal imaging are recommended for patients with locally advanced or suspected metastatic disease. At present, the role of positron emission tomography imaging in the diagnosis and staging of women with breast cancer is uncertain. In addition, serum tumor marker assays, including CA 15-3 and CEA, lack sensitivity and specificity and are not recommended in the initial assessment of women with early-stage or locally advanced breast cancer.

The implication of accurate staging at diagnosis is that breast cancer that remains localized to the breast and/or axilla is potentially curable, whereas metastatic disease is not. Consequently, the therapeutic goals for localized versus metastatic disease are vastly different. In the treatment of early-stage disease, potentially toxic regimens associated with higher cure rates may be considered. Conversely, the goal of treatment for metastatic disease is to optimize quality of life and extend survival.

EARLY-STAGE DISEASE

Rationale for Adjuvant Chemotherapy

A diagnosis of early-stage breast cancer denotes disease that is limited to the breast and/or axilla. However, despite early detection, a significant proportion of these women will experience a distant relapse and later die of recurrence-related complications. These distant recurrences indicate that some women have undetectable micrometastatic disease at diagnosis. Consequently, locoregional therapy with surgery and/or radiotherapy is inadequate for cure in some women. Systemic chemotherapy, aimed at eradicating these subclinical micrometastases has thus become an integral component of the treatment strategy for some women with early-stage breast cancer. Adjuvant systemic therapy decisions are typically made by adopting a risk-benefit calculus, whereby an individual's risk of recurrence is weighed against the potential toxicity of the proposed regimen. Risk estimates are primarily derived from information on tumor size, nodal involvement, hormone receptor status, and HER2 status (see below). Other patient characteristics considered when designing an appropriate adjuvant strategy include age, comorbid conditions, patient preference, the acceptability of anticipated toxicity, and the desire for the expected benefits.

Risk Stratification

Historically, prognostic estimates for disease that remains clinically localized to the breast and/or axilla have been derived primarily from information on tumor size and lymph node status. However, prognostic profiling in the modern era is now frequently augmented by biologic data. Consequently, the risk stratification paradigm has become increasingly sophisticated for some women and treatment strategies are increasingly tailored to the biology of an individual's tumor.

Tumor Size and Nodal Status

Tumor size and the extent of nodal involvement are well-established prognostic factors for patients with early-stage breast cancer (19). Although nodal status has historically conferred the most compelling prognostic information, the advent of SLNB techniques has presented new challenges in risk stratification. When compared with traditional axillary dissection techniques, SLNB typically yields fewer lymph nodes for evaluation. Because of the important decision that hinges on proving that the sentinel nodes are negative, a more detailed evaluation of a fewer number of nodes is permitted. Isolated tumor cells or micrometastases that were undetectable by traditional staining techniques are now detected by immunohistochemistry (IHC), but the prognostic significance of such findings in conventionally negative lymph nodes has not yet been fully elucidated (20–24).

Hormone Receptor Status

Hormone receptor status is a well-established prognostic and predictive factor. The risk of recurrence for women with estrogen receptor (ER)-negative breast cancer peaks as high as 18.5% approximately one to two years after surgery and declines rapidly thereafter to 1.4% in years 8 through 12 (Fig. 12.4) (19).

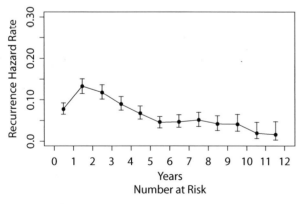

Number at Risk

3585 3226 2786 2443 2168 1972 1739 1428 1089 801 527 328

FIGURE 12.4

Annual hazard of breast cancer recurrence by estrogen receptor (ER) status. Reprinted with permission from the American Society of Clinical Oncology.

Most women, however, have breast cancers that are ER-positive. For these women, the recurrence pattern is unique from that of their ER-negative counterparts, with a smaller and later recurrence risk peak of 11.0% in years two to three and a significant rate of persistent recurrence (approximately 5%) through to year 12. Thus, ER-status provides important information about the anticipated natural history of an individual's breast cancer.

ER status also provides important predictive information, not only to response to hormonal therapy, but also to systemic chemotherapy. In a retrospective subset analysis of three cooperative group adjuvant chemotherapy trials, investigators demonstrated that for women with node-positive breast cancer, the absolute benefit of chemotherapy was more pronounced for the ER-negative cohort compared to the ER-positive cohort (25). Similar findings have been reported in a large collaborative meta-analysis of more than 145,000 women who participated in 194 trials conducted by the Early Breast Cancer Trialists' Collaborative Group (EBCTCG) (26).

HER2 Status

The HER2 receptor is a member of the transmembrane human epidermal growth factor receptor (EGFR) family and is overexpressed in approximately 20%–25% of human breast cancers. Although HER2 overexpression has historically conferred a worse prognosis compared with non-overexpressing cohorts, the prognostic significance has become less relevant with the advent of HER2-targeted therapy (27,28). HER2 status remains an important predictive factor, however, for responses not only to trastuzumab (Herceptin), a recombinant monoclonal HER2-targeted antibody, but also to other chemotherapeutic agents. The most notable of these is an increased sensitivity to anthracycline-containing regimens among women with HER2-overexpressing breast cancer (29,30). Synergy and/or additive effects have also been demonstrated with the combination of trastuzumab and taxanes or vinorelbine (31,32). HER2-overexpressing breast cancers are also relatively resistant to treatment with tamoxifen, but not aromatase inhibitors (AIs) (33,34).

Risk Calculation Tools

Multiple tools have been developed to increase the accuracy of clinical risk-benefit estimations. The most notable web-based prognostic tool is Adjuvant! Online (www.adjuvantonline.com), which estimates 10-year relapse and mortality rates based on various patient/tumor characteristics and estimates the expected benefit of various adjuvant systemic treatment strategies.

Hormonal maneuvers are the therapeutic cornerstone for women with hormone receptor positive early-stage breast cancer. However, for women with small, node-negative, ER-positive, early-stage breast cancer for whom adjuvant hormone therapy is anticipated, it is often difficult to ascertain the potential additional benefit to be derived from adjuvant systemic chemotherapy. Several multigene assays have been developed to facilitate risk-benefit estimations for these women (35–38). For example, the Oncotype DX assay utilizes a 21-gene expression profile to categorize a woman's risk of recurrence as low, intermediate, or high, with average associated 10-year distant recurrence rates of 6.8%, 14.3%, and 30.5%, respectively (35). This assay enables some women who are truly at low risk to forgo overtreatment and exposure to the deleterious effects of chemotherapy, while women at a higher risk of recurrence may be considered for a more aggressive therapeutic strategy. However, the ideal management strategy for women at intermediate risk remains uncertain. The TailorRx trial was designed to address this question and is currently randomizing women at intermediate risk Oncotype DX to hormone therapy alone or in combination with chemotherapy. This test is performed on paraffin-embedded tumor specimens. The MammaPrint assay, which stratifies women into low risk or high risk categories based on a 70-gene assay developed in Europe, received United States Food and Drug Administration (FDA) approval in 2007 (36). This test is performed on fresh frozen material. Additional gene profile assays are in development.

Adjuvant Chemotherapy for Early-stage Disease

Systemic chemotherapy has been an integral component of the adjuvant treatment strategy for many women with early-stage breast cancer since investigators first reported benefits with single agent chemotherapy after radical mastectomy in the 1970s. Systemic chemotherapy regimens have since undergone a number of refinements in formulations, schedules, and dosage. Polychemotherapy, whereby a minimum of two agents are administered in combination, was an early modification and represents an approach that has since been supported by a number of studies, including the Early Breast Cancer Trialists' Collaborative Group meta-analysis (26). Modern polychemotherapy regimens often incorporate an anthracycline and/or a taxane (Table 12.2). However, because many modern regimens have not been directly compared in randomized control trials, the superiority of any singular regimen has not been clearly established, nor have the benefits of any specific regimens for specific subgroups been clearly delineated.

One significant innovation in systemic chemotherapy administration is the dose dense strategy, developed from the Norton-Simon model, whereby the interval between treatments is decreased in order to optimize tumor cell, thus improving the overall impact of therapy (39). Another innovation is in drug delivery. For example, the paclitaxel (Taxol) solvent, Cremophor, is associated with potentially life-threatening hypersensitivity reactions, and consequently requires specialized equipment and steroid premedication. Albumin-bound paclitaxel (nab-paclitaxel, Abraxane), is a Cremophor-free preparation that does not require steroid premedication or specialized intravenous tubing. When compared to the conventional formulation, nab-paclitaxel demonstrated improved response rates and time to progression in the metastatic setting (40); in 2008 the drug was evaluated in the adjuvant setting. The improved activity demonstrated in the metastatic setting is postulated to reflect the ability to administer higher doses of the active agent and potentially, the preferential delivery of albumin-bound paclitaxel to cancer cells.

Biologic/Targeted Therapy for Early-stage Disease

Breast cancer is not homogeneous, as indicated by the mix of hormone responsive and unresponsive tumor cells. Another distinction can be made, as discussed above, on the basis of HER2. Recognition of specific subtypes is important because it holds the promise of targeted therapies. In this regard, one of the most significant advances in breast cancer management has been the development of trastuzumab. This humanized HER2-targeted monoclonal antibody is the most extensively studied biologic therapy (after anti-estrogens) in the adjuvant setting to date. HER2 status is determined by IHC evaluation of the protein and/or fluorescence in situ hybridization (FISH) assay of the HER2 gene sequence. The addition of trastuzumab to various adjuvant chemotherapy backbones has been associated with significant survival benefits and is now a standard component of the adjuvant paradigm for this subgroup (27,28,32,41). In 2008, adjuvant studies of other promising biologic agents included bevacizumab (Avastin), an anti-VEGF antibody, and lapatinib (Tykerb), an orally active tyrosine kinase inhibitor that targets both the HER1 and HER2 receptors. It is hoped that the incorporation of generally well-tolerated targeted therapy into the adjuvant treatment strategy may permit some women to forgo some of the potentially toxic chemotherapeutic agents comprising conventional strategies.

TABLE 12.2
Selected Modern Adjuvant Chemotherapy Regimens

REGIMEN	AGENTS	DOSE	DAY OF ADMINISTRATION	FREQUENCY OF ADMINISTRATION	TOTAL NUMBER OF CYCLES
AC-T[53,54]	Doxorubicin	60 mg/m² IV	Day 1	Every 3 weeks or every 2 weeks with G-CSF support	4
	Cyclophosphamide	600 mg/m² IV	Day 1		
	Paclitaxel	175 mg/m2 IV	Day 1		4
CEF[55,56] (with cotrimoxazole prophylaxis)	Cyclophosphamide	75 mg/m²/d PO	Days 1–14	Every 4 weeks	6
	Epirubicin	60 mg/m²/d IV	Days 1 & 8		
	5-Fluorouracil	500 mg/m²/d IV	Days 1 & 8		
CMF[57,58]	Cyclophosphamide	600 mg/m² IV	Day 1	Every 3 weeks	8
	Methotrexate	40 mg/m² IV	Day 1		
	5-Fluorouracil	600 mg/m² IV	Day 1		
FEC[59]	5-Fluorouracil	500 mg/m² IV	Day 1	Every 3 weeks	6
	Epirubicin	100 mg/m² IV	Day 1		
	Cyclophosphamide	500 mg/m² IV	Day 1		
FEC-D[60]	5-Fluorouracil	500 mg/m² IV	Day 1	Every 3 weeks	3
	Epirubicin	100 mg/m² IV	Day 1		
	Cyclophosphamide	500 mg/m² IV	Day 1		
	Docetaxel	100 mg/m² IV	Day 1	Every 3 weeks	3
TAC[61]	Docetaxel	75 mg/m² IV	Day 1	Every 3 weeks	6
	Adriamycin	50 mg/m² IV	Day 1		
	Cyclophosphamide	500 mg/m² IV	Day 1		

Abbreviations: AC-T, adriamycin/cyclophosphamide-paclitaxel; CEF, cyclophosphamide/epirubicin/5-fluorouracil; CMF, cyclophosphamide/methotrexate/5-fluorouracil; FEC, 5-fluorouracil/epirubicin/cyclophosphamide; FEC-D, 5-fluorouracil/epirubicin/cyclophosphamide-docetaxel; TAC, docetaxel/adriamycin/cyclophosphamide; G-CSF, granulocyte-colony stimulating factor; PO, by mouth; IV, intravenous.

Hormone Therapy for Early-stage Disease

Women with hormone-sensitive, early-stage breast cancer, as determined by estrogen and/or progesterone receptor status, are typically treated with adjuvant hormone therapy. The basic concept is that hormone-responsive cancers will not grow when estrogen-driven proliferation is inhibited. By "hormone therapy," we really mean anti-estrogen therapy, although the actual mechanisms of action for some hormone agents are too complex for such simple summation. Functionally, adjuvant hormone therapy for pre- or peri-menopausal women with hormone-sensitive tumors is comprised of tamoxifen or ovarian suppression. The efficacy of tamoxifen or an AI in combination with medical or surgical ovarian suppression is not well defined. The Sup-

pression of Ovarian Function Trial (SOFT) is currently randomizing pre-menopausal women with early-stage, hormone-sensitive breast cancer to tamoxifen, tamoxifen with ovarian suppression or an AI (exemestane, Aromasin) with ovarian suppression.

Prior to the early 2000s, tamoxifen was also considered the cornerstone of hormonal therapy for postmenopausal women with early-stage, hormone-sensitive disease. However, studies evaluating third-generation AIs in the adjuvant setting were reported as early as 2004. AIs inhibit the aromatase enzyme, which catalyzes the peripheral conversion of steroid precursors into active forms of estrogen. These drugs have been evaluated in a number of adjuvant strategies, including sequential strategies after two to three years of tamoxifen, upfront strategies, and extended strategies beyond five years of tamoxifen (42–47). Each of these demonstrated significant benefits; however, the superiority of any given strategy has not been determined. The most common AI-related toxicities include myalgias/arthralgias and decreased bone mineral density. However, AIs are not associated with the increased risk of thromboembolic events and new uterine cancers, which are associated with tamoxifen administration.

Adjuvant Radiotherapy

Because there is a significant risk of recurrence after breast conserving surgery, radiotherapy to the conserved breast is indicated in this setting to optimize local control (48). The addition of ipsilateral breast radiotherapy to breast conserving surgery is associated with a significantly lower rate of local recurrence (7% vs 26% at 15 years), and is thus an integral component of the breast conserving approach (12). Because of the increased risk of locoregional recurrence and the overall survival benefits demonstrated to date, radiotherapy post-mastectomy is indicated for women with large (5 cm or greater) tumors and/or four or more involved axillary lymph nodes (12,49). The benefits of radiotherapy for women with one to three involved lymph nodes is not well defined, and significant regional variability in practice patterns exist. By convention, radiotherapy is typically administered upon completion of adjuvant systemic therapy.

LOCALLY ADVANCED BREAST CANCER

Locally advanced breast cancer (LABC) is associated with a poorer prognosis than early-stage disease. The definition of LABC has not been consistent across clinical trials; however, the term generally denotes tumors that are large (greater than 5 cm), have extensive lymph node involvement, and/or involve the skin or chest wall. Inflammatory breast cancer (IBC) is a specific entity under the LABC umbrella, characterized by diffuse erythema, edema, and/or peau d'orange affecting the majority of the breast. IBC is primarily a clinical rather than pathological diagnosis, and portends a particularly poor prognosis.

LABC is represented by the stage III designation in the TNM classification system. LABC is typically treated with induction (neoadjuvant) chemotherapy followed by definitive locoregional therapy with surgery, radiotherapy or both. The practice of delivering neoadjuvant (preoperative) treatment (chemotherapy, hormone therapy, biologic therapy) affords a number of potential advantages. First, inoperable tumors can be rendered resectable. In addition, a neoadjuvant approach has the advantage of downstaging the cancer, thereby increasing the likelihood of a breast conserving approach as well as allowing procurement of pathologic specimens that may provide important correlative data regarding response to therapy. On the other hand, a number of potential benefits, including theoretically earlier eradication of micrometastases and the prevention of spontaneous somatic mutations postulated to lead to drug resistant cell populations, have not been observed. In research trials, response to neoadjuvant chemotherapy appeared to provide important prognostic information, which generally correlates with overall survival, but this form of treatment has not been generalized to standard practice (50).

Outside of a clinical trial, neoadjuvant chemotherapy is typically comprised of an anthracycline- and/or taxane-containing regimen followed by an assessment of response to therapy (46). Subsequent definitive locoregional therapy is indicated if a complete or near-complete clinical response is observed. However, in the absence of these findings, further neoadjuvant therapy with a non-cross-resistant chemotherapy regimen may be considered (ie, with a taxane if an anthracycline was previously administered, or vice versa). Although the optimal duration of trastuzumab administration in this setting is unknown, extrapolating from the survival benefits demonstrated with trastuzumab in the adjuvant setting, all women with HER2-overexpressing LABC should be considered for a 52-week course of trastuzumab therapy in the absence of any contraindication and regardless of whether treatment begins before or after surgery.

LOCOREGIONAL RECURRENCE

Despite adequate definitive therapy, a significant number of women with early-stage or LABC experience a locoregional recurrence, typically within the first 5 years after diagnosis (12). A recurrence in the ipsilateral preserved breast or chest wall is described as "local" whereas a recurrence in the ipsilateral axillary, supraclavicular, infraclavicular, and/or internal mammary nodes is described as "regional." If a locoregional recurrence is suspected, diagnostic re-evaluation with biopsy (including re-evaluation of hormone receptor and HER2 status) and repeat staging investigations to rule out distant recurrence should be considered. If recurrence occurs in the preserved breast after breast-conserving treatment, mastectomy is generally indicated. If recurrence occurs in the chest wall only, a wide local excision may be considered. Additional postexcision radiotherapy should also be considered, especially if postmastectomy radiotherapy was not previously administered. With regional recurrence after primary breast-conserving treatment or mastectomy, repeat axillary staging in the absence of clinically detectable nodal disease may be considered. ALND, if not previously performed, or resection (if ALND was previously performed) may be considered in the setting of clinically suspicious lymphadenopathy. The goal is to avoid under treating potentially curable second primary cancers that can arise in preserved duct epithelium. Very long-term disease control (and even cure) is reported for a subset of patients following local relapse only.

Systemic chemotherapy after definitive therapy for a locoregional recurrence is commonly recommended, although the benefits of this practice are not well defined. In a large, international, multicenter, phase III clinical trial led by International Breast Cancer Study Group and National Surgical Adjuvant Breast and Bowel Project investigators, women with a radically resected, locoregional breast cancer recurrence are currently being randomized to radiotherapy with or without chemotherapy. Until the results of this study are reported, systemic chemotherapy or in hormone-sensitive disease, hormone therapy, can be considered on an individual basis. As in the adjuvant setting, all women with HER2-overexpressing breast cancer should be considered for trastuzumab therapy.

METASTATIC BREAST CANCER

Metastatic breast cancer (MBC) represents approximately 5% of all new breast cancer diagnoses (1). In addition, the majority of women with early-stage or LABC who experience a relapse will relapse at a distant site. MBC is associated with a median survival of two to three years. Because MBC is generally incurable, the goals of therapy are to improve quality of life and ideally, improve survival. Consequently, the potential for treatment-related toxicity must be carefully weighed against the goals of therapy.

There is no consensus regarding the ideal treatment strategy for women with MBC; consequently, regional variations in practice patterns are observed. In general, however, reasonable MBC management strategies can be determined by considering a number of patient and tumor characteristics. The disease-free interval, prior adjuvant therapy prescription, number of metastatic sites, and potential for visceral crisis, as well as patient age, patient preference, comorbidities, performance status, hormone receptor status, and HER2 status, should all be considered when devising a treatment strategy. Bisphosphonate therapy should be considered in women with metastases to bone for the prevention of skeletal-related events (51). In general, endocrine therapies, which are generally well tolerated and associated with favorable toxicity profiles,

are recommended for women with hormone-responsive MBC who are not at risk for visceral crisis. Conversely, systemic chemotherapy is typically recommended for women with hormone-refractory disease, hormone-receptor negative disease, selected women with rapidly progressive disease, and/or women with significant cancer-related symptoms. All women with HER2-overexpressing MBC should be considered for trastuzumab therapy in the absence of any clear contraindication. In 2007, lapatinib, a small molecule tyrosine kinase inhibitor, was approved by the U.S. FDA for the treatment of anthracycline, taxane, and trastuzumab pretreated HER2-overexpressing MBC (40). For patients with HER2-normal disease, one trial suggested an advantage for the anti-angiogenic monoclonal antibody, bevacizumab, added to weekly paclitaxel as first-line therapy (52). The role of biologic therapy remains an active and promising area of investigation. Women should be considered for participation in clinical trials where appropriate.

CONCLUSIONS

Breast cancer is an important public health issue. The incidence and prevalence of breast cancer are significant. However, important strides in diagnosis and treatment have resulted in significant improvements in breast cancer-specific mortality rates (4,5). In the coming years, further improvements in screening and diagnostic technology are anticipated, with a particular focus on imaging modalities that exploit some of the biologic features of breast cancer. Similarly, clinical trials of promising biologic/targeted therapies as well as drug delivery and scheduling innovations continue in the adjuvant, neoadjuvant, and metastatic settings. It is hoped that these innovations in diagnosis and treatment will translate into ongoing improvements in breast cancer-specific outcomes.

References

1. American Cancer Society. *Cancer Facts & Figures.* http://www.cancer.org/docroot/STT/content/STT_1x_Cancer_Facts_and_Figures_2008.asp?from=fast
2. Claus EB, Schildkraut JM, Thompson WD, Risch NJ. The genetic attributable risk of breast and ovarian cancer. *Cancer.* 1996;77(11):2318–2324.
3. Chen S, Parmigiani G. Meta-analysis of BRCA1 and BRCA2 penetrance. *J Clin Oncol.* 2007;25(11):1329–1333.
4. Berry DA, Cronin KA, Plevritis SK, et al. Effect of screening and adjuvant therapy on mortality from breast cancer. *N Engl J Med.* 2005;353(17):1784–1792.
5. Elkin EB, Hurria A, Mitra N, Schrag D, Panageas KS. Adjuvant chemotherapy and survival in older women with hormone receptor-negative breast cancer: assessing outcome in a population-based, observational cohort. *J Clin Oncol.* 2006;24(18):2757–2764.

6. Smart CR, Hartmann WH, Beahrs OH, Garfinkel L. Insights into breast cancer screening of younger women. Evidence from the 14-year follow-up of the Breast Cancer Detection Demonstration Project. *Cancer.* 1993;72(4 Suppl):1449–1456.

7. Pisano ED, Gatsonis C, Hendrick E, et al. Diagnostic performance of digital versus film mammography for breast-cancer screening. *N Engl J Med.* 2005;353(17):1773–1783.

8. Soo MS, Rosen EL, Baker JA, Vo TT, Boyd BA. Negative predictive value of sonography with mammography in patients with palpable breast lesions. *AJR.* 2001;177(5):1167–1170.

9. Moy L, Slanetz PJ, Moore R, et al. Specificity of mammography and US in the evaluation of a palpable abnormality: retrospective review. *Radiology.* 2002;225(1):176–181.

10. Flobbe K, Bosch AM, Kessels AG, et al. The additional diagnostic value of ultrasonography in the diagnosis of breast cancer. *Arch Intern Med.* 2003;163(10):1194–1199.

11. Saslow D, Boetes C, Burke W, et al. American Cancer Society guidelines for breast screening with MRI as an adjunct to mammography. *CA Cancer J Clin.* 2007;57(2):75–89.

12. Early Breast Trialists' Collaborative Group. Effects of radiotherapy and of differences in the extent of surgery for early breast cancer on local recurrence and 15-year survival: an overview of the randomised trials. *Lancet.* 2005;366(9503):2087–2106.

13. Fisher ER, Land SR, Fisher B, Mamounas E, Gilarski L, Wolmark N. Pathologic findings from the National Surgical Adjuvant Breast and Bowel Project: twelve-year observations concerning lobular carcinoma in situ. *Cancer.* 2004;100(2):238–244.

14. Fisher B, Costantino JP, Wickerham DL, et al. Tamoxifen for the prevention of breast cancer: current status of the National Surgical Adjuvant Breast and Bowel Project P-1 study. *J Natl Cancer Inst.* 2005;97(22):1652–1662.

15. Chuba PJ, Hamre MR, Yap J, et al. Bilateral risk for subsequent breast cancer after lobular carcinoma-in-situ: analysis of surveillance, epidemiology, and end results data. *J Clin Oncol.* 2005;23(24):5534–5541.

16. Fisher B, Dignam J, Wolmark N, et al. Tamoxifen in treatment of intraductal breast cancer: National Surgical Adjuvant Breast and Bowel Project B-24 randomised controlled trial. *Lancet.* 1999;353(9169):1993–2000.

17. Houghton J, George WD, Cuzick J, Duggan C, Fentiman IS, Spittle M. Radiotherapy and tamoxifen in women with completely excised ductal carcinoma in situ of the breast in the UK, Australia, and New Zealand: randomised controlled trial. *Lancet.* 2003;362(9378):95–102.

18. American Joint Committee on Cancer (AJCC). *AJCC Cancer Staging Manual*, 6th ed. New York: Springer-Verlag; 2002.

19. Saphner T, Tormey DC, Gray R. Annual hazard rates of recurrence for breast cancer after primary therapy. *J Clin Oncol.* 1996;14(10):2738–2746.

20. Susnik B, Frkovic-Grazio S, Bracko M. Occult micrometastases in axillary lymph nodes predict subsequent distant metastases in stage I breast cancer: a case-control study with 15-year follow-up. *Ann Surg Oncol.* 2004;11(6):568–572.

21. Cummings MC, Walsh MD, Hohn BG, Bennett IC, Wright RG, McGuckin MA. Occult axillary lymph node metastases in breast cancer do matter: results of 10-year survival analysis. *Am J Surg Pathol.* 2002;26(10):1286–1295.

22. Millis RR, Springall R, Lee AH, Ryder K, Rytina ER, Fentiman IS. Occult axillary lymph node metastases are of no prognostic significance in breast cancer. *Br J Cancer.* 2002;86(3):396–401.

23. Elson CE, Kufe D, Johnston WW. Immunohistochemical detection and significance of axillary lymph node micrometastases in breast carcinoma. A study of 97 cases. *Anal Quant Cytol Histol.* 1993;15(3):171–178.

24. Herbert GS, Sohn VY, Brown TA. The impact of nodal isolated tumor cells on survival of breast cancer patients. *Am J Surg.* 2007;193(5):571–573; discussion 3–4.

25. Berry DA, Cirrincione C, Henderson IC, et al. Estrogen-receptor status and outcomes of modern chemotherapy for patients with node-positive breast cancer. *JAMA.* 2006;295(14):1658–1667.

26. Early Breast Cancer Trialists' Collaborative Group. Effects of chemotherapy and hormonal therapy for early breast cancer on recurrence and a 15-year survival: an overview of the randomised trials. *Lancet.* 2005;365:1687–1717.

27. Piccart-Gebhart MJ, Procter M, Leyland-Jones B, et al. Trastuzumab after Adjuvant Chemotherapy in HER2-Positive Breast Cancer. *N Engl J Med.* 2005;353(16):1659–1672.

28. Romond EH, Perez EA, Bryant J, et al. Trastuzumab plus adjuvant Chemotherapy for operable HER2-positive breast cancer. *N Engl J Med.* 2005;353(16):1673–1684.

29. Pritchard KI, Shepherd LE, O'Malley FP, et al. HER2 and responsiveness of breast cancer to adjuvant chemotherapy. *N Engl J Med.* 2006;354(20):2103–2111.

30. Paik S, Bryant J, Park C, et al. erbB-2 and response to doxorubicin in patients with axillary lymph node positive, hormone receptor-negative breast cancer. *J Natl Cancer Inst.* 1998;90(18):1361–1370.

31. Marty M, Cognetti F, Maraninchi D, et al. Randomized phase II trial of the efficacy and safety of trastuzumab combined with docetaxel in patients with human epidermal growth factor receptor 2-positive metastatic breast cancer administered as first-line treatment: the M77001 study group. *J Clin Oncol.* 2005;23(19):4265–4274.

32. Joensuu H, Kellokumpu-Lehtinen PL, Bono P, et al. Adjuvant docetaxel or vinorelbine with or without trastuzumab for breast cancer. *N Engl J Med.* 2006;354(8):809–820.

33. Schiff R, Chamness GC, Brown PH. Advances in breast cancer treatment and prevention: preclinical studies on aromatase inhibitors and new selective estrogen receptor modulators (SERMs). *Breast Cancer Res.* 2003;5(5):228–231.

34. Ellis MJ, Coop A, Singh B, et al. Letrozole is more effective neoadjuvant endocrine therapy than tamoxifen for ErbB-1- and/or ErbB-2-positive, estrogen receptor-positive primary breast cancer: evidence from a phase III randomized trial. *J Clin Oncol.* 2001;19(18):3808–3816.

35. Paik S, Shak S, Tang G, et al. A multigene assay to predict recurrence of tamoxifen-treated, node-negative breast cancer. *N Engl J Med.* 2004;351(27):2817–2826.

36. van de Vijver MJ, He YD, van't Veer LJ, et al. A gene-expression signature as a predictor of survival in breast cancer. *N Engl J Med.* 2002;347(25):1999–2009.

37. Buyse M, Loi S, van't Veer L, et al. Validation and clinical utility of a 70-gene prognostic signature for women with node-negative breast cancer. *J Natl Cancer Inst.* 2006;98(17):1183–1192.

38. Wang Y, Klijn JG, Zhang Y, et al. Gene-expression profiles to predict distant metastasis of lymph-node-negative primary breast cancer. *Lancet.* 2005;365(9460):671–679.

39. Norton L. A Gompertzian model of human breast cancer growth. *Cancer Res.* 1988;48:7067–7071.

40. Gradishar WJ, Tjulandin S, Davidson N, et al. Phase III trial of nanoparticle albumin-bound paclitaxel compared with polyethylated castor oil-based paclitaxel in women with breast cancer. *J Clin Oncol.* 2005;23(31):7794–7803.

41. Slamon D EW, Robert N, et al. Phase III randomized trial comparing doxorubicin and cyclophosphamide followed by docetaxel (ACT) with doxorubicin and cyclophosphamide followed by docetaxel and trastuzumab (ACTH) with docetaxel, carboplatin and trastuzumab (TCH) in HER2 positive early breast cancer patients: BCIRG 006 study. In: San Antonio Breast Cancer Symposium; San Antonio, TX; 2005.

42. Howell A, Cuzick J, Baum M, et al. Results of the ATAC (Arimidex, Tamoxifen, Alone or in Combination) trial after completion of 5 years' adjuvant treatment for breast cancer. *Lancet.* 2005;365(9453):60–62.

43. Coates AS, Keshaviah A, Thurlimann B, et al. Five years of letrozole compared with tamoxifen as initial adjuvant therapy for postmenopausal women with endocrine-responsive early breast cancer: update of study BIG 1-98. *J Clin Oncol.* 2007;25(5):486–492.

44. Coombes RC, Kilburn LS, Snowdon CF, et al. Survival and safety of exemestane versus tamoxifen after 2–3 years' tamoxifen treatment (Intergroup Exemestane Study): a randomised controlled trial. *Lancet.* 2007;369(9561):559–570.

45. Goss PE, Ingle JN, Martino S, Robert NJ, et al. Updated analysis of the NCIC CTG MA.17 randomized placebo (P) controlled trial of letrozole (L) after five years of tamoxifen in postmenopausal women with early stage breast cancer. *Proc Am Soc Clin Oncol.* 2004;23:87.

46. Schwartz GF, Hortobagyi GN. Proceedings of the consensus conference on neoadjuvant chemotherapy in carcinoma of the breast, April 26-28, 2003, Philadelphia, Pennsylvania. *Cancer.* 2004;100(12):2512–2532.

47. Boccardo F, Rubagotti A, Puntoni M, et al. Switching to anastrozole versus continued tamoxifen treatment of early breast cancer: preliminary results of the Italian Tamoxifen Anastrozole Trial. *J Clin Oncol.* 2005;23(22):5138–5147.

48. Eifel P, Axelson JA, Costa J, et al. National Institutes of Health Consensus Development Conference Statement: adjuvant therapy for breast cancer, November 1–3, 2000. *J Natl Cancer Inst.* 2001;93(13):979–989.

49. Harris JR, Halpin-Murphy P, McNeese M, Mendenhall NP, Morrow M, Robert NJ. Consensus Statement on postmastectomy radiation therapy. *Int J Rad Oncol Biol Phys.* 1999;44(5):989–990.

50. Buzdar AU, Singletary SE, Booser DJ, Frye DK, Wasaff B, Hortobagyi GN. Combined modality treatment of stage III and inflammatory breast cancer. M.D. Anderson Cancer Center experience. *Surg Oncol Clin N Am.* 1995;4(4):715–734.

51. Hillner BE, Ingle JN, Chlebowski RT, et al. American Society of Clinical Oncology 2003 update on the role of bisphosphonates and bone health issues in women with breast cancer. *J Clin Oncol.* 2003;21(21):4042–4057.

52. Miller K, Wang M, Gralow J, et al. A randomized phase III trial of paclitaxel versus paclitaxel plus bevacizumab as first-line therapy for locally recurrent or metastatic breast cancer: a trial coordinated by the Eastern Cooperative Oncology Group (E2100). In: 28th Annual San Antonio Breast Cancer Symposium 2005; San Antonio, Texas: Breast Cancer Research and Treatment; 2005; S6.

53. Henderson IC, Berry DA, Demetri GD, et al. Improved outcomes from adding sequential Paclitaxel but not from escalating Doxorubicin dose in an adjuvant chemotherapy regimen for patients with node-positive primary breast cancer. *J Clin Oncol.* 2003;21(6):976–983.

54. Citron ML, Berry DA, Cirrincione C, et al. Randomized trial of dose-dense versus conventionally scheduled and sequential versus concurrent combination chemotherapy as postoperative adjuvant treatment of node-positive primary breast cancer: first report of Intergroup Trial C9741/Cancer and Leukemia Group B Trial 9741. *J Clin Oncol.* 2003;21(8):1431–1439.

55. Levine MN, Bramwell VH, Pritchard KI, et al. Randomized trial of intensive cyclophosphamide, epirubicin, and fluorouracil chemotherapy compared with cyclophosphamide, methotrexate, and fluorouracil in premenopausal women with node-positive breast cancer. National Cancer Institute of Canada Clinical Trials Group. *J Clin Oncol.* 1998;16(8):2651–2658.

56. Ejlertsen B, Mouridsen HT, Jensen MB, et al. Improved outcome from substituting methotrexate with epirubicin: results from a randomized comparison of CMF versus CEF in patients with primary breast cancer. *Eur J Cancer.* 2007;43(5):877–884.

57. Fisher B, Dignam J, Mamounas EP, et al. Sequential methotrexate and fluorouracil for the treatment of node-negative breast cancer patients with estrogen receptor-negative tumors: eight-year results from National Surgical Adjuvant Breast and Bowel Project (NSABP) B-13 and first report of findings from NSABP B-19 comparing methotrexate and fluorouracil with conventional cyclophosphamide, methotrexate, and fluorouracil. *J Clin Oncol.* 1996;14(7):1982–1992.

58. Fisher B, Anderson S, Tan-Chiu E, et al. Tamoxifen and chemotherapy for axillary node-negative, estrogen receptor-negative breast cancer: findings from National Surgical Adjuvant Breast and Bowel Project B-23. *J Clin Oncol.* 2001;19(4):931–942.

59. French Epirubicin Study G. Benefit of a high-dose epirubicin regimen in adjuvant chemotherapy for node-positive breast cancer patients with poor prognostic factors: 5-year follow-up results of french adjuvant study group 05 randomized trial. *J Clin Oncol.* 2001;19(3):602–611.

60. Roché H, Fumoleau P, Spielmann M, et al. Sequential adjuvant epirubicin-based and docetaxel chemotherapy for node-positive breast cancer patients: the FNCLCC PACS 01 Trial. *J Clin Oncol.* 2006;24(36):5664–5671.

61. Martin M, Pienkowski T, Mackey J, et al. Adjuvant docetaxel for node-positive breast cancer. *N Engl J Med.* 2005;352(22):2302–2313.

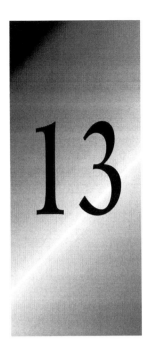

Evaluation and Treatment of Prostate and Genitourinary Cancer

13

Alexei Morozov
Susan F. Slovin

This chapter will begin with an overview of prostate cancer followed by a discussion of genitourinary cancers which include cancers of the urinary tract (bladder, urethra, and kidney) and the male genital tract (testis and penis). In the United States, it was estimated that over 186,000 new cases of prostate cancer would be diagnosed 2008, accounting for 29% of all new cancer diagnoses in men. For a man aged 70 or older, the estimated risk of developing prostate cancer is one in seven (1). Prostate cancer is the second largest cause of cancer mortality in men; in the United States, it was estimated that over 28,000 deaths from prostate cancer would occur in 2008. There has, however, been a steady decline in the prostate cancer death rate in the US since 1997 (1). Worldwide, there is wide variation in prostate cancer incidence rates among geographic and ethnic groups. The highest incidence of prostate cancer is seen in African-Americans and Caribbean men of African descent (2). Geographically, the highest rates are seen in North America and Western Europe, intermediate rates in Africa, and lowest rates in Asia. These trends were seen prior to the prostate-specific antigen (PSA) era as well (2,3). In addition to race and ethnicity, the presence of a first-degree relative with prostate cancer is a well-established risk factor for development of prostate cancer. Having an affected father confers a twofold risk of prostate cancer. The risk is further increased if multiple relatives are affected with prostate cancer, or if relatives with the disease were diagnosed before age 65 (4). Obesity was found to be positively associated with a risk of prostate cancer in a cohort

analysis involving 900,000 patients. Patients with a BMI older than aged 35 were found to be 34% more likely to die from prostate cancer (5).

DIAGNOSIS

Following the introduction of PSA testing in the mid-1980s, the incidence of prostate cancer more than doubled, reaching its peak in 1992. Whereas in the pre-PSA era 50% of prostate cancers presented with metastatic disease, more than 90% of prostate cancers are now detected at the organ-confined stage. The American Cancer Society and the American Urological Association recommend screening PSA testing in men aged 50 or older with a life expectancy of at least 10 years, or starting at age 45 if any risk factors are present (6–8). Urinary symptoms such as hesitancy, nocturia, diminished urinary stream, as well as any change in erectile or ejaculatory function, perineal pain, or abnormal digital rectal exam (DRE) may prompt PSA testing in the appropriate clinical setting. Age-specific normal limits of PSA values have been described (9). The differential diagnosis for elevated PSA includes benign prostatic hypertrophy, prostatitis, and prostate cancer. A low free (unbound) PSA was approved by the U.S. Food and Drug Administration (FDA) as an indicator of likely malignancy in the setting of normal DRE and PSA between 4 and 10. A trial of antibiotics may help exclude the diagnosis of prostatitis. Poorly differentiated prostate carcinomas may produce minimal or no

KEY POINTS

- Prostate cancer is the second largest cause of cancer mortality in men, predicted to cause more than 28,000 deaths in the United States in 2008.
- The American Cancer Society and the American Urological Association recommend screening prostate-specific antigen (PSA) testing in men aged 50 or older with a life expectancy of at least 10 years, or starting at aged 45 if any risk factors are present.
- Many patients die with prostate cancer rather than from it.
- Androgen deprivation therapy (ADT), usually with a gonadotropin-releasing hormone (GnRH) analog, alone or in combination with an anti-androgen to block the castration testosterone flare, is highly effective at slowing tumor growth.
- After anti-androgen withdrawal, second-line anti-androgens, and adrenal suppression have been exhausted, the combination of the anti-microtubule inhibitor docetaxel along with prednisone is the standard of care.
- Pretreatment electromyography is being evaluated as a tool to assess for preexisting neuropathy, which may be exacerbated by docetaxel or similar agents such as the vinca alkaloids or estramustine.
- Bladder cancer is the fourth most common cancer in men and the eighth most common cause of cancer-related death in men.

- Germ cell tumor of the testis is the most common malignancy in young men.
- Long-term toxicity of chemotherapy in testicular cancer includes infertility, bleomycin-associated pulmonary toxicity, Raynaud's phenomenon, peripheral neuropathy, increased risk of cardiovascular disease, and secondary malignancy risk, which is highest in those treated with chemotherapy and radiation.
- Cancer of the kidney and renal pelvis is the seventh most common in men and ninth most common in women; in the United States, it was estimated that 33,000 new cases in men and 21,000 in women would occur in 2008.
- The tyrosine kinase inhibitors induce partial and complete remissions in patients with clear cell renal cell carcinoma, making them the standard of care for the metastatic setting.
- A unique feature of renal cell carcinoma is that approximately 20% of patients present with paraneoplastic symptoms, including anemia or erythrocytosis, weight loss, malaise, hypercalcemia, hepatic dysfunction in the absence of metastases, glomerulonephritis, neuromyopathy, and dermatitis.
- Carcinoma of the penis comprises less than 1% of all malignancies in men.

PSA, which can mask the diagnosis of prostate cancer. If clinical suspicion of malignancy is high, a transrectal ultrasound-guided biopsy of the prostate is performed. Metastatic disease may present with bone pain, spinal cord compression, or symptoms of visceral organ involvement.

The most common histologic type of prostate cancer is adenocarcinoma. The Gleason grading system is a measure of glandular differentiation determined at low magnification. The primary (most prevalent) and the secondary (second most prevalent) glandular patterns are graded from 1 (most histologically similar to normal prostate) to 5 (most undifferentiated and therefore most aggressive) (Fig. 13.1). The sum of the two values (the Gleason score), as well as the order of individual components (eg, 4 + 3 vs 3 + 4, the first number indicating the most predominant pattern), are powerful predictors of outcome (10). If suspicion for metastatic disease is high, a computed tomography (CT) scan of the abdomen and pelvis is performed to evaluate for soft tissue disease in the liver, lung, and lymph nodes. A CT scan is insufficient to evaluate the prostate itself. A bone scan complements the CT scan in evaluating for bone metastases. Proton emission tomography (PET) scan can detect actively metaboliz-

ing disease. It is FDA-approved only for assessment of treatment response in patients receiving chemotherapy in the setting of a clinical trial. Magnetic resonance imaging (MRI) with an endorectal probe is useful to determine the extent of local disease (11). ProstaScint scan is an imaging modality using indium-111 oxine conjugated to a monoclonal antibody against prostate specific membrane antigen (PSMA). This imaging technique is FDA-approved for use in detecting occult recurrent disease. PSMA was originally thought to be a specific marker for prostate cancer. However, due to a high false positive rate, the use of this test remains controversial (12). The staging system for prostate cancer is presented in Table 13.1.

DEFINITIVE THERAPY

Prostate cancer is a heterogeneous disease. Many patients die with prostate cancer rather than from it (13). A clinical states model was proposed (14) to account for competing causes of death at any given state of cancer progression, and the likelihood of transitioning from one clinical state to the next (Fig. 13.2). For localized or regionally advanced prostate cancer, risk

PROSTATIC ADENOCARCINOMA
(Histologic Grades)

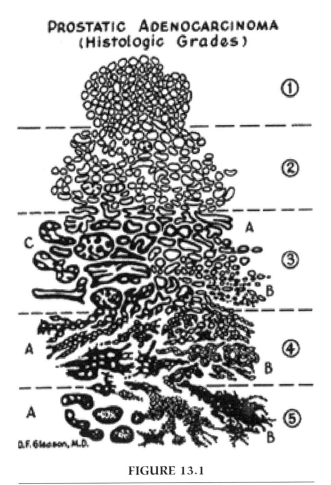

D.F. Gleason, M.D.

FIGURE 13.1

Gleason Grading System of Prostate Cancer. (From Ref. 42, with permission.)

stratification is performed using clinical stage, Gleason score, and pretreatment PSA (Table 13.2). Advantages, disadvantages, and contraindications of the treatment approaches for localized or regional prostate cancer are outlined in Table 13.3. Neoadjuvant, concomitant, or adjuvant hormonal therapy may be considered for high-risk disease (15,16). The decision regarding optimal therapy for early-stage prostate cancer is made in consultation with a urologic surgeon, medical oncologist, and radiation oncologist (17). Assessment tools to estimate the rate of self-reported side effects following definitive therapy have been developed and validated extensively (18,19) (Table 13.3).

RISING PSA FOLLOWING DEFINITIVE THERAPY

Since the introduction of PSA, it became possible to identify a new subgroup of patients; that is, those who develop rising PSA levels following definitive therapy

TABLE 13.1
2002 AJCC TNM Staging of Prostate Cancer

PRIMARY TUMOR, CLINICAL (T)

TX Primary tumor cannot be assessed

T0 No primary tumor

T1 Clinically inapparent, not palpable or visible by imaging

    T1a Incidental histologic finding, ≤5% of resected tissue

    T1b Incidental histologic finding, >5% of resected tissue

    T1c Tumor identified by needle biopsy, for any reason (eg, elevated PSA)

T2 Palpable or visible tumor, confined within the prostate

    T2a ≤½ one lobe

    T2b One lobe

    T2c Both lobes

T3 Tumor extends through the capsule

    T3a ECE, unilateral or bilateral

    T3b Seminal vesicle involvement

T4 Tumor is fixed or invades adjacent structures

    T4a Invades bladder neck, external sphincter or rectum

    T4b Invades levator muscles or fixed to pelvic sidewalls

PRIMARY TUMOR, PATHOLOGIC (T)

pT2 Organ-confined

    pT2a Unilateral, involving half of one lobe or less

    pT2b Unilateral, involving more than half of one lobe but not both lobes

    pT2c Bilateral

pT3 Extraprostatic extension

    pT3a Extraprostatic extension

    pT3b Seminal vesicle involvement

pT4 Invasion of bladder or rectum

Regional lymph nodes (N)

NX Regional lymph nodes cannot be assessed

N0 No regional lymph node metastasis

N1 Metastasis in regional lymph node or nodes

Distant metastases (M)

MX Distant metastasis cannot be assessed

M0 No regional lymph node metastasis

M1 Distant metastasis

    M1a: Nonregional lymph nodes

    M1b: Bone(s)

    M1c: Other site(s)

Source: From Ref. 43, with permission.

TABLE 13.2

Risk Stratification for Clinically Localized and Regional Prostate Cancer[a]

	LOW RISK	INTERMEDIATE RISK	HIGH RISK	VERY HIGH RISK
Clinical stage	T1a-T2a	T2b-T2c	T3a-T3b	T3c-T4 or any T, N1-3
Gleason score	2–6	7	8–10	Any
PSA, ng/ml	<10	10–20	>20	Any

[a]One of three criteria is sufficient for a given risk category.
Source: From Ref. 17, with permission.

for prostate cancer without any radiographic evidence of local recurrence or detectable metastatic disease. This clinical state is referred to as biochemical relapse, or "rising PSA, non-castrate" (14) (Fig. 13.2). Following definitive therapy for early prostate cancer, PSA nadir is an important prognostic factor. After prostatectomy, the PSA should become undetectable within 30 days. Causes of persistent detectable PSA levels following prostatectomy include residual normal prostate glandular tissue versus systemic micrometastatic disease. Following definitive radiotherapy, PSA is expected to fall below 0.5 ng/ml (20). Nomograms have been published to predict the likelihood of biochemical relapse as a surrogate for metastatic disease. Nomograms developed by Memorial-Sloan Kettering Cancer Center are available at www.nomograms.org. In 2005, nomograms using more clinically relevant endpoints were developed to assess the risk of metastatic disease in the setting of biochemical relapse (21). The initial workup of a rising PSA following definitive therapy includes digital rectal examination and imaging tests to rule out local recurrence and distant metastases. In patients with local recurrence following prostatectomy with node-negative disease, salvage radiotherapy is indicated. Conversely, salvage prostatectomy may be considered for recurrence within the prostate following radiotherapy, but is recommended only in selected cases. The presence of metastases necessitates the initiation of hormonal therapy. In the absence of documented local recurrence or metastatic disease, the remaining options include hormonal therapy, expectant monitoring or investigational approaches. PSA doubling time (based on the log slope of the PSA) becomes a powerful prognostic factor. Patients with a PSA doubling time of less than 3 months are candidates for hormonal therapy (22).

METASTATIC DISEASE

Prostate cancer, as well as normal prostate tissue, is highly sensitive to testosterone through the action of androgen receptor. Androgen deprivation therapy (ADT) usually with a gonadotropin-releasing hormone (GnRH) analog, alone or in combination with an anti-androgen to block the castration testosterone flare is therefore highly effective at slowing tumor growth. Several approaches to ADT have been developed (Table 13.4). ADT is highly effective at slowing progression of disease, but hormone-refractory disease usually develops within 18–24 months. After anti-androgen withdrawal (23), second-line anti-androgens, and adrenal suppression have been exhausted, cytotoxic chemotherapy may be necessary, although clinical trials are strongly advised in this setting. The combination of the anti-microtubule inhibitor, docetaxel, used along with prednisone, has been the standard of care (24,25). One of the main side effects of docetaxel is peripheral neuropathy (Table 13.5). Pretreatment electromyography (26) was evaluated in 2006 as a tool to assess for preexisting neuropathy, which may be exacerbated by docetaxel or similar agents, including the vinca alkaloids or estramustine. Mitoxantrone and prednisone (27,28) as well as estramustine are also approved by the FDA for hormone-refractory metastatic prostate cancer (see Table 13.5). Palliative measures include radiotherapy and ureteral stenting for urinary obstruction.

CARCINOMA OF THE BLADDER AND THE UPPER UROGENITAL TRACT

Epidemiology

It was projected that more than 68,000 (more than 51,000 in men and more than 18,000 in women) new cases of bladder cancer (including carcinoma in situ) would be reported in the United States in 2008. Projected death rates from bladder cancer numbered approximately 14,000 (almost 10,000 in men; more than 4,000 in women). Bladder cancer is the fourth most common cancer in men and the eighth most common cause of cancer-related death in men (1). There

TABLE 13.3
Main Treatment Options for Early Prostate Cancer

	ACTIVE OBSERVATION	RADICAL RETROPUBIC PROSTATECTOMY (RRP)	EXTERNAL BEAM RADIATION THERAPY (EBRT)	BRACHYTHERAPY
10-year PSA failure-free rate	Unknown	47%–78%	62%–83%	77%
Prevalence of side effects at 6 years follow-up[b]				
Urinary	N/A	8%	11%	16%
Bowel	N/A	3%	13%	10%
Sexual	N/A	39%	39%	55%
Other side effects	Anxiety side effects of surveillance re-biopsy	Perioperative complications (0%–5%)		Acute urinary retention (5%–34%) Rectal toxicity (2%–12%)
Advantages	Avoids or postpones treatment-related morbidity	■ Salvage radiation therapy remains an option ■ Improved prognosis based on pathologic features ■ Novel techniques (laparoscopic and robot-assisted) are being developed	■ Effective cancer control ■ Low risk of urinary incontinence ■ Available to patients with medical contra-indications to surgery	■ Equal cancer control rates for organ-confined tumors ■ Single treatment ■ Low risk of urinary incontinence (without prior TURP) ■ Available to patients with medical contra-indications to surgery
Disadvantages	■ Increased risk of metastases in intermediate-risk patients compared to prostatectomy ■ Anxiety-provoking	■ Significant risk of impotence ■ Risk of operative morbidity ■ Higher operator-dependence ■ Some risk of long-term incontinence	■ Significant risk of impotence ■ Lymph node involvement not determined ■ Salvage surgery is complicated by radiation changes ■ Prolonged treatment	■ Significant risk of impotence ■ Lymph node involvement not determined ■ Salvage surgery is complicated by radiation changes ■ Not appropriate for high-risk disease
Contraindications	■ High risk disease ■ Large prostate ■ Long life expectancy	■ Medical contra-indications to surgery ■ Neurogenic bladder	■ Previous pelvic XRT ■ Active inflammatory disease of rectum ■ Low bladder capacity ■ Chronic diarrhea	■ Previous pelvic XRT ■ Prior TURP ■ Large prostate ■ Significant voiding symptoms ■ Large tumor burden ■ Active inflammatory disease of rectum ■ Chronic diarrhea ■ Long life expectancy

[a]Retrospective study showed equivalent disease control rates with RRP and EBRT; randomized studies are in progress (44).
[b]Rates of adverse effects are unadjusted and therefore cannot be used to compare treatment modalities due to differences between groups(19)

Source: Modified from Ref. 17, with permission.

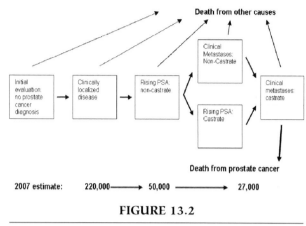

Death from other causes

2007 estimate: 220,000 ——→ 50,000 ————————→ 27,000

FIGURE 13.2

Clinical States Model of Prostate Cancer. (From Ref. 14 with permission.)

is a high degree of geographic and ethnic variation in the incidence rates, with the highest rates seen in non-Latino whites in the United States and Western Europe, and lowest rates in Asian-Americans (3). Cigarette smoking, occupational exposure to synthetic dyes, and prolonged use of an indwelling catheter are well-established risk factors for bladder cancer. Tumors of the upper urogenital tract, i.e. the renal pelvis and ureter, are about 17 times less common than bladder carcinoma, but have similar risk factors.

Diagnosis

Bladder cancer most commonly presents with total (present throughout the length of micturition), gross,

TABLE 13.4

Forms of Androgen Deprivation Therapy

APPROACH (Ref)	AGENTS USED	INDICATIONS	MECHANISM OF ACTION	SIDE EFFECTS
Nonsteroidal anti-androgen monotherapy[45,46]	Bicalutamide	Biochemical relapse as an alternative to combined androgen blockade	Competes with testosterone for binding to androgen receptor	■ Hot flashes ■ Breast tenderness ■ Anemia ■ LFT abnormalities
Combined androgen blockade (CAB)[16]	GnRH agonist (goserelin acetate, leuprolide acetate) combined with anti-androgen (bicalutamide)	■ Metastatic disease ■ Neoadjuvant, concomitant or adjuvant therapy for early prostate cancer ■ Biochemical relapse	■ Supra-physiologic levels of GnRH agonist inhibit the anterior pituitary and thereby reduce circulating testosterone levels ■ Anti-androgen blocks the action of remaining testosterone and adrenal androgens ■ Anti-androgen protects from flair in testosterone upon initiation of GnRH agonist	■ Impotence, loss of libido ■ Osteoporosis ■ Accelerated atherosclerosis ■ Personality change ■ Weight gain ■ Hot flashes ■ Anemia ■ LFT abnormalities
Anti-androgen withdrawal[23]	Discontinuation of anti-androgen	Rising PSA on CAB	Prolonged exposure to anti-androgens leads to mutations in androgen receptor which cause anti-androgen to act as an agonist	N/A
Second-line anti-androgen therapy[47]	Flutamide, Nilutamide, Bicalutamide, Abiraterone	Rising PSA following anti-androgen withdrawal	Resistance mutations in androgen receptor are specific to particular anti-androgen	■ Hot flashes ■ Breast tenderness ■ Anemia ■ LFT abnormalities ■ Impaired dark adaptation (Nilutamide)
Adrenal suppression therapy	Ketoconazole	Rising PSA following second-line anti-androgen therapy	Suppresses production of adrenal androgens	■ Adrenal suppression—may require steroid supplementation ■ Nausea, vomiting ■ Need to avoid antacids

TABLE 13.5
Commonly Used Chemotherapy Regimens in Hormone-refractory Prostate Cancer

REGIMEN (REF.)	MEDIAN SURVIVAL (MONTHS)	SHORT-TERM SIDE EFFECTS	LONG-TERM SIDE EFFECTS
Mitoxanthrone and prednisone (24,27)	16.5	Nausea, vomiting (40%) Bone marrow suppression (22%) Fatigue (35%) Stomatitis (8%)	Cardiotoxicity (22%) Sensory neuropathy (7%) Change in taste (7%)
Docetaxel and estramustine (28)	17.5	Nausea, vomiting (20%) Bone marrow suppression (16%) Fatigue Stomatitis	Cardiovascular events (15%) Neurologic events (7%)
Docetaxel and prednisone every three weeks (27)	18.9	Nausea, vomiting (40%) Bone marrow suppression (32%) Fatigue (50%) Stomatitis (20%)	Alopecia (65%) Sensory neuropathy (30%) Change in taste (18%)
Weekly docetaxel (27)	17.4	Nausea, vomiting (40%) Bone marrow suppression (2%) Fatigue (50%) Stomatitis (17%)	Alopecia (50%) Sensory neuropathy (24%) Change in taste (24%)

painless hematuria. Alternatively, microhematuria may be incidentally found on routine urinalysis. Although present in approximately 15% of the population, persistent microscopic hematuria on repeat evaluation should prompt further workup to exclude malignancy. In addition to urine cytology, new bladder tumor markers have been proposed for monitoring of patients with known bladder carcinoma (29). Cystoscopy or cystourethroscopy allow definitive diagnosis. For staging, transurethral resection of bladder tumor (TURBT) is required, along with CT scan of abdomen and pelvis, bone scan, and chest x-ray or CT of the chest. Staging of bladder cancer is reviewed in Table 13.6. The most common histological type of bladder cancer is transitional cell carcinoma.

Treatment

Low-risk superficial bladder cancer (Ta grade 1–2) is treated with TURBT with or without a single dose of intravesical mitomycin C (MMC). Other intravesical agents include interferon, gemcitabine, and cyclophosphamide (Cytoxan). High-risk superficial tumors are treated with a course of induction intravesical chemotherapy or immunotherapy with Bacillus Calmette-Guerin (BCG) vaccine. Intravesical therapy causes a local inflammatory reaction, resulting in a cytokine-mediated antitumor effect. Organ-confined disease (T2) is treated with radical cystectomy with possible neoadjuvant or adjuvant chemotherapy with methotrexate, vinblastine, doxorubicin, and cisplatin (MVAC) (30).

Bladder-sparing approaches have been developed. For non-organ-confined disease that is resectable, radical cystectomy is indicated (31). In unresectable disease, chemotherapy is administered and response is monitored with CT scan and cystoscopy. Postchemotherapy surgery may be feasible. For patients with advanced and metastatic disease, the choice of chemotherapy regimen depends on performance status and the presence of visceral metastases (32).

TESTIS CANCER

Epidemiology

Germ-cell tumor of the testis is the most common malignancy in young men. In 2008, approximately 8,000 cases were predicted in the United States, with only 380 deaths, illustrating relatively good prognosis and effective treatment of germ-cell tumors. Risk factors include undescended testis, which predisposes to bilateral testis cancer, albeit more likely in the undescended testis, as well as Klinefelter's syndrome.

Diagnosis

Testis cancer commonly presents with a painless or painful testicular mass. In addition to malignancy, differential diagnosis includes epididymitis, epididymo-orchitis, and testicular torsion as well as hernia, hydrocele, testicular torsion, varicocele, and spermatocele.

TABLE 13.6

*American Joint Committee on Cancer 2002
TNM Bladder Cancer Staging*

Primary tumor (T)

Tx primary tumor cannot be assessed

T0 No evidence of primary tumor

Tis Carcinoma in situ

Ta Noninvasive papillary tumor

T1 Tumor invades the subepithelial connective tissue

T2 Tumor invades muscle

  pT2a Tumor invades superficial muscle (inner half)

  pT2b Tumor invades deep muscle (outer half)

T3 Tumor invades perivesical tissue

  pT3a Microscopically

  pT3b Macroscopically (extravesical mass)

T4 Tumor invades any of the following: prostate, uterus, vagina, pelvis or abdominal wall

  T4a Tumor invades prostate, uterus, vagina

  T4b Tumor invades pelvis or abdominal wall

Regional lymph nodes (N)

NX Regional lymph nodes cannot be assessed

N0 No regional lymph node metastasis

N1 Metastasis in a single lymph node, 2 cm or less in greatest dimension

N2 Metastasis in a single lymph node >2 cm but <5 cm in greatest dimension, or multiple lymph nodes, none >5 cm in greatest dimension

N3 Metastasis in a lymph node >5 cm in greatest dimension

Distant metastasis (M)

MX Distant metastasis cannot be assessed

M0 No distant metastasis

M1 Distant metastasis

Source: From Ref. 43, with permission.

TABLE 13.7

*Testicular Cancer Staging System of the
American Joint Committee of Cancer*

Primary tumor (T)

pTX Primary tumor cannot be assessed (if no radical orchiectomy is performed, TX is used)

pT0 No evidence of primary tumor (histological scar in testis)

pTis Intratubular germ cell neoplasia (carcinoma-in-situ)

pT1 Tumor limited to the testis and epididymis and no vascular/lymphatic invasion

pT2 Tumor limited to the testis and epididymis with vascular/lymphatic invasion or tumor extending through the tunica albuginea with involvement of the tunica vaginalis

pT3 Tumor invades the spermatic cord with or without vascular/lymphatic invasion

pT4 Tumor invades the scrotum with or without vascular/lymphatic invasion

Regional lymph nodes (N): Clinical

Nx Regional lymph nodes cannot be assessed

N0 No regional lymph node metastasis

N1 Lymph node mass ≤2 cm in greatest dimension or multiple lymph node masses, none >2 cm in greatest dimension

N2 Lymph node mass >2 cm but not >5 cm in greatest dimension, or multiple lymph node masses, any one mass >2 cm but not >5 cm in greatest dimension

N3 Lymph node mass >5 cm in greatest dimension

Regional lymph nodes (N): Pathologic

pN0 No evidence of tumor in lymph nodes

pN1 Lymph node mass, ≤2 cm in greatest dimension and ≤5 nodes positive; none >2 cm in greatest dimension

pN2 Lymph node mass >2 cm but not >5 cm in greatest dimension, >5 nodes positive, none >5 cm, evidence of extranodal extension of tumor

pN3 Lymph node mass >5 cm in greatest dimension

Distant metastases (M)

M0 No evidence of distant metastases

M1 Nonregional nodal or pulmonary metastases

M2 Nonpulmonary visceral metastases

Ultrasound is the next diagnostic step. Gynecomastia may be present due to secretion of beta-human chorionic gonadotropin (hCG) by the tumor. Metastatic disease may present with supraclavicular adenopathy, abdominal or back pain, bone pain, or CNS manifestations of brain metastases. Serum alpha fetoprotein (AFP), beta-hCG, and lactate dehydrogenase (LDH) are measured both to monitor treatment and to make the distinction between seminoma (which never causes AFP elevation) and non-seminomatous germ cell tumors (NSGCT). Staging according to The International Germ Cell Cancer Collaborative Group (33) is shown in Tables 13.7–13.10. Seminomatous and NSGCT demonstrate different clinical behavior and are treated differently.

Treatment

Radical orchiectomy through the inguinal approach is required for diagnosis and staging. Early-stage seminoma (stage cI and cIIA) is treated with adjuvant radiotherapy with near-100% cure rate. For early non-seminomatous tumors (stage cI and cIIA) retroperitoneal relapse is common. Treatment options include surveillance, retroperitoneal lymph node dissection (RPLND), and adjuvant chemotherapy

TABLE 13.8
Testicular Cancer Stage Grouping

STAGE	T	N	M	S
0	pTis	N0	M0	S0
Ia	T1	N0	M0	S0
Ib	≥T2	N0	M0	S0
Is	T any	N0	M0	S any
IIa	T any	N1	M0	S0, S1
IIb	T any	N2	M0	S0, S1
IIc	T any	N3	M0	S0, S1
IIIa	T any	N any	M1	S0, S1
IIIb	T any	N any	M0, M1	S2
IIIc	T any	N any	M0, M1	S3

Source: From Ref. 43, with permission.

TABLE 13.9
The International Germ Cell Cancer Collaborative Group Staging System

RISK	SEMINOMA	NON-SEMINOMA
Good risk	Nonpulmonary visceral metastases absent; any S stage; any primary tumor site	S stage 0 or 1; nonpulmonary visceral metastases absent; gonadal or retroperitoneal primary tumor
Intermediate risk (any criterion)	Nonpulmonary visceral metastases present; any S stage; any primary tumor site	S stage 2; nonpulmonary visceral metastases absent; gonadal or retroperitoneal primary tumor
Poor risk (any criterion)	–	Mediastinal primary tumor site; nonpulmonary visceral metastases present; S stage 3

TABLE 13.10
Definitions of Serologic (S) Staging for Germ Cell Tumors

STAGE	LDH	HCG	AFP
S1	<1.5 × upper limit of normal	<5000 IU/L	<1000 ng/ml
S2	1.5–10 × upper limit of normal	5000–50,000 IU/L	1000–10,000 ng/ml
S3	>10 × upper limit of normal	>50,000 IU/L	>10,000 ng/ml

Abbreviations: LDH, lactate dehydrogenase; HCG, human chorionic gonadotropin; AFP, alpha fetoprotein.
Source: From Ref. 43, with permission.

(34). Features indicative of a high risk for retroperitoneal relapse, such as predominant embryonal carcinoma histology, the presence of lymphovascular invasion, or extension into the tunica or scrotum, necessitate a primary RPLND after normalization of markers. Patients with advanced disease are treated with chemotherapy, according to the risk-stratification scheme of The International Germ Cell Cancer Collaborative Group (1997) (Tables 13.8 and 13.9). Patients with good-risk disease are treated with three cycles of bleomycin, etoposide, and cisplatin (BEP) or four cycles of etoposide and cisplatin. High-risk patients are treated with four cycles of bleomycin, etoposide, and cisplatin. Long-term toxicity of chemotherapy includes infertility, bleomycin-associated pulmonary toxicity, Raynaud's phenomenon, peripheral neuropathy, increased risk of cardiovascular disease, and secondary malignancy risk, which is highest in those treated with chemotherapy and radiation (35).

RENAL CELL CARCINOMA

Epidemiology

Cancer of the kidney and renal pelvis is the seventh most common in men and ninth most common in women, with an estimated 33,000 new cases in men and 21,000 in women in predicted in the United States in 2008. Cigarette smoking, obesity, hypertension, and possibly, diuretic use have been linked to renal cell carcinoma. Two main genetic syndromes are associated with renal cell carcinoma. A germline mutation in the *VHL* gene predisposes to Von Hippel-Lindau (VHL) syndrome, which includes renal cell carcinoma of clear cell type. A germline mutation in the *MET* proto-oncogene is associated with hereditary renal cell carcinoma of papillary cell type.

Diagnosis

Over 50% of renal cell carcinoma cases are diagnosed incidentally on abdominal imaging. A unique feature of renal cell carcinoma is that approximately 20% of patients present with paraneoplastic symptoms including anemia or erythrocytosis, weight loss, malaise, hypercalcemia, hepatic dysfunction in the absence of metastases, glomerulonephritis, neuromyopathy, and dermatitis. The AJCC staging system for renal cell carcinoma is outlined in Tables 13.11 and 13.12.

Treatment

For localized renal cell carcinoma diagnosed by characteristic imaging appearance, biopsy is not

TABLE 13.11
AJCC Staging of Renal Cell Carcinoma

Primary tumor (T)
TX Primary tumor cannot be assessed
T0 No evidence of primary tumor
T1 Tumor 7 cm or less in greatest dimension, limited to the kidney
T1a Tumor 4 cm or less in greatest dimension, limited to the kidney
T1b Tumor more than 4 cm but not more than 7 cm in greatest dimension, limited to the kidney
T2 Tumor more than 7 cm in greatest dimension, limited to the kidney
T3 Tumor extends into major veins or invades adrenal gland or perinephric tissues but not beyond Gerota's fascia
T3a Tumor directly invades the adrenal gland or perirenal and/or renal sinus fat but not beyond Gerota's fascia
T3b Tumor grossly extends into the renal vein or its segmental (muscle-containing) branches, or vena cava below the diaphragm
T3c Tumor grossly extends into vena cava above diaphragm or invades the wall of the vena cava
T4 Tumor invades beyond Gerota's fascia
Regional lymph nodes (N)
NX Regional lymph nodes cannot be assessed
N0 No regional lymph node metastases
N1 Metastases in a single regional lymph node
N2 Metastases in more than one regional lymph node
MX Distant metastasis cannot be assessed
M0 No distant metastasis
M1 Distant metastasis

indicated. Radical nephrectomy is performed. Partial nephrectomy is performed for bilateral tumors or when radical nephrectomy would result in the need for dialysis. Renal cell carcinoma, thought to be an immunologically mediated disease, has shown spontaneous regressions over time including regression of metastatic lesions with removal of the primary renal mass. Low-volume metastatic disease can rarely be resected with curative intent. For the majority of patients with metastatic disease, systemic therapy remains the initial treatment of choice. Renal cell carcinoma is traditionally one of the most highly chemotherapy-resistant tumors. Metastatic renal cell carcinoma has a median survival of 9–15 months. Features associated with shortened survival include low Karnofsky performance status (1.5 times upper limit of normal), low hemoglobin (less than the lower limit of normal), high serum calcium, and

TABLE 13.12

Stage Grouping for Renal Cell Carcinoma

Stage I	T1 N0 M0
Stage II	T2 N0 M0
Stage III	T1 N1 M0
	T2 N1 M0
	T3 N0 M0
	T3 N1 M0
	T3a N0 M0
	T3a N1 M0
	T3b N0 M0
	T3b N1 M0
	T3c N0 M0
	T3c N1 M0
Stage IV	T4 N0 M0
	T4 N1 M0
	Any T N2 M0
	Any T Any N M1

Source: From Ref. 43, with permission.

absence of prior nephrectomy (36). Interferon and IL-2 are two traditional agents, with response rates of 10%–15%. In 2007, the standard of care for metastatic renal cell carcinoma changed with the introduction of sunitinib (Sutent) (37) as first-line therapy, demonstrating approximately 6-month prolongation of progression-free survival; and sorafenib (Nexavar) (38) showing three-month prolongation of progression-free survival in the second-line setting. Sunitinib and sorafenib are oral tyrosine kinase inhibitors designed to target the vascular endothelial growth factor VEGF pathway, which is activated in renal cell carcinoma due to loss of the VHL tumor suppressor gene (39).

PENILE CANCER

Carcinoma of the penis comprises less than 1% of all malignancies in men. Predisposing factors include the presence of foreskin and HPV exposure. The presenting lesion is usually painless. Squamous cell carcinoma is the most common histology. Penile conservation surgical techniques such as laser, Mohs surgery, and partial penectomy are used when feasible (40). Brachytherapy and external beam radiotherapy are alternatives to surgery for localized disease. Several chemotherapy agents are active for metastatic disease (41). This disease is most responsive to cisplatin. However, recurrent surgical resections are needed to debulk disease in regional lymph nodes.

References

1. American Cancer Society. *Cancer Facts and Figures*. Atlanta, GA: American Cancer Society; 2007.
2. Hsing AW, Tsao L, Devesa SS. International trends and patterns of prostate cancer incidence and mortality. *Int J Cancer*. 2000;85:60–67.
3. Parkin DM, Bray F, Ferlay J, Pisani P. Global cancer statistics, 2002. *CA Cancer J Clin*. 2005;55:74–108.
4. Giovannucci E, Platz EA. Epidemiology of prostate cancer. In: Vogelzang NJ, Scardino pT, Shipley WU, Debruyne FMJ, Linehan WM, eds. *Comprehensive Textbook of Genitourinary Oncology*. Philadelphia: Lippincott Williams and Wilkins; 2006:9.
5. Calle EE, Rodriguez C, Walker-Thurmond K, Thun MJ. Overweight, obesity, and mortality from cancer in a prospectively studied cohort of U.S. adults. *N Engl J Med*. 2003;348:1625–1638.
6. American Urological Association. Prostate-specific antigen (PSA) best practice policy. *Oncology*. 2000;14:267–272, 277–278, 280 passim.
7. Harris R, Lohr KN. Screening for prostate cancer: an update of the evidence for the U.S. Preventive Services Task Force. *Ann Intern Med*. 2002;137:917–929.
8. Smith RA, Cokkinides V, Eyre HJ. Cancer screening in the United States, 2007: a review of current guidelines, practices, and prospects. *CA Cancer J Clin*. 2007;57:90–104.
9. Oesterling JE. Age-specific reference ranges for serum PSA. *N Engl J Med*. 1996;335:345–346.
10. Gleason DF, Mellinger GT, Veterans Administration Cooperative Urological Research Group. Prediction of prognosis for prostatic adenocarcinoma by combined histological grading and clinical staging. 1974. *J Urol*. 2002;167:953–958; discussion 959.
11. Hricak H, Choyke PL, Eberhardt SC, Leibel SA, Scardino PT. Imaging prostate cancer: a multidisciplinary perspective. *Radiology*. 2007;243:28–53.
12. Thomas CT, Bradshaw PT, Pollock BH, et al. Indium-111-capromab pendetide radioimmunoscintigraphy and prognosis for durable biochemical response to salvage radiation therapy in men after failed prostatectomy. *J Clin Oncol*. 2003;21:1715–1721.
13. Sakr WA, Grignon DJ, Haas GP, Heilbrun LK, Pontes JE, Crissman JD. Age and racial distribution of prostatic intraepithelial neoplasia. *Eur Urol*. 1996;30:138–144.
14. Scher HI, Heller G. Clinical states in prostate cancer: toward a dynamic model of disease progression. *Urology*. 2000;55:323–327.
15. Messing EM, Manola J, Yao J, et al. Immediate versus deferred androgen deprivation treatment in patients with node-positive prostate cancer after radical prostatectomy and pelvic lymphadenectomy. *Lancet Oncol*. 2006;7:472–479.
16. Loblaw DA, Virgo KS, Nam R, et al. Initial hormonal management of androgen-sensitive metastatic, recurrent, or progressive prostate cancer: 2006 update of an American Society of Clinical Oncology Practice Guideline. *J Clin Oncol*. 2007;22(14):2927–2941.
17. Shipley WU, Scardino PT, Kaufman DS, Kattan MW. Treatment of early stage prostate cancer. In: Vogelzang NJ, Scardino pT, Shipley WU, Debruyne FMJ, Linehan WM, eds. *Comprehensive Textbook of Genitourinary Oncology*. Philadelphia: Lippincott Williams and Wilkins; 2006:153.
18. Talcott JA, Manola J, Clark JA, et al. Time course and predictors of symptoms after primary prostate cancer therapy. *J Clin Oncol*. 2003;21:3979–3986.
19. Miller DC, Sanda MG, Dunn RL, et al. Long-term outcomes among localized prostate cancer survivors: health-related quality-of-life changes after radical prostatectomy, external radiation, and brachytherapy. *J Clin Oncol*. 2005;23:2772–2780.
20. American Society for Therapeutic Radiology and Oncology. Consensus statement: guidelines for PSA following radiation

therapy. American Society for Therapeutic Radiology and Oncology Consensus Panel. *Int J Radiat Oncol Biol Phys.* 1997;37:1035–1041.

21. Slovin SF, Wilton AS, Heller G, Scher HI. Time to detectable metastatic disease in patients with rising prostate-specific antigen values following surgery or radiation therapy. *Clin Cancer Res.* 2005;11:8669–8673.

22. D'Amico AV. Management of rising PSA following surgery or radiation therapy. In: Vogelzang NJ, Scardino pT, Shipley WU, Debruyne FMJ, Linehan WM, eds. *Comprehensive Textbook of Genitourinary Oncology.* Philadelphia: Lippincott Williams and Wilkins; 2006:285.

23. Kelly WK, Scher HI. Prostate specific antigen decline after antiandrogen withdrawal: the flutamide withdrawal syndrome. *J Urol.* 1993;149:607–609.

24. Tannock IF, Osoba D, Stockler MR, et al. Chemotherapy with mitoxantrone plus prednisone or prednisone alone for symptomatic hormone-resistant prostate cancer: a Canadian randomized trial with palliative end points. *J Clin Oncol.* 1996;14:1756–1764.

25. Kantoff PW, Halabi S, Conaway M, et al. Hydrocortisone with or without mitoxantrone in men with hormone-refractory prostate cancer: results of the cancer and leukemia group B 9182 study. *J Clin Oncol.* 1999;17:2506–2513.

26. Stubblefield MD, Slovin S, MacGregor-Cortelli B, et al. An electrodiagnostic evaluation of the effect of pre-existing peripheral nervous system disorders in patients treated with the novel proteasome inhibitor bortezomib. *Clin Oncol (R Coll Radiol).* 2006;18:410–418.

27. Tannock IF, de Wit R, Berry WR, et al. Docetaxel plus prednisone or mitoxantrone plus prednisone for advanced prostate cancer. *N Engl J Med.* 2004;351:1502–1012.

28. Petrylak DP, Tangen CM, Hussain MH, et al. Docetaxel and estramustine compared with mitoxantrone and prednisone for advanced refractory prostate cancer. *N Engl J Med.* 2004;351:1513–1520.

29. Black PC, Brown GA, Dinney CP. Molecular markers of urothelial cancer and their use in the monitoring of superficial urothelial cancer. *J Clin Oncol.* 2006;24:5528–5535.

30. Grossman HB, Natale RB, Tangen CM, et al. Neoadjuvant chemotherapy plus cystectomy compared with cystectomy alone for locally advanced bladder cancer. *N Engl J Med.* 2003;349:859–866.

31. Herr HW, Donat SM. Role of radical cystectomy in patients with advanced bladder cancer. In: Vogelzang NJ, Scardino pT, Shipley WU, Debruyne FMJ, Linehan WM, eds. *Comprehensive Textbook of Genitourinary Oncology.* Philadelphia: Lippincott Williams and Wilkins; 2006:467.

32. Galsky M, Bajorin D. Chemotherapy for metastatic bladder, alone or in combination with other treatment. In: Vogelzang NJ, Scardino pT, Shipley WU, Debruyne FMJ, Linehan WM, eds. *Comprehensive Textbook of Genitourinary Oncology.* Philadelphia: Lippincott Williams and Wilkins; 2006:533.

33. International Germ Cell Cancer Collaborative Group. International Germ Cell Consensus Classification: a prognostic factor-based staging system for metastatic germ cell cancers. International Germ Cell Cancer Collaborative Group. *J Clin Oncol.* 1997;15:594–603.

34. Carver BS, Sheinfeld J. Germ cell tumors of the testis. *Ann Surg Oncol.* 2005;12:871–880.

35. Gilligan TD. Chronic toxicity from chemotherapy for disseminated testicular cancer. In: Vogelzang NJ, Scardino pT, Shipley WU, Debruyne FMJ, Linehan WM, eds. *Comprehensive Textbook of Genitourinary Oncology.* Philadelphia: Lippincott Williams and Wilkins; 2006:330.

36. Motzer RJ, Mazumdar M, Bacik J, Berg W, Amsterdam A, Ferrara J. Survival and prognostic stratification of 670 patients with advanced renal cell carcinoma. *J Clin Oncol.* 1999;17:2530–2540.

37. Motzer RJ, Hutson TE, Tomczak P, et al. Sunitinib versus interferon alfa in metastatic renal-cell carcinoma. *N Engl J Med.* 2007;356:115–124.

38. Escudier B, Eisen T, Stadler WM, et al. Sorafenib in advanced clear-cell renal-cell carcinoma. *N Engl J Med.* 2007;356:125–134.

39. Brugarolas J. Renal-cell carcinoma—molecular pathways and therapies. *N Engl J Med.* 2007;356:185–187.

40. Russo P, Horenblas S. Surgical management of penile cancer. In: Vogelzang NJ, Scardino pT, Shipley WU, Debruyne FMJ, Linehan WM, eds. *Comprehensive Textbook of Genitourinary Oncology.* Philadelphia: Lippincott Williams and Wilkins; 2006:809.

41. Pizzocaro G, Tan WW, Drieger R. Chemotherapy for penile cancer. In: Vogelzang NJ, Scardino pT, Shipley WU, Debruyne FMJ, Linehan WM, eds. *Comprehensive Textbook of Genitourinary Oncology.* Philadelphia: Lippincott Williams and Wilkins; 2006:827.

42. Tannenbaum MP. Histologic grading of prostate adenocarcinoma. In: Tannenbaum, M. (editor). *Urologic Pathology: The Prostate.* Philadelphia: Lea & Febiger; 1977:181.

43. Greene FL, American Joint Committee on Cancer. *AJCC Cancer Staging Atlas.* New York, NY: Springer; 2006.

44. Akakura K, Suzuki H, Ichikawa T, et al. A randomized trial comparing radical prostatectomy plus endocrine therapy versus external beam radiotherapy plus endocrine therapy for locally advanced prostate cancer: results at median follow-up of 102 months. *Jpn J Clin Oncol.* 2006;36:789–793.

45. Loblaw DA, Mendelson DS, Talcott JA, et al. American Society of Clinical Oncology recommendations for the initial hormonal management of androgen-sensitive metastatic, recurrent, or progressive prostate cancer. *J Clin Oncol.* 2004;22:2927–2941.

46. McLeod DG, Iversen P, See WA, et al. Bicalutamide 150 mg plus standard care vs standard care alone for early prostate cancer. *BJU Int.* 2006;97:247–254.

47. Beekman K, Tilley WD, Buchanan G, Scher HI. Beyond first-line hormones: options for treatment of castration-resistant disease. In: Vogelzang NJ, Scardino pT, Shipley WU, Debruyne FMJ, Linehan WM, eds. *Comprehensive Textbook of Genitourinary Oncology.* Philadelphia: Lippincott Williams and Wilkins; 2006:330.

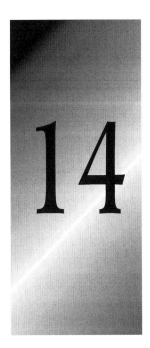

Evaluation and Treatment of Lung and Bronchus Cancer

Jorge E. Gomez

Approximately 213,380 cases of lung cancer were reported in 2007, accompanied by an estimated 160,390 deaths from the disease (1). The three other most common cancers, prostate, breast, and colon, were estimated at 511,740 cases, with 120,140 deaths. Lung cancer is the second most common cancer in men and women but is the leading cause of cancer mortality in both, surpassing prostate cancer in men and breast cancer in women. These statistics serve to emphasize the aggressive nature of lung cancer and the importance of efforts to both treat and prevent it. Although lung cancer incidence and death rates have been decreasing slightly in men, they have been increasing in women, likely related to increasing tobacco consumption.

EPIDEMIOLOGY

The majority of lung cancers are related to the consumption of tobacco products. Published studies have shown the association between smoking and the development of lung cancer. Smoking has also been strongly associated with an increased risk of death from lung cancer, which increases as the amount of tobacco consumption increases (2–4). However, approximately 15% of all lung cancers occur in nonsmokers. Asbestos and radon exposure has also been linked to the development of lung cancer (5,6), although their absolute contribution is difficult to calculate. Asbestos is a fibrous mineral used in many products including insulation, construc-

tion pipes, ceiling tiles, and other construction elements until the 1980s. Radon is a gas formed by the decay of radium that is naturally present in the environment, but can accumulate in homes. A meta-analysis published in 2004 showed a statistically significant increase in the risk of lung cancer with increased concentrations of radon (7). Although the major cause of lung cancer is likely environmental, some studies have suggested an inherited susceptibility to lung cancer. Specific genetic abnormalities have not been identified.

Lung cancer is a disease of the elderly and middle aged, with a median age at presentation of 70 (8). The incidence of lung cancer in women, which had traditionally been low, has been rapidly approaching the numbers seen in men. Approximately 46% of the estimated 213,380 lung cancers in 2007 occurred in women, along with 44% of the estimated deaths from this disease (1).

PATHOLOGY

Lung carcinoma is a pathologically heterogeneous tumor. The most important distinction is between small cell carcinoma and non-small cell carcinoma. Small cell carcinoma will be discussed later in this chapter. The World Health Organization (WHO) classification of lung tumors divides non-small cell lung cancer into different subtypes (Table 14.1) (9). The most common in order of incidence are adenocarcinoma, squamous cell

---

KEY POINTS

■ Lung cancer is the second most common cancer in men and women, but is the leading cause of cancer mortality in both, surpassing prostate cancer in men and breast cancer in women.

■ Smoking has been strongly associated with an increased risk of death from lung cancer, which increases as the amount of tobacco consumption increases.

■ Lung carcinoma is a pathologically heterogeneous tumor. The most important distinction is between small cell carcinoma and non-small cell carcinoma.

■ The most common non-small cell lung carcinomas, in order of incidence, are adenocarcinoma, squamous-cell carcinoma, and large-cell carcinoma.

■ Lung cancer is usually diagnosed through a workup initiated because of one of the multiple symptoms caused by the disease.

■ Treatment for early stage disease usually involves one or more modalities of treatment which include surgery, chemotherapy, and radiation therapy. Patients with advanced disease are treated with chemotherapy while other modalities are used for palliation of specific symptoms.

■ Small cell lung cancer is almost exclusively a disease of smokers and a diagnosis of small cell lung cancer in a nonsmoker should raise significant doubts.

■ As with non-small cell lung cancer, the treatment of small cell lung cancer depends on multiple modalities, mainly chemotherapy and radiation therapy. Surgery plays a minor role in this disease.

---

carcinoma, and large cell carcinoma. There are subtle clinical differences between these subtypes, but there is no clear evidence that tumor histology is an important prognostic variable in non-small cell lung cancer. Adenocarcinoma is the most common, making up approximately 30%–40% of lung cancers. It is more likely to be located in the periphery of the lung and to be associated with fibrous scarring. Squamous cell carcinoma tends to be centrally located, cavitates more commonly, and is more likely to be associated with hypercalcemia than most other lung cancers. Bronchoalveolar carcinoma is a subtype of adenocarcinoma characterized by slow growth and long periods of stable disease. (Fig. 14.1) Finding a mix of several of these histologies in a tumor sample is not uncommon.

SCREENING

Lung cancer is only curable in its early stages. Unfortunately, the majority of patients diagnosed with lung cancer have advanced disease that is incurable. Although there have been large strides in prevention of lung cancer by smoking cessation, smoking rates remain high in the United States and throughout the world. Therefore, early detection of lung cancer is important in subjects who are at high risk.

Three large, randomized controlled trials performed in the United States during the 1970s and 1980s were unable to prove a decrease in lung cancer mortality with chest x-ray and sputum cytology screening for lung cancer. These studies were, however, able to show a significant increase in the early detection of lung cancer lesions (10–12).

TABLE 14.1

1999 WHO Classification of Invasive Malignant Epithelial Lung Tumors

Squamous cell carcinoma
    Variants: papillary, clear cell, small cell, basaloid
Small cell carcinoma
    Variant: combined small cell carcinoma
Adenocarcinoma
    Acinar
    Papillary
Bronchioloalveolar carcinoma
    Nonmucinous (Clara cell/type II pneumocyte type)
    Mucinous (Goblet cell type)
    Mixed mucinous and nonmucinous (Clara cell/type II pneumocyte/goblet cell type) or indeterminate
    Solid adenocarcinoma with mucin formation
    Mixed
    Variants: well-differentiated fetal adenocarcinoma, mucinous ("colloid"), mucinous cystadenocarcinoma, signet ring, clear cell
Large cell carcinoma
    Variants: large cell neuroendocrine carcinoma, combined large cell neuroendocrine carcinoma, basaloid carcinoma, lymphoepithelioma-like carcinoma, clear cell carcinoma, large cell carcinoma with rhaboid phenotype
Adenosquamous carcinoma
Carcinomas with pleomorphic, sarcomatoid, or sarcomatous elements
    Carcinomas with spindle and/or giant cells
    Pleomorphic carcinoma
    Spindle cell carcinoma

Continued

TABLE 14.1
1999 WHO Classification of Invasive Malignant Epithelial Lung Tumors, Continued

Giant cell carcinoma
Carcinosarcoma
Blastoma (Pulmonary blastoma)
Carcinoid tumor
   Typical carcinoid
   Atypical carcinoid
Carcinomas of salivary gland type
   Mucoepidermoid carcinoma
   Adenoid cystic carcinoma
   Others
Unclassified carcinoma

Source: From Ref. 9.

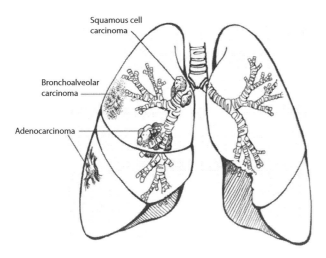

FIGURE 14.1

Illustration depicting several types of non-small cell lung carcinoma. Adenocarcinoma tends to be located in the periphery and associated with fibrous scarring; squamous-cell carcinoma is usually located centrally and may be associated with cavitation and with bronchoalveolar carcinoma, a subtype of adenocarcinoma that is often characterized by slow growth and potentially long periods of stable disease.

More recently, low-dose spiral CT has been shown to improve early detection of small lung cancer lesions over screening chest x-ray (13,14). Henschke at al. screened 1,000 subjects, aged 60 years or older and with at least 10 pack-years of cigarette smoking, with low-dose CT. Noncalcified pulmonary nodules were found in 233 subjects; of the 27 subjects found to have lung cancer, 26 had resectable lesions. The International Early Lung Cancer Action Program Investigators screened 31,567 asymptomatic persons at risk

for lung cancer with low-dose CT. Of the 484 lung cancers that were diagnosed, 85% were clinical stage I. High risk for lung cancer was defined as having a history of cigarette smoking, occupational exposure (asbestos, beryllium, uranium, or radon), or exposure to secondhand smoke. It is clear that screening with CT for lung cancer in individuals at high risk can diagnose early stage, curable lung cancers. However, there is concern that this screening may also be associated with finding noncancerous lesions and may lead to additional testing, which can be both costly and invasive. Although no improvement in the overall survival from lung cancer has been found to date, it is important to continue efforts to improve early detection and treatment in the context of clinical trials.

PREVENTION

While the cause of most human cancers is not clearly understood, it is well recognized that exposure to tobacco smoke is the major cause of lung cancer. Although not all lung cancer is related to tobacco consumption, approximately 85% of lung cancer patients have had significant exposure. The risk of lung cancer decreases in subjects who have stopped smoking when compared to current smokers (15), although this risk never returns to the levels of an individual who has never smoked. Therefore, the most important preventive measure for non-small cell lung cancer is never consuming tobacco products. In a close second place is smoking cessation for individuals who already smoke. This modifiable behavioral factor should be where the greatest preventive efforts should be made by government and nongovernment health institutions.

Multiple large clinical trials have been performed with different agents in an attempt to prevent lung cancer. Approximately 70,000 people have participated in chemoprevention trials with beta carotene. Two of these large trials suggested an increased risk of lung cancer in patients receiving beta carotene (16,17). Multiple trials of retinoids in patients who have had non-small cell lung cancer have not shown improvement in recurrences or survival.

DIAGNOSIS

Lung cancer is usually diagnosed through a workup initiated because of one of the multiple symptoms caused by the disease. A significant number of patients, however, are diagnosed incidentally through chest x-rays performed in a routine health evaluation or as part of an evaluation for another health issue. Symptoms of lung cancer are related to the location of the disease.

Symptoms of local disease are as follows:

Dyspnea and cough can be related to lung collapse due to obstructing lesions or pericardial or pleural effusion.

Hemoptysis is related to bleeding from bronchial lesions.

Hoarseness can be caused by recurrent laryngeal nerve involvement causing vocal cord paralysis.

Pain can be caused by involvement of pleura or chest wall.

Symptoms of superior vena cava syndrome are caused by compression by tumor or lymph nodes.

Symptoms of metastatic disease include the following:

Brain metastases can produce headaches, nausea, vomiting, confusion, seizures, and focal neurologic symptoms.

Bone metastases can produce pain or fractures.

Paraneoplastic syndromes can be indicated as follows:

Hypercalcemia can cause confusion, nausea, and vomiting.

Pulmonary hypertrophic osteoarthropathy causes pain and bone deformity. Clotting abnormalities are not uncommon, and can cause deep venous thromboses and pulmonary emboli.

The standard workup for non-small cell lung cancer may include the following studies:

1. Bronchoscopy may help with the initial diagnosis of lung cancer by providing easy access to tissue and can assist in adequately staging patients with lung cancer.
2. Fine needle aspiration biopsy of lung lesions can easily diagnose most of lung cancers.
3. CT scan of the chest, including adrenal glands, with intravenous contrast can help determine stage and can serve as a baseline for the evaluation of response to treatment.
4. Radiographic imaging of the brain in patients with either early or locally advanced disease can help identify patients who have asymptomatic metastatic disease. In patients with advanced disease who have neurologic symptoms it can help assess the extent of disease and plan treatment.
5. PET scan is essential for staging of early disease and is useful for evaluating sites of metastatic disease.

6. Bone scan is useful for detecting metastatic disease in patients with bone symptoms or elevated alkaline phosphatase.
7. Pulmonary function tests can help assess the adequacy of postoperative pulmonary function in patients who are surgical candidates.
8. Mediastinoscopy—the direct evaluation of the mediastinum—is important to adequately confirm or exclude mediastinal lymph node involvement.

PARANEOPLASTIC SYNDROMES

Paraneoplastic syndromes are a combination of symptoms produced by substances formed by the tumor or produced by the body in response to the tumor. In non-small cell lung cancer the most common paraneoplastic syndromes are:

Hypercalcemia. Severe hypercalcemia in non-small cell lung cancer is usually due to the production of a parathyroid hormone related peptide (PTH rP). This protein binds to the same receptors as parathyroid hormone (PTH) and increases bone resorption of calcium and reabsorption of calcium in the kidney. This syndrome can be treated with intravenous hydration, diuretics, and bisphosphonates, and is usually an indicator of poor prognosis. Hypercalcemia can also be caused by metastatic disease to the bone.

Hypertrophic pulmonary osteoarthropathy. This syndrome is more common in adenocarcinoma and is characterized by abnormal proliferation of bone tissue at the distal extremities. This can take the form of mild arthralgias, or a more severe form that presents with swelling and pain of the bones of the extremities caused by proliferative periostitis.

Thrombotic phenomenon. Cancer has been associated multiple clotting abnormalities, including migratory superficial thrombophlebitis, deep venous thrombosis and pulmonary embolism, nonbacterial thrombotic endocarditis, and disseminated intravascular coagulation (18,19). The causes of these thrombotic events are multifactorial and are related both to the biology of the tumor and the prothrombotic properties of chemotherapeutic agents. Although there are no large randomized clinical trials to support this management, patients with active lung cancer who have a first episode venous or arterial thromboembolism should most likely be treated with anticoagulants for the remainder of their lives.

STAGING

As in most other cancers, stages are among the most important prognostic factors in non-small cell cancer. Stage depends on several important factors, such as primary tumor size and characteristics (T), the presence or absence of lymph nodes (N), and the presence or absence of metastatic disease (M). This system, known as TNM, was developed by The International Staging System for NSCLC and is the most commonly used in the United States (Tables 14.2 and 14.3). Clinical staging is performed by means of the standard radiologic imaging performed during the diagnosis. Pathologic confirmation of enlarged mediastinal lymph nodes by mediastinoscopy is critical in planning treatment in early-stage non-small cell lung cancer.

TABLE 14.2
Staging of Non-Small Cell Lung Cancer

Staging
As in most other cancers, stage is one of the most important prognostic factors in non-small cell lung cancer. The TNM staging system of The International Staging System for NSCLC is the most commonly used in the United States. Stage depends on several important factors such as primary tumor size and characteristics (T), the presence or absence of lymph nodes (N), and the presence or absence of metastatic disease (M)

Tumor (T)
TX Primary tumor cannot be assessed, or tumor proven by the presence of malignant cells in sputum or bronchial washings but not visualized by imaging or bronchoscopy
T0 No evidence of primary tumor
Tis Carcinoma *in situ*
T1 Tumor 3 cm or less in greatest dimension, surrounded by lung or visceral pleura, without bronchoscopic evidence of invasion more proximal than the lobar bronchus
T2 Tumor with any of the following features of size or extent: More than 3 cm in greatest dimension; Involves main bronchus, 2 cm or more distal to the carina; Invades the visceral pleura; associated with atelectasis or obstructive pneumonitis that extends to the hilar region but does not involve the entire lung
T3 Tumor of any size that directly invades any of the following: chest wall (including superior sulcus tumors), diaphragm, mediastinal pleura, parietal pericardium; or tumor in the main bronchus, 2 cm distal to the carina, but without involvement of the carina; or associated atelectasis or obstructive pneumonitis of the entire lung
T4 Tumor of any size that invades any of the following: mediastinum, heart, great vessels, trachea, esophagus, vertebral body, carina; or tumor with a malignant pleural or pericardial effusion, or with satellite tumor nodule(s) within the ipsilateral primary-tumor lobe of the lung

Lymph Nodes (N)
NX Regional lymph nodes cannot be assessed
N0 No regional lymph node metastasis
N2 Metastasis to ipsilateral mediastinal and/or subcarinal lymph node(s)
N3 Metastasis to contralateral mediastinal, contralateral hilar, ipsilateral or contralateral scalene, or supraclavicular lymph node(s)

Metastasis (M)
MX Presence of distant metastasis cannot be assessed
M0 No distant metastasis
M1 Distant metastasis present
Stage Ia: a T1 lesion
Stage Ib: a T2 lesion
Stage IIa: a T1 lesion with N1 lymph nodes
Stage IIb: a T2 or T3 lesion with N1 lymph nodes
Stage IIIa: a T1-T3 lesion with N2 lymph nodes
Stage IIIb: any T lesion with N3 lymph nodes, or a T4 lesion
Stage IV: tumors with any metastatic disease

Source: Adapted from AJCC Cancer Staging Manual, 6th edition, New York, 2002.

TABLE 14.3
Stage Grouping for NSCLC

STAGE	T	N	M
Ia	T1	N0	M0
Ib	T2	N0	M0
IIa	T2	N1	M0
IIb	T2	N1	M0
	T3	N0	M0
IIIa	T3	N1	M0
	T1	N2	M0
	T2	N2	M0
	T3	N2	M0
IIIb	T4	N0	M0
	T4	N1	M0
	T4	N2	M0
	T1	N3	M0
	T2	N3	M0
	T3	N3	M0
	T4	N3	M0
IV	Any T	Any N	M1

Abbreviations: T, tumor; N, lymph nodes; M, metastasis.

Source: Adapted from: *AJCC Cancer Staging Manual*, 6th edition, New York, 2002.

TREATMENT

Non-small cell lung cancer is treated according to stage. Although the five-year overall survival for all patients diagnosed with non-small cell lung cancer is approximately 15%, the goal of treatment in early stages is to cure patients of their disease. Treatment for early stage disease usually involves one or more modalities of treatment, which include surgery, chemotherapy, and radiation therapy. Patients with advanced disease are treated with chemotherapy while other modalities are used for palliation of specific symptoms.

Stages I and II

Surgical resection is the best treatment for patients with stage I or II disease, with lobectomy producing a significantly decreased incidence of local recurrence over a limited resection (20). Although resection can be curative, many patients will recur within the first five years. Adjuvant chemotherapy has improved survival after surgery by 5%–12% in patients with stage II and III disease, and is a part of the standard treatment (21–24). Adjuvant chemotherapy is more controversial in stage I disease; one randomized trial showed improved disease-free survival but no improvement of

overall survival (25). A meta-analysis of adjuvant chemotherapy including 4,584 patients showed a 5.3% improvement in survival at five years for patients receiving adjuvant chemotherapy versus those who did not (26). The most important large randomized clinical trials of adjuvant chemotherapy have been performed with regimens containing cisplatin and either etoposide or a vinca alkaloid, with the abovementioned meta-analysis suggesting superiority of the cisplatin/vinorelbine regimen.

Stage IIIA

The standard treatment of stage IIIa non-small cell lung cancer is controversial. Accepted modalities include preoperative or neoadjuvant chemotherapy followed by surgery; neoadjuvant chemotherapy and radiation followed by surgery; or definitive chemotherapy and radiation. The main controversy is based on the poor survival—between 13% and 23% at five years (27)—of patients with ipsilateral mediastinal lymph nodes positive for cancer that are treated with surgery alone. Trials comparing neoadjuvant chemotherapy followed by surgery to surgery alone have been small, but have suggested an improved survival for patients receiving chemotherapy (28–32). A phase III randomized trial of concurrent chemotherapy and radiotherapy versus concurrent chemotherapy and radiotherapy followed by surgical resection in stage IIIA non-small cell lung cancer performed by Albain and colleagues was reported at the 2005 American Society of Clinical Oncology meeting (33). Randomized patients numbered 429, and 396 patients were eligible. The authors found an improvement in progression-free survival but no improvement in overall survival. This increase in progression-free survival is present in spite of increased mortality in patients undergoing pneumonectomy. These two approaches, chemotherapy versus chemotherapy and radiation, before surgery, are currently being compared in randomized clinical trials.

Stage IIIB

Stage IIIB non-small cell lung cancer is treated with a combination of chemotherapy and radiation. Several studies in the late 1980s and early 1990s showed improved survival for sequential chemotherapy and radiation therapy over radiation therapy alone (34–38). Subsequent trials compared sequential chemotherapy and radiation to concurrent chemotherapy and radiation, showing an improvement in survival for the concurrent treatment arms (39,40). The five-year overall survival for patients who receive concurrent treatment is approximately 15%, with a median survival of 16–17 months. The chemotherapy used in the multimodality treatment of stage IIIb in these clinical trials was a combination of cisplatin and either etoposide or a vinca alkaloid. The advantage of this chemotherapy regimen over others is the ability to deliver full doses of chemotherapy during concurrent treatment. Since the major cause of death in these patients is systemic recurrence of their cancer, systemic treatment with effective chemotherapy is extremely important.

Stage IV

The mainstay of treatment in stage IV disease is chemotherapy. Multiple trials that have compared chemotherapy to best supportive care have shown an improvement in survival and quality of life in patients receiving chemotherapy. The overall survival difference is approximately 1.5 months (41). Standard chemotherapy regimens are composed of platinum-based doublets. A randomized trial of four platinum based doublets (cisplatin and gemcitabine, cisplatin and docetaxel, cisplatin and paclitaxel, or carboplatin and paclitaxel) showed no improvement in survival for any one regimen (42). The response rate to chemotherapy is approximately 17%–20% and the median survival for patients receiving chemotherapy is approximately nine months. Two recent trials have shown an improvement in survival by the addition of bevacizumab to either paclitaxel/carboplatin or gemcitabine/cisplatin (43,44). Second-line chemotherapies like docetaxel, erlotinib (Tarceva), and pemetrexed (Alimta) can also improve survival and/or quality of life. Erlotinib is an EGFR tyrosine kinase inhibitor that has recently been approved for the second line treatment of non-small cell lung cancer. There is strong evidence suggesting that patients who have specific mutations in EGFR have a significantly higher response rate to EGFR tyrosine kinase inhibitors (45).

Radiation therapy plays an important palliative role in stage IV disease by alleviating symptoms when treating brain metastases or leptomeningeal involvement, painful bone metastases, obstructive bronchial lesions, and superior vena cava syndrome.

Surgery can play a role in stage IV disease. There are multiple anecdotal reports of patients enjoying long-term survival after resection of single metastatic lesions in the brain, adrenals, lung, and other areas.

SPECIAL CLINICAL SCENARIOS

Superior Sulcus Tumors

In the 1920s and 1930s, Pancoast described lung tumors in the apex of the lungs. These tumors are important because of their significant potential for local extension and invasion of vertebral bodies, brachial plexus, the sympathetic chain, and ribs. The typically described presentation of Horner syndrome, shoulder pain, and upper extremity muscle atrophy is called Pancoast syndrome. Because of the difficult local control issues, the treatment of this tumor is usually a multimodality treatment that includes chemotherapy, radiation therapy, and both thoracic and spinal surgery, and usually begins with concurrent chemotherapy and radiation followed by surgical resection (46).

Malignant Pleural Effusions

The presence of a pleural effusion is a common finding a non-small cell lung cancer (Fig. 14.2). All effusions should be tested to test for the possibility of malignant effusion, which can cause significant morbidity in the form of dyspnea and rarely disappear spontaneously. The drainage of a malignant pleural effusion by thoracentesis may often alleviate symptoms of dyspnea, but this symptomatic improvement will frequently be short lived. In patients with lung cancer, a tube thoracostomy with pleurodesis may be the best procedure to prevent re-accumulation of fluid. Pleurodesis may be performed with different sclerosing agents including tetracycline, bleomycin, and talc. Thoracoscopy is a good alternative to thoracostomy, given the possibility of clearing adhesions that cause loculation.

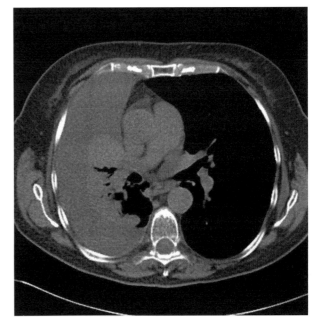

FIGURE 14.2

Computed tomography demonstrating pleural fluid surrounding a partially collapsed right lung.

Pericardial Effusion

The pericardial space is another area that can commonly accumulate fluid containing malignant cells (Fig. 14.3). Malignant cells can enter the pericardial space through the lymphatic drainage, through the arterial circulation, and by direct extension. Clinically, patients with pericardial effusion typically present with dyspnea, hypotension, tachycardia, and other signs of decreased cardiac output. The diagnosis is one that is suspected in patients with lung cancer and symptoms of shock. Most large pericardial effusions are readily visualized on CT scans of the chest; however, echocardiography is more specific and sensitive. Although pericardiocentesis can quickly relieve symptoms of shock and restore adequate circulation, fluid will quickly re-accumulate in patients with lung cancer. Open pericardiotomy can allow access to the pericardial sac for immediate drainage and placement of the drainage catheter. Sclerosis of the pericardial space can be performed with doxycycline, bleomycin, or thiotepa.

Superior Vena Cava Syndrome

Obstruction of the superior vena cava is a known complication of both small cell and non-small cell lung cancer (Fig. 14.4). In this disease, it is typically caused by compression or invasion of the superior vena cava by a right-sided tumor. The clinical presentation depends upon the length of evolution of the process. When there is an acute obstruction of the superior vena cava, patients present with facial, neck, and upper extremity swelling, dyspnea, orthopnea, and facial erythema. In a slow obstruction, symptoms of acute swelling are less apparent, and the symptoms of venous hypertension causing distention of collateral circulation are visible, in the form of dilated and prominent cutaneous veins. Superior vena cava syndrome can be adequately diagnosed in lung cancer through CT scan or MRI, although contrast venography is more accurate in identifying collateral circulation. In lung cancer, the treatment of severe vena cava syndrome is usually conservative, with radiation therapy being the best treatment for acute disease. Slowly progressive obstruction may sometimes respond to chemotherapy. In patients with complete obstruction who remain symptomatic after radiation therapy, stenting of the superior vena cava with a metallic stent can restore patency and adequately relieve obstructive symptoms (47).

SMALL CELL LUNG CANCER

Epidemiology

Small cell lung cancer is almost exclusively a disease of smokers, and a diagnosis of small cell lung cancer in a nonsmoker should raise significant doubts. This fact

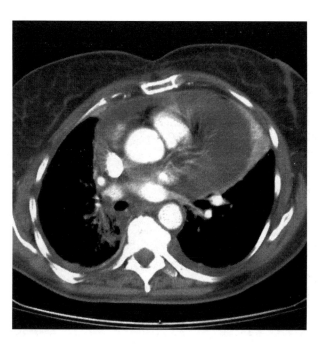

FIGURE 14.3

Computed tomography demonstrating fluid significantly dilating the pericardial sack.

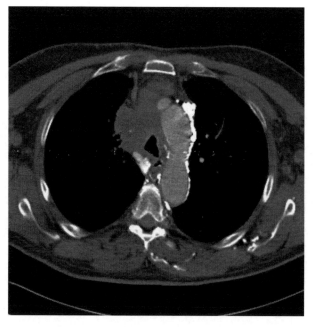

FIGURE 14.4

Computed tomography demonstrating tumor surrounding the superior vena cava. A pinpoint amount of contrast can be seen in the center of the collapsed vein.

may explain why the proportional incidence of small cell lung cancer in the United States has decreased over time. The Surveillance, Epidemiology, and End Results (SEER) database shows a decrease in the proportion of small cell lung cancer from 17% of all lung cancers in 1986 to 13% in 2002, parallel to a decrease in tobacco consumption in men. At the same time, the percentage of small cell lung cancer in women has increased from 28% in 1973 to 50% in 2002 (48).

Staging

The TNM staging system is generally not used for small cell lung cancer. Patients with small cell lung cancer are staged according to a classification developed by the Veterans Administration Lung Cancer Study Group in the 1970s. This classification divides patients into limited- or extensive-stage disease. Recent changes to this classification have improved its prognostic value.

Limited disease is defined as disease that is confined to one hemithorax with or without ipsilateral or contralateral mediastinal or supraclavicular lymph node metastases with or without ipsilateral pleural effusions independent of cytology. This has now been modified to exclude patients with a pleural or pericardial effusion, since these patients are unlikely to be cured with radiation therapy. Another modification that stresses the importance of radiation therapy in limited stage disease is that the tumor must be encompassed by a reasonable or tolerable radiation port.

Extensive disease is defined as any disease at sites beyond those defined in limited disease. The staging procedures and tests for small cell lung cancer are the same as those for non-small cell lung cancer. In patients with no radiographic signs of metastatic disease, but significant abnormalities in peripheral blood counts or elevation in alkaline phosphatase, a bone marrow biopsy may reveal metastases.

PROGNOSTIC FACTORS

Many groups have studied prognostic factors for small cell lung cancer. The most important prognostic factors found are performance status, stage of disease, age, and gender. The Southwest Oncology Group (SWOG) published a database of 2,580 patients with small cell lung cancer in 1990 showing that patients with good performance status, female sex, aged younger than 70 years, white race, and normal lactate dehydrogenase (LDH) were favorable independent predictors of outcome (49). In patients with limited disease, they found that high LDH, the presence of pleural effusion, and advanced age were important negative prognostic factors.

PARANEOPLASTIC SYNDROMES

Although paraneoplastic syndromes occur in non-small cell lung cancer, they are found more commonly in small cell lung cancer. Most of these syndromes are mediated by autoantibodies or by production of peptide hormones, allowing a classification into either endocrine or neurological syndromes. The most common endocrine syndrome is hyponatremia; it occurs in approximately 15% of patients, and has been linked to elevated levels of vasopressin (50) and atrial natriuretic factor in causing an SIADH like picture. Ectopic secretion of ACTH causing Cushing syndrome occurs in approximately 1%–3% of cases. Most neurological paraneoplastic syndromes are immune mediated. Multiple antibodies have been identified that are related to specific syndromes such as anti-Yo in cerebellar degeneration and anti-Hu in encephalomyelitis, sensory neuropathies, and autonomic dysfunction (51,52). The most common neurologic paraneoplastic syndrome is the Lambert–Eaton syndrome, believed to be related to antibodies against presynaptic voltage gated calcium channels, which occurs in approximately 3%–5% of small cell lung cancer patients, and causes a myasthenia syndrome.

TREATMENT

As with non-small cell lung cancer, the treatment of small cell lung cancer depends on multiple modalities, mainly chemotherapy and radiation therapy. Surgery plays a minor role in this disease.

Chemotherapy

Small cell lung cancer is an extremely chemotherapy-sensitive tumor. Response rates to standard agents are in the range of 60%–80%. The most accepted regimen in the United States is a common nation of etoposide (Eposin) and cisplatin, which has been the standard of care since the early 1990s (53). The median survival for patients with extensive disease in phase 3 trials is approximately 9–12 months. A trial by Noda showed superiority for a regimen containing irinotecan (Camptosar) and cisplatin, but subsequent trials have not shown the same results (54). Multiple high-dose chemotherapy strategies have not shown an advantage when compared to standard-dose treatments. Trials comparing etoposide and cisplatin with three drug combinations have either not shown a significant advantage, or have shown a small advantage at the cost of increased toxicity (53). The standard duration of treatment is approximately four cycles. The strategy of continuing treatment beyond four to six cycles has not been proven to be beneficial (55,56). In extensive disease, chemotherapy is given as a single modality. In limited disease it is given concurrently with radiation therapy.

Radiation Therapy

Radiation therapy as a single modality is not usually curative in small cell lung cancer. However, SCLC is highly sensitive to radiation therapy, and radiation therapy is an effective palliatives maneuver in many clinical situations, including:

Metastases causing pain
Obstructive bronchial lesions
Severe hemoptysis
Bone metastases at risk for fracture
Brain metastases

The most important use of radiation therapy in this disease is in combination with chemotherapy for limited stage disease. A meta-analysis published by Pignon et al. in 1992 showed a significant advantage in survival for patients receiving a combination of chemotherapy and radiation versus chemotherapy alone (57). Incorporating radiation therapy early in the course of chemotherapy confers a statistically significant survival advantage over incorporating radiation therapy in the latter cycles of chemotherapy (58–61). The median survival for patients with limited disease in phase III trials is 20–23 months with an overall five-year survival of approximately 20%.

Prophylactic Cranial Irradiation (PCI)

Isolated CNS metastases occur in approximately 15% of limited disease stage patients were treated with concurrent chemotherapy and radiation with curative intent. A meta-analysis published in 1999 showed a 5.4% increase in three-year survival in patients receiving PCI, as well as a 54% reduction in the risk of brain metastases (62). The PCI is delivered after completion of chemotherapy and radiation. A study presented at the American Society of Clinical Oncology meeting in 2007 showed an improvement in survival for patients with extensive disease receiving PCI after a documented response to chemotherapy compared to patients without PCI (63).

Surgery

Since small cell lung cancer is considered a systemic disease, with micrometastatic disease already present at the time of diagnosis, surgery as a single modality is not usually curative. A randomized trial studying the benefit of surgery in patients receiving both chemotherapy and radiation showed no increase in survival for patients who had a resection over patients who did not (64). Patients who are found to have small cell lung cancer at the time of surgery and have a complete resection, should receive adjuvant chemotherapy. Patients who do not have a complete resection should be treated with both chemotherapy and radiation.

References

1. Jemal A, Siegel R, Ward E, Murray T, Xu J, Thun MJ. Cancer statistics, 2007. *CA Cancer J Clin.* 2007;57(1):43–66.
2. Doll R, Peto R, Wheatley K, Gray R, Sutherland I. Mortality in relation to smoking: 40 years' observations on male British doctors. *BMJ (Clinical research ed).* 1994;309(6959):901–911.
3. Hammond EC. Smoking in relation to the death rates of one million men and women. *Natl Cancer Inst Monogr.* 1966;19:127–204.
4. McLaughlin JK, Hrubec Z, Blot WJ, Fraumeni JF, Jr. Smoking and cancer mortality among U.S. veterans: a 26-year follow-up. *Int J Cancer.* 1995;60(2):190–193.
5. Field RW, Steck DJ, Smith BJ, et al. Residential radon gas exposure and lung cancer: the Iowa Radon Lung Cancer Study. *Am J Epidemiol.* 2000;151(11):1091–1102.
6. van Loon AJ, Kant IJ, Swaen GM, Goldbohm RA, Kremer AM, van den Brandt PA. Occupational exposure to carcinogens and risk of lung cancer: results from The Netherlands cohort study. *Occup Environ Med.* 1997;54(11):817–824.
7. Darby S, Hill D, Auvinen A, et al. Radon in homes and risk of lung cancer: collaborative analysis of individual data from 13 European case-control studies. *BMJ (Clinical research ed).* 2005;330(7485):223.
8. Ries LAG MD, Krapcho M, Mariotto A, et al. SEER Cancer Statistics Review, 1975-2005, National Cancer Institute. Bethesda, MD, http://seer.cancer.gov/csr1975–2005/, based on November 2007 SEER data submission, posted to the SEER website, 2008.
9. The World Health Organization histological typing of lung tumors. *Am J Clin Pathol.* 1982;77:123–136.
10. Fontana RS, Sanderson DR, Taylor WF, et al. Early lung cancer detection: results of the initial (prevalence) radiologic and cytologic screening in the Mayo Clinic study. *Am Rev Respir Dis.* 1984;130(4):561–565.
11. Frost JK, Ball WC, Jr., Levin ML, et al. Early lung cancer detection: results of the initial (prevalence) radiologic and cytologic screening in the Johns Hopkins study. *Am Rev Respir Dis.* 1984;130(4):549–554.
12. Melamed MR. Lung cancer screening results in the National Cancer Institute New York study. *Cancer.* 2000;89(11 Suppl):2356–2362.
13. Henschke CI, McCauley DI, Yankelevitz DF, et al. Early Lung Cancer Action Project: overall design and findings from baseline screening. *Lancet.* 1999;354(9173):99–105.
14. Henschke CI, Yankelevitz DF, Libby DM, Pasmantier MW, Smith JP, Miettinen OS. Survival of patients with stage I lung cancer detected on CT screening. *N Engl J Med.* 2006;355(17):1763–1771.
15. Samet JM. Health benefits of smoking cessation. *Clin Chest Med.* 1991;12(4):669–679.
16. The effect of vitamin E and beta carotene on the incidence of lung cancer and other cancers in male smokers. The Alpha-Tocopherol, Beta Carotene Cancer Prevention Study Group. *N Engl J Med.* 1994;330(15):7.
17. Omenn GS, Goodman GE, Thornquist MD, et al. Effects of a combination of beta carotene and vitamin A on lung cancer and cardiovascular disease. *N Engl J Med.* 1996;334(18):1150–1155.

18. Blom JW, Vanderschoot JP, Oostindier MJ, Osanto S, van der Meer FJ, Rosendaal FR. Incidence of venous thrombosis in a large cohort of 66,329 cancer patients: results of a record linkage study. *J Thromb Haemost*. 2006;4(3):529–535.

19. Sack GH, Jr., Levin J, Bell WR. Trousseau's syndrome and other manifestations of chronic disseminated coagulopathy in patients with neoplasms: clinical, pathophysiologic, and therapeutic features. *Medicine*. 1977;56(1):1–37.

20. Ginsberg RJ, Rubinstein LV. Randomized trial of lobectomy versus limited resection for T1 N0 non-small cell lung cancer. Lung Cancer Study Group. *Ann Thorac Surg*. 1995;60(3):615–622; discussion 22–23.

21. Arriagada R, Bergman B, Dunant A, Le Chevalier T, Pignon JP, Vansteenkiste J. Cisplatin-based adjuvant chemotherapy in patients with completely resected non-small cell lung cancer. *N Engl J Med*. 2004;350(4):351–360.

22. Douillard J, Rosell R, Delena A, Legroumellec A, Torres F, Carpagnano F. ANITA: Phase III adjuvant vinorelbine (N) and cisplatin (P) versus observation (OBS) in completely resected (stage I-III) non-small cell lung cancer (NSCLC) patients (pts): Final results after 70-month median follow-up. On behalf of the Adjuvant Navelbine International Trialist Association. In: American Society of Clinical Oncology Annual Meeting; 2005; 2005.

23. Douillard JY, Rosell R, De Lena M, et al. Adjuvant vinorelbine plus cisplatin versus observation in patients with completely resected stage IB-IIIA non-small cell lung cancer (Adjuvant Navelbine International Trialist Association [ANITA]): a randomised controlled trial. *Lancet Oncol*. 2006;7(9):719–727.

24. Winton T, Livingston R, Johnson D, et al. Vinorelbine plus cisplatin vs. observation in resected non-small cell lung cancer. *N Engl J Med*. 2005;352(25):2589–2597.

25. Strauss Gea. Adjuvant chemotherapy in stage IB non-small cell lung cancer (NSCLC): Update of Cancer and Leukemia Group B (CALGB) protocol 9633. In: American Society of Clinical Oncology Annual Meeting; 2006.

26. Pignon JP. Lung Adjuvant Cisplatin Evaluation (LACE): a pooled analysis of five randomized clinical trials including 4,584 patients. In: American Society of Clinical Oncology Annual Meeting; 2006; Atlanta, GA; 2006.

27. Mountain CF. Revisions in the international system for staging lung cancer. *Chest*. 1997;111(6):1710–1717.

28. Depierre A, Milleron B, Moro D, Chevret D, Braun D, Quoix E. Phase III trial of neo-adjuvant chemotherapy (NCT) in resectable stage I (except T1N0), II, IIIa non-small cell lung cancer (NSCLC): the French experience. *Proc Am Soc Clin Oncol*. 1999;18:465a.

29. Depierre A, Milleron B, Moro-Sibilot D, et al. Preoperative chemotherapy followed by surgery compared with primary surgery in resectable stage I (except T1N0), II, and IIIa non-small cell lung cancer. *J Clin Oncol*. 2002;20(1):247–253.

30. Rosell R, Gomez-Codina J, Camps C, et al. A randomized trial comparing preoperative chemotherapy plus surgery with surgery alone in patients with non-small cell lung cancer. *N Engl J Med*. 1994;330(3):153–158.

31. Roth JA, Fossella F, Komaki R, et al. A randomized trial comparing perioperative chemotherapy and surgery with surgery alone in resectable stage IIIA non-small cell cancer. *J Natl Cancer Inst*. 1994;86:673–680.

32. Roth JA, Neely Atkinson E, Fossella F, et al. Long-term follow-up of patients enrolled in a randomized trial comparing perioperative chemotherapy and surgery with surgery alone in resectable stage IIIA non-small cell lung cancer. *Lung Cancer*. 1998;21:1–6.

33. Albain KS. Phase III study of concurrent chemotherapy and radiotherapy (CT/RT) vs CT/RT followed by surgical resection for stage IIIA(pN2) non-small cell lung cancer (NSCLC): outcomes update of North American Intergroup 0139 (RTOG 9309). . In: American Society of Clinical Oncology Annual Meeting; 2005; Orlando, FL; 2005.

34. Dillman R, Seagren S, Propert K, et al. A randomized trial of induction chemotherapy plus high-dose radiation versus radiation alone in stage III non-small cell lung cancer. *N Engl J Med*. 1990;323:940–945.

35. Dillman RO, Herndon J, Seagren SL, Eaton WL, Jr., Green MR.Improved survival in stage III non-small cell lung cancer: seven-year follow-up of cancer and leukemia group B (CALGB) 8433 trial [see comments]. *J Natl Cancer Inst*. 1996;88(17):1210–1215.

36. Le Chevalier T, Arriagada R, Quoix E, et al. Radiotherapy alone versus combined chemotherapy and radiotherapy in nonresectable non-small cell lung cancer: first analysis of a randomized trial in 353 patients. *J Natl Cancer Inst*. 1991;83:417–423.

37. Sause W, Kolesar P, Taylor SI, et al. Final results of phase III trial in regionally advanced unresectable non-small cell lung cancer: Radiation Therapy Oncology Group, Eastern Cooperative Oncology Group, and Southwest Oncology Group. *Chest*. 2000;117(2):358–364.

38. Sause WT, Scott C, Taylor S, et al. Radiation Therapy Oncology Group (RTOG) 88-08 and Eastern Cooperative Oncology Group (ECOG) 4588: preliminary results of a phase III trial in regionally advanced, unresectable non-small cell lung cancer. *J Natl Cancer Inst*. 1995;87(3):198–205.

39. Curran WJ, Scott C, Langer C, et al. Long term benefit is observed in a phase III comparison of sequential vs concurrent chemo-radiation for patients with unresected stage III nsclc: RTOG 9410. *Proc Am Soc Clin Oncol*. 2003;22:621.

40. Furuse K, Fukuoka M, Kawahara M, et al. Phase III study of concurrent versus sequential thoracic radiotherapy in combination with Mitomycin, Vindesine and Cisplatin in unresectbale stage III non-small cell lung cancer. *J Clin Oncol*. 1999;17:2692–2699.

41. Chemotherapy in non-small cell lung cancer: a meta-analysis using updated data on individual patients from 52 randomised clinical trials. Non-small Cell Lung Cancer Collaborative Group. *BMJ (Clinical research ed)*. 1995;311(7010):899–909.

42. Schiller JH, Harrington D, Belani CP, et al. Comparison of four chemotherapy regimens for advanced non-small cell lung cancer. *N Engl J Med*. 2002;346(2):92–98.

43. Manegold C. Randomised, double-blind multicentre phase III study of bevacizumab in combination with cisplatin and gemcitabine in chemotherapy-na 239;ve patients with advanced or recurrent non-squamous non-small cell lung cancer. In: American Society of Clinical Oncology Annual Meeting; 2007; Chicago, IL; 2007.

44. Sandler A, Gray R, Perry MC, et al. Paclitaxel-carboplatin alone or with bevacizumab for non-small cell lung cancer. *N Engl J Med*. 2006;355(24):2542–2550.

45. Paz-Ares Lea. A prospective phase II trial of erlotinib in advanced non-small cell lung cancer (NSCLC) patients (p) with mutations in the tyrosine kinase (TK) domain of the epidermal growth factor receptor (EGFR). In: American Society of Clinical Oncology Annual Meeting 2006; Chicago, IL; 2006.

46. Rusch VW, Giroux DJ, Kraut MJ, et al. Induction chemoradiation and surgical resection for non-small cell lung carcinomas of the superior sulcus: Initial results of Southwest Oncology Group Trial 9416 (Intergroup Trial 0160). *J Thorac Cardiovasc Surg*. 2001;121:472–483.

47. Nagata T, Makutani S, Uchida H, et al. Follow-up results of 71 patients undergoing metallic stent placement for the treatment of a malignant obstruction of the superior vena cava. *Cardiovasc Intervent Radiol*. 2007;30(5):959–67.

48. Govindan R, Page N, Morgensztern D, et al. Changing epidemiology of small cell lung cancer in the United States over the last 30 years: analysis of the surveillance, epidemiologic, and end results database. *J Clin Oncol*. 2006;24(28):4539–4544.

49. Albain KS, Crowley JJ, LeBlanc M, Livingston RB. Determinants of improved outcome in small cell lung cancer: an analysis of the 2,580-patient Southwest Oncology Group data base. *J Clin Oncol*. 1990;8(9):1563–1574.

50. Johnson BE, Chute JP, Rushin J, et al. A prospective study of patients with lung cancer and hyponatremia of malignancy. *Am J Respir Crit Care Med*. 1997;156(5):1669–1678.

51. Graus F, Keime-Guibert F, Rene R, et al. Anti-Hu-associated paraneoplastic encephalomyelitis: analysis of 200 patients. *Brain*. 2001;124(Pt 6):1138–1148.

52. Peterson K, Rosenblum MK, Kotanides H, Posner JB. Paraneoplastic cerebellar degeneration. I. A clinical analysis of 55 anti-Yo antibody-positive patients. *Neurology.* 1992;42(10):1931–1937.

53. Roth BJ, Johnson DH, Einhorn LH, et al. Randomized study of cyclophosphamide, doxorubicin, and vincristine versus etoposide and cisplatin versus alternation of these two regimens in extensive small cell lung cancer: a phase III trial of the Southeastern Cancer Study Group. *J Clin Oncol.* 1992;10(2):282–291.

54. Hanna N, Bunn PA, Jr., Langer C, et al. Randomized phase III trial comparing irinotecan/cisplatin with etoposide/cisplatin in patients with previously untreated extensive-stage disease small cell lung cancer. *J Clin Oncol.* 2006;24(13):2038–2043.

55. Giaccone G, Dalesio O, McVie GJ, et al. Maintenance chemotherapy in small cell lung cancer: long-term results of a randomized trial. European Organization for Research and Treatment of Cancer Lung Cancer Cooperative Group. *J Clin Oncol.* 1993;11(7):1230–1240.

56. Spiro SG, Souhami RL, Geddes DM, et al. Duration of chemotherapy in small cell lung cancer: a Cancer Research Campaign trial. *Br J Cancer.* 1989;59(4):578–583.

57. Pignon JP, Arriagada R, Ihde DC, et al. A meta-analysis of thoracic radiotherapy for small cell lung cancer. *N Engl J Med.* 1992;327(23):1618–1624.

58. De Ruysscher D, Pijls-Johannesma M, Bentzen SM, et al. Time between the first day of chemotherapy and the last day of chest radiation is the most important predictor of survival in limited-disease small cell lung cancer. *J Clin Oncol.* 2006;24(7):1057–1063.

59. De Ruysscher D, Pijls-Johannesma M, Vansteenkiste J, Kester A, Rutten I, Lambin P. Systematic review and meta-analysis of randomised, controlled trials of the timing of chest radiotherapy in patients with limited-stage, small cell lung cancer. *Ann Oncol.* 2006;17(4):543–552.

60. Fried DB, Morris DE, Poole C, et al. Systematic review evaluating the timing of thoracic radiation therapy in combined modality therapy for limited-stage small cell lung cancer. *J Clin Oncol.* 2004;22(23):4837–4845.

61. Murray N, Coy P, Pater JL, et al. Importance of timing for thoracic irradiation in the combined modality treatment of limited-stage small cell lung cancer. The National Cancer Institute of Canada Clinical Trials Group. *J Clin Oncol.* 1993;11(2):336–344.

62. Auperin A, Arriagada R, Pignon JP, et al. Prophylactic cranial irradiation for patients with small cell lung cancer in complete remission. Prophylactic Cranial Irradiation Overview Collaborative Group. *N Engl J Med.* 1999;341(7):476–484.

63. Slotman Bea. A randomized trial of prophylactic cranial irradiation (PCI) versus no PCI in extensive disease small cell lung cancer after a response to chemotherapy (EORTC 08993-22993). In: American Society of Clinical Oncology Annual Meeting; 2007; Chicago, Il; 2007.

64. Lad T, Piantadosi S, Thomas P, Payne D, Ruckdeschel J, Giaccone G. A prospective randomized trial to determine the benefit of surgical resection of residual disease following response of small cell lung cancer to combination chemotherapy. *Chest.* 1994;106(6 Suppl):320S–323S.

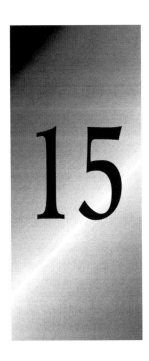

Evaluation and Treatment of Colorectal Cancer

Leonard B. Saltz
Austin G. Duffy

Approximately 150,000 people are diagnosed with colorectal cancer (CRC) annually in the United States, making it the fourth most common cancer diagnosis, behind lung, breast, and prostate (1). A number of factors have resulted in an improved, and improving, outlook for patients diagnosed with this disease, although colorectal cancer still remains the number two cause of cancer death in this country.

The major modality for management of local-regional CRC is surgical resection. With the exception of the introduction and widespread adoption of total mesorectal excision (TME) for rectal cancer—which substantially improved local control of this disease (2)—the standard surgical techniques have changed little in recent years. Laparoscopic surgery has emerged as a treatment option, but this has not altered outcome or prognosis. Therefore, we must look at other areas to uncover the causes of this improved prognosis.

The wide adoption of the use of colonoscopic screening for polyps has undoubtedly had a reductive effect on the incidence of CRC and, with the earlier diagnosis of established cancers (3), has also led to improved survival times, both spurious (as a result of lead-time bias) and real (earlier diagnosis of more curable lesions and the earlier implementation of curative adjuvant therapies). Undoubtedly the most important factor has been the advent of a greater number of active systemic chemotherapy agents. This has led not only to prolonged survival for metastatic disease, but also to some increases in the numbers of patients that are

actually cured, through the incorporation of some of these agents into the adjuvant treatment following complete surgical resection.

The improvement in systemic therapy has altered the landscape in a number of ways. Patients with stage IV (metastatic) disease are surviving for longer periods (4), often with good functionality and quality of life, at least in the initial phases of treatment. However, long-term treatment of metastatic disease does appear to be resulting in a changing pattern of treatment failure. These patients are more likely to suffer events such as bone or brain metastases, or spinal cord compression, which have heretofore been unusual occurrences in CRC. In a sense, the natural history of the disease has been altered. In addition, more patients will have been exposed to the increased toxicities of the new therapies in the adjuvant setting. These patients have a high probability of cure; therefore, both the known and unknown long-term toxicities of therapy are of enormous significance for them. In addition, the wider use of more effective but potentially more toxic therapies means that more patients will be at risk for acute hospitalizations, with all the attendant morbidities and rehabilitation issues associated with this.

The aim of this chapter is to outline the therapeutic paradigm as it currently pertains to CRC, referencing briefly the major clinical trial milestones. In previous times, a patient with CRC receiving chemotherapy had, almost by definition, a very limited life expectancy. The role of rehabilitation medicine in such a patient

KEY POINTS

- Approximately 150,000 people are diagnosed with colorectal cancer (CRC) annually in the United States, making it the fourth most common cancer diagnosis and the second leading cause of cancer death in the United States.
- The wide adoption of colonoscopic screening for polyps has had a reductive effect on the incidence of CRC and, with the earlier diagnosis of established cancers, improved survival times.
- The major modality for management of local-regional CRC is surgical resection, with the primary goal of removing the primary tumor and an adequate margin of healthy tissue along with the draining lymph nodes.
- A greater number of active systemic chemotherapy agents have led not only to prolonged survival for metastatic CRC, but also an increase in the numbers of patients that are cured.
- The postoperative management of CRC patients is dependent on two major factors—the performance status of the patient and the stage of the disease.

- The backbone of systemic therapy in this disease is 5-fluorouracil (5-FU) with two major cytotoxic additions being irinotecan and oxaliplatin.
- The addition of bevacizumab, a monoclonal antibody directed against vascular endothelial growth factor (VEGF)—an important mediator of tumor angiogenesis—to standard irinotecan-based chemotherapy improved the survival of patients by nearly five months.
- FOLFOX, the combination of oxaliplatin with the LV5FU2 (short-course infusion 5-FU with leucovorin incorporated into a 48-hour regimen given every other week) has been shown to be more effective than 5-FU therapy alone in patients with untreated metastatic colorectal cancer.
- The main toxicity of oxaliplatin, which is often dose-limiting, is neurotoxicity, which commonly manifests as a peripheral symmetrical cold sensitivity and paresthesias affecting the hands, feet, and throat.

was likely to be very minimal given the competing priorities of symptom control in the context of a terminal illness. The black/white duality of that previous era has now been replaced by a gradation of grays as CRC is increasingly viewed as a chronic illness, in which the goals of rehabilitation medicine and oncology are likely to have increasing areas of overlap.

CLINICAL OVERVIEW

Approximately 80% of patients present with localized and, therefore, potentially curable disease (5). Prior to undergoing resection, patients should have staging computed tomography (CT) imaging of the chest and abdomen, and in the pelvis (in patients with rectal cancer, those with intrapelvic primaries, and all females) to rule out metastatic disease. A preoperative serum carcinoembryonic antigen (CEA) level should be drawn, as this has prognostic value and may help dictate postoperative treatment choices. For cancers outside of the rectum, initial surgery (ie, without preoperative, or neoadjuvant, therapy) is standard practice. The main principle of surgical oncology in colorectal, as in other cancers, is to remove the primary tumor with adequate margins of healthy tissue, in association with removal of the draining lymph nodes. The overwhelming majority of patients can be expected to have a surgical resection without a permanent colostomy; irreversible colostomy procedures such as abdominal

perineal resection (APR) are reserved only for a small subset of patients with distal rectal tumors on or very close to the anal verge.

The postoperative management of patients with CRC is dependent on two major factors—the performance status of the patient and the stage of the disease. Performance status, a numeric quantitation of the patient's overall state of well-being, is most commonly quantitated according to either the Eastern Cooperative Oncology Group (ECOG) or Karnofsky scoring systems. In the postoperative patient, performance status is a fluid variable that may be affected by surgical wound healing and by complications, but may improve with time.

CRC is staged according to the American Joint Commission on Cancer (AJCC) Tumor-Node-Metastasis (TNM) system (Table 15.1), which is primarily based on the pathological findings postresection but also takes into account the surgical and radiological findings (primarily for the metastatic [M] portion of the staging). Median expected survival times correlate with pathological stage. The broad paradigm of therapy is outlined in Table 15.2.

TREATMENT OF METASTATIC DISEASE

A meta-analysis of seven trials (866 patients) demonstrated convincingly that palliative chemotherapy was associated with an improvement in overall survival (6).

TABLE 15.1
TNM Staging for CRC

Primary Tumor (T)
Carcinoma in situ; intraepithelial (within glandular basement membrane) or invasion of lamina propria (intramucosal)
Tumor invades submucosa
Tumor invades muscularis propria
Tumor invades through the muscularis propria into the subserosa, or into nonperitonealized pericolic or perirectal tissues
Tumor directly invades other organs or structures, and/or perforates visceral peritoneum
Regional Lymph Node (N)
Regional nodes cannot be assessed
No regional nodal metastases
Metastasis in 1–3 regional lymph nodes
Metastasis in 4 or more regional lymph nodes
Distant Metastasis (M)
Distant metastasis cannot be assessed
No distant metastasis
Distant metastasis

TABLE 15.2
Therapies for Gastrointestinal Cancer According to Stage

Stage I: surgery only
Stage II: surgery ± adjuvant chemotherapy (controversial)
Stage III: surgery + adjuvant chemotherapy
Stage IV: chemotherapy only (occasionally surgery if resectable oligo-metastatic disease)

The chemotherapy used in these trials would today be considered suboptimal and the authors commented that the overall quality of evidence relating to treatment toxicity, symptom control, and quality of life measurement was poor by current standards. The field has moved on from this; however, this meta-analysis represents proof of principle that active systemic therapy is superior (compared to best supportive care) in terms of providing a survival benefit in this disease.

The backbone of systemic therapy in this disease is 5-FU, a fluoropyrimidine that acts by inhibiting thymidylate synthase, a critical enzyme in DNA synthesis. This drug was first patented in 1957. For much of the 1960s through the mid-1990s, investigational energies were focused largely on the various methods of administering and/or modulating 5-FU (7). These included bolus schedules on a daily or weekly basis or short course and prolonged infusional schedules that employed the use of semipermanent venous access devices. 5-FU was also combined with putative "biomodulating" compounds, such as leucovorin (Wellcovorin) or levamisole (Ergamisol), in an attempt to increase its efficacy. It is a fair summation to say that these different schedules had somewhat different toxicity profiles, but had approximate equivalence in terms of efficacy. Infusional schedules had, if anything, a slightly superior efficacy, with less hematologic toxicity. Leucovorin, a biomodulator that enhances 5-FU cytotoxicity by interacting with the enzyme thymidylate synthase, thereby prolonging inhibition of the enzyme by 5-FU, has remained a frequent component of 5-FU-based regimens. The combination of bolus and short-course infusional 5-FU with leucovorin has been incorporated into a 48-hour regimen given every other week (the de Gramont, or LV5FU2 regimen). This regimen has formed the backbone of several modern chemotherapy schedules for this disease, to which newer, active drugs have been added as they emerge from development. Oral formulations of fluoropyrimidines have also been developed, and these have been shown to have similar efficacy to parenteral leucovorin-modulated 5-FU regimens (8).

For several decades, the median survival times remained static at approximately one year. Towards the end of 1990s, as newer drugs were incorporated into practice, median survival times began to improve. The two major cytotoxic additions were irinotecan and oxaliplatin.

Irinotecan is an inhibitor of the enzyme topoisomerase 1. After early phase studies established its efficacy as a single agent in 5-FU-refractory disease, three major trials demonstrated the superiority of irinotecan combined with 5-FU compared to 5-FU alone in the first-line metastatic setting (9–11). The main toxicities of irinotecan are diarrhea and neutropenia.

Oxaliplatin is a platinum derivative that has synergistic activity with 5-FU. The combination of oxaliplatin with the LV5FU2 regimen (given the epithet FOLFOX) has been shown to be more effective than 5-FU therapy alone in patients with untreated metastatic colorectal cancer (12). The main toxicity of oxaliplatin, which is often dose-limiting, is neurotoxicity, which most commonly manifests as a peripheral symmetrical cold sensitivity and paresthesias affecting the hands, feet, and throat.

The emergence of irinotecan and oxaliplatin has added layers of complexity to treatment decisions that were simple when 5-FU was the only therapy available. A question that rapidly emerged was: which drug is the more active, and is the combination of both drugs together more efficacious than sequential therapy? Although FOLFOX out-performed irinotecan when the irinotecan was given with bolus 5-FU (13), when irinotecan is given with the LV5FU2 method (and given the epithet FOLFIRI), the regimens appear to be equivalent in terms of efficacy in the metastatic setting (14,15).

The study by Tournigrand et al. also answers the question about whether the order in which the treatments are given matters. This trial treated patients with either FOLFOX or FOLFIRI and then allowed them to cross over to the other therapy upon progression of their disease. There was no difference in survival between the two groups. The combination of irinotecan and oxaliplatin together (IROX) as first-line therapy has not been shown to be superior, and in the Intergroup study performed inferiorly to FOLFOX (13).

While the addition of these two effective chemotherapies to the armamentarium has prolonged median survival times modestly, the outcomes for patients with metastatic colorectal cancer remain poor, with cure being a vanishingly rare phenomenon. Clearly, additional and better therapies are still needed. For this reason, the so-called "targeted" therapies, an approach derived from an understanding of tumour biology, wherein drugs are rationally designed with a specific biological purpose in mind, have been investigated in colorectal cancer. This approach has yielded some modest improvements in treatment, although the benefits have been far more modest than had been hoped for.

The first pivotal study of a biologic, or targeted, therapy in CRC was presented in 2003, when the addition of bevacizumab, a monoclonal antibody directed against vascular endothelial growth factor (VEGF)—an important mediator of tumor angiogenesis—to standard irinotecan-based chemotherapy, improved the survival of patients by nearly five months (16). This study not only represented a change in standard first-line therapy of metastatic colorectal cancer, but also represented a proof of principle for anti-VEGF therapy. The efficacy of adding bevacizumab to oxaliplatin-based therapy, oral fluoropyrimidines, and also in the second-line setting has also been proven in large randomized trials (17,18). Of note, however, the addition of bevacizumab to oxaliplatin-based therapy in front-line therapy was not associated with a significant survival advantage in a recent large study (19).

Initially it was felt that these rationally-derived therapies would be less toxic than the older, cytotoxic chemotherapies. In a sense this is true, but as has been the case with trastuzumab in breast cancer, serious and important toxicities have surfaced. In addition, since these drugs have only modest activity on their own, the toxicity of all the older chemotherapy that must be used in conjunction with the targeted therapy remains. Bevacizumab is associated with a small risk of large or small bowel perforation and an increased frequency of arterial thrombotic events (myocardial infarction, cerebrovascular accident, transient ischemic attack, or angina). It also causes hypertension in 15%–18% of individuals, and can interfere with wound healing.

The second major target in colorectal cancer therapeutics has been the epidermal growth factor receptor (EGFR). Cetuximab is a monoclonal antibody directed against EGFR, and was shown to have modest activity as a single agent in irinotecan-refractory colorectal cancer (20). Intriguingly, cetuximab appears to overcome irinotecan-refractoriness, as shown in two trials that demonstrated superiority for the combination of irinotecan and cetuximab over cetuximab alone in patients who had already progressed on irinotecan (20,21). The role of cetuximab in the first-line therapy of colorectal cancer has not yet been established. A recent study demonstrated a very modest benefit (under one month) for the combination of cetuximab with FOLFIRI versus FOLFIRI alone (22). This disappointing result makes it difficult to recommend routine use of this therapy in the first-line setting. Unlike the case of trastuzumab in breast cancer, there is no correlation between immunohistochemical staining of EGFR and response to anti-EGFR therapy; therefore, EGFR staining should not be used for clinical decision making (and in the authors' opinion should not be done) (23). The most common toxicity of cetuximab is an acneiform rash, which in up to 20% of patients can be quite severe. Interestingly, those who get the more severe rash are more likely to benefit from therapy. Recently, panitumumab, a fully humanized monoclonal antibody, has been approves by the U.S. Food and Drug Administration for therapy in refractory colorectal cancer. In the registration trial, it demonstrated an 8% single-agent response rate and a very modest improvement in progression-free survival over best supportive care alone (24).

The emergence of these new therapies in a relatively contracted period of time has engendered much optimism for the patient diagnosed with advanced colorectal cancer. There is a greater complexity to managing this disease, however, with more potential toxicities, and that optimism must be tempered by the reality that the advances, hard fought for though they have been, are modest. The relative placing of each new agent within the therapeutic paradigm has not been fully elucidated. Until that process occurs, we at least have data which tell us that the fact of exposure to the maximum amount of available active therapies is an important factor associated with prolonged survival (25).

Adjuvant Therapy

A certain proportion of patients will have a recurrence of their colorectal cancer in the months and years following surgery. Excluding de novo second primary colon cancers (so-called metachronous primary cancers, which occur in 1.5%–3% of colorectal cancer patients in the first five years) it is reasonable to assume that for patients who relapse, the tumor had already metastasized prior to (or at the time of) resection, and had existed at a microscopic level. The biological hypothesis underlying the strategy of adjuvant therapy is that the eradication of these micrometastases is achievable and that cure can be effected in patients who were otherwise destined to relapse.

Since 1990, the use of systemic chemotherapy following potentially curative resection has been standard practice in patients with stage III (local regional lymph node metastases only) and some stage II (full-thickness tumors, clean lymph nodes) disease, based on major trials which demonstrated a survival benefit for adjuvant chemotherapy compared to no treatment or ineffective treatment (26–28). The basic component of this therapy is 5-FU. As outlined above in the metastatic setting, a great deal of investigational energy was expended on the question of how best to administer the treatment in terms of method and duration of administration, and what best to combine it with. A large Intergroup study was among those that showed no additional benefit for prolonging chemotherapy beyond six months (29). As yet, there is no way to predict who will benefit from the addition of chemotherapy following curative surgery. It must be remembered that in evaluating studies in common diseases such as colorectal cancer or breast cancer, small differences in therapeutic arms often translate into large absolute numbers when applied to the population at large.

The clear survival gains demonstrated in the adjuvant trials apply to those with nodal involvement, for whom the risk of recurrence is higher. The use of chemotherapy in patients at stage II is more controversial. Most of the adjuvant studies have shown a trend towards improved survival, but have had insufficient power to detect statistically significant differences. It is accepted practice to offer adjuvant therapy to those with stage II disease who have high-risk features (high CEA, perforation, presentation with obstruction, or microvascular invasion). Molecular markers are not routinely used to delineate which patients in stage II would benefit from chemotherapy. An ECOG study in 2008 aimed to prospectively stratify stage II patients into risk categories based on microsatellite instability and loss of heterozygosity of 18q, assigning high-risk patients to randomization with FOLFOX with or without bevacizumab and low-risk patients to observation alone.

An important development in adjuvant studies has been the demonstration that three-year disease-free survival is a surrogate for five-year overall survival (30). This has the practical effect of shortening the length of time taken for questions to be answered by clinical trials, and in adjuvant studies where the majority of patients will be cured and the number of events are less, this is crucial to the development of the field. This is of particular importance in the current era of multiple active agents whose role(s) in the adjuvant setting need to be explored.

The rational belief that therapies which are effective in the metastatic setting should prove beneficial in the adjuvant setting is a dominant philosophy in the design of adjuvant studies in medical oncology. Logically, a therapy which is effective in the advanced setting should be even more effective where the disease burden is less (microscopic, if present at all), thus increasing the proportion of people cured with adjuvant treatment. Thus, some studies have focused on moving some of the treatments that have emerged in recent years to an earlier stage in the therapeutic paradigm, although some results have been quite disappointing.

Oxaliplatin-based therapy has been proven to be more effective than 5-FU/LV alone (31). In the pivotal study, 2,246 patients with resected colorectal cancer were randomized to de Gramont 5-FU with or without oxaliplatin. There was an absolute difference in disease-free survival of 7% reported at three years, which has persisted on longer follow-up (32). The NSABP C-07 trial has confirmed the benefits of adding oxaliplatin to 5-FU in the adjuvant setting (33).

Surprisingly, given its equivalent efficacy in the metastatic setting, irinotecan-based regimens have been shown to be ineffective in the adjuvant setting (34–36). Trials incorporating bevacizumab and cetuximab into adjuvant therapy are currently underway. The irinotecan experience should serve as a cautionary note that just because some benefit from these agents has been seen in the metastatic setting does not mean that they will be effective in the adjuvant setting. We must wait for the trial results. It should be noted that the long terms effects of any of the agents used in the treatment of CRC are not known. Even 5-FU has only been consistently given to patients with curable disease for less than two decades. Whether late sequelae from exposure to these drugs will be seen remains unknown at this time.

CONCLUSIONS

The field of treating gastrointestinal cancer has changed enormously in a short period of time and this has engendered much optimism. The unexpected toxicities of many of these new agents must sound a note of caution however. Likewise, the negative adjuvant data with irinotecan speaks to the importance of conducting well-designed clinical trials to rigorously evaluate the plethora of potential therapies in all settings before reaching conclusions regarding safety or efficacy. We urgently need predictive testing to prevent patients from being exposed to therapies from which they will not benefit. Microarray technology offers the possibility of profiling tumors according to their inherent biology, rather than our current pathological staging which is more a function of when the patient happens to present. The design of our clinical trials will need to incorporate these technologies so that they are evaluated in a prospective manner.

References

1. Jemal A, Siegel R, Ward E, Murray T, Xu J, Thun MJ. Cancer statistics, 2007. *CA Cancer J Clin.* 2007;57(1):43–66.
2. Tzardi M. Role of total mesorectal excision and of circumferential resection margin in local recurrence and survival of patients with rectal carcinoma. *Dig Dis.* 2007;25(1):51–55.
3. Winawer SJ, Zauber AG, Ho MN, et al. Prevention of colorectal cancer by colonoscopic polypectomy. The National Polyp Study Workgroup. *N Engl J Med.* 1993;329(27):1977–1981.
4. Goldberg RM. Advances in the treatment of metastatic colorectal cancer. *Oncologist.* 2005;10(Suppl 3):40–48.
5. Jessup JM, McGinnis LS, Steele GD, Jr., Menck HR, Winchester DP. The National Cancer Data Base. Report on colon cancer. *Cancer.* 1996;78(4):918–926.
6. Simmonds PC. Palliative chemotherapy for advanced colorectal cancer: systematic review and meta-analysis. Colorectal Cancer Collaborative Group. *BMJ.* 2000;321(7260):531–535.
7. Saltz LB. Another study of how to give fluorouracil? *J Clin Oncol.* 2003;21(20):3711–3712.
8. Hoff PM, Ansari R, Batist G, et al. Comparison of oral capecitabine versus intravenous fluorouracil plus leucovorin as first-line treatment in 605 patients with metastatic colorectal cancer: results of a randomized phase III study. *J Clin Oncol.* 2001;19(8):2282–2292.
9. Douillard JY, Cunningham D, Roth AD, et al. Irinotecan combined with fluorouracil compared with fluorouracil alone as first-line treatment for metastatic colorectal cancer: a multicentre randomised trial. *Lancet.* 2000;355(9209):1041–1047.
10. Saltz LB, Cox JV, Blanke C, et al. Irinotecan plus fluorouracil and leucovorin for metastatic colorectal cancer. Irinotecan Study Group. *N Engl J Med.* 2000;343(13):905–914.
11. Kohne CH, van Cutsem E, Wils J, et al. Phase III study of weekly high-dose infusional fluorouracil plus folinic acid with or without irinotecan in patients with metastatic colorectal cancer: European Organisation for Research and Treatment of Cancer Gastrointestinal Group Study 40986. *J Clin Oncol.* 2005;23(22):4856–4865.
12. de Gramont A, Figer A, Seymour M, et al. Leucovorin and fluorouracil with or without oxaliplatin as first-line treatment in advanced colorectal cancer. *J Clin Oncol.* 2000;18(16):2938–2947.
13. Goldberg RM, Sargent DJ, Morton RF, et al. A randomized controlled trial of fluorouracil plus leucovorin, irinotecan, and oxaliplatin combinations in patients with previously untreated metastatic colorectal cancer. *J Clin Oncol.* 2004;22(1):23–30.
14. Tournigand C, Andre T, Achille E, et al. FOLFIRI followed by FOLFOX6 or the reverse sequence in advanced colorectal cancer: a randomized GERCOR study. *J Clin Oncol.* 2004;22(2):229–237.
15. Colucci G, Gebbia V, Paoletti G, et al. Phase III randomized trial of FOLFIRI versus FOLFOX4 in the treatment of advanced colorectal cancer: a multicenter study of the Gruppo Oncologico Dell'Italia Meridionale. *J Clin Oncol.* 2005;23(22):4866–4875.
16. Hurwitz H, Fehrenbacher L, Novotny W, et al. Bevacizumab plus irinotecan, fluorouracil, and leucovorin for metastatic colorectal cancer. *N Engl J Med.* 2004;350(23):2335–2342.
17. Saltz LBea. Bevacizumab (Bev) in combination with XELOX or FOLFOX4: Efficacy results from XELOX-1/NO16966, a randomized phase III trial in the first-line treatment of metastatic colorectal cancer (MCRC). In: GI Cancer Symposium; 2007; Orlando, Florida; 2007.
18. Giantonio BJ, Catalano PJ, Meropol NJ, et al. High-dose bevacizumab improves survival when combined with FOLFOX4 in previously treated advanced colorectal cancer: Results from the Eastern Cooperative Oncology Group (ECOG) study E3200. *ASCO Meeting Abstracts.* 2005;23(16 Suppl):2.
19. Saltz LB. Bevacizumab (Bev) in combination with XELOX or FOLFOX4: Updated efficacy results from XELOX-1/NO16966, a randomized phase III trial in first-line metastatic colorectal cancer. In: ASCO; 2007; Chicago, IL; 2007.
20. Saltz LB, Meropol NJ, Loehrer PJ, Sr., Needle MN, Kopit J, Mayer RJ. Phase II trial of cetuximab in patients with refractory colorectal cancer that expresses the epidermal growth factor receptor. *J Clin Oncol.* 2004;22(7):1201–1208.
21. Cunningham D, Humblet Y, Siena S, et al. Cetuximab monotherapy and cetuximab plus irinotecan in irinotecan-refractory metastatic colorectal cancer. *N Engl J Med.* 2004;351(4):337–345.
22. Van Cutsem E. Randomized phase III study of irinotecan and 5-FU/FA with or without cetuximab in the first-line treatment of patients with metastatic colorectal cancer (mCRC): The CRYSTAL trial. In: ASCO; 2007; Chicago, IL; 2007.
23. Chung KY, Shia J, Kemeny NE, et al. Cetuximab shows activity in colorectal cancer patients with tumors that do not express the epidermal growth factor receptor by immunohistochemistry. *J Clin Oncol.* 2005;23(9):1803–1810.
24. Van Cutsem E, Peeters M, Siena S, et al. Open-label phase III trial of panitumumab plus best supportive care compared with best supportive care alone in patients with chemotherapy-refractory metastatic colorectal cancer. *J Clin Oncol.* 2007;25(13):1658–1664.
25. Grothey A, Sargent D, Goldberg RM, Schmoll HJ. Survival of patients with advanced colorectal cancer improves with the availability of fluorouracil-leucovorin, irinotecan, and oxaliplatin in the course of treatment. *J Clin Oncol.* 2004;22(7):1209–1214.
26. Wolmark N, Rockette H, Fisher B, et al. The benefit of leucovorin-modulated fluorouracil as postoperative adjuvant therapy for primary colon cancer: results from National Surgical Adjuvant Breast and Bowel Project protocol C-03. *J Clin Oncol.* 1993;11(10):1879–1887.
27. Efficacy of adjuvant fluorouracil and folinic acid in colon cancer. International Multicentre Pooled Analysis of Colon Cancer Trials (IMPACT) investigators. *Lancet.* 1995;345(8955):939–944.
28. O'Connell MJ, Mailliard JA, Kahn MJ, et al. Controlled trial of fluorouracil and low-dose leucovorin given for six months as postoperative adjuvant therapy for colon cancer. *J Clin Oncol.* 1997;15(1):246–250.
29. Haller DG, Catalano PJ, Macdonald JS, et al. Phase III study of fluorouracil, leucovorin, and levamisole in high-risk stage II and III colon cancer: final report of Intergroup 0089. *J Clin Oncol.* 2005;23(34):8671–8678.
30. Sargent DJ, Wieand HS, Haller DG, et al. Disease-free survival versus overall survival as a primary end point for adjuvant colon cancer studies: individual patient data from 20,898 patients on 18 randomized trials. *J Clin Oncol.* 2005;23(34):8664–8670.
31. Andre T, Boni C, Mounedji-Boudiaf L, et al. Oxaliplatin, fluorouracil, and leucovorin as adjuvant treatment for colon cancer. *N Engl J Med.* 2004;350(23):2343–2351.
32. de Gramont Aea. Oxaliplatin/5FU/LV in adjuvant colon cancer: updated efficacy results of the MOSAIC trial, including survival, with a median follow-up of six years. In: ASCO; 2007.
33. Wolmark N, Wieand S, Kuebler JP, Colangelo L, Smith RE. A phase III trial comparing FULV to FULV + oxaliplatin in stage II or III carcinoma of the colon: results of NSABP Protocol C-07. *ASCO Meeting Abstracts.* 2005;23(16 suppl):LBA3500.
34. Saltz LB, Niedzwiecki D, Hollis D, et al. Irinotecan plus fluorouracil/leucovorin (IFL) versus fluorouracil/

leucovorin alone (FL) in stage III colon cancer (intergroup trial CALGB C89803). *ASCO Meeting Abstracts.* 2004;22 (14 suppl):3500.

35. van Cutsem E, Labianca R, Hossfeld D, et al. Randomized phase III trial comparing infused irinotecan/5-fluorouracil (5-FU)/folinic acid (IF) versus 5-FU/FA (F) in stage III colon cancer patients (pts). (PETACC 3). *ASCO Meeting Abstracts.* 2005;23(16 suppl):LBA8.

36. Ychou M, Raoul JL, Douillard JY, et al. A phase III randomized trial of LV5FU2+CPT-11 vs. LV5FU2 alone in adjuvant high risk colon cancer (FNCLCC Accord02/FFCD9802). *ASCO Meeting Abstracts.* 2005;23(16 suppl):3502.

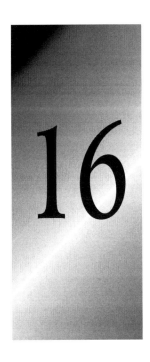

Evaluation and Treatment of Melanoma

Jedd D. Wolchok
Yvonne Saenger

Prominent clinical features of the "black cancer" were first recorded by physicians in the early 19th century. At that time, Dr. William Norris of Stourbridge of England noted that melanoma could spread rapidly and widely throughout the body, that patients generally remain in good health until the final stages, and that the disease affects individuals with fair complexions and many nevi (1). Unfortunately, despite tremendous advances in cancer biology, Dr. Norris' description of the natural history of melanoma remains essentially accurate at the present time. It has, however, long been known that melanoma is an unpredictable syndrome and that rare patients live for years and even decades in symbiosis with the disease. The reasons for this remain unclear, although genetic profiling is now beginning to sort out different melanoma subtypes (2). Melanoma, in this sense, is a cancer which has frustrated and mystified generations of patients and clinicians.

Melanoma is treated with surgery, chemotherapy, radiotherapy, and immunotherapy, as well as experimental targeted therapies in development. Surgery remains the mainstay of clinical management for limited disease. The observation, first documented by Dr. Alexander Breslow, that tumor depth is a key determinant of prognosis, allows surgeons to tailor surgery based on the patient's risk. Once the cancer has metastasized, however, conventional chemotherapy and radiotherapy provide clinical benefit only to a minority of patients. Immunotherapy plays an important role in the clinical management of melanoma and remains a highly active

area of ongoing research. Finally, an understanding of the genetic aberrations in the signaling pathways driving melanomas is beginning to emerge, and this lays the groundwork for the development of effective targeted therapies.

RELEVANT ASPECTS OF MELANOCYTE BIOLOGY

Melanoma is presumed to develop from melanocytes, cells whose normal physiologic role is to produce pigment. Precursor cells originate in the neural crest and during embryologic development they migrate to their target tissues, most prominently the skin. It has been hypothesized that this migratory developmental program may be reactivated in metastatic malignant melanoma (3). Once located in the skin, the melanocyte "stem cell" resides in hair follicles, while more differentiated progeny home to the dermal epidermal junction, where they associate with keratinocytes. Melanocytes are not only found in the skin, however, but are also present in the conjunctiva, gastrointestinal and genital mucosa, leptomeninges, and even the capsules of lymph nodes. This explains why primary melanomas occasionally arise in the eye and areas other than the skin.

The primary function of melanocytes is to modulate the organism's exposure to potentially damaging solar radiation. Melanocytes accomplish this by producing

KEY POINTS

- Prominent clinical features of the "black cancer" were first recorded by physicians in the early 19th century.
- Melanoma is treated with surgery, chemotherapy, radiotherapy, and immunotherapy, as well as experimental targeted therapies in development.
- Surgery remains the mainstay of clinical management for limited disease.
- Tumor depth is a key determinate of prognosis.
- Melanoma is presumed to develop from melanocytes found not only in the skin, but the conjunctiva, gastrointestinal and genital mucosa, leptomeninges, and even the capsules of lymph nodes.
- The incidence of melanoma among white populations has increased substantially over the past century.
- Children in particular should be protected from the sun, since there is some evidence that exposure early in life is more likely to lead to melanoma.

- The ABCD rule, which describes lesions that are *a*symmetric, have blurred *b*orders, are non-uniform in *c*olor, and have a *d*iameter greater than 5 mm. However, evolution (or enlargement) is the most sensitive indicator of a lesion in need of biopsy.
- In up to 20% of cases, the first melanoma symptom is from a metastatic lesion.
- One distinguishing feature of melanoma is the propensity to metastasize to the small bowel and manifest as gastrointestinal bleeding.
- Brain metastases are common and generally hemorrhagic, frequently causing seizures, which are occasionally the first manifestation of disease.
- Median survival for patients with metastatic disease is approximately 8.5–11 months, although there are occasional long-term survivors.
- There continues to be intense investigation of melanoma vaccines and other immunotherapies.

melanin which adsorbs light in the UV spectrum. Melanin is only produced by melanocytes, and there is unique enzymatic machinery involved in melanin synthesis. Melanin is produced from tyrosine in membrane bound vesicles called melanosomes, and these granules are then packaged and transferred to keratinocytes via export of the entire melanosome. Intriguingly, it has been observed that melanosomes are positioned in response to UV radiation within the keratinocyte to form a parasol-like structure protecting the nucleus (4). Importantly, skin pigmentation is determined by the number and quality of the melanosomes—not by the number of melanocytes. Darker skinned individuals are therefore better shielded from UV radiation but do not have a higher total number of melanocytes.

The molecular basis for the susceptibility of pale individuals to melanoma is partially understood at this time (5). Tanning is essentially an increase in pigment production triggered by sun exposure. The exact mechanism whereby this occurs is unclear, although there is significant evidence that DNA damage directly induces tanning (6). Mutations in the MC1R melanocortin 1 receptor (MC1R) gene are associated with poor tanning and predispose some fair-skinned individuals to melanoma. Over 30 MC1R gene alleles have been identified in human populations (7). MC1R is a membrane bound G-protein coupled receptor that activates cyclic adenosine monophosphate (AMP) responsive element binding protein (CREB) transcription factors (8). These in turn up-regulate multiple gene products including microphthalmia transcription factor (MITF), a master regulatory gene implicated in melanin production, melanocyte differentiation, and malignant transformation (9). Signaling via MC1R modulates pigmentation by increasing the relative levels of eumelanin (brown/black) versus pheomelanin (red/yellow). Pheomelanin both provides inferior UV adsorption and is a source of reactive oxidative byproducts which can cause DNA damage (10).

As a lineage, melanocytes appear in some aspects to be primed for tumorigenesis. They are constantly exposed to oxidative tyrosine metabolites, byproducts of melanin synthesis (11), and are remarkably resistant to apoptosis, perhaps due to high levels of expression of anti-apoptotic genes, including bcl-2 (12). Cultured melanocytes will grow and display some phenotypic features of melanomas before senescing (13). Melanocytes isolated from benign nevi, however, have been reported to form colonies in soft agar, an assay commonly used as a test for oncogenic transformation (14). Some of these features are suppressed by coculture with keratinocytes, highlighting the importance of tissue stroma in regulation of melanocyte growth and differentiation (15).

EPIDEMIOLOGY

The incidence of melanoma among white populations has increased very substantially over the past century.

This increase is now tapering off, although rates remain much higher than they were a generation ago. In the United States, the Surveillance, Epidemiology, and End Results program (SEER) estimated that in the period from2000 to 2004, the incidence of melanoma would reach 18.5/100,000 persons per year, with white men having the highest incidence of 27.2/100,000/year. This puts the average lifetime risk at about 1.7% (16). Incidence varies widely around the globe, and the high incidence rates seen in Australia (40.5 per 100,000/year) suggest that the combination of fair skin and a sunny tropical climate predisposes to melanoma (17). Other regions with relatively high incidence are Northern Europe and Israel. Comparisons between populations with differing generational demographics are complicated because melanoma, despite being among the most common cancers in young people, is in fact, like most other cancers, a disease of older adults (median age of diagnosis is 59 in the United States).

In general, there appear to be two major factors underlying trends in melanoma incidence over the past century. The first is increasing sun exposure due to cultural factors among white populations, including the partial abandonment of pallor as a symbol of status and an increased willingness to display naked skin. The evidence that melanoma is related to sun exposure is epidemiologically robust, and includes the correlation between incidence among whites in North America and Australia with proximity to the equator, the increased rates among European migrants to sunny regions, particularly if they migrated at an earlier age, and evidence that, with heightened awareness of the risk of sun exposure, rates are now starting to decline among younger people (18). Studies also suggest that intermittent sun exposure may be worse, partially accounting for increased melanoma incidence in higher socioeconomic groups (19).

The second major factor underlying the increase in melanoma incidence over the past century is heightened awareness and screening. Cancer registries around the world have reported that the average thickness of melanoma at diagnosis has decreased over recent decades (18). Mortality rates, meanwhile, have gradually stabilized in the United States and elsewhere. These trends in the absence of major therapeutic advances, suggest that early detection artificially elevated incidence rates over the past 20–30 years, and is now having an impact on mortality since lesions, which would have been causing deaths, were removed.

If sunlight is the primary environmental factor contributing to melanoma genesis in whites, genetic factors also play an important role. Accordingly, a reported family history of melanoma confers the same increase in risk, which is approximately a twofold increase, as

a reported history of intense sun exposure (20). A diagnosis of xeroderma pigmentosum meanwhile increases risk by 1,000-fold in individuals younger than aged 20. There are undoubtedly certain families in whom the increased risk is much higher than others, although the molecular basis for this is largely unknown. Mutation in CDKN2A has been associated with melanoma and pancreatic cancer, but genetic testing is generally not recommended, because individuals from families with a high incidence of melanoma should receive dermatologic screening regardless of genotype. Phenotypic features correlating most closely with melanoma risk in the white population include skin type (difficulty tanning and propensity to burn), frequency of atypical nevi, frequency of common nevi, freckling, and light skin and/or hair (16). Nevi and freckling, however, reflect childhood sun exposure as well as genetic factors. Ethnic African populations rarely develop melanoma, and when they do it is usually on the palms and soles of the feet. Risk factors for melanoma in Africans are unknown. Asians, even pale individuals, have an exceedingly low rate of melanoma (17).

PREVENTION

Given the scope of epidemiologic evidence that sun exposure causes melanoma, basic precautions aimed at minimizing sunburn are advisable. Children in particular should be protected from the sun, because there is some evidence that exposure early in life is more likely to lead to melanoma. Individuals with fair complexions and/or many moles, poor tanners, individuals with red hair, and members of families at high risk should be especially cautious. Patients should also be cognizant of any atypical moles and bring any rapidly changing or unusual appearing lesions to medical attention. While there is no definitive study proving that hats and sunscreen prevent melanoma, epidemiologic trends including declining incidence in younger populations, and a stabilization of the death rate from melanoma in the United States in the absence of significant therapeutic advances, suggests that public health prevention measures have had a positive impact.

There is controversy regarding routine screening for melanoma, but it seems eminently reasonable for individuals at high risk. This would include at a minimum, people with a personal history of melanoma, a strong family history or known genetic predisposition, and numerous or atypical moles. While there is no large scale population based study that conclusively proves that screening benefits patients, the fact that depth is critical to prognosis and that screening leads to detection of thinner melanomas is a logical justification for screening.

CLINICAL PRESENTATION

The diagnosis of cutaneous malignant melanoma is difficult even for experienced dermatologists. Several general principles are useful to physicians confronted with a suspicious lesion. First, if the lesion is worrisome to the patient, it should probably be excised. Patients may be more sensitive to the fact that a lesion is an "ugly duckling," different from their other moles, and there are many substantiated reports of patients reporting itching or other more nonspecific symptoms associated with subsequently confirmed melanomas. Second, the lesion is suspicious if it has changed over weeks or months in terms of size, shape, or pigmentation. Third, any lesion that appears disordered or unusual and does not fit the profile of any known benign skin lesion should be biopsied, particularly if it is ulcerated, bleeding, or pruritic. Fourth, lesions are more concerning if the patient has a personal or family history of melanoma, atypical nevi, a history of intense sun exposure, or visibly sun damaged skin. Fifth, it is important to remember that not all melanomas are pigmented. If a lesion is of questionable concern and there are reasons to avoid biopsy, photography can be useful for monitoring. Finally, the ABCD rule can be applied, as melanomas are generally *a*symmetric, have blurred *b*orders, are black in *c*olor, and have a *d*iameter greater than 5 mm.

Melanoma can arise in rare atypical locations that escape monitoring by patients or physicians, and male patients are less likely to notice abnormal skin lesions than are female patients. Melanoma arising on the scalp, soles of the feet, palms of the hand, nail beds, oral cavity, genitals, and ocular conjunctiva often escapes attention. Nailbed melanomas sometimes have the appearance of hematomas and the patient may even give a history of trauma to the nail, while lesions on the palms and feet may be camouflaged by thickened skin. Ocular melanomas usually present as visual disturbances or are detected incidentally on ophthalmologic exam. Mucosal melanoma of the head and neck generally presents with epistaxis, obstruction, or odynophagia, or they may be noticed by the patient because of their color. Vaginal melanomas are sometimes found incidentally on pelvic exam, but often present with bleeding.

In up to 20% of cases, the first melanoma symptom is from a metastatic lesion (16). Most commonly, the patient notices a swollen lymph gland. In 5% of these cases, a primary lesion is never identified and has presumably regressed. Melanoma with distant spread, similar to other advanced cancers, presents with organ dysfunction. One distinguishing feature of melanoma is the propensity to metastasize to the small bowel and manifest as gastrointestinal bleeding. Brain metastases are common and generally hemorrhagic, frequently causing seizures, which are occasionally the first manifestation of disease. Finally, in patients diagnosed with a second skin melanoma, it is important to confirm the presence of an in situ component within the pathologic specimen in order to exclude an epidermotrophic metastasis.

HISTOPATHOLOGIC DIAGNOSIS

When evaluating a suspicious cutaneous lesion, an excisional biopsy is best, preferably 1–3 mm in diameter so as not to obscure drainage patterns for sentinel lymph node sampling. Shave biopsies should generally be avoided when melanoma is suspected because they do not provide a good estimate of tumor thickness, the key prognostic variable. There are unfortunately no definitive criteria for microscopic interpretation of melanocytic lesions; therefore, an experienced pathologist is essential, particularly for difficult or uncertain cases. Cytologic features and tissue architecture must be interpreted within the clinical context. Essential information to be obtained from biopsy include status of peripheral and deep margins, Breslow thickness, histologic ulceration, Clark level (measures the penetration through epidermal and dermal layers), the presence or absence of satellite lesions, and the presence or absence of an in situ component. These factors are all critical in estimating prognosis in the setting of localized disease. The presence of satellite lesion(s), in particular, confer a higher risk of recurrence. Other features of interest include location, regression, mitotic rate, tumor infiltrating lymphocytes, vertical growth phase, angiolymphatic invasion, neurotropism, and histologic subtype.

CLINICAL MANAGEMENT

The clinical management of melanoma is summarized in Table 16.1 and is a function of tumor burden. Localized disease less than 1 mm in depth is treated by wide local excision (WLE) only unless adverse prognostic factors are present in which case a sentinel lymph node biopsy (SLNB) may be offered to the patient. Intermediate thickness melanomas are treated with WLE and SLNB; however, SLNB is controversial in deep lesions or in the presence of satellite lesion(s). If disease is detected in a lymph node, completion lymph node dissection (CLND) is generally recommended. Regional and/or systemic metastases are also resected if feasible. Regional recurrences may be treated with isolated limb perfusion and/or intralesional therapies. Radiation is used for brain metastases and occasionally to achieve

TABLE 16.1

Clinical Management of Malignant Melanoma

EXTENT OF DISEASE	TREATMENT PLAN
In situ melanoma	Wide local excision (WLE) with 0.5-cm margins
Melanoma <1 mm in depth	WLE with 1-cm margins. Consider sentinel lymph node biopsy (SNLB) if adverse pathologic features present
Melanoma >4 mm in depth	WLE with 2 cm margins. SNLB. Optional adjuvant therapy if >2 mm and ulcerated
Melanoma >4 mm in depth and/or with satellite lesion	WLE with 2-cm margins. Optional SNLB. Optional adjuvant therapy
Melanoma metastatic to lymph nodes	WLE of primary lesion. completion lymph node dissection (CLND). Optional adjuvant therapy
Melanoma with regional metastasis	Surgical excision of all lesions with clear margins if feasible, with optional adjuvant therapy. If lesions cannot be excised, consider alternative local therapies or systemic therapy as below
Melanoma with systemic metastasis	Surgical excision of isolated metastasis or low burden of disease or for palliation. Excision and/or irradiation of any brain metastasis. Systemic chemotherapy and/or immunotherapy

local control. Systemic therapies for non-resectable disease include chemotherapy and immunotherapy. More detailed explanations are provided below.

Clinical Management of Localized Disease

It was readily apparent to those physicians who first described melanoma in the 18th and 19th centuries that these dangerous pigmented lesions should be surgically eliminated. While these pioneering clinicians advocated radical procedures such as amputation, the scale of the recommended surgical intervention has gradually declined over the past 200 years. Current recommendations are for wide local excision (WLE) with margins of 0.5 cm for in situ disease, 1 cm for lesions less than 1 mm in thickness, and 2 cm for lesions greater than 2 mm (21).

The primary concern for patients diagnosed with melanoma is the potential for disease recurrence. For patients with lesions less than 1 mm in thickness, prognosis is excellent, with a five-year survival rate of 93%. If the primary lesion is greater than 1 mm, the five-year survival rate decreases to 68%. The predictive power of tumor thickness was confirmed in a multivariate analysis of 13,581 patients performed by The American Joint Committee on Cancer (AJCC) (22). Ulceration suggests that the malignant cells are able to cross tissue barriers, and was the most accurate secondary predictive factor for all tumors except for very thin melanomas. In these lesions, the Clark level was more highly prognostic. Other factors affecting prognosis include age (better in those younger than aged 60), site (better for lesions located in the extremities), and gender (prognosis is better for females).

Lymph node status, however, when known, is superior to all prognostic indicators. This was shown in a Cox regression analysis of 1,201 patients in the AJCC melanoma database, and is the primary rationale for SLNB (22). The prognostic value of SLNB was recently prospectively validated in the third interim analysis of the Multicenter Selective Lymphadenectomy Trial (MSLT), in which 1,347 patients with intermediate depth melanoma were randomized to WLE with or without SLNB (23). In this study, melanoma specific mortality was 26.2% in patients with a positive SLNB, as compared to 9.7% in patients with a negative SLNB. While SLNB has not been proven to improve overall survival, the procedure is generally well tolerated and consideration of SLNB is recommended for patients with intermediate thickness and/or ulcerated primaries, and may also be considered for some patients with high-risk thin melanomas, particularly if the patient is young and high-risk features are present (Clark level IV or V, regression, high mitotic rate). SLNB for patients with thick melanomas and/or satellite lesions is controversial.

Routine surveillance is recommended for patients with a history of localized cutaneous melanoma. All patients with more than in situ disease should receive follow-up physical examinations, and patients with deep primaries and/or positive lymph nodes should be seen at least every six months for two to three years of follow-up. The risk of recurrence decreases over time, with most patients experiencing recurrence within two years. Recurrences in patients with thin melanomas are rare and occur later on average. Recommendations for imaging to screen for metastatic disease vary by institution and are not grounded in epidemiologic evidence. Dermatologic screening and sun exposure precautions are advised for all patients.

Clinical Management of Local Recurrence and Regional Metastases

The distinction between local recurrence and regional metastasis has historically been subjective; traditionally, lesions within 2 cm of the scar were categorized as local recurrence. According to the more current definition, a lesion must contain in situ disease or a radial growth phase in order to be classified as a true local scar recurrence (21). In any case, recurrence near the site of a previously excised melanoma is predictive of a poor prognosis, and in the Intergroup Melanoma Surgical Trial was associated with a five-year survival of 9% (24). The detection of local recurrence or regional metastasis should therefore be followed by full body imaging prior to resection. If the lesion is a true local recurrence rather than a metastasis, and there is no evidence of systemic spread, surgical margins should be wide.

For regional and nodal metastases, surgery is the mainstay of treatment. If disease is bulky and not amenable to resection, alternative local and systemic therapies may be considered. Local therapies in current use include isolated limb perfusion or infusion with melphalan, intralesional injection with immune modulating agents and/or chemotherapy, radiation, and laser ablation. Systemic therapy using biologic agents and/or chemotherapy may also be employed in this setting.

In patients who have melanoma which has spread to the lymph nodes, the burden of disease in the nodes is highly prognostic (22). A patient with a micrometastasis in one node, for example, has a far better outcome than one with clinically palpable disease in many nodes. Removal of all lymph nodes in the affected basin is the standard of care, although a prospective randomized trial is underway to determine the value of this procedure in patients with a positive SLNB and no clinical evidence of residual nodal disease (MSLT II) (25). Radiation is generally given if there is suspicion that residual tumor remains after surgery, and adjuvant therapy may be considered as described below.

The Question of Adjuvant Therapy

Once the melanoma lesion has been excised and the patient has been educated about the risks of sun exposure and advised to visit the dermatologist for screening along with his or her immediate family members, the question of possible adjuvant therapy emerges. Adjuvant therapy is generally considered for patients with positive lymph nodes, satellite lesions, primary lesions greater than 4 mm in thickness or ulcerated lesions that are greater than 2 mm in thickness, or previously resected metastatic lesions. There is no therapy conclu-

sively proven to prevent disease recurrence; therefore, observation remains an acceptable choice for anyone with a history of melanoma and no evidence of disease.

High-dose interferon alpha is the only U.S. Food and Drug Administration (FDA)-approved adjuvant therapy for melanoma; however, there is considerable controversy surrounding its use because of limited efficacy and significant toxicity (26,27). There is no evidence that interferon improves overall survival, although there is some evidence that it does delay recurrence (28). Interferon may be more effective in patients who develop autoantibodies while on therapy, but these patients cannot be selected for prospectively (29). High-dose interferon is associated with many side effects, most prominently fatigue, flulike symptoms, depression, and liver toxicity. Low-dose interferon is less toxic, but it does not have established efficacy. There is no evidence that chemotherapy in the adjuvant setting is beneficial. A recent trial of biochemotherapy showed no advantage relative to high-dose interferon (30). Temozolomide (Temodar) is sometimes used in the adjuvant setting for patients at high risk of recurrence, but this is based on an extrapolation of data in patients with metastatic disease. Granulocyte-macrophage colony stimulating factor (GM-CSF), a stimulant of bone marrow production of immune cells, is sometimes offered based on a small study suggesting a possible benefit (31). Experimental vaccines may be given in the adjuvant setting, although none have been proven effective to date.

Clinical Management of Systemic Metastases

Median survival for patients with metastatic disease is approximately 8.5–11 months, although there are occasional long-term survivors. Survival correlates with site and number of metastases, remission duration, surgical resectability, response to systemic therapy, and serum lactic dehydrogenase (LDH) levels (32). Metastatic melanoma is highly aggressive, versatile, and grows in many organs, including lung, liver, bone, brain, gastrointestinal tract (small bowel in particular), spleen, kidney, heart, bone marrow, pancreas, peritoneum, adrenal glands, thyroid, breast, and placenta. Metastases are generally detected by clinical and radiologic criteria, as there are currently no reliable serum markers for metastatic disease.

Due to the diversity of sites of metastases, patients develop a variety of constellations of symptoms, many of which require palliative care. Prominent oncologic complications in melanoma include seizures and neurologic impairment due to hemorrhagic brain metastases and/or leptomeningeal disease, venous thrombosis and pulmonary embolism, GI bleeding and/or obstruction due to small bowel disease, liver necrosis and hemorrhage, rupture of a splenic metastasis, bony disease impinging on the spinal cord, marrow failure due to infiltration by melanoma, and urinary obstruction.

In many institutions, surgery remains the treatment of choice for patients who have resectable disease and a moderate rate of disease progression (tumor doubling time). There are multiple published studies documenting long-term survival, and even apparent cures, in selected patients after metastasectomy (33). The difficulty is that there are no large prospective randomized trials conclusively showing a benefit of surgery; however, it seems that patients who have limited metastases and more indolent disease do benefit from surgical intervention. Metastasectomy is particularly recommended for limited brain metastases, although stereotactic radiosurgery (SRS) is an excellent alternative. Partial or whole brain radiation may then be given as an adjuvant. Metastasectomy is also often used for a solitary lung metastasis where five-year survival rates of 20% have been reported (34).

Patients with widely disseminated disease are not candidates for surgical treatment and are treated with systemic medication, generally chemotherapy, immunotherapy, or a combination of both. Dacarbazine (DTIC) is the only FDA-approved cytotoxic agent for melanoma, and yields an estimated 7%–20% response rate (35). Temozolomide is an oral formulation of a similar drug, with a similar activity profile and an advantage of higher central nervous system penetrance (36). Response rates are higher with combination chemotherapy regimens such as the cisplatin, vinblastine, and DTIC regimen; the Dartmouth regimen, consisting of cisplatin, dacarbazine, carmustine (BiCNU), and tamoxifen; and the BHD regimen, consisting of BiCNU, hydroxyurea, and dacarbazine). However, none of these regimens have been shown to prolong overall survival. Biochemotherapy, a combination of chemotherapy and cytokine therapy with interleukin 2 (IL-2) and interferon, yielded highly promising results in phase II trials, but similar to chemotherapy did not yield reproducible improvements in overall survival. It is worth noting, however, that melanoma trials are smaller than breast cancer trials, for example, and therefore not powered to detect subtle differences in survival. Nonetheless, the choice of "aggressive" combination therapy versus single agent temozolomide or dacarbazine is often made based on the perceived need for rapid palliation.

Immunotherapy is an alternative to chemotherapy in metastatic melanoma, and yields similar therapeutic benefit. Interferon alpha, in the metastatic setting, produced a 16% response rate, with occasional durable responses (37), and improved response rates (although not overall survival) when given in combination with temozolomide (38). The most widely used immunotherapy in the metastatic setting is high dose IL-2, which in a trial conducted in the late 1980s yielded a 17% response rate with a small percentage of participants alive at five years, leading to speculation of possible cure (39). High-dose IL-2 is extremely toxic, and must be given in a monitored setting. Finally, the anti-angiogenic agent bevacizumab was recently shown to have some efficacy in metastatic melanoma (40).

EXPERIMENTAL IMMUNOTHERAPIES IN MELANOMA

A wide array of immune therapies is under development in both the adjuvant and metastatic setting. In the metastatic setting, the most promising for general application is checkpoint blockade with anti-CTLA-4 antibodies. CTLA-4 is a surface molecule expressed by activated T cells, and it functions as a "brake" on the immune system, signaling via an inhibitory tyrosine associated motif (ITIM) to down-regulate T-cell responses. By inhibiting CTLA-4, immune responses against melanoma can be generated. This strategy has been evaluated in several published phase I and phase II trials, with an overall response rate of 15% in pretreated patients (41). As was seen with IL-2, some of these responses appear to be quite durable. Anti-CTLA-4 therapy is associated in some patients with immune related adverse events, including rash, diarrhea, and more rarely, colitis, which can cause perforation (42). Therefore, extremely close monitoring of patients' bowel habits is essential. Responses to anti-CTLA-4 therapy appear to be different from responses to cytotoxic therapy; they may develop over weeks to months and sometimes "progression" is noted on scans prior to response. The development of inflammation in metastatic deposits complicates radiologic interpretation in these patients.

There continues to be intense investigation of melanoma vaccines. Vaccination against cancer is a difficult challenge because the immune systems of cancer patients are usually tolerant of the tumor and considers it self. Phase III trials of vaccines in melanoma patients have yielded disappointing results to date (43). Many strategies have been explored, including whole cell, protein, and, most recently, dendritic cell (DC)-based vaccines and DNA vaccines. DCs are the most potent antigen-presenting cell (APC) in the immune system, and multiple strategies are under investigation whereby they are generated ex vivo from the patient, coated with melanoma antigens, and reinfused. In DNA vaccination, cDNA encoding the antigen of interest is introduced into the skin, lymph node, or muscle, where it is taken up by APCs. DNA vaccination has advantages, both because CpG sequences in the DNA itself are inherently immunogenic, and because DNA is easy to manipulate to enhance the intrinsic immunogenicity of the encoded protein (44). One strategy to overcome self-tolerance is to vaccinate using xenogeneic (cross-species) antigen. It has been shown, for example, that vaccination against human melanoma antigens generate lymphocytes which are then cross reactive against mouse melanoma antigens (45).

Adoptive T-cell therapy using T cells isolated from tumor specimens, (tumor infiltrating T cells or TILs), has also been under intense investigation in recent years, and yielded a 51% response rate in a phase I study in selected pretreated patients (46). This study highlighted several factors which are important for the engraftment of transferred T cells. First, lymphodepletion with conditioning chemotherapy appears to be critical. This may be due to the phenomenon of homeostatic proliferation, whereby there is a compensatory proliferation of T cells when their numbers are low. Second, transfer of a combination of CD4+ and CD8+ T cells appears to be essential to the development of a robust CD8+ T-cell response, which was critical to efficacy. Third, the differentiation status of the CD8+ T cells is important for successful engraftment. Experimental approaches using transgenic T-cell receptors have also been used in this setting (47). Further studies in this area should yield better understanding of the antimelanoma T-cell response and to the development of newer and more widely applicable protocols for adoptive T-cell transfer in patients.

GENETIC LESIONS IN MELANOMA

It is evident from clinical and epidemiological data that melanoma is a genetically heterogeneous disease. Genetic profiling data has been used in the classification of melanomas into four different subtypes (2). These genetic profiles are characterized by distinct patterns of genetic aberration and correlate with melanomas arising in sun damaged skin, in normal skin, acral, and mucosal melanomas. Some of the defining mutations in these cancers are thought to be "driving mutations," in that they are required for the initiation of tumor growth. Moreover, the "oncogene addiction" hypothesis postulates that cancer cells become so dependent on the aberrant activation of particular signaling pathways that they cannot survive in their absence. The hope is that treatment with small molecule inhibitors targeted to particular signaling pathways can be tailored for individual patients based on melanoma genotype.

The RAS-RAF-MEK-ERK (MAP kinase) signaling pathway has received particular attention because it mediates diverse effects, including cell growth, and is frequently constitutively active in human tumors. In melanoma, mutations in B-Raf are reported in 66% of cases, while a further 15% have mutations in N-Ras (48). Mutations in these two signaling molecules are mutually exclusive, suggesting that two hits to this pathway would be redundant and confer no further selective advantage. Moreover, cell lines with a B-Raf mutation are sensitive to MEK inhibition, whereas cells with N-Ras are not, demonstrating that regulation of this pathway is highly complex (49). Phase I clinical trials of MEK and B-Raf inhibitors are underway. Amplification and mutations in the oncogenic tyrosine kinase, c-kit, have also been detected in a subset of melanomas and clinical trials with Imatinib, a c-kit inhibitor, are ongoing (50). Multiple other pathways including the Wnt pathway, the fibroblast growth factor pathway, and the PI3-AKT pathway, have been implicated in melanoma growth and metastasis (51). Further study of in vitro and in vivo models will deepen our understanding of the molecular biology of melanoma, leading to new biologic therapies for clinical application.

References

1. Norris W. *Eight Cases of Melanomsis with Pathological and Therapeutical Remarks on that Disease.* London: Longman, Brown, Green, Longman and Roberts; 1857.
2. Curtin JA, Fridlyand J, Kageshita T, et al. Distinct sets of genetic alterations in melanoma. *N Engl J Med.* 2005;353(20):2135–2147.
3. Gupta PB, Kuperwasser C, Brunet JP, et al. The melanocyte differentiation program predisposes to metastasis after neoplastic transformation. *Nat Genet.* 2005;37(10):1047–1054.
4. Boissy RE. Melanosome transfer to and translocation in the keratinocyte. *Exp Dermatol.* 2003;12(Suppl 2):5–12.
5. Lin JY, Fisher DE. Melanocyte biology and skin pigmentation. *Nature.* 2007;445(7130):843–850.
6. Eller MS, Yaar M, Gilchrest BA. DNA damage and melanogenesis. *Nature.* 1994;372(6505):413–414.
7. Healy E, Jordan SA, Budd PS, Suffolk R, Rees JL, Jackson IJ. Functional variation of MC1R alleles from red-haired individuals. *Hum Mol Genet.* 2001;10(21):2397–2402.
8. Mountjoy KG, Robbins LS, Mortrud MT, Cone RD. The cloning of a family of genes that encode the melanocortin receptors. *Science.* 1992;257(5074):1248–1251.
9. Steingrimsson E, Copeland NG, Jenkins NA. Melanocytes and the microphthalmia transcription factor network. *Annu Rev Genet.* 2004;38:365–411.
10. Hill HZ, Hill GJ. UVA, pheomelanin and the carcinogenesis of melanoma. *Pigment Cell Res.* 2000;13(Suppl 8):140–144.
11. Prota. Recent advances in the chemistry of melanogenesis in mammals. *J Invest Dermatol.* 1980;75(1):122–127.
12. McGill GG, Horstmann M, Widlund HR, et al. Bcl2 regulation by the melanocyte master regulator Mitf modulates lineage survival and melanoma cell viability. *Cell.* 2002;109(6):707–718.
13. Shih IM, Elder DE, Hsu MY, Herlyn M. Regulation of Mel-CAM/MUC18 expression on melanocytes of different stages of tumor progression by normal keratinocytes. *Am J Pathol.* 1994;145(4):837–845.
14. Mancianti ML, Herlyn M, Weil D, et al. Growth and phenotypic characteristics of human nevus cells in culture. *J Invest Dermatol.* 1988;90(2):134–141.

15. Scott GA, Haake AR. Keratinocytes regulate melanocyte number in human fetal and neonatal skin equivalents. *J Invest Dermatol.* 1991;97(5):776–781.

16. http://seer.cancer.gov/statfacts/html/melan.html?statfacts_page=melan.html&x=14&y=20. (Accessed at January 31, 2009).

17. Ferlay J, Bray F, Pisani P, Parkin DM. *GLOBOCAN 2000: Cancer Incidence, Mortality and Prevalence Worldwide, version 1.0.* IARC CancerBase No 5. In. Lyon: IARC Press; 2001.

18. Berwick M, Weinstock, M. Epidemiology: current trends. In: Balch CM HA, Sober AJ, Soong S, eds. *Cutaneous Melanoma.* St. Lousi, Missouri: QMP; 2003;15–23.

19. Elwood JM, Jopson J. Melanoma and sun exposure: an overview of published studies. *Int J Cancer.* 1997;73(2):198–203.

20. Cho E, Rosner BA, Feskanich D, Colditz GA. Risk factors and individual probabilities of melanoma for whites. *J Clin Oncol.* 2005;23(12):2669–2675.

21. Coit et al. Houghton Aea. NCCN Clinical Practice Guidelines in Oncology-Melanoma. (Accessed at January 31, 2009).

22. Balch CM, Soong SJ, Gershenwald JE, et al. Prognostic factors analysis of 17,600 melanoma patients: validation of the American Joint Committee on Cancer melanoma staging system. *J Clin Oncol.* 2001;19(16):3622–3634.

23. Morton DL, Thompson JF, Cochran AJ, et al. Sentinel-node biopsy or nodal observation in melanoma. *N Engl J Med.* 2006;355(13):1307–1317.

24. Karakousis CP, Balch CM, Urist MM, Ross MM, Smith TJ, Bartolucci AA. Local recurrence in malignant melanoma: long-term results of the multiinstitutional randomized surgical trial. *Ann Surg Oncol.* 1996;3(5):446–452.

25. Multicenter Selective Lymphadenectomy Triall II. 2007. (Accessed 2007, at http://www.clinicaltrials.gov/ct/show/NCT00297895?order=1.) (Accessed at January 31, 2009).

26. Hurley KE, Chapman PB. Helping melanoma patients decide whether to choose adjuvant high-dose interferon-alpha2b. *Oncologist.* 2005;10(9):739–742.

27. Tarhini AA, Shipe-Spotloe J, DeMark M, Agarwala SS, Kirkwood JM. Response to "helping melanoma patients decide whether to choose adjuvant high-dose interferon-alpha2b." *Oncologist.* 2006;11(5):538–539; author reply 9–40.

28. Kirkwood JM, Manola J, Ibrahim J, Sondak V, Ernstoff MS, Rao U. A pooled analysis of eastern cooperative oncology group and intergroup trials of adjuvant high-dose interferon for melanoma. *Clin Cancer Res.* 2004;10(5):1670–1677.

29. Gogas H, Ioannovich J, Dafni U, et al. Prognostic significance of autoimmunity during treatment of melanoma with interferon. *N Engl J Med.* 2006;354(7):709–718.

30. Kim KBea. A Phase III Randomized Trial of Adjuvant Biochemotherapy (BC) versus Interferon-alpha-2b (IFN) in Patients (pts) with High Risk for Melanoma Recurrence. *J Clin Oncol.* 2006; *ASCO Annual Meeting Proceedings Part I.* 24(18S):8003.

31. Spitler LE, Grossbard ML, Ernstoff MS, et al. Adjuvant therapy of stage III and IV malignant melanoma using granulocyte-macrophage colony-stimulating factor. *J Clin Oncol.* 2000;18(8):1614–1621.

32. Balch CM, Soong SJ, Murad TM, Smith JW, Maddox WA, Durant JR. A multifactorial analysis of melanoma. IV. Prognostic factors in 200 melanoma patients with distant metastases (stage III). *J Clin Oncol.* 1983;1(2):126–134.

33. Wong JH, Skinner KA, Kim KA, Foshag LJ, Morton DL. The role of surgery in the treatment of nonregionally recurrent melanoma. *Surgery.* 1993;113(4):389–394.

34. Friedel G, Pastorino U, Buyse M, et al. Resection of lung metastases: long-term results and prognostic analysis based on 5206 cases—the International Registry of Lung Metastases. *Zentralblatt fur Chirurgie.* 1999;124(2):96–103.

35. Anderson CM, Buzaid AC, Legha SS. Systemic treatments for advanced cutaneous melanoma. *Oncology.* 1995;9(11):1149–1158; discussion 63–64, 67–68.

36. Bleehen NM, Newlands ES, Lee SM, et al. Cancer Research Campaign phase II trial of temozolomide in metastatic melanoma. *J Clin Oncol.* 1995;13(4):910–913.

37. Keilholz U, Goey SH, Punt CJ, et al. Interferon alfa-2a and interleukin-2 with or without cisplatin in metastatic melanoma: a randomized trial of the European Organization for Research and Treatment of Cancer Melanoma Cooperative Group. *J Clin Oncol.* 1997;15(7):2579–2588.

38. Kaufmann R, Spieth K, Leiter U, et al. Temozolomide in combination with interferon-alfa versus temozolomide alone in patients with advanced metastatic melanoma: a randomized, phase III, multicenter study from the Dermatologic Cooperative Oncology Group. *J Clin Oncol.* 2005;23(35):9001–9007.

39. Rosenberg SA, Yang JC, Topalian SL, et al. Treatment of 283 consecutive patients with metastatic melanoma or renal cell cancer using high-dose bolus interleukin 2. *JAMA.* 1994;271(12):907–913.

40. Varker KA, Biber JE, Kefauver C, et al. A randomized phase 2 trial of Bevacizumab with or without daily low-dose interferon alfa-2b in metastatic malignant melanoma. *Ann Surg Oncol.* 2007;14(8):2367–2376.

41. Dranoff G. CTLA-4 blockade: unveiling immune regulation. *J Clin Oncol.* 2005;23(4):662–664.

42. Maker AV, Phan GQ, Attia P, et al. Tumor regression and autoimmunity in patients treated with cytotoxic T lymphocyte-associated antigen 4 blockade and interleukin 2: a phase I/II study. *Ann Surg Oncol.* 2005;12(12):1005–1016.

43. Parmiani G, Castelli C, Santinami M, Rivoltini L. Melanoma immunology: past, present and future. *Curr Opin Oncol.* 2007;19(2):121–127.

44. Weber LW, Bowne WB, Wolchok JD, et al. Tumor immunity and autoimmunity induced by immunization with homologous DNA. *J Clin Invest.* 1998;102(6):1258–1264.

45. Turk MJ, Wolchok JD, Guevara-Patino JA, Goldberg SM, Houghton AN. Multiple pathways to tumor immunity and concomitant autoimmunity. *Immunol Rev.* 2002;188:122–135.

46. Rosenberg SA, Dudley ME. Cancer regression in patients with metastatic melanoma after the transfer of autologous antitumor lymphocytes. *Proc Natl Acad Sci USA.* 2004;101(Suppl 2):14639–14645.

47. Morgan RA, Dudley ME, Wunderlich JR, et al. Cancer regression in patients after transfer of genetically engineered lymphocytes. *Science.* 2006;314(5796):126–129.

48. Davies H, Bignell GR, Cox C, et al. Mutations of the BRAF gene in human cancer. *Nature.* 2002;417(6892):949–954.

49. Solit DB, Garraway LA, Pratilas CA, et al. BRAF mutation predicts sensitivity to MEK inhibition. *Nature.* 2006;439(7074):358–362.

50. Curtin JA, Busam K, Pinkel D, Bastian BC. Somatic activation of KIT in distinct subtypes of melanoma. *J Clin Oncol.* 2006;24(26):4340–4346.

51. Kalinsky K, Haluska FG. Novel inhibitors in the treatment of metastatic melanoma. *Expert Rev Anticancer Ther.* 2007;7(5):715–724.

Evaluation and Treatment of Lymphoma

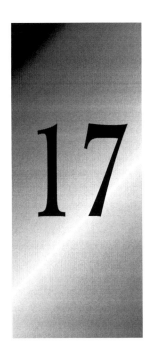

Enrica Marchi
Jasmine Zain
Owen A. O'Connor

The lymphomas represent one of the most heterogenous and diverse set of malignancies known to medicine. Underneath the umbrella of lymphoma exist some of the most rapidly growing cancers known to science, including diseases such as Burkitt lymphoma and lymphoblastic lymphoma/leukemia, as well as some of the slowest and most indolent cancers such as small lymphocytic lymphoma and follicular lymphoma. This remarkable diversity of diseases imposes significant challenges on pathologists and clinicians who seek to understand and elucidate what are sometimes subtle differences between the related subtypes of lymphoma. The understanding and diagnosis of lymphoma relies heavily on standard techniques of immunophenotyping, flow cytometry, cytogenetics, and the latest techniques in molecular biology, such as polymerase chain reaction (PCR) and fluorescent in situ hybridization (FISH). More recently, gene expression profiling of tumor samples has led to further understanding of these diseases. The improved understanding of the biological differences between the different forms of lymphoma has afforded us enormous opportunities to tailor specific treatments that are beginning to go well beyond simple CHOP-based chemotherapy.

All lymphomas are derived from lymphocytes, a form of white blood cell routinely generated by pluripotent hematopoietic stem cells, which reside in the intramedullary compartment of the bone marrow. There are three major lymphocyte populations that contribute to a functional immune system: B cells, T cells, and natural killer (NK) cells. These different types of lymphocytes mediate distinctly different immune effector functions. Surface proteins and receptors used in antigen recognition and mediating cellular immunity help differentiate these subsets of lymphocytes. For example, the B-cell receptor (BCR) and surface immunoglobulin (sIg) are found only on B cells, the T-cell receptor (TCR) is found on T cells, and clusters of differentiation (CD) are found on B cells, T cells, and NK cells. The variable expression of these and other proteins, form the basis for techniques in immunohistochemistry to differentiate the subpopulations of lymphocytes. While the details regarding the ontogeny of B cells and T cells is well beyond the scope of this chapter, the differentiation of these cells involves a multitude of steps in lymphoid organs, including the lymph node, spleen, thymus, and submucosal tissues (eg, Pyers patches in the gastrointestinal tract). During this complex process, lymphocytes "learn" to differentiate self from nonself, and in the process begin to form the major arms of our immune system: humoral immune responses, which are B-cell dependent, and cell mediated immunity, which is T-cell and NK-cell dependent. The type of lymphoma that develops typically depends on where in this ontogeny the cells become dysregulated. Figures 17.1 and 17.2 provide a schematic of B-cell and T-cell ontogeny, highlighting the different points in differentiation where different subtypes of lymphoma arise.

KEY POINTS

- All lymphomas are derived from lymphocytes, a form of white blood cell routinely generated by pluripotent hematopoietic stem cells.
- Non-Hodgkin lymphoma (NHL) comprises 5% of all malignancies and represents the fifth most common cancer in the United States. It is the most common hematologic malignancy in adults in the United States.
- Depending on the classification scheme used, there are considered to be more than 60 different subtypes of lymphoma.
- Immunosuppression, as a result of congenital or acquired medical conditions, a variety of autoimmune disorders, and certain infections is an acknowledged risk factor for the development of NHL.
- According to the WHO classification, NHLs are divided into: (1) B-cell neoplasms, which are further divided in *precursor* B-cell lymphoblastic leukemia/lymphoma and *mature* B-cell neoplasms; and (2) T-cell neoplasms, which are divided into the *immature* T-cell leukemia/lymphoma, and *mature* or post-thymic T-cell and natural killer (NK)-cell neoplasms such as peripheral T-cell lymphoma not otherwise specified (PTCL NOS) (Tables 17.1 and 17.2).
- The most common clinical presentation of NHL is painless and slowly progressive peripheral lymphadenopathy.

- Perhaps the most critical element in the diagnosis and treatment of a patient with lymphoma is making the right histopathologic assessment.
- Chemotherapy remains the most important modality for managing most patients with lymphoma, and different regimens are employed depending upon the disease. Radiotherapy still plays a critical role in selected cases.
- Rituximab, the first monoclonal antibody approved by the U.S. Food and Drug Administration for the treatment of any cancer, targets the CD20 molecule presents on the surface of B cells. Randomized studies have demonstrated its activity in follicular lymphoma (FL), mantle cell lymphoma, and diffuse large B-cell lymphoma (DLBCL) in untreated or relapsing patients.
- Approximately two-thirds of patients with advanced Hodgkin disease (HD) can be cured with the current approaches to treatment.
- Because most HD patients can be cured with modern treatment modalities and will have a life expectancy equivalent to age-matched healthy individuals, it is important in the formulation of the treatment strategy to take into account not just the acute treatment-related toxicities, but also the long-term side effects of the chemotherapy and radiotherapy.

NON-HODGKIN LYMPHOMA

Introduction

Non-Hodgkin lymphoma (NHL) refers to all malignancies of the lymphoid system, with the exception of Hodgkin disease. The development of the lymphoid system is a highly regulated process, characterized by differential expression of innumerable cell-surface and intracytoplasmic proteins. Dysregulation of either the number or function of the cells can result in humoral deficiency, autoimmunity, or malignancy. Despite the variability in cell of origin and clinical presentation of these diseases, there are several clinical and pathologic features common to many lymphoproliferative diseases. Lymphadenopathy and splenomegaly, as well as changes in circulating lymphocytes and quantitative immunoglobulins, can be seen in malignant and benign lymphoproliferative diseases alike. However, all malignant diseases are characterized by an accumulation of proliferating lymphocytes, a process that can take years or hours, depending on the discrete subtype of lymphoma.

Although not all lymphomas originate in lymph nodes, most will invariably involve them at some point during the course of the disease. Historically, the cell of origin and the clinical behavior of the different subtypes of lymphoma have formed the basis for the widely differing nomenclatures used to classify these diseases. Over the past 100 years, many classification schemes have been proposed, leading to considerable confusion in communicating a specific diagnosis to patients and colleagues, a conundrum that has made interpreting the literature across eras of time virtually impossible. These classifications have evolved in parallel to our understanding of lymphoma biology. They reflect and encompass the immunological, cytogenetic, and clinical data that is available to describe these different subtypes. The most recent classification of NHLs, the revised American-European lymphoma (REAL) classification (1), was proposed in 1994 (Table 17.1), and has recently been updated by the World Health Organization (WHO) (2). This classification essentially divides these diseases into B-cell or T-cell/NK-cell neoplasms, which are yet further subdivided into precursor (ie, less differentiated) or mature (ie, more differentiated)

B- and T- Cell Development

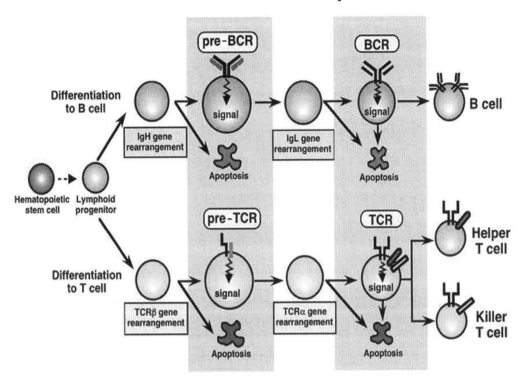

Schematic of B- and T-cell ontogeny.

FIGURE 17.1

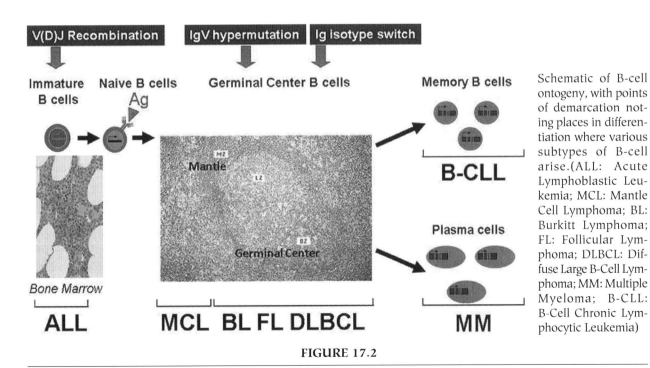

Schematic of B-cell ontogeny, with points of demarcation noting places in differentiation where various subtypes of B-cell arise.(ALL: Acute Lymphoblastic Leukemia; MCL: Mantle Cell Lymphoma; BL: Burkitt Lymphoma; FL: Follicular Lymphoma; DLBCL: Diffuse Large B-Cell Lymphoma; MM: Multiple Myeloma; B-CLL: B-Cell Chronic Lymphocytic Leukemia)

FIGURE 17.2

TABLE 17.1

Who Classification of Non Hodgkin Lymphomas

B-CELL NEOPLASMS

Precursor B-cell neoplasm
Precursor B-lymphoblastic leukemia/lymphoma (precursor B-cell acute lymphoblastic leukemia)
Mature (peripheral) B-cell neoplasms
B-cell chronic lymphocytic leukemia/small lymphocytic lymphoma
B-cell prolymphocytic leukemia
Lymphoplasmacytic lymphoma
Splenic marginal zone B-cell lymphoma (þ¹ villous lymphocytes)
Hairy cell leukemia
Plasma cell myeloma/plasmacytoma
Extranodal marginal zone B-cell lymphoma of MALT type
Nodal marginal zone B-cell lymphoma (þ¹ monocytoid B cells)
Follicular lymphoma
Mantle cell lymphoma
Diffuse large B-cell lymphoma
Burkitt lymphoma/ Burkitt cell leukemia

T- AND NK-CELL NEOPLASMS

Precursor T-cell neoplasm
Precursor T-lymphoblastic lymphoma/leukemia (precursor T-cell acute lymphoblastic leukemia)
Mature (peripheral) T-cell neoplasms
T-cell prolymphocytic leukemia
T-cell granular lymphocytic leukemia
Aggressive NK-cell leukemia
Adult T-cell lymphoma/leukemia (HTLV1þ)
Extranodal NK/T-cell lymphoma, nasal type
Enteropathy-type T-cell lymphoma
Hepatosplenic gd T-cell lymphoma
Subcutaneous panniculitis-like T-cell lymphoma
Mycosis fungoides/Sezary syndrome
Anaplastic large cell lymphoma, T/null cell, primary cutaneous type
Peripheral T-cell lymphoma, not otherwise characterized
Angioimmunoblastic T-cell lymphoma
Anaplastic large cell lymphoma, T/null cell, primary systemic type

forms of lymphoma. Depending on the classification scheme used, there are considered to be 30–35 different subtypes of lymphoma, comprising a diverse set of diseases with widely varying natural histories, each possessing its own subtleties in presentation, prognosis and management. Malignancies such as precursor B- or T-lymphoblastic leukemia/lymphoma evolve in the bone marrow, frequently giving rise to very high leukocyte counts (lymphocytosis) and generalized lymphadenopathy. Lymphoproliferative malignancies such as Burkitt lymphoma exhibit a penchant for involving the central nervous system. While potentially curable, these lymphomas are considered some of the most rapidly growing cancers known to science, and require aggressive chemotherapy that can continue for up to two years. In contrast, mature forms of B-cell and T-cell lymphoma, such as chronic lymphocytic leukemia (CLL) and mycosis fungoides, respectively, are more indolent diseases that often do not require treatment until they become symptomatic or threaten vital organ function.

Epidemiology and Etiology

NHL comprises 5% of all malignancies and represents the fifth most common cancer in the United States. It is the most common hematologic malignancy in adults in the United States. An estimated 66,000 cases of NHL were predicted for 2008, with an estimated 19,000 deaths, giving the disease a case fatality ratio of nearly 30%. Between 1950 and 1999, the incidence of NHL increased by about 3%–5% per year in the United States, accounting for a nearly 90% increase over those five decades. While the etiology for the increase in lymphoma is still poorly understood, HIV is thought to account for only a marginal component at best. Fortunately, this trend has changed over the recent past, with a nearly flat or decreasing incidence over the past five years. Despite the numerous claims, no specific etiology can explain these changes in incidence.

The overall incidence of lymphoma is higher in males (3). Irrespective of race, the incidence for males is approximately 23.5 per 100,000; in females, the incidence is approximately 16.3 per 100,000. The median age at the diagnosis across all forms of NHL is 67 years. Like many forms of cancer, there is a trend of increasing incidence as a function of age. Approximately 1.7% of cases of NHL are diagnosed under age 20; 4.1% of cases between ages 20 and 34; 7.4% of cases between ages 35 and 44; 14.0%–19% of cases between ages 45 and 64. The highest percentage, and approximately 23% of cases, are seen between ages 65 and 84. Interestingly, there is a significant decrease in NHL incidence for those older than age 85, where the incidence is only 8.5% of all cases. As noted earlier, the incidence of NHL has been rising over the past several decades (4), increasing from an age-adjusted rate of 11.1 per 100,000 in 1975 to 20.4 in 2004. Increases were seen in both nodal and extranodal subtypes of lymphoma. While increases were seen across both genders, the increase was greatest for female patients, with the male to female ratio changing from 1.26 in 1990–1992 to 1.13 in 2002–2004. Increases have been observed over time in the percentage of low-grade and T-cell/NK-cell subtypes compared with other aggressive histologic subtypes. Not surprisingly, incidence also varies significantly by race, with whites exhibiting a much higher risk of lymphoma compared to African-Americans and Asian Americans. In whites, the incidence rate is 24.3 and 17.1 per 100,000 males and females, respectively; while in African Americans, the incidence is 18.4 (males) and 12.1 (females) per 100,000; and 19.2 and 14.6 per 100,000 Hispanic males and females respectively. These differences in incidence across different ethnic groups are not uniform across all histologies. For example, the indolent lymphomas are far less common in African Americans, while diseases such as peripheral T-cell lymphoma, mycosis fungoides, and Sezary Syndrome are more common in African American populations.

The prognosis for patients with NHL improved significantly between 1990–1992 and 2002–2004 for both overall survival and age-specific survival. Overall, 5- and 10-year survival improved from 50.4% and 39.4%, respectively, in 1990–1992, to 66.8% (+16.4 percentage points) and 56.3% (+16.9 percentage points), respectively, in 2002–2004 ($P < .001$ for both). The greatest gains were seen in patients aged 15–44 years, for whom five-year relative survival increased by over 25%. NHL mortality rates peaked in 1997 at 8.9, after which they slowly decreased, reaching a rate of 7.0 in 2004.

While the etiologic factors contributing to lymphoma are generally not well defined, a number of risk factors have been described. Immunosuppression as a result of congenital or acquired medical conditions is an acknowledged risk factor. Immunosuppression associated with solid organ transplant is a well-known risk factor for lymphomas, in particular post-transplantation lymphoproliferative disorders (PTLD) (5,6). The overall incidence of PTLD is approximately 2%–8%, being highest in patients undergoing lung, gastrointestinal tract, and heart transplants, and lowest in patients receiving renal and liver transplants. For most of these patients, the disease develops approximately one or two years following the solid organ transplant, and it is frequently positive for Epstein-Barr virus (EBV), which is believed to result from impaired host immune surveillance of latently infected B cells. PTLD manifesting later is frequently EBV-negative, and carries a worse prognosis. Each transplant subtype has distinct features including organ source, duration and extent of immunosuppression, patient selection, risk of allograft involvement with PTLD, and variable merits for reduction of immunosuppression following a new diagnosis of PTLD. Consequently, each different type of transplant is unique with regard to the features of the associated PTLD (7).

Multiple autoimmune disorders (8,9), including Sjögren's disease (10), lupus, and rheumatoid arthritis, have also been linked with NHL. Most rheumatologists and oncologists consider autoimmune disorders and lymphoproliferative malignancies to exist on either end of a spectrum of lymphocyte dysregulation. That is, patients with autoimmune disorders are at higher risk for developing lymphoma, and patients with lymphoma are at higher risk for developing concomitant autoimmune disorders. Because many autoimmune disorders are treated with immunosuppressive therapy, it is often difficult to determine whether the underlying autoimmune disorder, or its immunosuppressive treatment, is responsible for the lymphoma.

Another increasingly important risk factor for lymphoma is infection, especially viral and bacterial infections. Patients who are HIV positive have a 59- to 104-fold higher risk of developing lymphoma compared to those who are HIV negative, with aggressive forms of NHL such as Burkitt and diffuse large B-cell lymphoma being the most likely (11–13). Variations in the geographic distribution of lymphoma have led to an improved understanding of many viral risk factors. Some lymphoma subtypes demonstrate marked geographic variation and association with very specific viruses. EBV is known to be a causal agent of a nasal subtype of NK-cell lymphoma in South America and Asia as well as endemic Burkitt lymphoma in Africa. These diseases, both very aggressive, require distinctly different treatments. Another retrovirus, human T-cell lymphotropic virus-1 (HTVL-1), is known to cause adult T-cell leukemia/lymphoma (HTLV-1 ATLL) in Caribbean, Asian, and African populations. Hepatitis C has been associated with B-cell lymphoma in northern Italy and Japan. In addition to viruses, other infectious agents have clear links to the development of NHL. For example, Helicobacter pylori is likely the etiologic agent leading to gastric mucosa-associated lymphoid tissue (MALT) lymphomas (14). MALT lymphomas were first described by Isaacson and Wright in 1983 in a small series of patients with low-grade B-cell gastrointestinal lymphomas. In H. pylori-related MALT lymphomas of the stomach, a course of antibiotics can not only eradicate the infection, but can induce cure of the lymphoma in approximately 75% of cases. The 25% that are unresponsive to antibiotics either carry a chromosomal translocation t(11;18)(q21;q21) or demonstrate a clinically advanced stage of the disease (15–17). Some studies suggest that eradication rates achieved by the first-line treatment with a proton pump inhibitor (PPI), clarithromycin, and amoxicillin have decreased to 70%–85%, in part due to increasing clarithromycin resistance in new strains of H. pylori. Eradication rates may also be lower with 7- versus 14-day regimens. Bismuth-containing quadruple regimens for 7–14 days are another first-line treatment option. Sequential therapy for 10 days has shown promise in Europe, but requires validation in North America. The most commonly used salvage regimen in patients with persistent *H. pylori* infection is bismuth quadruple therapy, though more recent data from Europe suggests that a PPI, levofloxacin, and amoxicillin for 10 days is more effective and better tolerated than bismuth quadruple therapy for persistent *H. pylori* infection (18).

Although MALT lymphomas occur most frequently in the stomach, they have also been described in various nongastrointestinal sites, such as the salivary gland, conjunctiva, thyroid, orbit, lung, breast, kidney, skin, liver, uterus, and prostate; some of these locations have also been linked to a specific infectious etiology. For example, *Borrelia burgdorferi*, transmitted by a tick, has been associated with some forms of extranodal marginal zone lymphoma of the skin (frequently referred to as skin-associated lymphoid tissue or SALT) (19), which has been successfully treated with doxycycline. Interestingly, however, nodal forms of these lymphomas do not appear to be associated with any infectious agents and may represent a genetically distinct subcategory of the marginal zone lymphomas.

Besides infectious etiologies, a number of different environmental factors have been associated with lymphoma, including exposure to pesticides and herbicides in farmers, and an array of occupational chemical exposures for those working in specific industries, such as chemists, dry cleaners, printing workers, wood workers, beauticians, and cosmetologists. While some of these associations are stronger than others, most links between lymphoma and a discrete environmental factor remain uncertain at best.

Classification

The histopathologic classification of lymphoma has evolved over the years as our understanding of the disease has improved. Despite this progress, lymphoma classification has been a source of confusion for clinicians and pathologists alike. In the last decade or so, much new information has become available regarding the morphological features, immunophenotype, and cytogenetic differences between many forms of lymphoma. This refined understanding has resulted in recognition of new entities and refinement of previously recognized disease categories. Prior to 1994, the National Cancer Institute (NCI) Working Formulation (20) and the Kiel (21,22) classification were used in the United States and in Europe, respectively. However, these classification schemes inadequately differentiated important subtypes of lymphoma, and were associated with a generally poor concordance among different hematopathologists. In 1994, the REAL classification was proposed as a mutually acceptable system, based on morphologic, immunophenotyping, and cytogenetic characteristics. The classification of NHLs has become a list of well-defined disease entities, each with its own distinctive clinical and biological features. Refinements of the REAL classification were recently incorporated into the WHO classification, in which morphologic, genetic, immunophenotypic, and clinical features are all used in defining discrete disease entities. According to the WHO classification, NHLs are divided into: (1) B-cell neoplasms, which are further divided in *precursor* B-cell lymphoblastic leukemia/lymphoma and *mature* B-cell neoplasms; and (2) T-cell neoplasms, which are divided into the *immature* T-cell leukemia/lymphoma, and *mature* or post-thymic T-cell and NK-cell neoplasms such as peripheral T-cell lymphoma not-otherwise-specified (PTCL NOS) (Tables 17.1 and 17.2).

Signs and Symptoms

Two-thirds of patients with any form of lymphoma present with lymphadenopathy; however, extranodal disease is common and can involve any organ. The presentation can be varied, depending on the subtype and location of the disease. In the case of indolent lymphomas (ie, chronic lymphocytic leukemia/lymphoma [CLL], follicular lymphoma, or marginal zone lymphoma), the most common clinical presentation is painless and slowly progressive peripheral lymphadenopathy. Primary extranodal presentation and symptoms including fever (ie, temperature higher than 38°C for three consecutive days, weight loss exceeding 10% of body weight in six months, and drenching night sweats, a grouping of symptoms known as B symptoms). B symptoms frequently arise as a consequence of cytokines released by the malignant disease; these symptoms might bring the disease to the physician's attention. However, B symptoms are uncommon at presentation, although both extranodal presentation and B symptoms can become common in patients with advanced stages of the disease. In the case of aggressive lymphoma, the clinical presentation can be more varied. Symptoms can be related to the rapid growth of the disease in a particular part of the body, causing compromise of some vital organ function (dyspnea in patients with primary mediastinal lymphoma; hydronephrosis or lower extremity edema in patients with diffuse large B-cell or Burkitt lymphoma in the pelvis). Alternatively, symptoms may be associated with an acutely enlarging lymph node associated with pain, or with a cosmetic finding. While superior vena cava syndrome is unusual in patients with lymphoma, even those with large bulky mediastinal disease, the development of pleural and pericardial effusions can be common in those with thoracic disease. These presentations are due to the presence of bulky lymphoma, or to its involvement of the parietal or visceral pleura. The very rapidly growing Burkitt

TABLE 17.2

Immunophenotypic Features and Molecular Characteristics of Non Hodgkin Lymphomas

Subtype	Frequency	Immunophenotype	Molecular lesions
DLBCL	31	CD20+	Bcl2, Bcl6,cMYC
FL	22	CD20+,CD10+,CD5-	Bcl2
SLL/CLL	6	CD20 weak, CD5+, CD23+	+12,del(13q)
MCL	6	CD20+,CD5+,CD23-	Cyclin D1
PTCL	6	CD20-,CD3+	Variable
MZL (MALT)	5	CD20+,CD5-,CD23-	Bcl10,+3,+18
PML	2	CD20+	Variable
ALCL	2	CD20-,CD3+,CD30+,CD15-,EMA+	ALK
LL (T/B)	2	T cell CD3+,B cell CD19+	Variable,TCL-3
Burkitt-like	2	CD20+,CD10-,CD5-	cMYC,Bcl2
MZL (Nodal)	1	CD20+,CD10-,CD23-,CD5-	+3,+18
SLL,PL	1	CD20+,cIg=,CD5-,CD23-	Pax-5
BL	1	CD20+,CD10+,CD5-	c-MYC
TOTAL	88		

DLBCL: Diffuse Large B-Cell Lymphoma; FL: Follicular Lymphoma; SLL: Small Lymphocytic Lymphoma; CLL: Chronic Lymphocytic Leukemia; MCL: Mantle Cell Lymphoma; PTCL: Peripheral T-Cell Lymphoma; MZL: Marginal Zone Lymphoma; PML: Primary Mediastinal Lymphoma; ALCL: Anaplastic Large Cell Lymphoma; LL: Lymphocytic Leukemia; PL: Prolymphocytic Leukemia; BL: Burkitt Lymphoma.

lymphoma (doubling time in a range of 36–48 hours) commonly presents as massive intra-abdominal disease, leading patients to experience a host of symptoms, ranging from bowel obstruction to hydronephrosis to lower extremity edema. Bone marrow involvement is more frequent in the indolent lymphomas, but can be seen in up to 25% of cases in diffuse large B-cell lymphoma (DLBCL). Patients presenting with intramedullary involvement of the bone marrow will often develop cytopenias, which are frequently detected incidentally on routine complete blood counts (CBC). The presence of B symptoms is considered an ominous sign, although it is not part of the International Prognostic Index (IPI), as discussed below.

Diagnosis and Staging

Perhaps the most critical element in the diagnosis and treatment of a patient with lymphoma is making the right histopathologic assessment. This requires consultation with an expert hematopathologist familiar with the latest techniques in immunophenotyping and cytogenetics. For this reason, it is imperative that every diagnosis of lymphoma be based on an adequate specimen, which should ideally include an excisional biopsy of an involved lymph node or an incisional biopsy of a large mass. Under no circumstances should a fine needle aspiration (FNA) be used to document a first-time diagnosis of lymphoma. In select cases, a bone marrow biopsy can be sufficient for a diagnosis in a patient with

CLL or acute lymphoblastic leukemia (ALL). Evaluation of lymph node architecture plays a crucial role in aiding the hematopathologist in differentiating normal from malignant cells.

NHL often involves discontiguous lymph node sites and extranodal areas. For this reason, total body computed tomography (CT) imaging of the neck, chest, abdomen, and pelvis are required to fully appreciate the extent of disease. CT imaging provides clear interpretation of anatomy and is best used to measure changes in size of abnormal lymph nodes or extranodal masses. However, given the "normal" presence of lymphatic tissue throughout the body, CT imaging can be unsatisfactory for delineating an enlarged fibrotic node that has resolved its lymphomatous infiltration from one with active NHL and cannot differentiate viable from dead disease. The (18)F-fluoro-deoxyglucose positron emission tomography (FDG-PET) has emerged as an important imaging tool in many forms of lymphoma based on the increased accumulation of FDG in the sites of active lymphoma (23). The increased sensitivity of PET imaging is capable of providing additional detail regarding extent of disease, and is especially useful in differentiating viable disease from fibrotic tissue. Unfortunately, it cannot distinguish lymphoma from sites of active inflammation, which also represents a collection of highly metabolically active, nonmalignant cells. Most recently, PET imaging has begun to play a major role in the prognostication of patients with diffuse large B-cell lymphoma and Hodgkin disease receiving active therapy. The PET scan in these cases serves as a means to evaluate true in vivo chemosensitivity. Patients who are able to convert their PET scan from positive to negative at the interim restaging analysis have been demonstrated to have superior outcomes compared to those patients who fail to convert their PET scan (25). This type of information is now being used to tailor and individualize therapy for patients based upon their functional imaging studies (26).

Almost all patients with NHL require a bone marrow biopsy at diagnosis. While there are some exceptions to this rule, a bone marrow biopsy will determine the presence of disease in the marrow before starting treatment, and can be important in determining whether a patient is responding or progressing through a particular treatment. Certainly, a patient with lymphoma presenting with cytopenia deserves a bone marrow biopsy to ascertain the cause of the bone marrow suppression. Evaluation of the gastrointestinal tract and examination of Waldeyer's ring might be warranted in patients MALT and mantle cell lymphoma, two diseases that frequently involve these particular sites. Although its use in this setting is controversial, lumbar puncture should be performed in patients with Burkitt lymphoma, patients with testicular or Waldeyer's Ring involvement, and certainly in any patient presenting with a focal neurological exam.

Compared to the solid tumor malignancies, the staging of lymphoma is relatively straightforward, and employs the Ann Arbor classification shown in Table 17.3. Staging is based on the involvement of broad lymph node regions. For example, stage I is comprised of involvement of a single lymph node region, whereas stage II disease involves more than one lymph node region on the same side of the diaphragm. Stage III disease is defined as disease both above and below the diaphragm, and stage IV disease is characterized by involvement of one or more extralymphatic organs, with or without associated lymph node involvement. The letter 'E' is added to the stage to denote involvement of an extranodal sites, the letter 'S' when there is the splenic involvement, and the letter 'X' when there is bulky disease (eg, <10 cm in greatest transverse diameter). Frequently, the letters A or B will denote the absence or presence of constitutional or B symptoms.

Prognostic Factors

Unlike most solid tumors, stage alone does not define the complete risk of a particular patient, an observation that should be intuitive when dealing with a malignancy born in the bone marrow and disseminated via hematogenous and lymphatic spread. Clearly, patients with similar diagnoses can have varied clinical presentations and outcomes. Reliable prognostic markers play

\multicolumn{2}{c}{TABLE 17.3}
\multicolumn{2}{c}{*Ann Arbor Staging Classification for Non Hodgkin Lymphomas*}
STAGE	**AREA OF INVOLVEMENT**
I	One lymph node region
IE	One extralymphatic organ or site
II	Two or more lymph node regions on the same side of the diaphragm
IIE	One extralymphatic organ or site (localized) in addition to criteria for stage II
III	Lymph node regions on both sides of the diaphragm
IIIE	One extralymphatic organ or site (localized) in addition to criteria for stage III
IIIS	Spleen in addition to criteria for stage III
IIISE	Spleen and one extralymphatic organ or site (localized) in addiction to criteria for stage III
IV	One or more extralymphatic organs with or without associated lymph node involvement (diffuse or disseminated); involved organs should be designed by subscript letters

a valuable role in aiding the clinician in discriminating these various subgroups of patients, sometimes by leading to different treatment recommendations based on the prognostic score. Historically, a large number of clinical and molecular prognostic factors have been reported in the literature (27–33). However, the recent introduction of monoclonal antibody-based therapies such as rituximab (Rituxan) have revolutionized the outcome of patients and reduced the reliability of the older prognostic scores, which were largely developed in the pre-rituximab era. As such, many of these prognostic models have had to be revalidated given the change in the standard treatment (34). Perhaps the most universally applied prognostic model is the IPI (35). This score was developed based upon 2,031 patients in 16 different institutions and cooperative groups in United States, Europe, and Canada, and has become the primary means by which clinicians predict outcome of patients with aggressive NHL. Based on the number of negative prognostic features present at the time of the diagnosis (aged 60 or older; Ann Arbor Stage III or IV; serum LDH level above normal; two or more extranodal sites; and performance status greater than or equal to ECOG 2), four prognostic groups were identified. The four risk groups (low, low-intermediate, high-intermediate, and high risk) had distinctly different rates of complete response, relapse-free survival, and overall survival. For example, the low-risk group exhibited a complete-response rate of 87% and a 5-year overall survival of 73%, whereas the high-risk group had a complete-response rate of only 44% and a 5-year overall survival of only 26%. Since the publication of the IPI, other groups have formulated their own more disease specific prognostic models. For example, in follicular lymphoma (FL), the Follicular Lymphoma International Prognostic Index (FLIPI) (36) stratifies patients similar to the IPI. In this case, a disease-specific prognostic index makes intuitive sense given the widely different behavior of these two diseases. Application of the IPI to patients with the FL does not differentiate the different prognostic categories well (ie, there is an over-representation of patients with low to low-intermediate risk). Again, based on a retrospective review of a large collection of patients with FL, a multivariate analysis led to the development of the following five independent risk factors: hemoglobin level lower that 12 g/dl, serum LDH higher than the upper normal value, Ann Arbor Stage III-IV, number of nodal sites higher than four, and aged older than 60 years. The FLIPI index defines three risk groups: low (0–1 risk factor), intermediate (2 risk factors), and high (≥3 risk factors). Similar to the IPI in aggressive lymphoma, the risk category effectively stratified patients; those patients in the low-risk group exhibited a five year overall survival of 90.6%; the intermediate-risk group exhibited a five year overall survival of 77.6%, and the high-risk group had a 5-year overall survival of only 52.5%.

This approach is gradually being applied to many individual subtypes of lymphoma, including the peripheral T-cell lymphomas. The concept is that the varying biological the 3 basis for different lymphomas will be reflected differentially across the diverse subtypes of the disease. For example, a prognostic index in peripheral T-cell lymphoma unspecified (PTCLU) called the Prognostic Index for PTCLU (PIT) (37) is based on four clinical variables: age (older than 60 years), PS (≥2), LDH level (more than 1× normal) and bone marrow involvement. The PIT differs from IPI because the variables related to the extension of the disease (stage and number of extranodal sites involved) do not seem to adversely affect prognosis. The PIT identified four groups of patients: group 1, with no adverse factors; group 2, with one factor; group 3, with two factors; and group 4, with three or four factors, and was successful in identifying groups with different clinical outcome. For the patients in the group 1, the 5-year survival rate was 62.3%; for patients in group 2, 52.9%; for patients in group 3, 32.9%; and for patients in group 4, 18.6%. The PIT does not include tumor-specific factors, and a new score was developed that integrates both clinical and tumor-specific characteristics (eg, Ki-67 marking ≥80%) (38). These prognostic scores are useful for designing risk-adapted therapy that is personalized to an individual's particular disease. Based on the fact that aggressive lymphomas are considered curable and indolent lymphomas generally are not, the therapeutic approach for each kind of lymphoma, let alone specific patients, can differ dramatically. As such, for patients with generally curable disease, the tolerance for toxicity is higher given the return for possible cure, whereas for patients with an incurable disease, the tolerance for toxicity is typically much lower given the goals of treatment are oriented towards chronic management.

PRINCIPLES OF THERAPY

Chemotherapy remains the most important modality for managing most patients with lymphoma, and different regimens are employed depending upon the disease. While a detailed discussion of these different regimens is well beyond the scope of this chapter, suffice it to say that the selection of any given therapy is based upon an assessment of host morbidities and toxicity, with the goal of selecting the optimal treatment associated with the most favorable side effect profile (Table 17.4). Despite the implementation of various newer strategies, radiotherapy still plays a critical role in selected cases. However, modern treatment strategies, including monoclonal antibodies targeting lymphoma-associated antigens, radioimmunotherapy, therapeutic vaccination, high-dose chemotherapy combined with autologous stem-cell transplantation (ASCT), and allogenic hematopoietic stem cell transplantation, have the potential to profoundly impact clinical outcomes in lymphoma therapy. Rituximab, for example, the first monoclonal antibody approved by the U.S. Food and Drug Administration (FDA) for the treatment of any cancer, targets the CD20 molecule presents on the surface of B cells. Randomized studies have demonstrated its activity in follicular lymphoma (FL), mantle cell lymphoma, and DLBCL (39), in untreated or relapsing patients. Noncomparative studies have shown activity in all other subtypes of B-cell lymphoma. Because of its high activity and low toxicity ratio, rituximab has transformed the outcome of patients with B-cell lymphoma. A combination regimen consisting of chemotherapy, rituximab, cyclophosphamide, doxorubicin, vincristine, and prednisone (R-CHOP), has been found to have the highest efficacy ever described with any chemotherapy in DLBCL and FL. The role of rituximab in the treatment of B-cell lymphomas has rapidly emerged from the relapsed setting to the front line for virtually every B-cell subtypes of NHL. Presently, the role of maintenance rituximab in indolent lymphomas after first-line therapy is being defined as is the integration of radioimmunotherapy into the first-line therapeutic regimens.

Radioimmunotherapy (RIT) combines radiation delivered by radioisotopes with the targeting effect of

TABLE 17.4
Chemotherapeutic Regimens for Non Hodgkin Lymphoma

REGIMEN	DOSE	ROUTE	FREQUENCY
CVP ± Rituximab			Every 21 days
Cyclophosphamide	750–1,000 mg/m²	IV	Day 1
Vincristine	1.4 mg/m	IV	Day 1
Prednisone	100 mg or 100 mg/m²	PO	Day 1–5
Rituximab	375 mg/m²	IV	Day 1
CHOP ± Rituximab			Every 21 or 14 days (with G-CSF)
Cyclophosphamide	750 mg/m²	IV	Day 1
Doxorubicin	50 mg/m²	IV	Day 1
Oncovin (Vincristine)	1.4 mg/mL (max 2 mg)	IV	Day 1
Prednisone	40 mg/m² or 100 mg/d	PO	Day1–5
Rituximab	or 100mg/m²/d	IV	Day 1
	375 mg/m²		
CHOEP ± Rituximab			Every 21 days
Cyclophosphamide	750 mg/m²	IV	Day 1
Doxorubicin	50 mg/m²	IV	Day 1
Etoposide	100 mg/m²	IV	Day 1–3
Oncovin (Vincristine)	1.4 mg/mL (max 2 mg)	IV	Day 1
Prednisone	100 mg/m²	PO	Day1–5
Rituximab	375 mg/m²	IV	Day 1
FND			Every 21–28 days (depending on hematologic recovery)
Fludarabine	25 mg/m²	IV	Day 1–3
Novantrone	10 mg/m²	IV	Day 1
Dexamethasone	20 mg	PO/ IV	Day1–5

monoclonal antibodies (40). Two radioimmunocon-jugates are currently approved for relapsed/resistant low-grade or transformed lymphoma: iodine-131 tositumomab and yttrium-90 ibritumomab tiuxetan. These agents are also effective in aggressive lymphoma, a transformed lymphoma arising from a preexisting low grade lymphoma. Their major toxicity is myelosuppression, although patients can also experience significant periods of thrombocytopenia following treatment with either of these agents. High-dose chemotherapy and ASCT has an established therapeutic role in the treatment of chemo-sensitive relapsed aggressive lymphoma, but has limited to no merit in chemorefractory disease. Recurrent disease is the major cause of treatment failure in all patient subsets not cured with the primary therapy. Methods for better eradication of underlying lymphoma are needed to improve outcome. Few effective treatment options exist for chemotherapy-refractory indolent or transformed NHL. Nonmyeloablative allogeneic stem cell transplantation can produce durable disease-free survival in patients with relapsed or refractory indolent NHL, even in those patients who have relapsed following an ASCT. Generally, outcomes were good in patients with untransformed disease and related donors, whereas patients with transformed disease did poorly. Long-term survivors report good overall functional status. Allogeneic SCT has usually been employed in patients with relapsed or refractory disease, with the aim of providing both a tumor-free graft and the postulated graft-versus-lymphoma (GVL) effect. In support of the latter, the first retrospective studies comparing progression-free survival curves of patients undergoing autologous or allogeneic SCT showed a statistically significant difference in favor of allografted patients. Most retrospective studies on this issue showed that patients treated with allogeneic

SCT were usually affected by more advanced or refractory disease, thus suggesting the existence of immune-mediated antitumor activity (41–43). The additional evidence of clinical and molecular responses following the withdrawal of immunosuppressive therapy or donor lymphocyte infusions further supported the idea of an underlying GVL effect (44,45). However, the main obstacle to a wide application of myeloablative allogeneic SCT as a salvage strategy was the high incidence of transplant-related mortality (TRM) that offset the benefit of the GVL effect in terms of overall survival (46,47). Reduced intensity or nonmyeloablative allogeneic transplant have been developed to decrease the up-front mortality associated with an allogeneic transplant while maintaining the graft versus leukemia effect. While this approach allows the application of this modality to patients who are older than age 60, graft versus host disease remains a major challenge, with an incidence of 60%–70%.

IMPLICATION FOR REHABILITATION MEDICINE

There remains a host of concerns regarding the long-term management of patients who either have been cured of, or are being chronically managed for, their lymphoma that are significant for the practicing physiatrist. First of all, lymphoma patients are often elderly, entering a treatment program with an already compromised functional or performance status. In addition, many drugs used for the treatment of NHL exhibit toxicities that more often than not can have deleterious effects on a host of different organ systems. Many agents exhibit neurotoxicity, which may affect sensory, motor, or proprioceptive nerve fibers in a manner that contributes to a compromise in performance status. Many of these drugs render virtually all patients areflexive, the collective effects of which can lead to increase falls or tripping. Some patients with lymphoproliferative malignancies may experience involvement of the spinal cord or CNS, leading to pain, or compromised motor function, with lower or upper extremity weakness. These patients will obviously require more focused attention to address the collection of issues associated with spinal cord compression syndromes (48). An often overlooked side-effect of both the disease and its treatment involves the tendency for enhanced bone loss, leading to osteopenia and osteoporosis. Virtually every patient with lymphoma will require steroids, some for long-term management, which will further accelerate osteoporosis. Treatment-related bone loss is well recognized in prostate cancer, due to overt hypogonadism, and in breast cancer, but few studies have evaluated the effect of chemotherapy alone on bone mineral density (BMD) compared to the same population cross matched by age. The association of chemotherapy and an increased risk of fracture and osteoporosis in elderly patients with NHL is well described (49). At the very least, assuming no contraindications to therapy, these patients should all be on calcium, vitamin D, and a bisphosphonate.

Bone marrow toxicity is the most common side effect of chemotherapy. It might present as anemia, leucopenia, or thrombocytopenia. Many elderly patients already have some compromise in their normal hematopoietic function, and following treatment may be left with some compromise in their blood counts. In addition, most patients who receive chemotherapy may incur compromise in their normal immune function that can last for 9–12 months, and may be at risk for various infections. Collectively, these patients may present with symptoms attributable to one cell lineage or another, including asthenia, tachycardia, and fatigue and dyspnea in anemic patients; fever, tachycardia, pain, dyspnea, and cellulitis in patients with leucopenia; and ecchymosis or epistaxis in patients with thrombocytopenia. The use of cytokines such as granulocyte-colony stimulating factor (GCSF) may be indicated for those patients with neutropenia, although recently, the use of erythropoietic stimulating factors has not been recommended for patients who are not actively receiving chemotherapy due to the increased risk of mortality (50,51).

HODGKIN LYMPHOMA

Introduction

In 1832, Sir Thomas Hodgkin presented the clinical history and the postmortem findings of the massive enlargement of the lymph nodes and spleens of seven patients in the first description of the disease (52). As late as 1865, Sir Samuel Wilks linked Thomas Hodgkin's name to the disease that he described as "Cases of the Enlargement of the Lymphatic Glands and Spleen (or Hodgkin's Disease)." In 1878, Greenfield was the first to publish a drawing of the pathognomonic "giant cells" that would later become known as the Reed-Sternberg cells, named after Carl Sternberg and Dorothy Reed (1902), who contributed the first definitive microscopic descriptions of Hodgkin disease. Despite the very strong evidence for the malignant nature of HD over the past century, it was not until 1998 that Reed-Sternberg cells were shown to be clonally expanding, pre-apoptotic, germinal center-derived B lymphocytes that resemble true malignant lymphoid cells (53).

Epidemiology and Etiology

Hodgkin disease (HD) is an uncommon lymphoid malignancy that represents about 1% of all de novo neoplasms occurring every year worldwide, with an annual incidence of two or three cases per 100,000 persons in Europe and the United States. Between 2001 and 2005, the age-adjusted incidence rate was 2.8 per 100,000 men and women per year, while the age-adjusted death rate was 0.4 per 100,000 men and women per year. These rates are based on cases diagnosed from 17 SEER geographic areas (54). In industrialized countries, the onset of HD has a bimodal distribution, with a first peak occurring in the third decade of life and a second peak occurring after age 50 years. The age-specific incidence differs markedly in various countries; moreover, the incidence of HD by age also differs by histologic subtypes. In the group of young adults, the most common subtype is nodular sclerosis HD, which occurs at a higher frequency than the others subtypes as discussed below. More men than women (1.4:1) develop the disease. Compared to whites, HD is less common in African Americans.

The cause of HD remains unknown, and there are no clearly defined risk factors for the disease. However, familial factors and viruses seem to play a role in its development. For example, same-sex siblings of patients with HD have a 10 times higher risk for the disease, whereas the monozygotic twin sibling of patients with HD have a 99 times higher risk than a dizygotic twin sibling of developing HD. Familial aggregation may implicate genetic factors, but other epidemiologic findings suggest an abnormal reaction to a possible infectious agent, and both aspects have been implicated in the pathogenesis of HD. EBV has been implicated in the development of HD; however, the link of the relationship between symptomatic primary infection and HD remain unclear. The association of infectious mononucleosis and HD is strongest in young adults, but virus in tumor cells is least frequently detected in tumors in young adults. Finally, there are no conclusive studies regarding the possible increased incidence of HD in patients who are HIV positive (55), although several series have been reported that suggest a higher risk in these patients.

Signs and Symptoms

HD commonly presents as asymptomatic lymphadenopathy. However, about 30% of patients exhibit systemic symptoms, including night sweats, fever, weight loss, and pruritus at the beginning of the disease. More than 80% of patients with HD present with lymphadenopathy above the diaphragm, often involving the anterior mediastinum; in contrast, less than 20%–30% of patients present with a lymphadenopathy limited to regions below the diaphragm. The most commonly involved peripheral lymph nodes are located in the cervical, supracervical, and axillary regions. In contrast to NHL, lymphadenopathy tends to be contiguous in patients with HD.

Diagnosis and Staging

The initial diagnosis of HD can be made only by incisional or excisional biopsy of an enlarged lymph node. Because of the importance of the architecture, fine needle aspiration should never be used to make the diagnosis. The diagnosis is based on the identification of the characteristic multinucleate giant cells within an inflammatory milieu. As mentioned above, these multinucleate giant cells, termed Reed-Sternberg (RS) cells, are diagnostic. These RS cells are the malignant component of HD and are its diagnostic hallmark. Unique to HD, these malignant RS cells comprise approximately 1% or less of the cellular mass of the tumor mass. The remainder of the tumor consists of a variable number of mononuclear elements, including normal B cells and T cells. In 1994, based on many morphologic, phenotypic, genotypic, and clinical findings, HD was described in the REAL classification system and subdivided into two main types: lymphocyte-predominant HD and classical HD. The latter further included the following subtypes: (1) nodular sclerosis classical HD; (2) mixed cellularity classic HD; (3) lymphocyte depletion classic lymphoma; and (4) the lymphocyte-rich classical HD. This approach has been approved by the recently developed WHO scheme, which has promoted lymphocyte-rich classic HD from a provisional entity to an accepted entity (Table 17.5).

The assignment of stage is critical for the selection of the proper treatment in HD. The stage is based on the following characteristics: (1) number of involved sites; (2) presence of lymphadenopathy both above and below the diaphragm; (3) presence of bulky disease (?10 cm); (4) presence of contiguous extranodal involvement or disseminated disease; and (5) presence of B-symptoms. The classical staging system is the Cotswald staging classification, which describes four stages as follows: stage I describes the involvement of a single lymph node region or lymphoid structure (eg, spleen, thymus,

TABLE 17.5 *Classification of Hodgkin Disease*	
Lymphocyte-predominant Hodgkin lymphoma	**Classic Hodgkin lymphoma** 1. Nodular sclerosis 2. Mixed cellularity 3. Lymphocyte depletion 4. Lymphocite-rich

Waldeyer's ring); stage II describes the involvement of two or more lymph node regions on the same side of the diaphragm, where the number of anatomic sites should be indicated by a subscript; stage III refers to the involvement of lymph node or structures on both sides of the diaphragm, and can be divided into III_1 with or without involvement of splenic, hilar, celiac, or portal nodes; and stage III_2 denotes involvement of para-aortic, iliac, or mesenteric nodes. Finally, stage IV is defined as involvement of extranodal site(s) beyond that designated E. In the absence of B symptoms, the stage is defined A; in presence of B symptoms, it is defined as B (Table 17.6).

Prognostic Factors

Approximately two-thirds of patients with advanced Hodgkin disease can be cured with the current approaches to treatment. Prediction of outcome is important to avoid over treating some patients and to identify others in whom standard treatment is likely to fail. The international database on Hodgkin disease was used to develop a parametric model for predicting survival. The model was based on data from 5,023 patients who represented different stages of the disease. In brief, seven prognostic factors were identified based on a multivariate analysis, and included: (1) a serum albumin level of less than 4 g per deciliter; (2) a hemoglobin level less that 10.5 g per deciliter; (3) leukocytosis (white-cell count of at least 15,000/mm³); (4) a lymphopenia (a lymphocyte count of less than 600/

mm³); (5) male gender; (6) aged 45 years or older; and (7) stage IV disease. The score predicted the 5-year rate of freedom from progression of disease as follows: zero factors, 84%; one risk factor, 77%; two risk factors, 67%; three risk factors, 60%; four risk factors, 51%; and five or more risk factors, 42%. The international prognostic score, called the IPSS or Hasenclever (56), can be useful in establishing enrollment criteria in clinical trial, to describe study population, and to support decisions about treatment in individual patients.

Treatment

HD is typically considered a chemotherapy and radiation sensitive disease. However, up until the beginning of the 21st century, patients with advanced stages of HD were considered incurable. With the advent of more effective drugs, De Vita and colleagues at the NCI pioneered new treatment regimens with remarkable success, achieving a 50% cure rate for patients with advanced-stage disease with the drug combination MOPP (Mechlorethamine, Oncovin, Procarbazine, Prednisone). Despite the promising results with MOPP therapy, many investigators continued to identify other novel regimens and used different chemotherapy programs to improve the efficacy and reduce the toxicities (57–59). Over time, it was realized that the MOPP regimen was associated with significant acute toxicities and a high risk of sterility and acute leukemia secondary to the alkylating agents (namely the nitrogen mustard mechlorethamine). In 1975, Bonadonna and colleagues (60) introduced the doxorubicin,

---

TABLE 17.6
Cotswolds Staging Classification

STAGE	DESCRIPTION
Stage I	Involvement of a single lymph node region or lymphoid structure or involvement of a single extralymphatic region (IE)
Stage II	Involvement of two or more lymph node regions on the same side of the diaphragm; localized contiguous involvement of only one extra nodal organ or site and lymph node on the same side of the diaphragm
Stage III	Involvement of lymph node regions on both sides of the diaphragm (III), which may also be accompanied by involvement of the spleen (IIIS) or by localized contiguous involvement of only one extranodal organ site (IIIE) or both (IIISE)
Stage IV	Diffuse or disseminate involvement of one or more extra nodal organs or tissues, with or without associated lymph node involvement
Designation applicable to any disease stage:	
A	No symptoms
B	Fever, drenching night sweats, unexplained loss of > 10% of body weight within the preceding 6 months
X	Bulky disease (>10 cm)
E	Involvement of a single extranodal site that is contiguous or proximal o the known nodal site

bleomycin, vincristine, and dacarbazine (DTIC-Dome) (ABVD) regimen. Direct comparison of the MOPP and ABVD regimens revealed both to be highly active, though ABVD was associated with significantly less germ-cell and hematopoietic toxicity, and a lower risk of developing acute leukemia. Presently, the treatment is tailored to the stage of the disease. In North America, cooperative group trials have defined limited-stage disease in patients with clinical stage I-IIA and an absence of bulky disease (≥10 cm). Patients with stage IIB or those with stage I-II bulky disease are treated with the same protocols as those with stage III-IV disease, typically receiving full course of chemotherapy, and are collectively referred to as having advanced stage disease. In addition, patients with bulky disease are considered for radiation therapy to the site to bulky disease. Generally, a number of principles have emerged regarding the management of HD, including:

1. Surgical staging (eg, splenectomy) is no longer necessary.
2. Treatment with combined modality therapy is superior to treatment with radiation therapy as a single agent.
3. Inclusion of chemotherapy as a part of combined modality therapy allows for a reduction in the magnitude of radiation therapy.
4. Chemotherapy as a single modality in patients with limited-stage disease is effective.

In brief, the treatment of choice for early-stage classical HD consists of combination chemotherapy (ABVD) sometimes followed by involved-field radiotherapy (IFRT) for patients with bulky disease. On the other hand, for the treatment of stage III/IV disease or patients with high-risk disease based on Hasenclever score, combination chemotherapy regimens and dose-intense regimens such as BEACOPP (Bleomycin, Etoposide, Adriamycin, Cyclophosphamide Oncovin, Procarbazine, Prednisone) are increasingly recommended. Table 17.7 summarizes some of these chemotherapeutic regimens routinely used for the treatment of Hodgkin lymphoma, and Table 17.8 summarizes the toxicities associated with the combination chemotherapy and radiation therapy. Generally, the use of extended field radiotherapy is being abandoned by most groups, being replaced by the increasing use of involved field radiotherapy. The one-year relative survival rate is 93%, the five-year survival is 86%, and after 10 years the survival rate decreases slightly to 81%.

Late Complications of Therapy

Because most HD patients can be cured with modern treatment modalities and will have a life expectancy equivalent to age-matched healthy individuals, it is of importance to take into account not just the acute treatment-related toxicities, but also the long-term side

---

TABLE 17.7
Chemotherapeutic Regimens

REGIMEN	DOSAGE	SCHEDULE	FREQUENCY
MOPP			Every 28 days
Mechlorethamine	6 mg/m²	IV	Day 1
Oncovin	1.4 mg/m²	IV (max dose 2 mg)	Day 1
Procarbazine	100 mg/m²	PO	Day 1–7
Prednisone	40 mg/m²	PO	Day 1–14
ABVD			Every 28 days
Adriamycin	25 mg/m²	IV	Days 1,15
Bleomycin	10 mg/m²	IV	Days 1,15
Vinblastine	6 mg/m²	IV	Days 1,15
Dacarbazine	375 mg/m²	IV	Days 1,15
BEACOPP			Every 21 days
Bleomycin	10 mg/m²	IV	Day 8
Etoposide	100 mg/m²	IV	Days 1–3
Adriamycin	25 mg/m²	IV	Day 1
Cyclophosphamide	650 mg/m²	IV	Day 1
Oncovin	1.4 mg/mL	IV	Day 8
Procarbazine	100 mg/m²	PO	Days 1–7
Prednisone	40 mg/m²	PO	Days 1–14
G-CSF (Granulocyte-Colony Stimulating Factor) from day 8			

| | TABLE 17.8 |
| | *Toxicities* |

ACUTE TOXICITIES	DELAYED TOXICITIES
Alopecia	Secondary malignancies (AML, ALL, NHL, melanoma, sarcoma, breast, gastric, lung, and thyroid cancer)
Nausea and vomiting	
Diarrhea	
Mucositis	
Paresthesias and neuropathies	Endocrine complications (infertility, hypothyroidism)
CNS confusion	
Anemia, leucopenia, thrombocytopenia	Pulmonary complication (pulmonary fibrosis)
Disulfiram like reaction following alcohol while taking procarbazine	Cardiac complications (cardiomyopathy, accelerated atherosclerotic heart disease, pericardial fibrosis)
Bleomycin-related lung toxicity	

effects of the chemotherapy and radiotherapy. The complications of the treatment could be mild, severe, or life-threatening, even for those cured of lymphoma. During the period from 1960s to the 1990s, the number of late-occurring sequelae of chemotherapy affected between 25% to 30% of patients after 10–20 years. This rate of complication balanced the initial success rates due to deaths that were consequences of treatment and not caused by the primary disease.

Modern combined-modality treatment strategies with reduced radiation fields, and declining intensities of induction chemotherapy have diminished the rate of late complications. Time will tell whether the still-aggressive drug combinations used in the early 21st century will be superior to the older treatment programs. Long-term complications of irradiation, including lung, heart, and thyroid dysfunction, in addition to secondary cancers of breast and lung, all remain important hurdles in our effort to not just cure the disease, but to decrease the morbidity and mortality of therapy. Some specific examples of these morbidities are discussed below.

Pneumonitis typically occurs 1–6 months after completion of mantle radiation therapy. The overall incidence of symptomatic pneumonitis is less than 5% after mantle irradiation. Patients with large mediastinal adenopathy or who received combined chemotherapy and radiation therapy have twofold or threefold greater risk (10%–15%) of developing this complication (61). After it resolves, there are usually no long-term sequelae. A mild nonproductive cough, low grade fever, and dyspnea characterize symptomatic radiation pneumonitis. Bleomycin-induced pneumonitis is typically an acute toxicity, though pulmonary fibrosis can be seen as a late complication.

Chemotherapy and radiotherapy have overlapping toxic effects on the heart. Modern treatment strategies

now avoid large radiation fields involving the heart, while efforts to limit excessive doses of cardiotoxic drugs such as anthracyclines have been incorporated into many new treatment programs. While these sequelae have become less common, they still affect 2%–5% of the patients. The risk of chronic cardiomyopathy increases as the cumulative dose of doxorubicin exceeds 400–450 mg/m². A careful cardiac evaluation using multi gated acquisition scans or echocardiograph patients treated with combined chemotherapy and radiotherapy is required, and probably should be performed as a workup for patients who developed unresolving dyspnea years after treatment.

The decline of the historical survival curves in HD in the second half of the 20th century was mainly attributed to the increasing number of secondary tumors. In the first three to five years after therapy, acute leukemias and lymphomas predominantly occur, whereas after 8–10 years, the number of solid tumors increases. The increasing incidence of secondary malignancies is potentiated by the administration of carcinogenic alkylating agents such as nitrogen mustard, procarbazine, and cyclophosphamide. Physicians should be aware that HD patients are at higher risk for developing secondary cancers, possibly because of some intrinsic genetic susceptibility to develop cancer compared to patients with other types of cancer. The incidence of solid tumors in treated HD patients increases with time and does not reach a plateau, even in the second decade after the treatment. The major risks appear to be lung and breast cancer (62–64). Other cancers include sarcomas, melanomas, connective tissue and bone marrow tumors, and skin cancers (65,66).

Gonadal dysfunction is another treatment-related disturbance that often occurs in young, sexually active HD patients. Loss of libido, sexual discomfort, impotence, and sterility are the major problems, and these symptoms afflict about 80% of the HD population (67,68). C-MOPP or C-MOPP-like chemotherapy induce azoospermia (69,70) in 50%–100% of male patients, and only 10%–20% will eventually recover after a long interval. A full course of C-MOPP chemotherapy causes approximately 50% of women (71) to have amenorrhea, with age-dependant premature ovarian failure. ABVD produces only limited and transient germ-cell toxicities in the men and rarely causes drug-induced amenorrhea.

CONCLUSIONS

Clearly, advances in the treatment of lymphoma have been significant, and may be among the most successful of any malignancy. As new drugs and new treatment paradigms emerge, our probability of curing or managing these patients will improve still further. The challenge moving forward is to make sure that we can nurture our elderly patients sufficiently enough that they are able to tolerate the noxious effects of our sometimes crude therapies. As the population ages, it is likely that the patients we treat will get older and older. These realities will most assuredly increase our reliance on those subspecialties of medicine that will be able to assist medical oncologists in formulating treatments that will allow for optimal outcomes.

References

1. Harris NL, Jaffe ES, Stein H, et al. A revised European-American classification of lymphoid neoplasms: a proposal for the international lymphoma study group. *Blood*. September 1, 1994;84(5):1361–1392.
2. Jaffe ES, Harris NL, Stein H, Vardiman J. World Health Organization classification: tumours of hematopoetic and lymphoid tissues. In: Jaffe ES, Harris NL, Stein H, Vardiman JW, eds. Lyon: IARC Press; 2001.
3. Surveillance, Epidemiology, and End Results (SEER) Program. SEER*Stat Database: Mortality—All COD, Public-Use With State, Total US (1969–2004), National Cancer Institute, DCCPS, Surveillance Research Program, Cancer Statistics Branch, released April 2007. http://www.seer.cancer.gov. Underlying mortality data provided by NCHS (http://www.cdc.gov/nchs). Accessed May 1, 2007.
4. Pulte D, Gondos A, Brenner B. Ongoing improvement in outcomes for patients diagnosed as having Non-Hodgkin lymphoma from the 1990s to the early 21st century. *Arch Intern Med*. 2008;168(5):469–476.
5. Armitage JM, Kormos RL, Stuardt RS, et al. Posttransplant lymphoproliferative disease in thoracic organ transplant patients: ten years of cyclosporine-based immunosuppression. *J Heart Lung Transplant*. November–December 1991;10(6):877–886; discussion 886–887.
6. Leblonde V, Sutton L, Doren R, et al. Lymphoproliferative disorders after organ transplantation: a report of 24 cases observed in a single center. *J Clin Oncol*. April 1995;13(4):961–968.
7. Hourigan MJ, Doecke J, Molee PN, et al. A new prognosticator for post-transplant lymphoproliferative disorders after renal transplantation. *Br J Haematol*. April 13, 2008.
8. Ekstrom Smedby K, Vajdic CM, et al. Autoimmune disorders and risk of non-Hodgkin lymphoma subtypes: a pooled analysis within the InterLymph Consortium. *Blood*. April 15, 2008;111(8):4029–4038. Epub 2008 Feb 8.
9. Mellemkjaer L, Pfeiffer RM, et al. Autoimmune disease in individuals and close family members and susceptibility to non-Hodgkin's lymphoma. *Arthritis Rheum*. March 2008;58(3):657–666.
10. Fain O, Aras N, et al. Sjögren's syndrome, lymphoma, cryoglobulinemia. *Rev Prat*. June 30, 2007;57(12):1287.
11. Beral V, Peterman T, et al. AIDS-associated non-Hodgkin lymphoma. *Lancet*. April 6, 1991;337(8745):805–809.
12. Rabkin CS, Biggar RJ, et al. Increasing incidence of cancers associated with the human immunodeficiency virus epidemic. *Int J Cancer*. March 12, 1991;47(5):692–696.
13. Ross R, Dworsky R, et al. Non-Hodgkin's lymphomas in never married men in Los Angeles. *Br J Cancer*. November 1985;52(5):785–787.
14. Wotherspoon AC. Gastric lymphoma of mucosa-associated lymphoid tissue and Helicobacter pylori. *Annu Rev Med*. 1998;49:289–299.
15. Parsonnet J, Isaacson PG. Bacterial infection and MALT lymphoma. *N Engl J Med*. January 15, 2004;350:213
16. Jaffe ES. Common threads of mucosa-associated lymphoid tissue lymphoma pathogenesis: from infection to translocation. *J Natl Cancer Inst*. April 21, 2004;96(8):571–573.
17. Ye H, Liu H, Attygalle A. Variable frequencies of t(11;18)(q21;q21) in MALT lymphomas of different sites: significant association with CagA strains of H pylori in gastric MALT lymphoma. *Blood*. August 1, 2003;102(3):1012–1018. Epub April 3, 2003.
18. University of Michigan Medical Center, Ann Arbor, Michigan 48109, USA American College of Gastroenterology Guideline on the Management of *Helicobacter pylori* Infection. *Am J Gastroenterol*. August 2007;102(8):1808–1825. Epub June 29, 2007.
19. Cerroni L, Zochling N, et al. Infection by Borrelia burgdorferi and cutaneous B-cell lymphoma. *J Cutan Pathol*. September 1997;24(8):457–461.
20. Krueger GR, Medina JR, Klein HO, et al. A new working formulation of non-Hodgkin's lymphomas. A retrospective study of the new NCI classification proposal in comparison to the Rappaport and Kiel classifications. *Cancer*. September 1, 1983;52(5):833–840.
21. Gerard-Marchant R, Hamlin I, Lennert K, et al. Classification of non Hodgkin lymphomas. *Lancet*. 1974;2:406–408.
22. Lukes RJ, Collins RD. Immunologic characterization of human malignant lymphomas. *Cancer*. October 1974;34(4 Suppl):1488–1503.
23. Cheson BD, Pfistner B, et al. Revised response criteria for malignant lymphoma. *J Clin Oncol*. February 10, 2007;25(5):579–586.
24. Castellucci P, Zinzani PL, Pourdehnad M. 18F-FDG PET in malignant lymphoma: significance of positive findings. *Eur J Nucl Med Mol Imaging*. July 2005;32(7):749–756. Epub March 23, 2005.
25. Spaepen K, Stroobants S, Dupont P, et al. Early restaging positron emission tomography with (18)F-fluorodeoxyglucose predicts outcome in patients with aggressive non-Hodgkin's lymphoma. *Ann Oncol*. September 2002;13(9):1356–1363.
26. Gallamini A, Hutchings M, Rigacci S. Early interim 2-[18F] fluoro-2-deoxy-D-glucose positron emission tomography is prognostically superior to international prognostic score in advanced-stage Hodgkin's lymphoma: a report from a joint Italian-Danish study. *J Clin Oncol* August 20, 2007;25(24):3746–3752. Epub July 23, 2007.
27. Rosenberg SA. Validity of the Ann Arbor staging classification for the non-Hodgkin's lymphomas. *Cancer Treat Rep*. 1977;61:1023–1027.
28. Fisher RI, Hubbard SM, DeVita VT, et al. Factors predicting long-term survival in diffuse mixed, histiocytic, or undifferentiated lymphoma. *Blood*. 1981;58:45–51.

29. Shipp MA, Harrington DP, Klatt MM, et al. Identification of major prognostic subgroups of patients with large-cell lymphoma treated with m-BACOD or M-BACOD. *Ann Intern Med.* 1986;104:757–765.

30. Jagannath S, Velasquez WS, Tucker SL, et al. Tumor burden assessment and its implication for a prognostic model in advanced diffuse large-cell lymphoma. *J Clin Oncol.* 1986;4:859–865.

31. Coiffier B, Lepage E. Prognosis of aggressive lymphomas: a study of five prognostic models with patients included in the LNH-84 regimen. *Blood.* 1989;74:558–564.

32. Velasquez WS, Jagannath S, Tucker SL, et al. Risk classification as the basis for clinical staging of diffuse large-cell lymphoma derived from 10-year survival data. *Blood.* 1989;74:551–557.

33. Coiffier B, Gisselbrecht C, Vose JM, et al. Prognostic factors in aggressive malignant lymphomas: description and validation of a prognostic index that could identify patients requiring a more intensive therapy. *J Clin Oncol.* 1991;9:211–219.

34. Sehn L. Optimal use of prognostic factors in non-Hodgkin lymphoma. *Hematology Am Soc Hematol Educ Program.* 2006;295–302.

35. The International Non-Hodgkin's Lymphoma Prognostic Factors Project. A predictive model for aggressive non-Hodgkin's lymphoma. *N Engl J Med.* 1993;329:987–994.

36. Solal-Céligny P, Roy P, Colombat P. Follicular lymphoma international prognostic index. *Blood.* September 1, 2004;104(5):1258–1265.

37. Gallamini A, Stelitano C, Calvi R, et al. Peripheral T-cell lymphoma unspecified (PTCL-U): a new prognostic model from a retrospective multicentric clinical study. *Blood.* April 1, 2004;103(7):2474–2479. Epub November 26, 2003.

38. Went P, Agostinelli C, Gallamini A. Marker expression in peripheral T-cell lymphoma: a proposed clinical-pathologic prognostic score. *J Clin Oncol.* June 1, 2006;24(16):2472–2479. Epub April 24, 2006.

39. Coiffier B, Lepage E, Briere J, et al. CHOP chemotherapy plus rituximab compared with CHOP alone in elderly patients with diffuse large-B-cell lymphoma. *N Engl J Med.* January 24, 2002;346(4):235–242.

40. Press OW, Leonard JP, Coiffier B. Immunotherapy of non-Hodgkin's lymphomas; hematology. *Am Soc Hematol Educ Program.* 2001;221–240.

41. Chopra R, Goldstone AH, Pearce R, et al. Autologous versus allogeneic bone marrow transplantation for non-Hodgkin's lymphoma: a case-controlled analysis of the European Bone Marrow Transplant Group Registry data. *J Clin Oncol.* 1992;10:1690–1695.

42. Ratanatharathorn V, Uberti J, Karanes C, et al. Prospective comparative trial of autologous versus allogeneic bone marrow transplantation in patients with non-Hodgkin's lymphoma. *Blood.* 1994;84:1050–1055.

43. Verdonck LF, Dekker AW, Lokhorst HM, et al. Allogeneic versus autologous bone marrow transplantation for refractory and recurrent low-grade non-Hodgkin's lymphoma. *Blood.* 1997;90:4201–4205.

44. van Besien KW, de Lima M, Giralt, et al. Management of lymphoma recurrence after allogeneic transplantation: the relevance of graft-versus-lymphoma effect. *Bone Marrow Transplant.* 1997;19:977–982.

45. Mandigers CM, Verdonck LF, Meijerink JP, et al. Graft-versus-lymphoma effect of donor lymphocyte infusion in indolent lymphomas relapsed after allogeneic stem cell transplantation. *Bone Marrow Transplant.* 2003;32:1159–1163.

46. Peniket AJ, Ruiz de Elvira MC, Taghipour G, et al. European Bone Marrow Transplantation (EBMT) Lymphoma Registry. An EBMT registry matched study of allogeneic stem cell transplants for lymphoma: allogeneic transplantation is associated with a lower relapse rate but a higher procedure-related mortality rate than autologous transplantation. *Bone Marrow Transplant.* 2003;31:667–678.

47. Farina L, Corradini P. Current role of allogeneic stem cell transplantation in follicular lymphoma. *Haematologica.* May 2007;92(5):580–582.

48. Chahal S, Lagera JE, Rider J, et al. Hematological neoplasms with first presentation as spinal cord compression syndromes: a 10-year retrospective series and review of the literature. *Clin Neuropathol.* November–December 2003;22(6):282–290.

49. Cabanillas ME, Lu H, Fans S, et al. Elderly patients with non-Hodgkin lymphoma who receive chemotherapy are at higher risk for osteoporosis and fractures. *Leuk Lymphoma.* August 2007;48(8):1514–1521.

50. Morrison VA. Non-Hodgkin's lymphoma in the elderly. Part 2: treatment of diffuse aggressive lymphomas. *Oncology.* September 2007;21(10):1191–1198; discussion 1198–1208, 1210.

51. Balducci L, Al-Halawani H, et al. Elderly cancer patients receiving chemotherapy benefit from first-cycle pegfilgrastim. *Oncologist.* December 2007;12(12):1416–1424.

52. Hodgkin T. On same morbid appearances of the absorbent glands and spleen. *Medico-Chirurgical Trans.* 1832;17:68–97.

53. Kuppers R, Rajewsky K. The origin of Hodgkin and Reed/Sternberg cells in Hodgkin's disease. *Annu Rev Immunol.* 1998;16:471–493.

54. Surveillance, Epidemiology, and End Results (SEER) Program. SEER*Stat Database: Mortality—All COD, Public-Use With State, Total US (1969–2004), National Cancer Institute, DCCPS, Surveillance Research Program, Cancer Statistics Branch, released April 2007. http://www.seer.cancer.gov. Underlying mortality data provided by NCHS (http://www.cdc.gov/nchs). Accessed May 1, 2007.

55. Engels EA, Biggar RJ, hall HI, et al. Cancer risk in people infected with human immunodeficiency virus in the United States. *Inter J Cancer.* July 1, 2008;123(1):187–194.

56. Hasenclever D, Diehl, et al. A prognostic score for advanced Hodgkin's disease. *N Engl J Med.* November 19, 1998; 339:1506.

57. Nissen NI, Pajak TF, Glidewell O. A comparative study of a BCNU containing 4-drug program versus MOPP versus 3-drug combinations in advanced Hodgkin's disease: a cooperative study by the Cancer and Leukemia Group B. *Cancer.* January 1979;43(1):31–40.

58. Bakemeier RF, Anderson RJ, Costello W, et al. BCVPP chemotherapy for advanced Hodgkin's disease: evidence for greater duration of complete remission, greater survival, and less toxicity than with a MOPP regimen. Results of the Eastern Cooperative Oncology Group study. *Ann Intern Med.* October 1984;101(4):447–456.

59. Hancock BW. Randomised study of MOPP (mustine, Oncovin, procarbazine, prednisone) against LOPP (Leukeran substituted for mustine) in advanced Hodgkin's disease. British National Lymphoma Investigation. *Radiother Oncol.* November 1986;7(3):215–221.

60. Bonadonna G, Zucali R, Monfardini S, et al. Combination chemotherapy of Hodgkin's disease with adriamycin, bleomycin, vinblastine, and imidazole carboxamide versus MOPP. *Cancer.* July 1975;36(1):252–259.

61. Tardell N, Thompson L, Mauch P. Thoracic irradiation in Hodgkin's disease: disease control and long-term complications. *Int J Radiat Oncol Biol Phys.* February 1990;18(2):275–281.

62. Van leeuwen FE, Swerdlow AJ, et al. *Second Cancers after Treatment of Hodgkin's Disease.* Philadelphia: Lippincott Williams & Wilkins; 1999:607–632.

63. Tucker MA. Solid second cancers following Hodgkin's disease. *Hematol Oncol Clin North Am.* April 1993;7(2):389–400.

64. Valagussa P. Second neoplasms following treatment of Hodgkin's disease. *Curr Opin Oncol.* September 1993;5(5):805–811.

65. Van leeuwen FE, Somers R, et al. Increased risk of lung cancer, non-Hodgkin's lymphoma, and leukemia following Hodgkin's disease. *J Clinic Oncol.* August 1989;7(8):1046–1058.

66. Hancock LS, Hoppe RT. Long-term complications of treatment and causes of mortality after Hodgkin's disease. *Semin Radiat Oncol.* July 1996;6(3):225–242.

67. Bokemeyer C, Schmoll HJ, et al. Long-term gonadal toxicity after therapy for Hodgkin's and non-Hodgkin's lymphoma. *Ann Hematol.* March 1994;68(3):105–110.

68. Ortin TT, Shostak CA. Gonadal status and reproductive function following treatment for Hodgkin's disease in

childhood: the Stanford experience. *Int J Radiat Oncol Biol Phys.* October 1990;19(4):873–880.

69. Tempest HG, Ko E. Sperm aneuploidy frequencies analysed before and after chemotherapy in testicular cancer and Hodgkin's lymphoma patients. *Hum Reprod.* February 2008;23(2): 251–258. Epub December 14, 2007.

70. Blumenfeld Z. Gender difference: fertility preservation in young women but not in men exposed to gonadotoxic chemotherapy. *Minerva Endocrinol.* March 2007;32(1):23–34.

71. Giuseppe L, Attilio G, et al. Ovarian function after cancer treatment in young women affected by Hodgkin disease (HD). *Hematology.* April 2007;12(2):141–147.

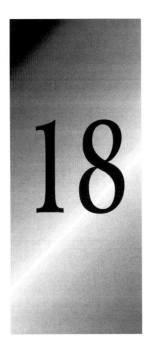

Evaluation and Treatment of Leukemia and Myelodysplasia

Heather J. Landau
Stephen D. Nimer

This chapter covers the common leukemias (AML, ALL, and CLL) and the myelodysplastic syndromes. We will describe the key features of these disorders and discuss how the various treatments affect the disease as well as the function of other organs, at times leading to acute or chronic organ dysfunction. With the advent of imatinib, dasatinib, and nilotinib, tyrosine kinase inhibitor therapy has dramatically changed the treatment of CML. Many excellent reviews have described the optimal approach to using these agents in CML, addressed how to best manage their side effects, and monitor the response to treatment (1,2). Therefore, CML will not be covered in this chapter.

ACUTE MYELOGENOUS LEUKEMIA (AML)

Unfortunately, the treatment of AML has not changed significantly in the past three to four decades (3,4), except for the treatment of acute promyelocytic leukemia (APL), a subtype of AML that is now eminently curable (5). The treatments for AML were initially designed based on the principles of nonoverlapping toxicities and, to some degree, different mechanisms of action. In the case of APL, the use of the vitamin A derivative all-trans retinoic acid (ATRA) has been a remarkable clinical advance. ATRA was also shown to represent targeted therapy, as the genetic abnormality underlying

APL involves translocation of the retinoic acid receptor alpha (RARa) gene (reviewed in Ref. 6).

Prognostic Features

The prognosis of AML depends on the age of the patient, the cytogenetic abnormalities detected, whether it occurs de novo or secondary to chemotherapy or environmental toxin exposure, and whether certain mutations or cell surface markers are found in the leukemia cell (7,8).

Specific cytogenetic abnormalities are associated with specific clinical syndromes, such as t(15;17) and with AML, M3 and t(8;21) with AML, M2. The core binding factor (CBF) leukemias are characterized by chromosomal translocations that involve either the CBFa gene (better known as the AML1 gene or the RUNX1 gene) or the CBFb gene. These genes encode proteins that form a complex at target gene promoters that can either turn on or turn off gene expression. The AML1 protein binds to DNA via its Runt domain, which is so named because of its homology to the drosophila gene Runt (9,10). It binds with a low affinity and is subject to ubiquitin-mediated proteasomal degradation, unless CBFb is also present. CBFb increases the affinity of AML1 for its DNA recognition sequence, and it protects AML1 from proteasomal degradation (11,12). The t(8;21) and the inv (16) or t(16;16), which is associated with AML, M4-Eo), generate the

KEY POINTS

- Acute leukemia manifests itself largely by its effects on normal hematopoiesis. Anemia, thrombocytopenia, and neutropenia, the result of marrow replacement by malignant cells, lead to increased fatigue, bruising or bleeding, and infection.

- Unfortunately, the treatment of acute myelogenous leukemia (AML) has not changed significantly in the past three to four decades, except for the treatment of acute promyelocytic leukemia (APL), a subtype of AML that is now eminently curable.

- The prognosis of AML depends on the age of the patient, the cytogenetic abnormalities detected, whether it occurs de novo or secondary to chemotherapy or environmental toxin exposure, and whether certain mutations or cell surface markers are found in the leukemia cell.

- Myelodysplastic disorders (MDS) are characterized by ineffective hematopoiesis, which most commonly manifests as a hypercellular bone marrow with peripheral blood cytopenias, but also by a variable tendency to progress to acute myelogenous leukemia.

- The clinical approach to patients with MDS should be based on (1) whether the patient has anemia only or also has significant neutropenia and/or thrombocytopenia; and (2) whether the patient has increased blasts and is therefore at risk for developing acute leukemia.

- Acute lymphoblastic leukemia (ALL) is the most common malignancy in children, but it is relatively uncommon in adults, with about 2,000 cases per year in the United States. Childhood ALL is cured with modern treatment regimens in approximately 80% of patients; however, only 20%–40% of adult patients are cured.

- Treatment of adult ALL is typically divided into four phases: induction, consolidation, maintenance, and central nervous system (CNS) prophylaxis.

- Treatment of ALL is complicated by toxicity, especially in older adults. Patients with diabetes, hypertension, or heart disease, which are common in the general population, are at increased risk for steroid-induced complications, vincristine-induced neuropathy, and anthracycline-associated cardiotoxicity.

- Chronic lymphocytic leukemia (CLL) is the most common leukemia in adults; approximately 10,000 new cases are diagnosed each year in the United States. The median age at diagnosis is approximately 70 years, with 80% of patients diagnosed at 60 years or older. Although the disease course is often indolent, each year approximately 4,600 patients die from complications of CLL, most commonly from infection.

- Conventional therapy for CLL is not curative and there is no evidence that patients with low or intermediate risk disease benefit from the early initiation of therapy. However, treatment is indicated for patients who have symptomatic progressive disease, bulky disease, or cytopenias.

---

leukemia-associated fusion proteins, AML1-ETO and CBFB-SMMHC, respectively. These AML subtypes tend to have a more favorable prognosis.

Treatment of AML

The treatment of AML in adults generally consists of combination therapy that includes an anthracycline (eg, Daunorubicin or Idarubicin) and cytosine arabinoside (Cytarabine). This treatment is often referred to as 7+3 because the cytosine arabinoside is given daily for seven days and the anthracycline given daily for three days. Once the diagnosis of AML is made, patients are quickly hospitalized, and treatment is initiated. Hydration and administration of allopurinol are started to prevent the infrequent occurrence of tumor lysis syndrome. The presence of an infection at the time of first presentation is a negative prognostic feature. It also complicates the initiation of treatment.

The most essential goal of therapy for AML is to achieve a complete remission (CR), which is defined by the disappearance of the leukemic blasts from the peripheral blood and the bone marrow (blasts must be less than 5%) and the return of the peripheral blood counts to normal levels (13). All of these features must last for at least one month to document a CR. In an attempt to induce a CR, induction chemotherapy may be given once or twice. Generally, the same chemotherapy drugs are repeated when leukemic cells persist after the first course of chemotherapy. As the rate of inducing a CR with a third course of induction chemotherapy is as low as 3%, a third course of similar chemotherapy is not recommended. Rather a distinct approach, using investigational agents (given the paucity of available drugs that have activity against AML blasts) is often considered for younger patients. For the elderly patients, who comprise the majority of patients with AML, a second course of induction chemotherapy is often not given because of concerns about toxicity. Additional myelosuppressive therapy can result in profound neutropenia and prolonged infection in these patients who are already quite compromised.

Once remission is achieved, further treatment is needed to prolong the remission duration and to offer the possibility of cure (which occurs in approximately 30%–40% of patients aged younger than 60 years). This treatment, called consolidation therapy, is intensive, although generally not as intensive as induction therapy. The optimal number of cycles of consolidation therapy is not known; however, patients who receive at least one cycle have a measurable cure rate (14). In general, patients are given two to four courses of consolidation therapy (15). In addition, both autologous and allogeneic transplantation can be offered to AML patients in first remission as a form of consolidation therapy, in an attempt to increase the cure rate. Several randomized trials (biologically randomized, based upon the availability of a suitable allogeneic donor, which historically meant an HLA-identical sibling) have been conducted and show better relapse-free survival but generally not better overall survival for patients who undergo autologous or allogeneic transplantation "upfront" (16–19). These studies suggest that patients aged younger than 60 years with poor prognosis AML seem to derive the greatest benefit from an allotransplant in first remission. Studies have shown that the CBF leukemia patients do best if given high dose cytosine arabinoside based consolidation therapy rather than a standard dose cytosine arabinoside based regimen (20).

What must be remembered when interpreting these studies is that the cure rates with the non-allotransplant approaches must include not only the cure rate from the initial therapy, but also the salvage rate when the allogeneic transplant is used to treat patients with relapsed disease (21).

Complications of AML Therapy

The side effects of induction chemotherapy include myelosuppression (which generally lasts weeks), GI toxicities due to breaking down of mucosal barriers, total alopecia, and the small possibility of long-term cardiac toxicity from the repeated administration of anthracycline-containing therapies. Patients with high risk AML often receive high dose cytabine as part of an induction regimen. Neurotoxicity (generally, cerebellar toxicity) occurs can, especially in the elderly or those with an elevated serum creatinine (ie, diminished renal function). Other than avoiding the use of the 3 gm/m² q12 hr dosing regimen for these types of patients, evaluating the patient's signature before each dose has been suggested as a way to avoid triggering severe cerebellar toxicity. Because cytosine arabinoside is excreted in tears, patients given high dose cytosine arabinoside require steroid eye drops before each dose of chemotherapy in order to avoid chemical conjunctivitis.

The toxicity of autologous transplantation is largely limited to the immediate post-transplant period, when patients have profound neutropenia. The transplant conditioning regimens for AML patients often include total body irradiation, which can cause severe mucositis, prolonged myelosuppression (nearly myeloablation), pulmonary toxicity (both acute and chronic), and premature cataract formation. High dose etoposide can cause profound hypotension during the prolonged drug infusion. Hemorrhagic cystitis and rarely, cardiopulmonary toxicity, can be seen with high dose cyclophosphamide.

The toxicity of allogeneic transplantation persists well beyond the initial 100 days post-transplant (22). In addition to complications from the profound immunosuppression that occurs post-transplant, both acute and chronic graft versus host disease (GVHD) result in liver, GI, and skin abnormalities that can also be severe. Chronic GVHD resembles an autoimmune disorder and can be very difficult to treat (23,24). Veno-occlusive disease of the liver (perhaps better described as sinusoidal obstruction syndrome, or SOS) is uncommon with autologous, but not allogeneic, transplantation (reviewed in 25).

Treatment of Acute Promyelocytic Leukemia (APL)

The most striking advances in the treatment of acute leukemia over the past decades have taken place in the treatment of APL, largely because of the use of all-trans retinoic acid (ATRA). APL has been more successfully treated than other subtypes of AML for years, but because patients with APL often present with disseminated intravascular coagulation (DIC), they can die from hemorrhage (or less commonly from thrombosis) before or during their induction chemotherapy, prior to achieving a complete remission (26). The remarkable ability of ATRA to both eliminate the leukemia cells, largely by triggering their differentiation into more mature myeloid cells, and to rapidly arrest the DIC process, has allowed more patients to survive induction chemotherapy and achieve a complete remission (27).

The diagnosis of APL may be obvious from the morphology of the cells involved and the presence of DIC, but the diagnosis is not always apparent during the initial workup of newly diagnosed AML. Detection of the PML-RARa fusion transcript in the leukemia cells not only confirms the diagnosis, but also confers an excellent prognosis because of the high response rate to ATRA plus chemotherapy (28). APL is classically accompanied by the t(15;17), which generates the PML-RARA fusion product, as well as a RARA-PML fusion protein. There are variant molecular forms of APL, including the t(5;17), which generates the PLZF-RARA fusion transcript and protein. Identifying this translocation is of great clinical importance because patients with the t(5;17) do not respond to ATRA based therapy. APL is a disease that is quite sensitive to anthracyclines; thus, many trials have focused on giving more anthracycline therapy (both for induction and consolidation) (29) rather than more cytosine arabinoside in an attempt to adequately treat the disease without causing repeated episodes of profound cytopenias. Nonetheless, cytosine arabinoside has clinical activity in APL (30).

Studies from the larger cooperative groups such as the Eastern Cooperative Oncology Group have shown that the inclusion of ATRA in the treatment of APL, either during the induction, consolidation, or maintenance phase of treatment, leads to a significant improvement in overall survival (31). Thus, the current standard approach to APL includes ATRA as part of an induction regimen, usually with chemotherapy using a regimen first reported by an Italian Leukemia Group, followed by consolidation therapy (two to four cycles of anthracycline containing treatment), followed by intermittent ATRA therapy given for 14 days every three months (32–34).

The relapse rate from this approach is perhaps 15%. For these patients, their disease can be very effectively treated with arsenic trioxide (ATO) (35). Relapsed APL patients are usually treated with an autologous transplant if their disease becomes undetectable by PCR, or with an allogeneic transplant, if PCR positivity persists despite various salvage treatments (36).

The most dramatic (and life threatening) side effect of ATRA therapy in APL is the retinoic acid (RA) syndrome (37). This side effect tends to occur in patients with higher baseline white blood cell (WBC) counts. Patients with APL tend to have low WBC counts, but in most patients treated with ATRA, the WBC count will begin to increase with the initiation of treatment. At times, the WBC count can reach very high levels, but even in patients who have only a modest rise in WBC count, the neutrophils and other earlier myeloid cells can infiltrate the lungs and cause a capillary leak syndrome that manifests itself with pulmonary infiltrates and hypoxia, and can progress to respiratory failure. This complication can be mitigated by the use of chemotherapy, and also by the use of corticosteroids, which are given at the first sign of pulmonary involvement (reviewed in Patatanian and Thompson) (38). This syndrome appears to be due to the differentiation and death of the APL cells, as it also occurs following treatment with ATO (39). Patients who develop leukocytosis from ATO (>10,000 cells/ml) are significantly more likely to develop the RA syndrome, but among patients with leukocytosis, there is no observed relation between the leukocyte peak and the probability of developing the syndrome. Given these findings, the syndrome has been renamed the "APL differentiation syndrome."

Side effects from ATO therapy include bradycardia and conduction disturbances, including prolonged QT interval. For this reason, it is particularly important to monitor electrolyte levels in patients receiving ATO, and to maintain serum potassium and magnesium levels at the high end of the normal range. Peripheral neuropathy, hyperglycemia, and skin rash are also seen in patients receiving ATO.

TREATMENT OF MYELODYSPLASTIC SYNDROMES

Over the past four years, three different drugs have been approved by the FDA for the treatment of patients with myelodysplastic syndromes (40–42). These disorders are characterized by ineffective hematopoiesis, which most commonly manifests as a hypercellular bone marrow with peripheral blood cytopenias, but also by a variable tendency to progress to acute myelogenous leukemia (43). Patients are classified by either the French-American-British (FAB) or the WHO classification systems, and prognosis is assigned using a score based on the key variables that predict survival. The most commonly used prognostic scoring system is the International Prognostic Scoring System (IPSS), which assigns a weighted score to each the following variables: cytogenetic abnormalities, percent bone marrow blasts, and the number of cytopenias (44). Other factors not taken into account in the IPSS but captured in the WHO classifications based prognostic scoring system (WPSS) are the transfusion requirements of the patients (those who require transfusion of either red blood cells or platelets have a poorer prognosis than transfusion-independent patients), and the influence of time on the course of the disease (45). In general, these classification systems separate myelodysplastic disorders (MDS) patients into relatively low-risk and high-risk groups. Because MDS is a disease of the elderly (with a median age of 70 or so), supportive care—meaning prompt administration of antibiotics and transfusions to provide symptomatic relief—has been the mainstay of therapy. However, the landscape of treatment options for MDS patients has changed, and so have the treatment algorithms.

The clinical approach to patients with MDS should be based on (1) whether the patient has anemia only or also has significant neutropenia and/or thrombocytopenia and (2) whether the patient has increased blasts and is therefore at risk for developing acute leukemia. If only anemia is present, patients may be given an erythropoietic stimulating agent (ESA) (46), immune modulatory therapy with lenalidomide, especially for 5q-patients (40) or ATG (47), or hypomethylating agents such as 5-azacytidine (42) or decitabine

(41). Patients who do not respond to these agents may be transfused on a regular basis. Patients at with low risk transfusion-dependent MDS are at risk for iron overload and should receive iron chelation therapy, using criteria such as those endorsed by the National Comprehensive Cancer Network or other organizations (48). Patients with significant thrombocytopenia or neutropenia can be treated with hypomethylating agents; however, for the younger patient with cytopenias and "refractory anemia" (by FAB classification), ATG can be used. At times, AML-like therapy may be the most appropriate form of therapy for some patients, despite its toxicity. Patients whose disease does not respond to these measures should be considered for an allogeneic transplant. MDS patients should be treated on clinical protocols whenever possible.

Patients with increased blasts are generally given hypomethylating agents, which seem to work best in patients with more advanced forms of MDS. These patients should not be given ATG, because they do not respond, and because it triggers prolonged immunosuppression. Allogeneic transplantation should be considered early for these patients.

ACUTE LYMPHOBLASTIC LEUKEMIA (ALL)

Although ALL is the most common malignancy in children, it is relatively uncommon in adults, with about 2,000 cases per year in the United States (49). Childhood ALL is cured with modern treatment regimens (50) in approximately 80% of patients; however, only 20%–40% of adult patients are cured (50,51). This large discrepancy in outcome reflects differences in the biology of the disease, with an increased incidence of unfavorable cytogenetic subgroups in adult patients (particularly Philadelphia chromosome-positive ALL patients) (52), along with an increased incidence of comorbidities that potentially limit the use of intensive therapy in adults.

Clinical Presentation and Diagnosis

Acute leukemia manifests itself largely by its effects on normal hematopoiesis. Anemia, thrombocytopenia, and neutropenia, the result of marrow replacement by malignant cells, lead to increased fatigue, bruising or bleeding, and infection. Although a marked elevation in WBC count is the classic hallmark of leukemia, pancytopenia is also common in adult patients with ALL. Mild hepatosplenomegaly and lymphadenopathy are seen in many cases.

Classification

While the FAB classification of ALL recognized three distinct subtypes (L1–L3) based on morphology and cytochemistry, most groups now characterize ALL based on immunophenotype and genetic features. Flow cytometric analysis defines three distinct subgroups that show considerable differences in presentation, clinical course, and prognosis.

Pre-B-cell ALL represents approximately 70% of patients and is manifested by immunoglobulin gene rearrangement and expression of an early B-cell markers such as CD19. Pro-B-cell disease is a more primitive B-cell leukemia that can be distinguished from the more common pre-B-cell ALL by the expression of CD10 (common ALL antigen or CALLA). Pre-B-cell and pro-B-cell ALL cells do not express surface immunoglobulin, the hallmark of the mature B cell. Pro-B-cell disease correlates with t(4;11). Overall, this subgroup has an intermediate prognosis when treated with standard chemotherapy regimens.

T-cell ALL is the second most common subtype, occurring in 20%–30% of patients. These lymphoblasts typically express T-cell antigens, including CD7, and variably express CD2, CD5, CD1a, and CD3. TdT is frequently expressed. CD4 and CD8 are sometimes expressed and are typically co-expressed, a pattern not found in mature T cells. The disease most often affects adolescents and young adults, and there is a significant male predominance. Patients typically present with mediastinal disease and there is a high frequency of central nervous system (CNS) involvement. With modern treatment regimens, patients with T-cell ALL have the most favorable prognosis of the ALL subtypes.

Mature B-cell disease is the least common ALL subtype representing less than 5% of adult ALL. The leukemic cells can be distinguished immunophenotypically from pre-B-cell lymphoblasts by surface immunoglobulin (Ig) expression. Karyotypically, these cells demonstrate t(8;14); rarely, the alternate translocations t(2;8) and t(8;22) can be seen. Adult patients typically present with extranodal disease, with the abdomen being the most frequent site of involvement. There is often early dissemination to the bone marrow and CNS infiltration occurs in up to 20% of adult patients (53). Patients who present with significant bone marrow involvement are said to have mature B-cell ALL, while those without bone marrow infiltration are said to have Burkitt lymphoma. Traditional ALL therapy is not appropriate for these patients; instead, a treatment regimen designed specifically for Burkitt lymphoma/leukemia should be used (54,55). Using regimens designed specifically for this rare disease, approximately 50% of adults with mature B-cell ALL can achieve long-term disease-free survival (55).

Prognostic Features

In general, older age is a continuous variable associated with a worse prognosis (56). The increased frequency of unfavorable cytogenetic subgroups such as Philadelphia chromosome-positive (Ph+) ALL, t(9;22) and t(4;11) in older patients with ALL contributes to their poor prognosis. Conversely, there is an increased incidence of favorable cytogenetic subgroups such as hyperdiploidy and t(12;21) in children compared to adults. A high WBC count at diagnosis is associated with a reduced likelihood of achieving a CR and decreased overall survival. Although a variety of WBC counts have been used to assign adults to a poor risk category, the most commonly used values are greater than 20,000/μl (57) or 30,000/μl (58).

The immunophenotype of the malignant cell is another prognostic factor (59). The rapidity of the response to therapy also has a significant impact on prognosis. Patients who require more than 4 or 5 weeks to achieve a CR during induction therapy have a lower likelihood of ultimately being cured (57, 58).

Treatment of ALL

Treatment of adult ALL is typically divided into four phases: induction, consolidation, maintenance, and CNS prophylaxis. With modern intensive therapy, complete responses are observed in 65%–90% of adults; however, most patients relapse, and only 20%–40% of adults with ALL are cured of their disease (60–68).

A combination of vincristine and prednisone has been the cornerstone of induction therapy for ALL, and achieves a complete response in approximately 50% of patients. The addition of an anthracycline increases the likelihood of achieving a complete response (83% compared to 47% without the anthracycline) (69). Further intensification with cyclophosphamide or L-asparaginase is widely accepted as improving remission induction rates. Therefore, most modern induction regimens contain four drugs (vincristine, glucocorticoid, anthracycline, and cyclophosphamide or asparaginase) or five drugs (vincristine, glucocorticoid, anthracycline, cyclophosphamide, and asparaginase). It has not yet been demonstrated that one multidrug regimen is superior to another. A novel approach to ALL induction combining cytosine arabinoside, an active agent most commonly used in the consolidation phase of ALL therapy, with a single very high-dose of mitoxantrone (80 mg/m^2) has been compared to a standard four-drug induction regimen. Early results have been reported in abstract form and indicate an improved frequency of CR but similar overall survival at five years for the patients who received the cytosine arabinoside and high-dose mitoxantrone induction regimen (68).

Postinduction consolidation (sometimes called intensification) involves giving a combination of drugs, usually cytosine arabinoside combined with other active agents, such as anthracyclines, alkylators, epidophillotoxins, or antimetabolites. The clinical trials investigating intensive multidrug consolidation therapy have demonstrated superior outcomes with this strategy. In a phase III trial reported by Fiere et al., patients were randomized to receive cytosine arabinoside, doxorubicin, and asparaginase as consolidation therapy or to immediately receive maintenance therapy following remission induction. The three-year disease-free survival was markedly improved in the patients who received multiagent consolidation compared to no consolidation at 38% versus 0%, respectively (70).

Prolonged maintenance therapy is a feature unique to the treatment of ALL. In pediatric patients, the value of prolonged maintenance has clearly been established and attempts to shorten the duration of maintenance to 18 months or less has resulted in a higher rate of relapse (71,72). Extending maintenance beyond three years has not been shown to be beneficial, thus two years of maintenance therapy has become standard (73). In adults with ALL, the data to support maintenance therapy is less direct. Several phase II studies in which maintenance therapy was omitted reported poor long-term results suggesting that maintenance is important (74–76). A combination of methotrexate and mercaptopurine, typically administered orally, constitute the backbone of maintenance therapy. While these drugs alone are often sufficient for pediatric patients, most adult regimens incorporate other active agents such as vincristine, prednisone, anthracyclines, and cyclophosphamide (77).

Although CNS leukemia is uncommon in adults at diagnosis (5%–10%), patients who do not receive prophylactic therapy have a cumulative CNS risk of 35% during the course of their disease (77). Risk factors for developing CNS disease include a high WBC count or an elevated LDH at initial presentation, and either T-cell or mature B-cell immunophenotype (59,78). CNS directed prophylactic therapy (intrathecal chemotherapy with or without whole brain irradiation) has been demonstrated to reduce the cumulative incidence of CNS relapse to approximately 10% (79); it is now universally recommended.

Allogeneic transplants have been used in adults with ALL. This dose-intense treatment has the ability to eradicate leukemia in a small subset of patients with disease refractory to conventional chemotherapy, and is the only potentially curative option in the relapsed setting (87). However, the lack of availability of HLA-matched donors and the mortality (20%–40%) seen with its use has limited this approach in patients with ALL in first CR.

Two large studies comparing allogeneic transplant to standard chemotherapy for patients in first CR failed to demonstrate a survival benefit for the transplant group (80,81). However, in one study a subset analysis suggested a benefit in certain high-risk patients and this has been confirmed for patients with Ph+ ALL (80). Currently, patients with Ph+ disease or t(4;11) are recommended to undergo an allogeneic transplant for ALL in first CR. Recent data suggesting that matched unrelated-donor transplantation may yield similar results to matched related-donor transplantation in adults with ALL has expanded donor availability for these patients at high risk (83). Autologous transplantation has no established role in treating patients with ALL.

Treatment of Philadelphia Chromosome–Positive ALL

The outcome of patients with Ph+ ALL is extremely poor when treated with conventional chemotherapy and five-year overall survival is less than 10%. Thus, allogeneic transplantation is currently recommended as standard therapy. Imatinib, a potent bcr-abl tyrosine kinase inhibitor, induces responses in a substantial proportion of Ph+ ALL patients, although the responses are not durable (84). While studies investigating the combination of imatinib in addition to chemotherapy in Ph+ ALL patients are ongoing, initial reports suggest that this combination results in superior outcomes when compared to historical controls (82,85,86). A high proportion of patients (50%–75%) have been able to be transplanted in first CR, the best current option for long-term survival. Durable remissions have also been observed with imatinib and chemotherapy alone without allograft, although longer follow-up is required to determine the effect on survival. The role of allogeneic transplantation in Ph+ disease for patients with the era of effective BCR-ABL inhibitors may be redefined.

Treatment of Relapsed ALL

Treatment of relapsed adult ALL is a major challenge. Because most initial treatment protocols incorporate multiple active agents with different cytotoxic mechanisms, a selection for drug resistance occurs. The complete remission rate in the salvage setting is much lower than with initial therapy, approximately 30%–40%, and the median remission duration is only six months. Salvage strategies typically include reinduction with the initial regimen in patients with late relapse or high-dose cytosine arabinoside or methotrexate in those who relapse early. Clofarabine, another effective agent, is FDA approved for treating childhood ALL; while it

induces CRs in adults as well, its role in this setting is not yet clear. If a second CR is achieved, allogeneic transplantation has resulted in long-term, disease-free survival in a small subset of patients (87). Outcomes with high-dose therapy and autologous stem cell support have been poor. Experimental approaches include treating patients with monoclonal antibodies directed against leukemia-specific antigens, novel transplantation strategies, and investigational agents that target key abnormalities such as gamma secretase inhibitors in T-cell ALL that have activating Notch mutations.

Complications of ALL Therapy

Treatment of ALL is complicated by toxicity, especially in older adults. Patients with diabetes, hypertension or heart-disease, which are common in the general population, are at increased risk for steroid-induced complications, vincristine-induced neuropathy and anthracycline-associated cardiotoxicity.

Vincristine induces cytotoxicity by binding to tubulin, resulting in microtubule depolymerization, metaphase arrest, and ultimately, apoptosis of cells. Vincristine also binds to neuronal tubulin and interferes with axonal microtubule function, leading to neurotoxicity characterized by a peripheral, symmetric, mixed sensory-motor, and autonomic polyneuropathy. Patients initially develop symmetric sensory impairment and paresthesias of the distal extremities. With continued treatment, neuritic pain and loss of deep tendon reflexes may occur followed by foot drop, wrist drop, motor dysfunction, ataxia, and paralysis. Rarely, cranial nerves are affected, resulting in hoarseness, diplopia, and facial palsies. Autonomic neurotoxicity often manifests as constipation. High doses of vincristine (>2 mg/m^2) can lead to acute, severe neurologic dysfunction leading to paralytic ileus, urinary retention, and orthostatic hypotension (88).

Anthracyclines are associated with acute and chronic cardiac toxicity (89). The susceptibility of cardiac muscle to anthracyclines remains unclear, but it appears to be due, at least in part, to the interaction of these drugs with oxygen free radicals and intracellular iron. Acute effects include nonspecific ECG changes; however, rarely a pericarditis-myocarditis syndrome can occur. More commonly, dose-dependent cardiac myopathy occurs, which leads to congestive heart failure associated with high mortality. Monitoring for the onset of cardiomyopathy with serial measurement of the left ventricular ejection fraction allows for earlier detection of subclinical cardiac toxicity. The iron chelator, Dexrazoxane provides effective cardioprotection and its use is advocated when the cumulative doxorubicin dose exceeds 300 mg/m^2.

Conclusions

Despite more than three decades of experience with various potentially curative treatment strategies in adult ALL, no single regimen yields superior results. Although there is wide variation in reported outcomes, interpretation of the literature is complicated by the differences in patient mix and the duration of follow-up of patients enrolled in studies (50). Several studies observed an apparent survival advantage for adolescents treated on pediatric regimens rather than adult regimens (90,91). These findings have led some researchers to promote more aggressive treatment, even for older adults. Risk-adapted strategies are being investigated in children. The limited success of current regimens in adults suggests that novel agents and new treatment approaches will be required to improve the outcomes for these patients.

CHRONIC LYMPHOCYTIC LEUKEMIA (CLL)

Approximately 10,000 new cases of chronic lymphocytic leukemia (CLL) are diagnosed each year in the United States (92). The median age at diagnosis is approximately 70 years, with 80% of patients diagnosed at 60 years or older (93). Although the disease course is often indolent, each year approximately 4,600 patients die from complications of CLL, most commonly from infection. There are no clearly identifiable risk factors for developing CLL, and it is the only leukemia that has not been linked with previous exposure to radiation (104). Although family members do have a slight genetic predisposition to develop CLL and other lymphoproliferative disorders, no specific genetic predisposition has been elucidated (94).

Clinical Presentation

Approximately 50% of patients with CLL are asymptomatic at presentation, and these patients are usually identified based on finding an isolated peripheral lymphocytosis on blood work for obtained for an unrelated indication (95). Constitutional symptoms such as night sweats, weight loss, and fatigue are present in 15% of patients at diagnosis (96). The most common presenting complaint is lymphadenopathy that may wax and wane. Other physical findings include splenomegaly, and less frequently, hepatomegaly. Although the lymphocyte count in CLL can often exceed 100,000/μL, patients do not typically experience symptoms from leukostasis due to the small size of the malignant lymphocytes (97).

Diagnosis

The most updated diagnostic criteria from the International Workshop on Chronic Lymphocytic Leukemia (IWCLL) requires (1) an absolute lymphocyte count of 5,000 lymphocytes/μL or greater; (2) a blood smear showing small mature lymphocytes without visible nucleoli (often with smudge cells that are characteristic of CLL); and (3) a minimal panel of cell surface markers to distinguish CLL from other B cell malignancies including CD19, CD 20, CD 23, CD 5, Fmc7, and cell-surface Ig staining, which shows light chain restriction (105). A bone marrow evaluation, while not needed for the diagnosis, is useful to determine the extent of involvement and the etiology of cytopenias.

The natural history of CLL is highly variable, but survival has been shown to correlate with clinical staging (Table 18.1) (106–108), and patients with Rai intermediate-risk disease or Binet stage B, as a group, have a median life expectancy of five to eight years. Patients with Rai low-risk disease have a life expectancy comparable to age- and sex-matched controls with traditional therapy. Other prognosis features including chromosomal abnormalities, as determined by fluorescent in-situ hybridization (FISH) (109), mutational status of the IgV gene (110), surface expression of CD38 (111), and cytoplasmic expression of ZAP70 (112). These allow patients to be placed into various prognostic groups.

Management of CLL

Conventional therapy for CLL is not curative, and there is no evidence that patients with low- or intermediate-risk disease benefit from the early initiation of therapy. Therefore, the standard of care is to treat patients when the disease is symptomatic or progressive as defined by the National Cancer Institute Working Group 1996 criteria (113); the 2008 update of these criteria is now available online (99). Criteria for therapy include B symptoms (ie, fever, chills, night sweats), obstructive adenopathy, rapidly progressive enlargement of lymph nodes or hepatosplenomegaly, development of or worsening thrombocytopenia and anemia, and a rapid lymphocyte doubling time. A high lymphocyte count in the absence of a rapid doubling time or the above features is not an indication for treatment.

Patients with low- or intermediate-risk disease (approximately 75% of patients) at diagnosis should be educated about complications of CLL including the high risk for infection, the possibility of developing a Richter's transformation, and the risk of autoimmune phenomena, specifically autoimmune hemolytic anemia and immune thrombocytopenia. They should be

TABLE 18.1
Modified Rai and Binet Staging Systems for Chronic Lymphocytic Leukemia with Approximate Median Survival Data by Stage

STAGE	CLINICAL FEATURES	MEDIAN SURVIVAL (YRS)
Modified Rai Staging System		
Low Risk	Lymphocytosis in blood and bone marrow	12.5
Intermediate Risk	Enlarged lymph nodes, spleen, or liver	7.2
High Risk	Anemia or thrombocytopenia	1.6
Binet Staging System		
A	Lymphocytosis + lymphadenopathy in <3 nodal groups	>10
B	Lymphadenopathy in >3 nodal groups	5
C	Anemia or thrombocytopenia	2

followed by clinical evaluation and complete blood count every three to six months to determine the pace of the disease and to monitor for complications. In the setting of progressive cytopenias, a bone marrow evaluation is necessary in order to distinguish immune-mediated cytopenias from progressive CLL because immune-mediated cytopenias may require different therapy than cytopenias due to progressive CLL.

Treatment is indicated for patients who have symptomatic progressive disease, bulky disease, or cytopenias. Oral chlorambucil monotherapy, which is usually well tolerated, was the standard of care for many years but rarely led to complete responses (~5%), and ultimately, patients succumbed to progressive resistant disease (114). A large, randomized, multicenter trial demonstrated that treatment with the purine analog fludarabine was superior to chlorambucil based on a higher frequency of response and longer duration of remission (114). Thus, fludarabine has formed the basis of subsequent combination studies. Combining fludarabine with corticosteroids and chlorambucil led to significant toxicity, which precluded any real improvement in response frequency (115–117). However, the use of fludarabine with cyclophosphamide and/or rituximab has shown significant activity with acceptable toxicity (118–121). The combination of a purine analog, an alkylating agent, and rituximab—fludarabine, cyclophosphamide, and rituximab (FCR) or pentostatin, cyclophosphamide, and rituximab (PCR)—results in very high overall and complete response rates when used as initial therapy; response rates are between 90% and 96%, with complete responses seen in 50%–70% of patients (121–122). Based on the observation that patients who achieve complete responses are more likely to have improved progression-free and overall survival (123) combination regimens are often given as initial therapy, even though it is not yet known whether

patients who are treated with this approach upfront will ultimately live longer.

For patients with relapsed and/or refractory CLL, the choice of salvage therapy is based on response to prior therapies. Re-treatment with combination therapies using purine analogs, alkylating agents, and rituximab can be effective, but typically is associated with lower response rates and shorter response duration than is achieved with initial therapy. In patients with purine analog refractory disease, alemtuzumab used alone or in combination with rituximab, achieves responses, but these are rarely complete or durable (124). In October 2008, Bendamustine was approved by the FDA for the treatment of CLL. It has single agent activity and has been given with rituximab alone or with mitoxantrone.

Cyclophosphamide, vincristine, and prednisone (CVP), as well as cyclophosphamide, vincristine, adriamycin, and prednisone (CHOP)-based regimens (125–126) also have activity and are often used in patients with autoimmune complications of CLL or transformed disease, respectively. However, more effective salvage strategies are needed for patients with relapsed/refractory CLL.

Traditionally, stem cell transplantation has not played a significant role in treating CLL patients because the risk of transplant-related complications was considered too high for patients who had a relatively indolent disease and a favorable prognosis or were elderly and had other comorbidities. The role of transplantation is now being reevaluated to define its curative potential in CLL.

Complications of CLL

CLL can affect both humeral and cellular immunity and some patients will relate a history of frequent infections that precede the diagnosis of CLL.

Hypogammaglobulinemia is associated with an increased susceptibility to severe infections (often with encapsulated organisms), and patients with documented low levels of Ig or recurrent infections are given intravenous Ig, which has been shown to decrease the incidence of serious bacterial infections. Defective cellular immunity often becomes evident as CLL progresses and patients receive cytotoxic therapy. Patients receiving treatment with purine analogs or alemtuzumab should receive herpes virus and pneumocystis pneumoniae prophylaxis (127). All patients should be advised to obtain early and aggressive antimicrobial therapy for symptomatic infection.

Immune dysregulation in patients with CLL is associated with an increased incidence of autoimmune phenomena, such as autoimmune hemolytic anemia (AIHA), immune thrombocytopenia (ITP), and pure red cell aplasia. These can occur at any time during the disease course, and their treatment is similar to the recommended therapy for de novo autoimmune disease. While treatment for the underlying CLL may also improve blood counts, treatment with purine analogs such as fludarabine has been associated with the development or worsening of AIHA or ITP and should be used with caution in these patients. The occurrence of these autoimmune conditions should be considered when monitoring the response to therapy with these agents. Other autoimmune disorders that have been reported in association with CLL include rheumatoid arthritis, Sjögren syndrome, systemic lupus erythematosus, ulcerative colitis, bullous pemphigoid, and Grave disease (128).

Patients with CLL have an increased risk of developing additional lymphoid malignancies as well as nonhematologic second malignancies. CLL transforms into a large cell lymphoma (Richter's transformation) in between 3% and 10% of patients. More rarely, CLL can transform into prolymphocytic leukemia (with >55% circulating prolymphocytes) and is associated with progression of cytopenias, splenomegaly, and refractoriness to therapy. Second malignancies such as Hodgkin lymphoma, lung, prostate, colon, and bladder cancers are increased in patients with CLL compared to the general population, and this risk is independent of initial treatment (129–130).

CLL is a common form of adult leukemia that causes considerable morbidity and mortality in some patients. Our understanding of CLL is evolving. Newer prognostic studies still do not influence the timing or type of treatment, and indications for therapy remain disease-related symptoms or significant cytopenias. Combination therapy with purine analogs, alkylating agents, and monoclonal antibodies have improved the likelihood of achieving complete remission and overall response rates, but no clear benefits in overall survival have been shown. Current research is focused on addressing these issues, and on establishing the role of stem cell transplantation in altering the natural history of this disease.

CONCLUSIONS

Signifiant advances have been made in our treatment of (APL), MDS, ALL, CML and CLL over the Past decade Hopefully in the decede to come we will better understand the basis of these designe and have better transplant and non-transplant oopptions to treat them.

References

1. Hughes T, Deininger M, Hochhaus A, Branford S, Radich J, Kaeda J, Baccarani M, Cortes J, Cross NC, Druker BJ, Gabert J, Grimwade D, Hehlmann R, Kamel-Reid S, Lipton JH, Longtine J, Martinelli G, Saglio G, Soverini S, Stock W, Goldman JM. Monitoring CML patients responding to treatment with tyrosine kinase inhibitors: review and recommendations for harmonizing current methodology for detecting BCR-ABL transcripts and kinase domain mutations and for expressing results. *Blood.* 2006;108:28-37.
2. Deininger MW. Optimizing therapy of chronic meyloid leukemia. *Exp Hematol.* 2007;35:144-154.
3. Gale RP, Cline MJ. High remission-induction rate in acute myeloid leukaemia. *Lancet.* 1977;1:497-499.
4. Rees JK, Sandler RM, Challener J, Hayhoe FG. Treatment of acute myeloid leukaemia with a triple ctyotoxic regime: DAT. *Br J Cancer.* 1977;36:770-776.
5. Wang ZY, Chen Z. Acute promyelocytic leukemia: from highly fatal to highly curable. *Blood.* 2008;111:2505-2515.
6. Scaglioni PP, Pandolfi PP. The theory of APL revisited. *Curr Top Microbiol Immunol.* 2007;313:85-100.
7. Estey E, Dohner H. Acute myeloid leukaemia. *Lancet.* 2006;368:1894-1907.
8. Lowenberg B. Prognostic factors in acute myeloid leukaemia. *Best Pract Res Clin Haematol.* 2001;14:65-75.
9. Peterson LF, Zhang DE. The 8;21 translocation in leukemogenesis. *Oncogene.* 2004;23:4255-4262.
10. Nimer SD, Moore MA. Effects of the leukemia-assocaited AML1-ETO protein on hematopoietic stem and progenitor cells. *Oncogene.* 2004;23:4249-4254.
11. Huang G, Shigasada K, Ito K, Wee HJ, Yokomizo T, Ito Y. Dimerization with PEBP2beta protects RUNX1/AML1 from ubiquitin-proteasome-mediated degradation. *Embo J.* 2001;20:723-733.
12. Wang Q, Stacy T, Miller JD, Lewis AF, Gu TL, Huang X, Bushweller JH, Bories JC, Alt FW, Ryan G, Liu PP, Wynshaw-Boris A, Binder M, Marin-Padilla M, Sharpe AH, Speck NA. The CBF-beta subunit is essential for CBFalpha2 (AML1) function in vivo. *Cell.* 1996;87;697-708.
13. Bruce D. Cheson, John M. Bennett, Kenneth J. Kopecky, Thomas Büchner, Cheryl L. Willman, Elihu H. Estey, Charles A. Schiffer, Hartmut Doehner, Martin S. Tallman, T. Andrew Lister, Francesco Lo-Coco, Roel Willemze, Andrea Biondi, Wolfgang Hiddemann, Richard A. Larson, Bob Löwenberg, Miguel A. Sanz, David R. Head, Ryuzo Ohno, Clara D. Bloomfield. Revised recommendations of the International Working Group for Diagnosis, Standardization of Response Criteria, Treatment Outcomes, and Reporting Standards for Therapeutic Trials in Acute Myeloid Leukemia. *J Clin Oncol.* 2003; 21:4642-4649.

14. Rowe JM. Consolidation therapy: what should be the standard of care? *Best Pract Res Clin Haematol*. 2008;21:53-60.

15. Mayer RJ, Davis RB, Schiffer CA, Berg DT, Powell BL, Schulman P, Omura GA, Moore JO, McIntyre OR, Frei E. Intensive postremission chemotherapy in adults with acute myeloid leukemia. Cancer and Leukemia Group B. *N Engl J Med*. 1994;331:896-903.

16. Reiffers J, Stoppa AM, Attal M, Michallet M, Marit G, Blaise D, Huguet F, Corront B, Cony-Makhoul P. Gastaut JA, Laurent G, Molina L, Broustet A, Maraninchi D, Pris J, Hollard D, Faberes C. Allogeneic vs autologous stem cell transplantation vs chemotherapy in patients with acute myeloid leukemia in first remission: the BGMT 87 study. *Leukemia*. 1996;10:1874-1882.

17. Burnett AK, Goldstone AH, Stevens RM, Hann IM, Rees JK, Gray RG, Wheatly K. Randomised comparison of addition of autologous bone-marrow transplantation to intensive chemotherapy for acute meyloid leukaemia in first remission: results of MRC AML 10 trial. UK Medical Research Council Adult and Children's Leukaemia Working Parties. *Lancet*. 1998;351: 700-708.

18. Zittoun RA, Mandelli F, Willemze R, de Witte T, Labar B, Resegott L, Leoni F, Damasio E, Visani G, Papa G, Caronia F, Hayat M, Stryckmans P, Rotoli B, Leoni P, Peetermans M, Dardenne M, Vegna ML, Petti MC, Solbu G, Suciu S. Autologous or allogeneic bone marrow transplantation compared with intensive chemotherapy in acute myelogenous leukemia. European Organization for Research and Treatment of Cancer (EORTC) and the Gruppo Italiano Malattie Ematologiche Maligne dell'Adulto(GIMEMA) Leukemia Cooperative Groups. *N Engl J Med*. 1995;332:217-223.

19. Cassileth PA, Harrington DP, Appelbaum FR, Lazarus HM, Rowe JM, Paietta E, Willman C, Hurd DD, Bennett JM, Blume KG, Head DR, Wiernik PH. Chemotherapy compared with autologous or allogeneic bone marrow transplantation in the management of acute myeloid leukemia transplantation in the management of acute myeloid leukemia in first remission. *N Engl J Med*. 1998;339:1649-1656.

20. Bloomfield CD, Lawrence D, Byrd JC, Carroll A, Pettenati MJ, Tantravahi R, Patil SR, Davey FR, Berg DT, Schiffer CA, Arthur DC, Mayer RJ. Frequency of prolonged remission duration after high-dose cytarabine intensification in acute myeloid leukemia varies by cytogenetic subtype. *Cancer Res*. 1998;58:4173-4179.

21. Oliansky DM, Appelbaum F, Cassileth PA, Keating A, Kerr J, Nieto Y, Stewart S, Stone RM, Tallman MS, McCarthy PL Jr, Hahn T. The role of cytotoxic therapy with hematopoietic stem cell transplantation in the therapy of acute myelogenous leukemia in adults: an evidence-based review. *Biol Blood Marrow Transplant*. 2008;14:137-180.

22. Kansu E, Sullivan KM. Late effects of hematopoietic stem cell transplantation; bone marrow transplantation. *Best Pract Res Clin Haematol*. 2007;4:209-222.

23. Holler E. Risk assessment in haematopoietic stem cell transplantation: GvHD prevention and treatment. *Best Pract Res Clin Haematol*. 2007;20:281-294.

24. Pavletic SZ, Lee SJ, Socie G, Vogelsang G. Chronic graft-versus host disease: implications of the National Institutes of Health consensu development project on criteria for clinical trials. *Bone Marrow Transplant*. 2006;38:645-651.

25. McDonald GB. Review article: management of hepatic disease following haematopoeitic cell transplant. *Ailment Pharmacol Ther*. 2006;24:441-452.

26. Tallman MS, Abutalib SA, Altman JK. The double hazard of thrombophilia and bleeding in acute promyelocytic leukemia. *Semin Thromb Hemost*. 2007;33:330-338.

27. Sanz MA. Treatment of acute promyelocytic leukemia. *Hematology Am Soc Hematol Educ Program*. 2006;147-155.

28. Reiter A, Lengfelder E. Grimwade D. Pathogenesis, diagnosis and monitoring of residual disease in acute promyelocytic leukaemia. *Acta Haematol*. 2004;112:55-67.

29. Sanz MA, Vellenga E, Rayon C, Diaz-Mediavilla J, Rivas C, Amutio E, Arias J, Deben G, Novo A, Bergua J, de la Serna J, Bueno J, Negri S, Beltran de Heredia JM, Marin G. All-trans retinoic acid and anthracycline monochemotherapy for the treatment of elderly patients with acute promyelocytic leukemia. *Blood*. 2004; 104:3490-3493

30. Ades L, Chevret S, Raffoux E, de Botton S, Guerci A, Pigneux A, Stoppa AM, Lamy T, Rigal-Huguet F, Vekhoff A, Meyer-Monard S, Maloisel F, Deconinck E, Ferrant A, Thomas X, Fegueux N, Chomienne C, Dombret H, Degos L, Fenaux P. Is cytarabine useful in the treatment of acute promyelocytic leukemia? Results of a randomized trail from the European Acute Promelocytic Leukemia Group. *J Clin Oncol*. 2006;24:5703-5710.

31. Tallman MS, Andersen JW, Schiffer CA, Appelbaum FR, Feusner JH, Ogden A, Shepherd L, Willman C, Bloomfield CD, Rowe JM, Wiernik PH. All-transretinoic acid in acute promyelocytic leukemia. *N Engl J Med*. 1997;337:1021-1028.

32. Sanz MA, Tallman MS, Lo-Coco F. Tricks of the trade for the appropriate management of newly diagnosed acute promyelocytic leukemia. *Blood*. 2005;105:3019-3025.

33. Fenaux P, Chastang C, Chevret S, Sanz M, Dombret H, Archimbaud E, Fey M, Rayon C, Huguet F, Sotto JJ, Gardin C, Makhoul PC, Travade P, Solary E, Fegueux N, Bordessoule D, Miguel JS, Link H, Desablens B, Stamatoullas A, Deconinck E, Maloisel F, Castaigne S, Preudhomme C, Degos L. A randomized comparison of all transretinoic acid (ATRA) followed by chemotherapy and ATRA plus chemotherapy and the role of maintenance therapy in newly diagnosed acute promyelocytic leukemia. the Eruopean APL Group. *Blood*. 1999;94: 1192-1200.

34. Mandelli F, Diverio D, Avvisati G, Luciano A, Barbui T, Bernasconi C, Broccia G, Cerri R, Falda M, Fioritoni G, Leoni F, Liso V, Petti MC, Rodeghiero F, Saglio G, Vegna ML, Visani G, Jehn U, Willemze R, Muus P, Pelicci PG, Biondi A, Lo Coco F. Molecular remission in PML/RAR alpha-positive acute promyelocytic leukemia by combined all-trans retinoic acid and idarubicin (AIDA) therapy. Gruppo Italiano-Malattie Ematologiche Maligne dell'Adulto and Associazione Italiana di Ematologia ed Oncologia Pediatrica Cooperative Groups. *Blood*. 1997;90:1014-1021.

35. Soignet SL, Maslak P, Wang ZG, Jhanwar S, Calleja E, Dardashti LJ, Corso D, DeBlasio A, Gabrilove J, Scheinberg DA, Pandolfi PP, Warrell RP Jr. Complete remission after treatment of acute promyelocytic leukemia arsenic trioxide. *N Engl J Med*. 1998; 339:1341-1348.

36. de Botton S, Fawaz A, Chevret S, Dombret H, Thomas X, Sanz, M, Guerci A, San Miguel J, de la Serna J, Stoppa AM, Reman O, Stamatoulas A, Fey M, Cahn JY, Sotto JJ, Bourhis JH, Parry A, Chomienne C, Degos L, Fenaux P. Autologous and allogeneic stem-cell transplantation as salvage treatment of acute promyelocytic leukemia initially treated with alltrans-retinoic acid: a retrospective analysis of the European acute promyelocytic leukemia group. *J Clin Oncol*. 2005;23:120-126.

37. Frankel SR, Eardley A, Lauwers G, Weiss M, Warrell RP, Jr. The "retinoic acid syndrome" in acute promyelocytic leukemia. *Ann Intern Med*. 1992;117:292-296.

38. Patatanian E, Thompson DF. Retinoic acid syndrome: a review. *J Clin Pharm Ther*. 2008;33:331-338.

39. Soignet SL, Frankel SR, Douer D, Tallman MS, Kantarjian H, Calleja E, Stone RM, Kalaycio M, Scheinberg DA, Steinherz P, Sievers EL, Coutre S, Dahlberg S, Ellison R, Warrell RP Jr. United States multicenter study of arsenic trioxide in relapsed acute promyelocytic leukemia. *J Clin Oncol*. 2001;19: 3852-3860.

40. List A, Dewald G, Bennett J, Giagounidis A, Raza A, Feldman E, Powell B, Greenberg P, Thomas D, Stone R, Reeder C, Wride K, Patin J, Schmidt M, Zeldis J, Knight R; Myelodysplastic Syndrome-003 Study Investigators. Lenalidomide in the myelodysplastic syndrome with chromosome 5q deletion. *N Engl J Med*. 2006;355:1456-1465.

41. Kantarjian H, Issa JP, Rosenfeld CS, Bennett JM, Albitar M, DiPersio J, Klimek V, Slack J, de Castro C, Ravandi F, Helmer R 3rd, Shen L, Nimer SD, Leavitt R, Raza A, Saba H. Decitabine improves patient outcomes in myelodysplastic

syndromes: results of a phase III randomized study. *Cancer.* 2006;106:1794-1803.

42. Silverman LR, Demakos EP, Peterson BL, Kornblith AB, Holland JC, Odchimar-Reissig R, Stone RM, Nelson D, Powell BL, DeCastro CM, Ellerton J, Larson RA, Schiffer CA, Holland JF. Randomized controlled trail of azacitidine in patients with the myelodysplastic syndrome: a study of the cancer and leukemia group B. *J Clin Oncol.* 2002;20:2429-2440.

43. Nimer SD. Myelodysplastic syndromes. *Blood.* 2008;111: 4841-4851.

44. Greenberg P, Cox C, LeBeau MM, Fenaux P, Moral P, Sanz G, Vallespi T, Hamblin T, Oscier D, Ohyashiki K, Toyama K, Aul C, Mufti G, Bennett J. International scoring system for evaluating prognosis in myelodysplastic syndromes. *Blood.* 1997;89:2079-2088.

45. Malcovati L, Germing U, Kuendgen A, Della Porta MG, Pascutto C, Invernizzi R, Giagounidis A, Hildebrandt B, Bernasconi P, Knipp S, Strupp C, Lazzarino M, Aul C, Cazzola M. Time dependent prognostic scoring system for predicting survival and leukemic evolution in myelodysplastic syndromes. *J Clin Oncol.* 2007;25:3503-3510.

46. Hellstrom-Lindberg E, Malcovati L. Supportive care and use of hematopoietic growth factors in myelodysplastic syndromes. *Semin Hematol.* 2008;45:14-22.

47. Sloand EM, Wu CO, Greenberg P, Young N, Barrett J. Factors affecting response and survival in patients with myelodysplasia treated with immunosuppressive therapy. *J Clin Oncol.* 2008;26:2505-2511.

48. Gattermann N. Guidelines on iron chelation therapy in patients with myelodysplastic syndromes and transfusional iron overload. *Leuk Res.* 2007;31(Suppl 3):S10-S15.

49. Jemal A, Murray T, Ward E, Samuels A, Tiwari RC, Ghafoor A, Feuer EJ, Thun MJ. Cancer statistics, 2005. *CA Cancer J Clin* 2005;55:10-30.

50. Lamanna N, Weiss M. Treatment options for newly diagnosed patients with adult acute lymphoblastic leukemia. *Curr Hematol Rep* 2004;3:40-6.

51. Hoelzer D, Gokbuget N, Digel W, Faak T, Kneba M, Reutzel R, Romejko-Jarosinska J, Zwolinski J, Walewski J. Acute lymphoblastic leukemia. *Hematology (Am Soc Hematol Educ Program)* 2002:162-92.

52. Pui CH, Relling MV, Downing JR. Acute lymphoblastic leukemia. *N Engl J Med* 2004;350:1535-48.

53. Soussain C, Patte C, Ostronoff M, Delmer A, Rigal-Huguet F, Cambier N, Leprise PY, Francois S, Cony-Makhoul P, Harousseau JL. Small noncleaved cell lymphoma and leukemia in adults. A retrospective study of 65 adults treated with the LMB pediatric protocols. *Blood* 1995;85:664-74.

54. Thomas DA, Cortes J, O'Brien S, Pierce S, Faderl S, Albitar M, Hagemeister FB, Cabanillas FF, Murphy S, Keating MJ, Kantarjian H. Hyper-CVAD program in Burkitt's-type adult acute lymphoblastic leukemia. *J Clin Oncol* 1999;17:2461-70.

55. Lee EJ, Petroni GR, Schiffer CA, Freter CE, Johnson JL, Barcos M, Frizzera G, Bloomfield CD, Peterson BA. Brief-duration high-intensity chemotherapy for patients with small noncleaved-cell lymphoma or FAB L3 acute lymphocytic leukemia: results of cancer and leukemia group B study 9251. *J Clin Oncol* 2001;19:4014-22.

56. Ohno R. Current progress in the treatment of adult acute leukemia in Japan. *Jpn J Clin Oncol* 1993;23:85-97.

57. Gaynor J, Chapman D, Little C, McKenzie S, Miller W, Andreeff M, Zalmen A, Berman E, Kempin S, Gee, T, Clarkson B. A cause-specific hazard rate analysis of prognostic factors among 199 adults with acute lymphoblastic leukemia: the Memorial Hospital experience since 1969. *J Clin Oncol* 1988;6:1014-30.

58. D Hoelzer, E Thiel, H Loffler, T Buchner, A Ganser, G Heil, P Koch, M Freund, H Diedrich and H Ruhl. Prognostic factors in a multicenter study for treatment of acute lymphoblastic leukemia in adults. *Blood* 1988;71:123-31.

59. C Boucheix, B David, C Sebban, E Racadot, MC Bene, A Bernard, L Campos, H Jouault, F, Sigaux and E Lepage. Immunophenotype of adult acute lymphoblastic leukemia, clinical parameters, and outcome: an analysis of a prospective trial including 562 tested patients (LALA87). French Group on Therapy for Adult Acute Lymphoblastic Leukemia. *Blood* 1994;84:1603-12.

60. Schauer P, Arlin ZA, Mertelsmann R, Cirrincione C, Friedman A, Gee TS, Dowling M, Kempin S, Straus DJ, Koziner B, McKenzie S, Thaler HT, Dufour P, Little C, Dellaquila C, Ellis S, Clarkson B. Treatment of acute lymphoblastic leukemia in adults: results of the L-10 and L-10M protocols. *J Clin Oncol* 1983;1:462-70.

61. Hoelzer D, Thiel E, Loffler H, Bodenstein H, Plaumann L, Buchner T, Ubanitz D, Kock P, Heimpel H, Engelhardt R. Intensified therapy in acute lymphoblastic and acute undifferentiated leukemia in adults. *Blood* 1984;64:38-47.

62. **This article does not exist**

63. Linker C, Damon L, Ries C, Navarro W. Intensified and shortened cyclical chemotherapy for adult acute lymphoblastic leukemia. *J Clin Oncol* 2002;20:2464-71.

64. Larson RA, Dodge RK, Burns CP, Lee EJ, Stone RM, Schulman P, Duggan D, Davey FR, Sobol RE, Frankel SR. A five-drug remission induction regimen with intensive consolidation for adults with acute lymphoblastic leukemia: cancer and leukemia group B study 8811. *Blood* 1995;85:2025-37.

65. Thomas X, Danaila C, Le QH, Sebban C, Troncy J, Charrin C, Lheritier V, Michallet M, Magaud JP, Fiere D. Long-term follow-up of patients with newly diagnosed adult acute lymphoblastic leukemia: a single institution experience of 378 consecutive patients over a 21-year period. *Leukemia* 2001;15:1811-22.

66. Annino L, Vegna ML, Camera A, Specchia G, Visani G, Fioritoni G, Ferrara F, Peta A, Ciolli S, Deplano W, Fabbiano F, Sica S, Di Raimondo F, Cascavilla N, Tabilio A, Leoni P, Invernizzi R, Baccarani M, Rotoli B, Amadori S, Mandelli F; GIMEMA Group. Treatment of adult acute lymphoblastic leukemia (ALL): long-term follow-up of the GIMEMA ALL 0288 randomized study. *Blood* 2002;99:863-71.

67. Takeuchi J, Kyo T, Naito K, Sao H, Takahashi M, Miyawaki S, Kuriyama K, Ohtake S, Yagasaki F, Murakami H, Asou N, Ino T, Okamoto T, Usui N, Nishimura M, Shinagawa K, Fukushima T, Taguchi H, Morii T, Mizuta S, Akiyama H, Nakamura Y, Ohshima T, Ohno R. Induction therapy by frequent administration of doxorubicin with four other drugs, followed by intensive consolidation and maintenance therapy for adult acute lymphoblastic leukemia: the JALSG-ALL93 study. *Leukemia* 2002;16:1259-66.

68. Weiss M.A., Heffner L, Lamanna N, Kataycio M, Schiller G, Coutre S, Maslak P, Jurcic J, Panageas K, Scheinberg D.A.. A randomized trial of cytoarabine with high-dose mitoxantrone compared to a standard vincristine/prednisone-based regimen as induction therapy for adult patients with ALL. *Journal of Clinical Oncology.* 2005; 23:6516.

69. Gottlieb AJ, Weinberg V, Ellison RR, Henderson ES, Terebelo H, Rafia S, Cuttner J, Silver RT, Carey RW, Levy RN. Efficacy of daunorubicin in the therapy of adult acute lymphocytic leukemia: a prospective randomized trial by cancer and leukemia group B. *Blood* 1984;64:267-74.

70. Fiere D, Extra JM, David B, Witz F, Vernand JP, Gastaut JA, Dauriac C, Pris J, Marty M. Treatment of 218 adult lymphoblastic leukemias. *Semin Oncol* 1987;14:64-6.

71. Toyoda Y, Manabe A, Tsuchida M, Hanada R, Ikuta K, Okimoto Y, Ohara A, Ohkawa Y, Mori T, Ishimoto K, Sato T, Kaneko T, Maeda M, Koike K, Shitara T, Hoshi Y, Hosoya R, Tsunematsu Y, Bessho F, Nakazawa S, Saito T. Six months of maintenance chemotherapy after intensified treatment for acute lymphoblastic leukemia of childhood. *J Clin Oncol* 2000;18:1508-16.

72. Schrappe M, Reiter A, Zimmermann M, Harbott J, Ludwig WD, Henze G, Gadner H, Odenwald E, Riehm H. Long-term results of four consecutive trials in childhood ALL performed by the ALL-BFM study group from 1981 to 1995. Berlin-Frankfurt-Munster. *Leukemia* 2000;14:2205-22.

73. Duration and intensity of maintenance chemotherapy in acute lymphoblastic leukaemia: overview of 42 trials involving 12 000

randomised children. Childhood ALL Collaborative Group. Lancet 1996;347:1783-8.

74. Cassileth PA, Andersen JW, Bennett JM, Hoagland HC, Mazza JJ, O'Connell MC, Paietta E, Wiernik P. Adult acute lymphocytic leukemia: the Eastern Cooperative Oncology Group experience. Leukemia 1992;6 Suppl 2:178-81.

75. Cuttner J, Mick R, Budman DR, Mayer RJ, Lee EJ, Henderson ES, Weiss RB, Paciucci PA, Sobol R, Davey F, Bloomfield C, Schiffer C. Phase III trial of brief intensive treatment of adult acute lymphocytic leukemia comparing daunorubicin and mitoxantrone: a CALGB Study. Leukemia 1991;5:425-31.

76. Dekker AW, van't Veer MB, Sizoo W, Haak HL, van der Lelie J, Ossenkoppele G, Huijgens PC, Schouten HC, Sonneveld Wellemze R, Verdonck LF, van Putten WL, Lowenberg B. Intensive postremission chemotherapy without maintenance therapy in adults with acute lymphoblastic leukemia. Dutch Hemato-Oncology Research Group. J Clin Oncol 1997;15:476-82.

77. Scheinberg DA MP, Weiss M. Acute Leukemias. 7th ed. Philadelphia: Lipincott Williams and Wilkins; 2004.

78. Kantarjian HM, Walters RS, Smith TL, Keating MJ, Barlogie B, McCredie KB, Freireich EJ. Identification of risk groups for development of central nervous system leukemia in adults with acute lymphocytic leukemia. Blood 1988;72:1784-9.

79. Omura GA, Moffitt S, Vogler WR, Salter MM. Combination chemotherapy of adult acute lymphoblastic leukemia with randomized central nervous system prophylaxis. Blood 1980;55:199-204.

80. Sebban C, Lepage E, Vernant JP, Gluckman E, Attal M, Reiffers J, Sulton L, Racadat E, Michallet M, Maraninchi D, Dreyfus F, Fiere D. Sebban C, Lepage E, Vernant JP, et al. Allogeneic bone marrow transplantation in adult acute lymphoblastic leukemia in first complete remission: a comparative study. French Group of Therapy of Adult Acute Lymphoblastic Leukemia. J Clin Oncol 1994;12:2580-7.

81. Zhang MJ, Hoelzer D, Horowitz MM, Gale RP, Messerer D, Klein JP, Loffler H, Sobocinski KA, Thiel E, Weisdorf DJ. Long-term follow-up of adults with acute lymphoblastic leukemia in first remission treated with chemotherapy or bone marrow transplantation. The Acute Lymphoblastic Leukemia Working Committee. Ann Intern Med 1995;123:428-31.

82. Thomas X, Boiron JM, Huguet F, Dombret H, Bradstock K, Vey N, Kovacsovics T, Delannoy A, Fegueux N, Fenaux P, Stamatoullas A, Vernant JP, Tournilhac O, Buzyn A, Reman O, Charrin C, Boucheix C, Gabert J, Lhéritier V, Fiere D Outcome of treatment in adults with acute lymphoblastic leukemia: analysis of the LALA-94 trial. J Clin Oncol. 2004; 22: 4075-86.

83. Kiehl MG, Kraut L, Schwerdtfeger R, Hertenstein B, Remberger M, Kroeger N, Stelljes M, Bornhaeuser M, Martin H, Scheid C, Ganser A, Zander AR, Kienast J, Ehninger G, Hoelzer D. Diehl V, Fauser AA, Ringden O. Outcome of allogeneic hematopoietic stem-cell transplantation in adult patients with acute lymphoblastic leukemia: no difference in related compared with unrelated transplant in first complete remission. J Clin Oncol 2004;22:2816-25.

84. Ottmann OG, Druker BJ, Sawyers CL, Goldman JM, Reiffers J, Silver RT, Tura S, Fischer T, Deininger MW, Schiffer CA, Baccarani M, Gratwohl A, Hochhaus A, Hoelzer D, Fernandes-Reese S, Gathmann I, Capdeville R, O'Brian SG. A phase 2 study of imatinib in patients with relapsed or refractory Philadelphia chromosome-positive acute lymphoid leukemias. Blood 2002;100:1965-71.

85. Yanada M, Tekeuchi J, Sugiura I, Akiyama H, Usui N, Yagasaki F, Kobayashi T, Ueda Y, Takeuchi M, Miyawaki S, Maruta A, Emi N, Miyazaki Y, Ohtake S, Jinnai I, Matsuo K, Naoe T, Ohno R, Japan Adult Leukemia Study Group. High complete remission rate and promising outcome by combination of imatinib and chemotherapy for newly diagnosed BCR-ABL-positive acute lymphoblastic leukemia: a phase II study by the Japan Adult Leukemia Study Group. J Clin Oncol 2006; 24:460-6.

86. Lee KH, Lee JH, Choi SJ, Lee JH, Seol M, Lee YS, Kim WK, Lee JS, Seo EJ, Jang S, Park CJ, Chi HS. Clinical effect of imatinib added to intensive combination chemotherapy for newly diag-

nosed Philadelphia chromosome-positive acute lymphoblastic leukemia. Leukemia 2005;19:1509-16.

87. Doney K, Fisher LD, Appelbaum FR, Buckner CD, Storb R, Singer J, Fefer A, Anasetti C, Beatty P, Bensinger W, Clift R, Hansen J, Hill R, Loughran TP Jr, Martin P, Petersen FB, Sanders J, Sullivan KM, Stewart P, Weiden P, Witherspoon R, Thomas ED. Treatment of adult acute lymphoblastic leukemia with allogeneic bone marrow transplantation. Multivariate analysis of factors affecting acute graft-versus-host disease, relapse, and relapse-free survival. Bone marrow transplantation 1991;7:453-9.

88. Haim N, Epelbaum R, Ben-Shahar M, Yarnitsky D, Simri W, Robinson E. Full dose vincristine (without 2-mg dose limit) in the treatment of lymphomas. Cancer 1994;73:2515-9.

89. Barry E, Alvarez JA, Scully RE, Miller TL, Lipshultz SE. Anthracycline-induced cardiotoxicity: course, pathophysiology, prevention and management. Expert Opin Pharmacother 2007;8:1039-58.

90. Boissel N, Auclerc MF, Lheritier V, Perel Y, Thomas X, Leblanc T, Rousselot P, Cayuela JM, Gabert J, Fegueux N, Piguet C, Huguet-Rigal F, Berthou C, Boiron JM, Pautas C, Michel G, Fiere D, Leverger G, Dombret H, Baruchel A. Should adolescents with acute lymphoblastic leukemia be treated as old children or young adults? Comparison of the French FRALLE-93 and LALA-94 trials. J Clin Oncol 2003;21:774-80.

91. de Bont JM, Holt B, Dekker AW, van der Does-van den Berg A, Sonneveld P, Pieters R. Significant difference in outcome for adolescents with acute lymphoblastic leukemia treated on pediatric vs adult protocols in the Netherlands. Leukemia 2004;18:2032-5.

92. Jemal A, Siegel R, Ward E, Murray T, Xu J, Smigal C, Thun MJ. Cancer statistics, 2006. CA Cancer J Clin 2006;56:106-30.

93. Jaffe ES HN, Stein H, Vardiman JW, editors. World Health Organization classification of tumours. Pathology and genetics of tumours of hematopoeitic and lymphoid tissues. Lyon (France): IARC Press; 2001.

94. Goldin LR, Pfeiffer RM, Li X, Hemminki K. Familial risk of lymphoproliferative tumors in families of patients with chronic lymphocytic leukemia: results from the Swedish Family-Cancer Database. Blood 2004;104:1850-4.

95. Molica S, Levato D. What is changing in the natural history of chronic lymphocytic leukemia? Haematologica 2001;86:8-12.

96. Pangalis GA, Vassilakopoulos TP, Dimopoulou MN, Siakantaris MP, Kontopidou FN, Angelopoulou MK. B-chronic lymphocytic leukemia: practical aspects. Hematol Oncol 2002;20:103-46.

97. Cukierman T, Gatt ME, Libster D, Goldschmidt N, Matzner Y. Chronic lymphocytic leukemia presenting with extreme hyperleukocytosis and thrombosis of the common femoral vein. Leukemia & lymphoma 2002;43:1865-8.

98. Kantarjian HM, O'Brian S, Smith TL, Cortes J, Giles FJ, Beran M, Peirce S, Huh Y, Andreeff M, Koller C, Ha CS, Keating MJ, Murphy S, Freireich EJ. Results of treatment with hyper-CVAD, a dose-intensive regimen, in adult acute lymphocytic leukemia. J Clin Oncol. 2000; 18: 547-561.

99. Hallek M, Cheson BD, Catovsky D, Caligaris-Cappio F, Dighiero G, Dohner H, Hillmen P, Keating MJ, Montserrat E, Rai KR, Kipps TJ; International Workshop on Chronic Lymphocytic Leukemia. Guidelines for the diagnosis and treatment of chronic lymphocytic leukemia: a report from the International Workshop on Chronic Lymphocytic Leukemia updating the National Cancer Institute-Working Group 1996 guidelines. Blood. 2008; 111: 5446-5456.

100. Group CAC. Duration and intensity of maintenance chemotherapy in acute lymphoblastic leukaemia: Overview of 42 trials involving 12,000 randomized children. Lancet. 1996; 347: 1783-1788.

101. Scheinberg DA MP, Weiss M. Acute Leukemias. Philadelphia: Lipincott-Raven; 2005.

102. Sandherr M, Einsele H, Hebart H, Kahl C, Kern W, Kiehl M, Massenkeil G, Penack O, Schiel X, Schuettrumpf S, Ullmann AJ, Cornely OA; Infectious Diseases Working Party, German Society for Hematology and Oncology. Antiviral prophy-

laxis in patients with haematological malignancies and solid tumours: Guidelines of the Infectious Diseases Working Party (AGIHO) of the German Society for Hematology and Oncology (DGHO). *Ann Oncol.* 2006; 17: 1051-1059.

103. Hamblin TJ. Autoimmune complications of chronic lymphocytic leukemia. *Semin Oncol.* 2006; 33: 230-239.

104. Preston DL, Kusumi S, Tomonaga M, Izumi S, Ron E, Kuramoto A, Kamuda N, Dohy H, Matsui T, Nonaka H, Thompson DE, Soda M, Mabuchi K. Cancer incidence in atomic bomb survivors. Part III. Leukemia, lymphoma and multiple myeloma, 1950-1987. Radiat Res 1994;137:S68-97.

105. Diehl LF, Karnell LH, Menck HR. The American College of Surgeons Commission on Cancer and the American Cancer Society. The National Cancer Data Base report on age, gender, treatment, and outcomes of patients with chronic lymphocytic leukemia. Cancer 1999;86:2684-92.

106. Rai KR, Sawitsky A, Cronkite EP, Chanana AD, Levy RN, Pasternack BS. Clinical staging of chronic lymphocytic leukemia. Blood 1975;46:219-34.

107. Binet JL, Auquier A, Dighiero G, Chastang C, Piguet H, Goasguen J, Vaugier G, Potron G, Colona P, Oberling F, Thomas M, Tchernia G, Jacquillat C, Boivin P, Lesty C, Duault MT, Monconduit M, Belabbes S, Gremy F. A new prognostic classification of chronic lymphocytic leukemia derived from a multivariate survival analysis. Cancer 1981;48: 198-206.

108. Rai: K. A critical analysis of staging in CLL, in Gale RP, Rai KR (eds): Chronic Lymphocytic Leukemia. Recent Progress and Future Direction. . New York, NY: Liss; 1987.

109. Dohner H, Stilgenbauer S, Benner A, Leupolt E, Krober A, Bullinger L, Dohner K, Bentz M, Lichter P. Genomic aberrations and survival in chronic lymphocytic leukemia. The New England journal of medicine 2000;343:1910-6.

110. Hamblin TJ, Davis Z, Gardiner A, Oscier DG, Stevenson FK. Unmutated Ig V(H) genes are associated with a more aggressive form of chronic lymphocytic leukemia. Blood 1999;94:1848-54.

111. Damle RN, Wasil T, Fais F, Ghiotto F, Valetto A, Allen SL, Buchbinder A, Budman D, Dittmar K, Kolitz J, Lichtman SM, Schulman P, Vinciguerra VP, Rai KR, Ferrarini M, Chiorazzi N. Ig V gene mutation status and CD38 expression as novel prognostic indicators in chronic lymphocytic leukemia. Blood 1999;94:1840-7.

112. Crespo M, Bosch F, Villamor N, Bellosillo B, Colomer D, Rozman M, Marcé S, López-Guillermo A, Campo E, Montserrat E.. ZAP-70 expression as a surrogate for immunoglobulin-variable-region mutations in chronic lymphocytic leukemia. The New England journal of medicine 2003;348:1764-75.

113. Cheson BD, Bennett JM, Grever M, Kay N, Keating MJ, O'Brian S, Rai KR. National Cancer Institute-sponsored Working Group guidelines for chronic lymphocytic leukemia: revised guidelines for diagnosis and treatment. Blood 1996;87:4990-7.

114. Rai KR, Peterson BL, Appelbaum FR, Kolitz J, Elias L, Shepherd L, Hines J, Threatte GA, Larson RA, Cheson BD, Schiffer CA . Fludarabine compared with chlorambucil as primary therapy for chronic lymphocytic leukemia. The New England journal of medicine 2000;343:1750-7.

115. O'Brien S, Kantarjian H, Beran M, Smith T, Koller C, Estey E, Robertson LE, Lerner S, Keating M. Results of fludarabine and prednisone therapy in 264 patients with chronic lymphocytic leukemia with multivariate analysis-derived prognostic model for response to treatment. Blood 1993;82:1695-700.

116. Elias L, Stock-Novack D, Head DR, Grever MR, Weick JK, Chapman RA, Godwin JE, Metz EN, Appelbaum FR. A phase I trial of combination fludarabine monophosphate and chlorambucil in chronic lymphocytic leukemia: a Southwest Oncology Group study. Leukemia 1993;7:361-5.

117. Weiss M, Spiess T, Berman E, Kempin S. Concomitant administration of chlorambucil limits dose intensity of fludarabine in previously treated patients with chronic lymphocytic leukemia. Leukemia 1994;8:1290-3.

118. Flinn IW, Byrd JC, Morrison C, Jamison J, Diehl LF, Murphy T, Piantadosi S, Seifter E, Ambinder RF, Vogelsang G, Grever MR. Fludarabine and cyclophosphamide with filgrastim support in patients with previously untreated indolent lymphoid malignancies. Blood 2000;96:71-5.

119. Byrd JC, Peterson BL, Morrison VA, Park K, Jacobson R, Hoke E, Vardiman JW, Rai K, Schiffer CA, Larson RA. Randomized phase 2 study of fludarabine with concurrent versus sequential treatment with rituximab in symptomatic, untreated patients with B-cell chronic lymphocytic leukemia: results from Cancer and Leukemia Group B 9712 (CALGB 9712). Blood 2003;101:6-14.

120. Wierda W, O'Brien S, Wen S, Faderl S, Garcia-Manero G, Thomas D, Do KA, Cortes Jk, Koller C, Beran M, Ferrajoli A, Giles F, Lerner S, Albitar M, Kantarjian H, Keating M. Chemoimmunotherapy with fludarabine, cyclophosphamide, and rituximab for relapsed and refractory chronic lymphocytic leukemia. J Clin Oncol 2005;23:4070-8.

121. Keating MJ, O'Brien S, Albitar M, Lerner S, Plunkett W, Giles F, Andreeff M, Cortes J, Faderl S, Thomas D, Koller C, Wierda W, Detry MA, Lynn A, Kantarjian H. Early results of a chemoimmunotherapy regimen of fludarabine, cyclophosphamide, and rituximab as initial therapy for chronic lymphocytic leukemia. J Clin Oncol 2005;23:4079-88.

122. Kay NE, Geyer SM, Call TG, Shanafelt TD, Zent CS, Jelinek DF, Tschumper R, Bone ND, Dewald GW, Lin TS, Heerema NA, Smith L, Grever MR, Byrd JC. Combination chemoimmunotherapy with pentostatin, cyclophosphamide, and rituximab shows significant clinical activity with low accompanying toxicity in previously untreated B chronic lymphocytic leukemia. Blood 2007;109:405-11.

123. Keating MJ, O'Brien S, Lerner S, Koller C, Beran M, Robertson LE, Freireich EJ, Estey E, Kantarjian H. Long-term follow-up of patients with chronic lymphocytic leukemia (CLL) receiving fludarabine regimens as initial therapy. Blood 1998;92:1165-71.

124. Faderl S, Thomas DA, O'Brien S, Garcia-Manero G, Kantarjian HM, Giles FJ, Koller C, Ferrajoli A, Verstovsek S, Pro B, Andreeff M, Beran M, Cortes J, Wierda W, Tran N, Keating MJ. Experience with alemtuzumab plus rituximab in patients with relapsed and refractory lymphoid malignancies. Blood 2003;101:3413-5.

125. Chemotherapeutic options in chronic lymphocytic leukemia: a meta-analysis of the randomized trials. CLL Trialists' Collaborative Group. J Natl Cancer Inst 1999;91:861-8.

126. Leporrier M, Chevret S, Cazin B, Boudjerra N, Feugier P, Desablens B, Rapp MJ, Jaubert J, Autrand C, Divine M, Dreyfus B, Maloum K, Travade P, Dighiero G, Binet JL, Chastang C; French Cooperative Group on Chronic Lymphocytic Leukemia. Randomized comparison of fludarabine, CAP, and ChOP in 938 previously untreated stage B and C chronic lymphocytic leukemia patients. Blood 2001;98:2319-25.

127. Sandherr M, Einsele H, Hebart H, Kahl C, Kern W, Kiehl M, Massenkeil G, Penack O, Schiel X, Schuettrumpf S, Ullmann AJ, Cornely OA; Infectious Diseases Working Party, German Soceity for Hematology and Oncology. Antiviral prophylaxis in patients with haematological malignancies and solid tumours: Guidelines of the Infectious Diseases Working Party (AGIHO) of the German Society for Hematology and Oncology (DGHO). Ann Oncol 2006;17:1051-9.

128. Hamblin TJ. Autoimmune complications of chronic lymphocytic leukemia. Seminars in oncology 2006;33:230-9.

129. Hisada M, Biggar RJ, Greene MH, Fraumeni JF, Jr., Travis LB. Solid tumors after chronic lymphocytic leukemia. Blood 2001;98:1979-81.

130. Kyasa MJ, Hazlett L, Parrish RS, Schichman SA, Zent CS. Veterans with chronic lymphocytic leukemia/small lymphocytic lymphoma (CLL/SLL) have a markedly increased rate of second malignancy, which is the most common cause of death. Leukemia & lymphoma 2004;45:507-13.

131. Doney K, Fisher LD, Appelbaum FR, et al. Treatment of adult acute

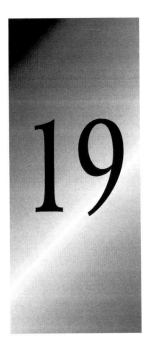

Evaluation and Treatment of Primary Central Nervous System Tumors

Sean A. Grimm
Lisa M. DeAngelis

Primary central nervous system (CNS) tumors encompass a heterogenous mix of histologies and sites of origin. Table 19.1 lists primary CNS tumors based on the World Health Organization (WHO) Classification. In this chapter, we will limit discussion to the presentation (Table 19.2), diagnosis, and treatment (Table 19.3) of the most common brain tumors: gliomas, meningiomas, and primary central nervous system lymphoma (PCNSL).

EPIDEMIOLOGY

Data concerning the incidence of primary CNS tumors are available from the American Cancer Society (ACS) and the Central Brain Tumor Registry of the United States (CBTRUS). Malignant tumors (excluding PCNSL) represented 1.4% of all CNS cancers diagnosed in 2007, but were projected to be the cause of death in 2.3% of all cancers (1). The incidence of brain tumors in 2006 was 20 cases per 100,000 adults (2). In adult men aged 20–39 years, CNS tumors were the second leading cause of death in 1998, 1999, 2001, and 2002, and the leading cause of death in 2000. The prevalence of CNS tumors in 2000 was: malignant 29.5 per 100,000; benign 97.5 per 100,000; and uncertain behavior 3.8 per 100,000 (3).

The most common types are gliomas (40% of all tumors and 78% of malignant tumors) and meningiomas (30% of all tumors) (2). Risk factors for the development of CNS tumors include ionizing radiation (4,5), familial syndromes (6), and immunosuppression (for PCNSL) (7).

CLINICAL PRESENTATION

CNS tumors can present with localized or generalized neurological dysfunction. Generalized symptoms and signs include headaches, seizures, and personality changes. Localized findings include focal weakness, sensory symptoms, gait ataxia, visual changes, or language dysfunction. Table 19.2 lists the relative frequency of each presenting symptom for the brain tumors discussed in this chapter. The neuro-anatomical location of the tumor determines the presenting symptoms and signs.

Contrary to popular perception, headache as the sole presenting symptom is rare. According to one prospective study of patients newly diagnosed with a brain tumor, isolated headache was the presenting symptom in only 8% (8). When associated with other symptoms or signs, headaches occurred at presentation in 37%–62% (9). Concurrent nausea, vomiting, an abnormal neurological examination, or significant change in a prior headache pattern, suggest a structural abnormality that warrants further investigation (10).

Seizures are the presenting symptom in 15%–30% of patients with a brain tumor (11). The location and histologic grade of a tumor correlate with seizure risk. Low-grade, slow growing tumors, and those located in

---

TABLE 19.1

World Health Organization Classification of Tumors of the Central Nervous System

Tumors of Neuroepithelial Tissue

Astrocytic tumors
  Astrocytoma
  Anaplastic astrocytoma
  Glioblastoma multiforme
  Pilocytic astrocytoma
  Subependymal giant-cell astrocytoma

Oligodendroglial tumors
  Oligodendroglioma
  Anaplastic oligodendroglioma

Mixed gliomas
  Oligoastrocytoma
  Anaplastic oligoastrocytoma

Ependymal tumors
  Ependymoma
  Anaplastic ependymoma
  Myxopapillary ependymoma
  Subependymoma

Choroid-plexus tumors
  Choroid-plexus papilloma
  Choroid-plexus carcinoma

Neuronal and mixed neuronal-glial tumors
  Gangliocytoma
  Dysembryoplastic neurepithelial tumor
  Ganglioglioma
  Anaplastic ganglioglioma
  Central neurocytoma

Pineal parenchymal tumors
  Pineocytoma
  Pineoblastoma

Embryonal tumors
  Medulloblastoma
  Primitive neuroectodermal tumor

Meningeal tumors
  Meningioma
  Hemangiopericytoma
  Melanocytic tumor
  Hemangioblastoma

Primary central nervous system lymphoma

Germ cell tumors
  Germinoma
  Embryonal carcinoma
  Yolk-sac tumor (endodermal-sinus tumor)
  Choriocarcinoma
  Teratoma
  Mixed germ-cell tumors

Tumors of the sellar region
  Pituitary adenoma
  Pituitary carcinoma
  Craniopharyngioma

Metastatic tumors

TABLE 19.2

Symptoms and Signs at Presentation

Symptom	High-Grade Glioma	Low-Grade Glioma	PCNSL	Meningioma
Seizures	++	+++	+	+++
Focal neurological dysfunction (eg, hemiparesis, visual field cut, hemisensory loss, aphasia)	+++	+	++	+
Cognitive/ behavioral changes	++	-	+++	+

the gray matter, are associated with the highest risk. Seizures are usually of focal onset, although secondary generalization often occurs. The clinical manifestation of focal seizures varies widely and is sometimes bizarre, but examples include isolated limb movements, tonic posturing, sensory symptoms, unpleasant smell, alteration of consciousness, déjà vu, or a sensation of fear.

DIAGNOSIS

In a patient suspected of harboring a CNS tumor, magnetic resonance imaging (MRI) scan with intravenous (I.V.) contrast is the preferred and only diagnostic test necessary. Head computerized tomography (CT) scan and non-contrast MRI are not adequate for a full evaluation, but CT must suffice for those unable to undergo an MRI (eg, patients who have a pacemaker). A normal contrast enhanced brain MRI essentially excludes a diagnosis of brain tumor. Once a tumor is identified, surgical biopsy or resection is necessary for histologic diagnosis because imaging characteristics are not definitive. Occasionally, positron emission tomography (PET) imaging, MR perfusion, or MR spectroscopy (MRS) are used to guide surgical biopsy to the most potentially malignant region of the tumor.

GLIOMAS

The gliomas are a morphologically and biologically heterogeneous group of primary CNS tumors that arise from neuroepithelial tissue. They are divided into two main histologic subgroups, astrocytoma and oligodendroglioma, and some tumors have mixed features that include both histologies. Both types can be low or high grade. High-grade tumors arise from previously low-grade lesions (secondary) or de novo (primary). Even though the low-grade tumors can be slow growing, most neuro-oncologists do not consider them benign because of diffuse infiltration of normal brain and confinement within the bony calvarium, limiting space for growth. In time (months to years), virtually all low-grade tumors will develop biologic characteristics and histologic features of aggressive gliomas. Although an individual tumor can have areas of low-grade and high-grade pathology, treatment is dictated by the highest grade identified. The third subgroup of gliomas, ependymoma, is less common and will not be discussed in this chapter.

Even when astrocytomas and oligodendrogliomas appear as discrete masses on neuroimaging, surgical cure usually is not possible because of diffuse microscopic infiltration of normal brain tissue. The most common classification and grading system used by neuropathologists is the WHO scheme, which grades gliomas based on nuclear atypia, mitosis, microvascular proliferation, and necrosis (12). The high-grade tumors are anaplastic astrocytoma, anaplastic oligodendroglioma, anaplastic oligoastrocytoma, and glioblastoma multiforme (GBM).

Astrocytic Tumors

Astrocytes are star-shaped supporting cells of the brain and spinal cord. In addition to forming a key component of the blood-brain barrier via their foot processes, they are thought to play an active role in creating and maintaining the microenvironment for neurons. The process by which an astrocyte transforms into a neoplastic cell is unknown, although several genetic abnormalities have been identified. Histologically, tumors of astrocytic origin can be identified by staining for glial fibrillary acidic protein (GFAP), a cytoplasmic fibrillary protein characteristic of astrocytes.

Glioblastoma Multiforme (GBM)

GBM (WHO grade IV) is thought to arise from astrocytes or their precursors (because GFAP can be identified in the cell cytoplasm), although the tumor cells are usually undifferentiated and have a bizarre morphology. It is the most common malignant primary brain tumor, and has a very poor prognosis; despite best treatment, most patients will not survive one year.

Cures are rare and overall survival rates at two and three years are 26% and 5%, respectively, in highly selected patients receiving the best treatment (13,14). The annual incidence in the United States is approximately 13,000 cases, making it the second most common primary brain tumor, representing 20% of all intracranial tumors. It is a tumor of the elderly, with a median age at onset of 64 years (2), although children and young adults are also affected.

GBM is usually localized to the cerebral hemispheres and presents with symptoms of increased intracranial pressure and focal neurological dysfunction. Seizures occur, but with less frequency than in low-grade tumors. On MRI (Fig. 19.1), the tumor appears as a heterogeneous contrast enhancing mass, with associated edema and mass effect. There is often a central area of necrosis, surrounded by a rim of contrast enhancement. The lesion is hypointense on T1- and hyperintense on T2-weighted sequences. The tumor often grows along white matter tracts and can cross the corpus callosum leading to the classic "butterfly" appearance. Although the MRI appearance may be characteristic, tissue diagnosis is essential. The surgical goal is to remove as much tumor as possible, although sometimes only a stereotactic biopsy is feasible when the tumor involves critical brain structures.

Grossly, the tumor appears as a necrotic, yellowish mass that diffusely infiltrates the normal brain. Microscopic features include increased cellularity, pleomorphism, atypia, mitoses, pseudo-palisading necrosis, and microvascular proliferation. Necrosis and vascular hyperplasia are the characteristic features that distinguish GBM from anaplastic astrocytoma.

Prognostic variables include age, extent of resection, performance status, and treatment. Although not curative, neurosurgery is the initial treatment modality. The goals of surgical resection are to improve patient function by decreasing mass effect and edema and to decrease the tumor volume to optimize the effectiveness of radiotherapy and chemotherapy (Table 19.3).

Following surgery, the standard of care is focal radiotherapy to a total dose of 60 Gy in combination with temozolomide (Temodar) chemotherapy (75 mg/m^2 daily during radiation), followed by 6–18 cycles of adjuvant temozolomide (150–200 mg/m^2 on a 5/28 day schedule). This treatment regimen is based on a phase III cooperative trial published by Stupp et al. in 2005, which was the first to demonstrate improved overall survival for GBM treated with radiotherapy plus chemotherapy versus radiotherapy alone (14). Patients in this study were randomized to radiotherapy alone (total dose of 60 Gy given as 2 Gy fractions, five days per week over six weeks) or concomitant daily temozolomide

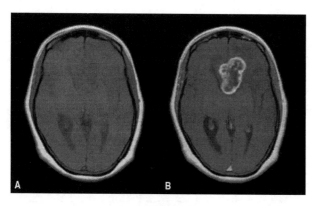

FIGURE 19.1

Glioblastoma multiforme. T1-weighted MRI pre- (A) and post- (B) contrast displaying a heterogeneous enhancing mass with associated edema and mass effect. Note the central area of necrosis, surrounded by a rim of contrast enhancement.

TABLE 19.3
Brain Tumor Initial Treatment

Low-Grade Glioma
　　Maximal tumor resection and/or follow without
　　treatment
　　Focal radiotherapy
　　Temozolomide for oligodendrogliomas
**Anaplastic Astrocytoma, Anaplastic
Oligoastrocytoma**
　　Maximal surgical resection
　　Focal radiotherapy +/- concurrent temozolomide
　　Adjuvant temozolomide chemotherapy
Glioblastoma Multiforme
　　Maximal surgical resection
　　Focal radiotherapy + concurrent temozolomide
　　Adjuvant temozolomide
Primary Central Nervous System Lymphoma
　　Methotrexate-based chemotherapy
　　Whole brain radiotherapy
Meningioma
　　Surgical resection
　　Focal radiotherapy
　　Stereotactic radiosurgery

(75 mg/m^2/day) with standard radiotherapy followed by six cycles of adjuvant temozolomide (150–200 mg/m^2/day on days 1–5 every 28 days). The important prognostic factors were equally balanced between the two groups. The group receiving chemoradiotherapy experienced significantly improved survival compared to the group receiving radiation therapy (RT) alone (median of 14.6 versus 12.1 months), with two-year survival rates of 26% and 10%, respectively.

At recurrence or progression, treatment options are limited. Re-resection can be helpful and probably extends survival about four to six months on average. Patients are not eligible for additional radiation treatment, and approved chemotherapeutic options are few. Active research is being conducted to discover and test promising agents. The current trend favors targeting specific cellular pathways thought to be important in tumor proliferation and survival. One example is the vascular endothelial growth factor (VEGF) pathway, which is important in tumor neovascularization. VEGF overproduction is commonly observed in gliomas, and the supporting vasculature is rich in VEGF receptors. A recent small phase II trial combined bevacizumab, an anti-VEGF antibody, with the cytotoxic agent irinotecan in patients with recurrent malignant gliomas. The authors of this study reported an impressive radiographic response in 63% of patients, a six-month progression-free survival probability of 38%, and six-month overall survival probability of 72% (15). Whether these results will be reproduced in larger trials remains to be seen.

Anaplastic Astrocytoma (AA) and Anaplastic Oligoastrocytoma

Anaplastic astrocytoma (WHO grade III astrocytoma) is a malignant tumor with a median survival of less than three years from diagnosis and estimated five-year survival of 28% despite best treatment (2). It is usually localized to the cerebral hemispheres and presents with seizures, symptoms of increased intracranial pressure and focal neurological dysfunction. The median age of onset is 41 years (16).

On MRI, the tumor presents as an ill-defined T1 hypointense and T2/FLAIR hyperintense mass. Heterogeneous contrast enhancement is usually present, although up to one-third of tumors may not enhance (17). PET imaging, MRS, and MRI with perfusion may assist in making a diagnosis but do not take the place of histology. Resection is advantageous therapeutically and diagnostically because a stereotactic biopsy may not be representative of the entire tumor.

Histologically, AAs are characterized by increased cellularity, nuclear atypia, marked mitotic activity, and microvascular proliferation. Although not curative, maximal resection is a positive prognostic factor. It reduces the mass effect responsible for neurological symptoms and the tumor burden for the subsequent chemotherapy and RT.

Standard treatment for AA consists of maximal surgical resection followed by focal radiotherapy. The standard radiotherapy approach is to treat the tumor bed and a surrounding margin to a total dose of 60 Gy in fractions. Higher doses and hyperfractionated/accelerated schedules have not shown benefit. The role of adjuvant chemotherapy in AAs is controversial. Based on the large randomized trial in GBM, many neuro-oncologists treat AA patients with concurrent temozolomide chemotherapy and RT followed by adjuvant temozolomide chemotherapy. This practice has not been studied in randomized trials for AA. At recurrence, temozolomide has shown efficacy in AA that was treated initially with radiotherapy alone (18). Other options at recurrence include carmustine (BiCNU) or enrollment on an experimental protocol.

Astrocytoma

Diffuse fibrillary astrocytoma (WHO grade II) is the most common low-grade astrocytoma and should be distinguished from the more benign pilocytic astrocytoma (WHO grade I) and pleomorphic xanthoastrocytoma (WHO grade II). The discussion in this section is limited to fibrillary astrocytoma. Fibrillary astrocytomas can originate anywhere in the CNS, but show a preference for the white matter of the cerebral hemispheres. Mean age at diagnosis is 35–40 years, and only a small percentage of patients are younger than 19 years or older than 65 (19). Seizures occur in approximately 80% of patients, and are the most common presenting symptom (20–22). Other, less common presentations include focal neurological deficits and mental changes. Presentation with symptoms and signs of raised intracranial pressure (headache, vomiting, and papilledema) is rare.

On MRI (Fig. 19.2), low-grade astrocytomas are usually hyperintense on T2/FLAIR and hypointense on T1 sequences. Upon administration of I.V. contrast, there is usually no to little enhancement, and the presence of contrast enhancement is a poor prognostic factor (20,22). Because astrocytomas are highly infiltrative, tumor always extends beyond the abnormality observed on neuroimaging.

Fluorodeoxyglucose or methionine PET imaging, MRS, and MR perfusion assist in assessing tumor grade, but histopathology is necessary for diagnosis. Tissue can be obtained via craniotomy or stereotactic biopsy, although maximal resection is preferable if the lesion can be removed safely. Stereotactic biopsies may be confounded by sampling error and may miss regions of high-grade tumor intermixed with low-grade areas. In contrast, a resection provides more tissue for analysis, may treat focal neurological symptoms and seizures, and may prolong survival.

Grossly, the tumor is slightly discolored yellow or grey, with indistinct margins from normal brain. Under the microscope, there is increased cellularity compared to normal brain tissue with mild to moderate nuclear

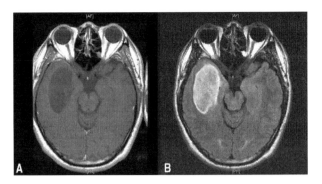

FIGURE 19.2

Astrocytoma. T1-weighted MRI post contrast (A) and FLAIR (B) sequence displaying a nonenhancing lesion in the right temporal lobe. Note that there is minimal mass effect or edema.

pleomorphism and no evidence of mitotic activity, vascular proliferative changes, or necrosis.

The type and timing of treatment for low-grade astrocytoma is controversial. The clinical course is difficult to predict, because tumor progression is highly variable among patients. Furthermore, studies are difficult to interpret because they are mostly retrospective in nature and include variable proportions of low-grade glioma subgroups.

RT is the most effective nonsurgical treatment, although the appropriate timing of its use has not been established. A large prospective study has shown that early radiotherapy prolongs progression-free survival but has no effect on overall survival, compared to reserving radiotherapy until disease progression. Clinically, it is difficult to predict whether early disease progression or the side effects of radiotherapy cause more disability to an individual patient. Consequently, some neuro-oncologists recommend treating early, while others advocate close monitoring, reserving treatment for disease progression.

Traditionally, chemotherapy has played a limited role in the treatment of low-grade astrocytoma because of the slow tumor growth rate. Since temozolomide has been shown efficacious in high-grade gliomas, enthusiasm for its use in low-grade gliomas has increased. To date, there are no good prospective trials to support its use, although it is the first choice for recurrent low-grade astrocytoma after radiotherapy.

Low-grade gliomas in patients aged 45 years or older tend to be biologically aggressive and often require immediate treatment consisting of maximum tumor resection followed by radiotherapy. Aggressive treatment may also be recommended for younger patients with medically intractable seizures, symptoms of increased intracranial pressure, or focal neurological deficits. Younger patients whose seizures are well controlled with anticonvulsant medications and who are neurologically normal may be followed closely and treatment held until there is clinical or radiographic progression. However, progression is often associated with transformation to a higher grade glioma.

The range of survival times for low-grade astrocytoma is large and unpredictable; some patients die early and others live for more than a decade. Most patients will die from their brain tumor once it progresses to a high-grade malignant glioma.

Oligodendroglioma

Oligodendroglioma makes up the other prominent category of glial cell tumors. Its cell of origin, the oligodendrocyte, is the glial cell that myelinates CNS axons. Oligodendroglioma is classified as low (WHO grade II) or high (anaplastic oligodendroglioma, WHO grade III) grade. They are less common than the astrocytic tumors, comprising only 3.7% of all primary brain tumors (2).

The oligodendrogliomas are usually supratentorial, arising in the frontal lobes. They also arise primarily in the white matter, but tend to infiltrate the cortex more than astrocytomas of similar grade. Diffuse infiltration of normal brain usually prohibits surgical cure.

On neuroimaging (Fig. 19.3), oligodendrogliomas cannot be distinguished from astrocytomas. Characteristically, the tumor is usually hypointense on T1- and hyperintense on T2-weighted sequences. The low-grade tumors typically do not enhance post-contrast, although the anaplastic tumors do. Contrast enhancement was a poor prognostic factor in several series. Oligodendrogliomas may be heavily calcified, which is often best appreciated on CT scan. MRS and PET imaging can help differentiate low-grade from high-grade lesions, although only histology is definitive.

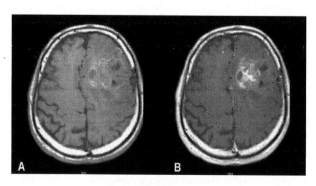

FIGURE 19.3

Anaplastic oligodendroglioma. T1-weighted MRI pre- (A) and post- (B) contrast displaying an enhancing lesion in the left frontal lobe. Note the hyperintense signal on the pre-contrast image consistent with hemorrhage or calcification, both of which are common findings in oligodendroglial tumors.

On gross pathology, they appear similar to astrocytomas, although calcification is a more frequent finding. Microscopically, the tumor cells have a classic "fried egg" appearance—uniform basophilic cells with cleared cytoplasm (perinuclear halos), distinct cell borders, and small bland hyperchromatic nuclei (23). Delicately branching vessels ("chicken wire" pattern) and microcalcifications are also common. Anaplastic oligodendrogliomas are characterized by high mitotic activity and microvascular proliferation.

Both low-grade and high-grade oligodendroglioma may show loss of heterozygosity for chromosomes (LOH) 1p and 19q. This genetic feature may predict a favorable response to chemotherapy or treatment in general. It is considered a positive prognostic factor and should be tested in all oligodendroglioma patients.

Low-Grade Oligodendroglioma

Low-grade oligodendroglioma presents most commonly as a focal seizure in a young adult (median age of onset is 41 years) (2). Because they grow more slowly than astrocytic tumors, there is often a prolonged period of symptoms (usually focal seizures) prior to diagnosis. Before modern neuroimaging, there are a few isolated case reports of patients experiencing seizures for decades, prior to a diagnosis of tumor. Presentation with focal neurological symptoms, such as hemiparesis or hemisensory symptoms occurs, although with lower frequency.

Young age, extent of resection, seizures as initial presenting symptom, high functional status, and presence of 1p and 19q LOH are all positive prognostic factors. In one study, patients diagnosed at younger than age 30 years had a 10-year survival of 75%, whereas those older than 50 years had a 10-year survival of 21%.

Treatment of low-grade oligodendrogliomas follows a paradigm similar to low-grade astrocytic tumors. If located in an accessible brain region, maximal resection is recommended. Asymptomatic patients or those with controlled focal seizures can be followed closely after surgery. Resection specimens should be sent for chromosomal analysis for prognostic considerations.

If the tumor is not resectable and the patient is asymptomatic (except for medically controlled seizures) a PET scan and MRS should be performed. If these confirm a low-grade tumor, the patient can be followed closely as above. If the patient is symptomatic, a biopsy or debulking should be performed followed by chemotherapy with temozolomide or radiotherapy. Oligodendroglioma, particularly associated with 1p and 19q LOH, often shows marked shrinkage of tumor and resolution of symptoms following chemotherapy. If chemotherapy fails, conformal radiotherapy to a total dose of 54 Gy is administered.

At recurrence, patients are treated with surgery if feasible, followed by RT (if not previously administered) and/or chemotherapy. Over time, low-grade oligodendrogliomas transform to anaplastic oligodendrogliomas, which is the cause of death in most patients.

Median overall survival is 16 years and not influenced by the sequence of chemotherapy or radiotherapy.

Anaplastic Oligodendroglioma

Anaplastic oligodendrogliomas present more commonly with focal neurological symptoms and signs than their low-grade counterparts. Seizures occur, but are often associated with hemiparesis, cognitive change, or hemisensory loss. The median age at diagnosis is 48 years (2) and median survival is three to five years (24,25).

Treatment of anaplastic oligodendroglioma is similar to AA. Like low-grade oligodendroglioma, 1p and 19q analysis may predict response to chemotherapy. Following maximal resection, patients are usually treated with conformal radiotherapy and adjuvant chemotherapy. The combination of procarbazine (Matulane), vincristine (Oncovin), and lomustine (CeeNU) in a regimen designated PCV is the only regimen that has been studied in prospective phase III trials of newly diagnosed patients (26,27). The addition of chemotherapy significantly prolongs progression-free survival but had no effect on overall survival. Because of the significant toxicity associated with PCV, most clinicians now use temozolomide, which is much better tolerated. The optimal number of chemotherapy cycles has not been established, but 6–18 cycles of adjuvant temozolomide are often used. Because oligodendroglioma can be exquisitely sensitive to chemotherapy, experimental protocols are underway to study treatment strategies using upfront chemotherapy and deferring radiotherapy. At recurrence, chemotherapeutic options include PCV, carboplatin, cisplatin, and carmustine. The 10-year survival rate is 29.6% (2).

MENINGIOMA

The term *meningioma* was coined by Harvey Cushing in 1922 to describe a tumor proximal to the meninges. Meningiomas are intracranial tumors that are thought to arise from the meningothelial arachnoid cap cells of the meninges. The overwhelming majority are benign, slow-growing tumors that compress the underlying brain but rarely invade it. They often invoke an osteoblastic response in surrounding bone, producing hyperostosis, which can be observed on head CT.

Meningiomas are the most common intracranial tumor, representing 30% (population-based studies) to 40% (autopsy studies) of all cases. They are diagnosed most often in late middle age; the median age is 64 years (2). Women (3:2 to 2:1) and African Americans predominate. Meningiomas are rare in children, accounting for less than 2% of pediatric brain tumors. Genetic predisposition (neurofibromatosis type 2) and prior exposure to ionizing radiation are the only definite predisposing risk factors. Sex hormones, history of breast cancer, and trauma have been proposed as risk factors, but evidence is incomplete.

Grossly, meningiomas are lobulated tumors with a rubbery consistency. When benign, they separate easily from brain tissue, although they can invade the sinuses and encase the cerebral arteries making surgical resection difficult. The tumor can penetrate the bone and present as a scalp mass. Growth patterns include a flat en plaque mass, infiltrating substantial portions of the meninges or, as a spherical mass lesion.

Microscopically, there is a wide range of benign pathologies (eg, meningothelial, fibrous, transitional, secretory, etc.), but most of the histologic subtypes do not have a clinical significance. In contrast, atypical (WHO grade 2), and anaplastic (WHO grade 3) meningiomas are aggressive tumors. Meningioma grading is based primarily on the mitotic count. High-grade meningiomas frequently invade the brain and can rarely metastasize (mostly to liver or bone).

Although there are a variety of presentations depending on tumor location, focal seizures and neurological deficits from brain or cranial nerve compression are most common. Other presenting symptoms and signs include anosmia, hemianopsia, cranial nerve dysfunction (II, III, IV, V, and VI), nuchal or suboccipital

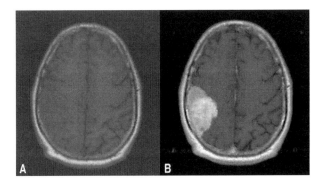

FIGURE 19.4

Meningioma. T1-weighted MRI pre- (A) and post- (B) contrast display an intensely enhancing mass in the right parietal region. Note that the lesion appears isointense prior to contrast administration, a differentiating feature from hemorrhage and metastasis, which are usually hyperintense and hypointense respectively.

pain, tongue atrophy, monoparesis, behavioral change, urinary incontinence, and hearing loss.

MRI (Fig. 19.4) is the preferred neuroimaging test. Because meningiomas do not lie behind the blood-brain barrier, they demonstrate intense, homogenous contrast enhancement, often with an enhancing dural tail. Meningiomas are usually hyperintense on T2 and isointense on T1-weighted imaging (a differentiating feature from metastases, hemorrhage, and schwannoma).

The differential diagnosis for a dural-based mass includes meningioma, lymphoma, metastases (commonly breast and prostate), myeloma, hematoma, inflammatory lesion (sarcoid, syphilis, or granulomatous infection), hemangiopericytoma, and hemangioblastoma.

If a patient is asymptomatic or has medically controlled seizures, meningiomas can be followed closely. If treatment is indicated, surgery is the mainstay and can be curative if the entire tumor is removed. In patients with unresectable tumors, conformal RT is the primary treatment modality. It is used following surgery in all instances of anaplastic meningioma, even if total resection was achieved. Radiosurgery is another option for recurrent benign, atypical, or anaplastic meningioma 3 cm or less in diameter.

There is no established chemotherapy for meningiomas. Isolated reports suggest that hydroxyurea, tamoxifen (Nolvadex), doxorubicin (Adriamycin), interferon-α, and mifepristone (RU486) may have efficacy in some patients.

Survival is widely variable and influenced by meningioma location and grade. In most patients, the tumor will not be the cause of their death.

PRIMARY CENTRAL NERVOUS SYSTEM LYMPHOMA (PCNSL)

PCNSL is a non-Hodgkin lymphoma that arises within and is restricted to the CNS (brain, spinal cord, meninges, and eye). It should be distinguished from metastatic systemic lymphoma because treatment differs. PCNSL occurs in two distinct patient populations—immunocompromised (HIV, transplant, etc.) and immunocompetent. The discussion in this chapter is limited to the immunocompetent group. During the period 1998–2002, PCNSL represented 3% of all primary brain tumors (2). The incidence rate increased more than 10-fold between 1973 and 1992 in presumably immunocompetent patients (28). Immunodeficiency is the only known risk factor; one study reported a 3,600-fold higher incidence rate in HIV patients than in the general population (29). Although prognosis is poor for most patients, survival has also improved in the last decade. The tumor is usually exquisitely sensitive to chemotherapy and radiation and

approximately 20%–30% of patients may be cured with current strategies.

PCNSL is predominately a diffuse large B-cell (CD20+) tumor that is indistinguishable from high-grade, non-Hodgkin lymphoma occurring elsewhere in the body. Microscopically, there is a multifocal, angiocentric pattern of growth. As these areas of perivascular lymphocytes become confluent, a solid mass is formed. The diagnosis can be confused with an inflammatory process since a large number of reactive T-lymphocytes may coexist within the tumor, or a glioma, when a prominent astrocytic or microglial response accompanies the tumor.

The median age at diagnosis is 60 years (2). PCNSL appears multifocal on neuroimaging in 30% and predominately involves the frontal lobes, corpus callosum, and deep periventricular brain structures. As a consequence of this deep localization, cognitive impairment or behavioral changes are the most common presenting features; seizures are rare. Other symptoms include headache, hemiparesis, and hemisensory loss. Symptoms often progress over weeks to months before a diagnosis is made. Patients do not experience the classic "B" symptoms such as fever, night sweats, and weight loss associated with systemic lymphoma; therefore, the

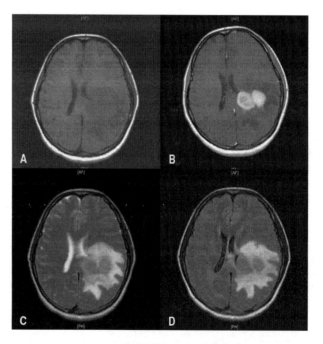

FIGURE 19.5

Primary central nervous system lymphoma. MRI, displaying T1 hypointense (A) a homogenously enhancing mass (B) in the deep left parietal lobe with associated edema and mass effect. The lesion is hypointense on T2 (C) and FLAIR (D) weighted sequences, a differentiating feature from glioma.

presence of these symptoms should prompt a careful investigation for systemic disease.

On MRI (Fig. 19.5), PCNSL is hypointense on T1 and hypo- to iso-intense on T2/FLAIR sequences, with variable surrounding edema. There is usually homogenous enhancement with IV contrast. Ring enhancement is uncommon, except in immunocompromised patients. The appearance on T2 sequences and lack of central necrosis help to differentiate PCNSL from glioma.

Even with a "classic" MRI appearance, histology is essential for diagnosis. At presentation, corticosteroids should not be administered unless absolutely necessary (eg, impending brain herniation). With steroid treatment, PCNSL can transiently disappear (due to apoptosis), delaying diagnosis. In a patient suspected of harboring PCNSL, stereotactic needle biopsy is the best approach because, unlike other primary brain tumors, extensive resection does not improve survival.

Once a diagnosis of CNS lymphoma has been established, an extent-of-disease evaluation should be performed. At diagnosis, ocular and spinal fluid involvement are present in 20% and 25% of patients, respectively. Current staging recommendations include an enhanced cranial MRI, lumbar puncture for cytology, slit lamp examination (to look for ocular lymphoma), enhanced spine MRI (if spinal symptoms are present), HIV serology, body CT scan, and bone marrow biopsy to look for systemic lymphoma (30). Body PET may uncover a systemic site not appreciated by conventional imaging.

As previously mentioned, corticosteroids can decrease edema and induce apoptosis of lymphoid cells. There is a complete resolution of tumor in 15% and greater than 50% shrinkage in 25% of patients after dexamethasone administration and before use of definitive therapy. Eventually, the disease recurs despite continued steroids, usually within a few months. Without more definitive treatment, rapid tumor growth usually occurs, and median survival is three to four months.

PCNSL is exquisitely sensitive to radiotherapy and chemotherapy. In contrast to the gliomas, whole brain radiotherapy (WBRT) is more effective than focal radiotherapy because of the extensive infiltration of the disease throughout the brain. The optimal dose is 40–50 Gy, and there is no benefit of adding a boost to the tumor site (31,32). With WBRT alone, median survival is 12–18 months and the five-year survival rate is only 4%.

The standard systemic lymphoma chemotherapeutic regimens are ineffective for PCNSL. Four prospective trials failed to show any advantage of cyclophosphamide-doxorubicin-vincristine-prednisone (CHOP) or the modified regimen with dexamethasone instead of prednisone (CHOD) plus WBRT over WBRT alone (33–35). High-dose systemic methotrexate is the most effective and widely used drug. It is the only agent that has demonstrated significant advantage over WBRT alone. Protocols utilizing this agent have reported median survivals of 30–60 months (36). To achieve sufficient drug concentrations in the CNS by overcoming the blood-brain barrier, IV methotrexate must be administered at a high-dose with a rapid infusion.

A median overall survival of 60 months was achieved in a prospective trial utilizing a regimen of five cycles of IV methotrexate 3.5 gm/m², vincristine, procarbazine (Matulane), and intrathecal methotrexate, followed by WBRT 45 Gy, and consolidation therapy with I.V. cytarabine (Cytosar) (37). With this treatment protocol, 87% of patients achieved a complete response. Unfortunately, the response is often short-lived with an approximately 50% relapse rate and a high incidence of treatment-related delayed neurotoxicity.

Neurotoxicity after PCNSL treatment is characterized by dementia, ataxia, and urinary incontinence occurring at a mean of seven months from diagnosis. Both methotrexate and radiotherapy can cause this syndrome, and the combination is synergistic. The risk is greatest in patients aged 60 years or older at diagnosis and when methotrexate is administered concurrently or following radiotherapy. In the trial mentioned above, patients 60 years or younger had a 100% incidence of neurotoxicity at 24 months, while those younger than 60 years had a 30% incidence at 96 months (37).

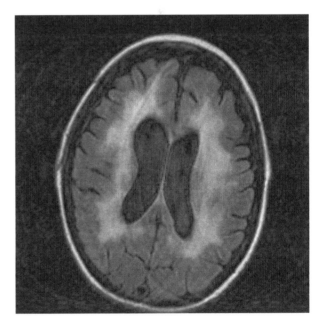

FIGURE 19.6

Leukoencephalopathy. MRI. FLAIR sequence displaying confluent periventricular white matter hyperintensity and large lateral ventricles.

On MRI (Fig. 19.6), treatment-related neurotoxicity is characterized by confluent periventricular T2/FLAIR hyperintensity and enlarged ventricles. There is no effective treatment for this complication, although some patients may benefit from ventriculoperitoneal shunt placement, even though intracranial pressure is not elevated; the situation is comparable to normal pressure hydrocephalus.

Recent work has focused on treatment strategies that reduce relapse risk and prevent neurotoxicity. In one PCNSL trial, withholding radiotherapy in patients aged 60 years and older did not worsen survival, eliminated treatment-related neurotoxicity but resulted in a higher relapse rate (41% vs 17%) (38). In 2008, studies investigated whether high-dose chemotherapy with autologous stem cell transplant can be a substitute for radiotherapy, and if lower dose WBRT can reduce the relapse rate without causing neurotoxicity. Rituximab (Rituxin), a monoclonal antibody to the CD-20 receptor of B-cells, is also being studied as an addition to methotrexate-based protocols.

More than 50% of patients who achieve a remission will eventually relapse. At recurrence, patients should undergo a repeat extent of disease evaluation. Chemotherapeutic options at relapse include a re-trial of high dose methotrexate, temozolomide, topotecan (Hycamtin), or the three drug regimen of procarbazine, vincristine, and lomustine. Some patients have an excellent response and prolonged survival to salvage therapy, but most will eventually die of tumor progression.

References

1. Jemal A, Siegel R, Ward E, Murray T, Xu J, Thun MJ. Cancer statistics, 2007. *CA Cancer J Clin.* 2007;57(1):43–66.
2. CBTUS. *Statistical Report: Primary Brain Tumors in the United States, 1998–2002.* Published by the Central Brain Tumor Registry of the United States; 2005.
3. Davis FG, Kupelian V, Freels S, McCarthy B, Surawicz T. Prevalence estimates for primary brain tumors in the United States by behavior and major histology groups. *Neurooncology.* 2001;3(3):152–158.
4. Amirjamshidi A, Abbassioun K. Radiation-induced tumors of the central nervous system occurring in childhood and adolescence. Four unusual lesions in three patients and a review of the literature. *Childs Nerv Syst.* 2000;16(7):390–397.
5. Ron E, Modan B, Boice JD, Jr., et al. Tumors of the brain and nervous system after radiotherapy in childhood. *N Engl J Med.* 1988;319(16):1033–1039.
6. Bondy M, Wiencke J, Wrensch M, Kyritsis AP. Genetics of primary brain tumors: a review. *J Neurooncology.* 1994;18(1):69–81.
7. Schabet M. Epidemiology of primary CNS lymphoma. *J Neurooncology.* 1999;43(3):199–201.
8. Vázquez-Barquero A, Ibáñez FJ, Herrera S, Izquierdo JM, Berciano J, Pascual J. Isolated headache as the presenting clinical manifestation of intracranial tumors: a prospective study. *Cephalalgia.* 1994;14(4):270–272.
9. Purdy RA, Kirby S. Headaches and brain tumors. *Neurol Clin.* 2004;22(1):39–53.
10. Forsyth PA, Posner JB. Headaches in patients with brain tumors: a study of 111 patients. *Neurology.* 1993;43(9):1678–1683.
11. Sperling MR, Ko J. Seizures and brain tumors. *Semin Oncol.* 2006;33(3):333–341.
12. Kleihues P, Cavenee WK. *International Agency for Research on Cancer. International Society of Neuropathology. Pathology and genetics of tumours of the nervous system.* Lyon: International Agency for Research on Cancer; 1998.
13. Scott JN, Rewcastle NB, Brasher PM, et al. Which glioblastoma multiforme patient will become a long-term survivor? A population-based study. *Ann Neurol.* 1999;46(2):183–188.
14. Stupp R, Mason WP, van den Bent MJ, et al. Radiotherapy plus concomitant and adjuvant temozolomide for glioblastoma. *N Engl J Med.* 2005;352(10):987–996.
15. Vredenburgh JJ, Desjardins A, Herndon JE, et al. Phase II trial of bevacizumab and irinotecan in recurrent malignant glioma. *Clin Cancer Res.* 2007;13(4):1253–1259.
16. See SJ, Gilbert MR. Anaplastic astrocytoma: diagnosis, prognosis, and management. *Semin Oncol.* 2004;31(5):618–634.
17. Henson JW, Gaviani P, Gonzalez RG. MRI in treatment of adult gliomas. *Lancet Oncol.* 2005;6(3):167–175.
18. Yung WK, Prados MD, Yaya-Tur R, et al. Multicenter phase II trial of temozolomide in patients with anaplastic astrocytoma or anaplastic oligoastrocytoma at first relapse. Temodal Brain Tumor Group. *J Clin Oncol.* 1999;17(9):2762–2771.
19. Wessels PH, Weber WEJ, Raven G, Ramaekers FCS, Hopman AHN, Twijnstra A. Supratentorial grade II astrocytoma: biological features and clinical course. *Lancet Neurol.* 2003;2(7):395–403.
20. Kreth FW, Faist M, Rossner R, Volk B, Ostertag CB. Supratentorial World Health Organization Grade 2 astrocytomas and oligoastrocytomas. A new pattern of prognostic factors. *Cancer.* 1997;79(2):370–379.
21. Leighton C, Fisher B, Bauman G, et al. Supratentorial low-grade glioma in adults: an analysis of prognostic factors and timing of radiation. *J Clin Oncol.* 1997;15(4):1294–1301.
22. Lote K, Egeland T, Hager B, et al. Survival, prognostic factors, and therapeutic efficacy in low-grade glioma: a retrospective study in 379 patients. *J Clin Oncol.* 1997;15(9):3129–3140.
23. Bruner JM. Neuropathology of malignant gliomas. *Semin Oncol.* 1994;21(2):126–138.
24. Cairncross G, Seiferheld W, Shaw E, et al. An intergroup randomized controlled trial (RCT) of chemotherapy plus radiation (RT) versus RT alone for pure and mixed anaplastic oligodendrogliomas: Initial report of RTOG 94-02. In: ASCO; 2004. *J Clin Oncol.* 2004;107S.
25. van den Bent MJ, Chinot O, Boogerd W, et al. Second-line chemotherapy with temozolomide in recurrent oligodendroglioma after PCV (procarbazine, lomustine and vincristine) chemotherapy: EORTC Brain Tumor Group phase II study 26972. *Ann Oncol.* 2003;14(4):599–602.
26. Cairncross G, Macdonald D, Ludwin S, et al. Chemotherapy for anaplastic oligodendroglioma. National Cancer Institute of Canada Clinical Trials Group. *J Clin Oncol.* 1994;12(10):2013–2021.
27. van den Bent MJ, Carpentier AF, Brandes AA, et al. Adjuvant procarbazine, lomustine, and vincristine improves progression-free survival but not overall survival in newly diagnosed anaplastic oligodendrogliomas and oligoastrocytomas: a randomized European Organisation for Research and Treatment of Cancer phase III trial. *J Clin Oncol.* 2006;24(18):2715–2722.
28. Corn BW, Marcus SM, Topham A, Hauck W, Curran WJ, Jr. Will primary central nervous system lymphoma be the most frequent brain tumor diagnosed in the year 2000? *Cancer.* 1997;79(12):2409–2413.
29. Coté TR, Manns AA, Hardy CR, Yellin FJ, Hartge P. Epidemiology of brain lymphoma among people with or without acquired immunodeficiency syndrome. AIDS/Cancer Study Group. *J Natl Cancer Inst.* 1996;88(10):675–679.
30. Abrey LE, Batchelor TT, Ferreri AJ, et al. Report of an international workshop to standardize baseline evaluation and

response criteria for primary CNS lymphoma. *J Clin Oncol.* 2005;23(22):5034–5043.

31. DeAngelis LM, Yahalom J, Thaler HT, Kher U. Combined modality therapy for primary CNS lymphoma. *J Clin Oncol.* 1992;10(4):635–643.

32. Nelson DF, Martz KL, Bonner H, et al. Non-Hodgkin's lymphoma of the brain: can high dose, large volume radiation therapy improve survival? Report on a prospective trial by the Radiation Therapy Oncology Group (RTOG): RTOG 8315. *Int J Radiat Oncol Biol Phys.* 1992;23(1):9–17.

33. Lachance DH, Brizel DM, Gockerman JP, et al. Cyclophosphamide, doxorubicin, vincristine, and prednisone for primary central nervous system lymphoma: short-duration response and multifocal intracerebral recurrence preceding radiotherapy. *Neurology.* 1994;44(9):1721–1727.

34. Schultz C, Scott C, Sherman W, et al. Preirradiation chemotherapy with cyclophosphamide, doxorubicin, vincristine, and dexamethasone for primary CNS lymphomas: initial report of radiation therapy oncology group protocol 88-06. *J Clin Oncol.* 1996;14(2):556–564.

35. Shibamoto Y, Tsutsui K, Dodo Y, Yamabe H, Shima N, Abe M. Improved survival rate in primary intracranial lymphoma treated by high-dose radiation and systemic vincristine-doxorubicin-cyclophosphamide-prednisolone chemotherapy. *Cancer.* 1990;65(9):1907–1912.

36. Shah GD, DeAngelis LM. Treatment of primary central nervous system lymphoma. *Hematol Oncol Clin North Am.* 2005;19(4):611–627, v.

37. Abrey LE, Yahalom J, DeAngelis LM. Treatment for primary CNS lymphoma: the next step. *J Clin Oncol.* 2000;18(17):3144–3150.

38. Gavrilovic IT, Hormigo A, Yahalom J, DeAngelis LM, Abrey LE. Long-term follow-up of high-dose methotrexate-based therapy with and without whole brain irradiation for newly diagnosed primary CNS lymphoma. *J Clin Oncol.* 2006; 24(28):4570–4574.

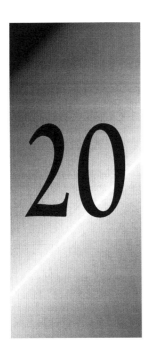

Evaluation and Treatment of Gynecologic Cancer

Meena J. Palayekar
Dennis S. Chi

Gynecologic cancers can originate from the uterus, ovaries, cervix, vulva, vagina, fallopian tubes, or peritoneum. Uterine cancers are the most common. They frequently arise from the endometrial lining of the uterus, and are usually diagnosed early, when the disease is confined to the uterus. Ovarian cancer is the second most frequent gynecologic malignancy. Its signs and symptoms are nonspecific; consequently, most ovarian cancers are not diagnosed until after the disease has spread to the upper abdomen or more distant sites. Invasive cervical cancer is one of the most common malignancies in developing countries, but has become increasingly more uncommon in the United States due to widespread screening using Papanicolaou (Pap) smears. Table 20.1 shows the stage at diagnosis and prognosis of the three most common gynecologic cancers. In this chapter, we will focus on these three gynecologic cancers, namely endometrial, ovarian, and cervical carcinomas. The interested reader is referred elsewhere for a more detailed description of these cancers and for information on the other less common gynecologic malignancies.

ENDOMETRIAL CANCER

Epidemiology

Endometrial cancer is the most common gynecologic malignancy in the United States, with an estimated 39,000 newly diagnosed cases expected in 2007 (1). It is most commonly diagnosed in affluent, obese, post-menopausal women of low parity. The incidence of endometrial cancer is higher in Western countries compared to developing countries. In the United States, white women have a twofold higher incidence of endometrial cancer compared to black women.

Etiology and Risk Factors

Endometrial adenocarcinoma is a cancer arising from the lining of the uterus. Two mechanisms are generally believed to be involved in the development of endometrial cancer. In approximately 75% cases, endometrial cancer develops in a background of endometrial hyperplasia due to exposure to unopposed estrogen, either endogenous or exogenous (type I). In these cases, the tumors tend to be well differentiated and associated with a favorable prognosis. Factors increasing exposure to estrogen, such as unopposed estrogen replacement therapy, obesity, anovulation, and estrogen-secreting tumors, increase the risk of type I endometrial cancer, whereas factors decreasing exposure to estrogens or causing an increase in progesterone levels, such as oral contraceptives and smoking, tend to be protective. Tamoxifen, used in the management of breast cancer, increases the risk of endometrial cancer two- to threefold due to its mild estrogenic effect on the female genital tract. Patients taking tamoxifen should be counseled about this risk,

KEY POINTS

- Gynecologic cancers can originate from the uterus, ovaries, cervix, vulva, vagina, fallopian tubes, or peritoneum.
- Endometrial cancer is the most common gynecologic malignancy in the United States, with an estimated 39,000 newly diagnosed cases expected in 2007.
- Tamoxifen, used in the management of breast cancer, increases the risk of endometrial cancer two- to threefold due to its mild estrogenic effect on the female genital tract.
- Patients with endometrial cancer commonly present with abnormal vaginal bleeding, usually, but not always, after menopause.
- Approximately 22,430 American women will be diagnosed with ovarian cancer in 2007, and an estimated 15,280 will die of the disease, making it the fifth most common cancer in women and the most common cause of gynecologic cancer mortality.
- Approximately 8%–13% of ovarian cancers are due to inherited mutations in the cancer susceptibility genes *BRCA1* and *BRCA2*.

- The majority of women with ovarian cancer present with advanced-stage disease, and these women are best treated in centers of excellence.
- State-of-the-art treatment for advanced ovarian cancer includes optimal primary tumor cytoreduction followed by systemic and intraperitoneal chemotherapy.
- Postoperative chemotherapy is known to significantly prolong survival in ovarian cancer, and the current data support the use of platinum and taxane-based regimens.
- Due to the widespread use of cervical cancer screening in the United States since the mid-1940s, the incidence of cervical cancer has steadily declined, with only 11,150 new cases expected in 2007.
- In June 2006, the Food and Drug Administration (FDA) approved Gardasil, the first quadrivalent vaccine to prevent cervical cancer and precancerous cervical lesions due to HPV-6, -11, -16, and -18.

and any abnormal vaginal bleeding should be investigated by an endometrial biopsy. In the other 25% of cases, endometrial adenocarcinoma appears relatively spontaneously without any clear transition from endometrial hyperplasia. These type II endometrial carcinomas generally arise in a background of atrophic endometrium, tend to be associated with a more undifferentiated cell type, and carry a worse prognosis.

Signs and Symptoms

Patients with endometrial cancer commonly present with abnormal vaginal bleeding, usually, but not always,

after menopause. Uncommonly, a hematometra may develop due to cervical stenosis, especially in elderly, estrogen-deficient patients, which may further progress to a pyometra, leading to a purulent vaginal discharge. Intermenstrual bleeding or prolonged heavy menstrual bleeding in premenopausal women should also arouse suspicion and should be further investigated with an endometrial biopsy.

Screening and Diagnosis

The American Cancer Society does not recommend routine screening for women with no risk factors or

TABLE 20.1					
Stage at Diagnosis and Five-Year Survival Rate of Gynecologic Cancers, United States, 1995–2001[1]					
SITE	STAGE AT DIAGNOSIS (%)			FIVE-YEAR SURVIVAL RATE (%)		
	Localized	Regional	Distant	Localized	Regional	Distant
Uterine corpus	72	16	8	96	66	25
Cervix	55	32	8	92	55	17
Ovary	19	7	68	94	69	29

Source: From Ref. 1.

for those at increased risk of endometrial cancer due to a history of exposure to unopposed estrogen (hormone replacement therapy, late menopause, tamoxifen therapy, nulliparity, infertility, obesity). However, these women should be educated about the symptoms of endometrial cancer, and any abnormal bleeding should be evaluated with an endometrial biopsy. Women with hereditary nonpolyposis colon cancer (HNPCC) syndrome have a 10-fold increased risk of endometrial cancer, with a cumulative risk for the disease of 43% by age 70. Therefore, it is recommended that these patients be offered annual screening with an endometrial biopsy starting at 35 years of age. On completion of childbearing, women with HNPCC who are undergoing surgery for colorectal cancer treatment or prevention should be offered the option of having a concurrent prophylactic hysterectomy. Prophylactic oophorectomy should also be considered, as these patients also have an increased risk of ovarian cancer.

Pathology

Adenocarcinoma

Endometrioid adenocarcinoma accounts for 75%–80% of endometrial carcinomas and is the most common type of endometrial cancer. It varies from well differentiated, with 95% glandular differentiation, to poorly differentiated, with less than 5% glandular differentiation. If the tumor has a malignant squamous component, it is called an adenosquamous carcinoma. Adenosquamous carcinomas are frequently associated with a poorly differentiated glandular component and therefore tend to have a worse prognosis.

Papillary Serous Carcinoma

Papillary serous carcinoma represents an aggressive form of endometrial cancer and accounts for 5%–10% of cases. It is usually found in older postmenopausal women. It has a tendency toward early myometrial invasion, extensive lymphatic space invasion, and early dissemination beyond the uterus.

Clear Cell Carcinoma

Clear cell carcinoma represents 1%–5% of endometrial carcinomas. Like serous carcinoma, it occurs in older postmenopausal women, presents at a higher stage, and has a poor prognosis due to its propensity for early intraperitoneal spread.

Secretory and Ciliary Adenocarcinoma

These are rare but well-differentiated types of endometrial carcinoma, with a good prognosis.

Mucinous Adenocarcinoma

Mucinous adenocarcinomas are tumors of low grade and stage, and are frequently seen in women treated with tamoxifen.

Sarcomas

Carcinosarcomas and other uterine sarcomas are uncommon tumors, accounting for less than 4% of all cancers of the uterine corpus.

Staging

In 1971, the International Federation of Gynecology and Obstetrics (FIGO) instituted clinical staging guidelines for endometrial cancer. Subsequently, seminal studies conducted by the Gynecologic Oncology Group (GOG) showed that information obtained at the time of surgery had significant impact on the accuracy of predicting prognosis and survival (2,3). Therefore, in 1988, FIGO introduced a surgical-pathologic staging system for endometrial cancer (Table 20.2). The surgical

TABLE 20.2
FIGO Surgical Staging for Endometrial Cancer

STAGE	GRADE	CHARACTERISTICS
IA	G1,2,3	Tumor limited to endometrium
IB	G1,2,3	Tumor invasion to less than half of the myometrium
IC	G1,2,3	Tumor invasion to more than half of the myometrium
IIA	G1,2,3	Endocervical glandular involvement only
IIB	G1,2,3	Cervical stromal invasion
IIIA	G1,2,3	Tumor invades serosa or adnexa or positive peritoneal cytology
IIIB	G1,2,3	Vaginal metastases
IIIC	G1,2,3	Metastases to pelvic or para-aortic lymph nodes
IVA	G1,2,3	Tumor invades the bladder and/or bowel mucosa
IVB		Distant metastases, including intra-abdominal and/or inguinal lymph nodes
		Histopathology: degree of differentiation
	G1	<5% of a nonsquamous or nonmorular solid growth pattern
	G2	6%–50% of a nonsquamous or nonmorular solid growth pattern
	G3	>50% of a nonsquamous or nonmorular solid growth pattern

Abbreviation: F160, International Federation of Gynecology and obstetrics.

staging procedure includes an abdominal exploration, peritoneal washings, biopsies of any suspicious lesions, total abdominal hysterectomy (TAH), bilateral salpingo-oophorectomy (BSO), and bilateral retroperitoneal pelvic and para-aortic lymph node dissection. In patients who are poor surgical candidates, the clinical staging system is still utilized.

Treatment

The cornerstone of treatment for endometrial cancer is a TAH-BSO, and this operation should be performed in all cases when feasible. Prospective surgical staging studies by the GOG have demonstrated that the incidence of lymph node metastasis is associated with the endometrial tumor grade and depth of invasion. With higher tumor grades and increasing depth of myometrial penetration, the likelihood of nodal metastasis increases (2,3). Given these findings, numerous authors have reported various preoperative and intraoperative strategies or algorithms that attempt to select patients for complete surgical staging based on tumor grade, depth of myometrial invasion, or intraoperative palpation of nodal areas. However, these strategies fail to detect at least 5%–10% of patients with high-risk factors who should have undergone comprehensive staging, and this inaccuracy could then lead to a second surgical procedure or the administration of unnecessary postoperative therapy (4). Therefore, we feel that comprehensive surgical staging should be considered for all patients with endometrial cancer when feasible. In patients with papillary serous and clear cell carcinoma, surgical staging also includes an omentectomy, as intra-abdominal disease is often found at this site.

Advances in minimally invasive surgical techniques have enabled surgeons to utilize laparoscopy to comprehensively stage patients with early-stage disease. A recently completed large, prospective, randomized trial conducted by the GOG (GOG LAP-2) confirmed prior studies that demonstrated that in well-trained hands, the laparoscopic approach, as compared to laparotomy, is associated with similar oncologic outcomes but decreases hospital stay and length of recovery time.

In patients who undergo surgical exploration for endometrial carcinoma and are found to have bulky retroperitoneal nodes or intra-abdominal metastasis, numerous studies have demonstrated a survival advantage to surgically debulking the metastasis to minimal residual disease prior to the initiation of postoperative therapy (5–7).

Stage I and II

Patients with stage IA/grade 1 or 2 tumors have an excellent prognosis, and no adjuvant therapy is necessary for this group. Patients with stage IA/grade 3 or stage IB disease of any grade are generally offered adjuvant vaginal vault radiation therapy to help prevent vaginal vault recurrence. For patients with stage IC, IIA, or IIB occult disease, postoperative therapy is tailored, usually involving whole-pelvic radiation therapy and/or vaginal brachytherapy, based on risk factors such as tumor grade, lymph-vascular space invasion, depth of myometrial penetration, and the patient's age (8). Patients with gross cervical involvement should undergo a radical hysterectomy instead of a simple hysterectomy, along with a BSO and pelvic and para-aortic lymphadenectomy. Postoperatively, adjuvant therapy is individualized.

Stage III and IV

The GOG recently reported the results of a randomized phase 3 trial of whole-abdominal radiation versus chemotherapy with doxorubicin and cisplatin in advanced endometrial carcinoma (9). Patients on the chemotherapy arm had significantly improved progression-free and overall survival rates. Distal recurrences were less for patients treated with chemotherapy. However, acute toxicity was greater with chemotherapy, and numerous prior studies have demonstrated excellent results with pelvic radiation therapy for isolated nodal and adnexal metastasis. In an attempt to improve efficacy and reduce toxicity, current studies are investigating combined radiation therapy and chemotherapy and other potentially less toxic chemotherapy regimens.

Recurrent Disease

Treatment for recurrent endometrial cancer needs to be tailored according to site of recurrence and prior therapy. Radiation therapy, surgery, endocrine therapy, or cytotoxic chemotherapy can be used alone or in combination. Patients who have not previously received radiation can be treated with radiation therapy. Surgical resection of isolated recurrences can be done. In patients with isolated, centrally located pelvic recurrence, pelvic exenteration can be considered (10,11).

OVARIAN CANCER

Epidemiology

Ovarian cancer is primarily a disease of postmenopausal women, with the majority of cases occurring in women between 50 and 75 years of age. Approximately 22,430 American women will be diagnosed with ovarian cancer in 2007, and an estimated 15,280 will die of the disease, making it the fifth most common cancer in women and the most common cause of gynecologic cancer mortality (1). Ovarian cancer is more common in Northern European and North American countries than in Asia, developing countries, or southern continents.

Etiology and Risk Factors

The etiology of ovarian cancer is unknown. Various risk factors have been reported, such as advancing age, infertility, endometriosis, use of assisted reproductive technologies, and application of perineal talc. Approximately 8%–13% of ovarian cancers are due to inherited mutations in the cancer susceptibility genes *BRCA1* and *BRCA2* (12,13). Women with mutations in *BRCA1* have a 35%–60% risk of developing ovarian cancer by the age of 70, whereas *BRCA2* mutation carriers have a 10%–27% risk of developing ovarian cancer by the age of 70. Approximately 1%–2% of ovarian cancers are associated with inherited defects in the mismatch repair genes *MLH1*, *MSH2*, and *MSH6*, associated with HNPCC syndrome. Carriers of this mutation have a 9%–12% risk of developing ovarian cancer by the age of 70. A family history of ovarian cancer is associated with a three- to fivefold increased risk of developing ovarian cancer compared with the general population (14). Multiple studies have shown multiparity and the use of oral contraceptives to be protective against ovarian cancer.

Signs and Symptoms

Ovarian cancer produces vague symptoms of abdominal pain, discomfort, and bloating. At a later stage, patients may present with weight loss, abdominal distension due to ascites, or a pleural effusion. Some patients may have menstrual irregularity or postmenopausal bleeding.

Screening and Diagnosis

Routine screening for ovarian cancer is not recommended. Women at an increased risk due to a family history of ovarian cancer but no proven genetic predisposition should be offered genetic counseling to help better clarify the risk of ovarian cancer. For this group, there is no clear evidence that currently available screening tests decrease mortality from ovarian cancer; therefore, routine screening is not recommended. Women with inherited mutations in *BRCA1* or the mismatch repair genes *MLH1*, *MSH2*, and *MSH6* should begin ovarian cancer screening between the ages of 30 and 35. For mutations in *BRCA2*, screening is initiated between the ages of 35 and 40.

Serum CA-125 and transvaginal ultrasound can be used for ovarian cancer screening, along with annual pelvic exams. Several studies have shown that a combination of transvaginal ultrasound and CA-125 results in a higher sensitivity for detection of ovarian cancer. A newer technology, proteomics, which involves evaluation of dozens to hundreds of low-molecular proteins simultaneously, is being developed. Newer serum markers, including osteopontin, YKL-40, prostasin, and lysophosphatidic acid (LPA), are being evaluated alone or in combination for ovarian cancer screening.

The diagnosis of ovarian cancer is generally made by histopathologic study following surgical evaluation. The stage of the disease can only be determined by surgery, as discussed next.

Pathology

Ovarian tumors are classified according to their tissue of origin. Eighty-five percent of ovarian cancers arise from the coelomic epithelium lining the ovary; 10% arise from germ cells; and approximately 5% are sex cord-stromal tumors, arising from ovarian mesenchymal tissue.

Epithelial Ovarian Tumors

Of the malignant epithelial ovarian tumors, 40%–50% are serous, 15%–25% are endometrioid, 6%–16% are mucinous, and 5%–11% are clear cell tumors. Less common types of epithelial cell tumors include transitional cell (Brenner), mixed epithelial, and undifferentiated carcinomas. Epithelial ovarian tumors can be benign, of low-malignant potential (borderline tumors), or frankly malignant. Borderline tumors have a much better prognosis than malignant epithelial cancers, but they are malignant and can result in death.

Germ Cell Tumors

Germ cell tumors are most commonly seen in the first two decades of life. The most common germ cell tumor is the mature cystic teratoma (dermoid), which is a benign tumor. Dysgerminoma is the most common malignant germ cell tumor, followed in incidence by the endodermal sinus tumor and the immature teratoma.

Sex Cord-Stromal Tumors

Sex cord-stromal tumors can either arise from the granulosa cells or the Sertoli-Leydig cells, and are named accordingly. More than 90% of malignant stromal tumors are granulosa cell tumors. These tumors can occur at any age, but are more common before menopause.

Staging and Prognosis

Ovarian cancer is surgically staged according to the FIGO staging system (Table 20.3). Surgical staging includes a complete abdominal and pelvic exploration with peritoneal washings, TAH-BSO, an infracolic omentectomy, and bilateral pelvic and para-aortic lymph node sampling. Peritoneal biopsies are taken from various peritoneal surfaces, and any suspicious lesions or adhesions are also sampled.

TABLE 20.3
FIGO Surgical Staging for Ovarian Cancer

STAGE	CHARACTERISTICS
I	Growth limited to the ovaries
IA	Growth limited to one ovary; no ascites; no tumor on the external surfaces; capsule intact
IB	Growth limited to both ovaries; no ascites; no tumor on the external surfaces; capsule intact
IC	Tumor either stage IA or IB present on the surface of one or both ovaries; capsule ruptured; ascites containing malignant cells or positive peritoneal washings
II	Growth involving one or both ovaries with pelvic extension of disease
IIA	Extension of disease and/or metastases to the uterus and/or fallopian tubes
IIB	Extension of disease to other pelvic tissues
IIC	Tumor either stage IIA or IIB but present on the surface of one or both ovaries; capsule ruptured; ascites containing malignant cells or positive peritoneal washings
III	Tumor involving one or both ovaries with peritoneal implants outside the pelvis and/or positive retroperitoneal or inguinal nodes; superficial liver metastases equals stage III; tumor is limited to the true pelvis, but with histologically verified extension to small bowel or omentum
IIIA	Tumor grossly limited to the true pelvis with negative nodes but with histologically confirmed microscopic seeding of abdominal peritoneal surfaces
IIIB	Tumor of one or both ovaries; histologically confirmed implants on abdominal peritoneal surfaces, none >2 cm in diameter; nodes negative
IIIC	Abdominal implants >2 cm in diameter and/or positive retroperitoneal or inguinal nodes
IV	Growth involving one or both ovaries with distant metastases; if pleural effusion is present, there must be positive cytology to allot case to stage IV; parenchymal liver metastases equals stage IV

Laparoscopic surgical staging can be done in patients whose cancer is diagnosed during laparoscopy or in patients with apparently early cancer who are referred for evaluation after inadequate initial surgery (15). If laparoscopic staging is attempted but cannot be adequately performed, an open laparotomy must be performed for comprehensive staging.

Treatment

Surgery followed by postoperative chemotherapy is standard treatment for all patients with advanced-stage disease (stages III and IV) and for most patients with early-stage disease (stages I and II). Postoperative chemotherapy is known to significantly prolong survival, and the current data support the use of platinum- and taxane-based regimens.

Stage I and II

After a systematic and complete surgical staging is performed, the patient's appropriate stage, prognosis, and treatment can be established. In general, a patient with stage IA/grade 1 epithelial ovarian cancer (low risk) will not benefit from adjunctive chemotherapy. It is debatable as to whether stage IA/grade 2 cancer requires adjunctive chemotherapy. In other early-stage disease (high risk), some type of adjunctive treatment is usually required. Table 21.4 shows the classification of ovarian cancer patients within broad categories and their recommended treatment. In low-risk patients who wish to maintain fertility, a unilateral salpingo-oophorectomy with uterine preservation is acceptable.

Stage III and IV

In these patients with metastatic disease, the goal of surgery is to surgically remove or "debulk" all visible and palpable tumor. This level of "cytoreduction" is not always achievable, as there can be more than 1,000 tumor nodules encountered at the time of exploration. In cases in which all tumor cannot be completely removed, studies have shown that there still is a survival benefit if all disease is removed such that the largest tumor nodule remaining measures 1 cm or less in maximal dimension (16). Attaining this level of residual disease status is currently defined as "optimal cytoreduction," and these patients may be candidates for treatment with intraperitoneal chemotherapy in addition to systemic chemotherapy (17). However, if disease is identified outside of the peritoneal cavity (stage IV disease) or if cytoreduction is suboptimal, patients are treated with systemic chemotherapy without an intraperitoneal component.

Chemotherapy

In the 1960s, single alkylating agents were the chemotherapy of choice for epithelial ovarian cancer. The most commonly used drugs were melphalan and chlorambucil. Overall response rates were 45%–55%, and complete clinical response was seen in 15%–20% of cases. Median survival was approximately 12 months. In the 1970s, multidrug regimens resulted in an improvement in overall response rates, complete clinical responses, and increased median survival of approximately 14 months. The introduction of cisplatin in the late 1970s resulted in combination chemotherapy regimens that achieved overall response rates

of 70%–80%, with complete clinical response rates of approximately 50%. The median survival increased to approximately 24–28 months with cisplatin and cyclophosphamide. The replacement of cyclophosphamide with paclitaxel further increased the median survival to 36 months in patients with suboptimally cytoreduced advanced-stage disease.

The GOG then evaluated the combination of carboplatin and paclitaxel and found survival to be equivalent to the combination of cisplatin and paclitaxel (18). Toxicity (particularly neurotoxicity) was less in the carboplatin arm. Based on these studies, the standard primary chemotherapy regimen for advanced ovarian cancer then became carboplatin and paclitaxel.

The GOG recently published the results of a prospective randomized phase 3 trial that compared intravenous paclitaxel plus cisplatin to intravenous paclitaxel plus intraperitoneal cisplatin and paclitaxel in patients with optimally cytoreduced stage III ovarian cancer (17). The study arm receiving the intravenous/intraperitoneal regimen had a 16-month improvement from 50–66 months in median overall survival compared to the intravenous-only control arm. This trial, along with others that have demonstrated improved survival for the intravenous/intraperitoneal approach, led the National Cancer Institute (NCI) to issue an NCI Clinical Announcement in January 2006 that recommended that women with optimally debulked stage III ovarian cancer be counseled about the clinical benefit associated with combined intravenous and intraperitoneal administration of chemotherapy. Due to concerns regarding increased toxicity, however, studies are ongoing to determine the best drug dosing and the safest and efficacious combined intravenous/intraperitoneal regimen.

TABLE 20.4
Recommended Therapy for Epithelial Ovarian Cancer

CATEGORY OF OVARIAN CANCER	RECOMMENDED (STANDARD) THERAPY
Early Ovarian Cancer	
Low risk (stages IA and IB, grade 1[a])	TAH, BSO, full surgical staging
High risk (stages IA and IB, grades 2 and 3; stages IC, IIA, IIB, and IIC)	TAH, BSO[b] full surgical staging
	Adjunctive therapy with combination carboplatin/paclitaxel chemotherapy
Advanced Ovarian Cancer	
Stage III with optimal residual disease[c]	Maximal surgical cytoreduction
	Combination chemotherapy with systemic carboplatin/paclitaxel or systemic/intraperitoneal cisplatin and paclitaxel
Stage IV and/or suboptimal[d]	Maximal surgical cytoreduction
	Combination chemotherapy with carboplatin/paclitaxel

Abbreviations: BSO, bilateral salpingo-oophorectomy; TAH, total abdominal hysterectomy.
[a]Some investigators include grade 2 in the low-risk category.
[b]Unilateral salpingo-oophorectomy is permissible in patients who desire further childbearing.
[c]Optimal (≤1 cm residual tumaor).
[d]Suboptimal (stage III or IV, >1 cm residual tumor).

Recurrent Disease

Patients who develop recurrent disease are generally divided into one of two categories. Platinum-sensitive patients are defined as those who develop recurrent disease six months or more after completion of their primary platinum-based chemotherapy. Platinum-resistant patients relapse within six months of completion of their primary therapy. Patients with platinum-sensitive recurrent disease are usually retreated with platinum-based chemotherapy. These patients are frequently treated with combination chemotherapy with a taxane or gemcitabine added to the platinum compound. Some patients with platinum-sensitive recurrent disease may benefit from a second debulking surgery. The selection of patients for secondary cytoreduction should be based on the disease-free interval from completion of primary therapy, the number of recurrence sites, and the probability of achieving cytoreduction to minimal residual disease (19). Patients with platinum-resistant recurrence are generally not candidates for retreatment with platinum therapy or secondary cytoreduction. These patients are usually offered salvage chemotherapy with other agents or a clinical trial.

CERVICAL CANCER

Epidemiology

Due to the widespread use of cervical cancer screening in the United States since the mid-1940s, the incidence of cervical cancer has steadily declined, with only 11,150 new cases expected in 2007 (1). Cervical cancer still continues to be a significant health problem worldwide, especially in developing countries, where it is a leading cause of death among middle-aged women, primarily from the lower socioeconomic classes, with poor access to medical care and routine screening facilities. The peak age for developing cervical cancer is 47 years. Approximately 47% of women with invasive cervical cancer are aged <35 years at the time of diagnosis. Older women, aged >65 years represent only 10% of the patient population, but they are more likely to succumb to their disease due to more advanced stage at the time of diagnosis.

ETIOLOGY AND RISK FACTORS

Sexual Activity

Invasive cervical cancer can be viewed as a sexually transmitted disease. Early age-of-onset of sexual activity, especially before 16 years of age; onset of sexual activity within one year of menarche; multiple sexual partners; a history of genital warts; and multiparity increase the risk of invasive cervical carcinoma. This is because in early reproductive life, the cervical transformation zone is more susceptible to the oncogenic agent human papillomavirus (HPV). HPV-16 and HPV-18 are the types most commonly associated with cervical cancer. In June 2006, the FDA approved Gardasil, the first quadrivalent vaccine to prevent cervical cancer and precancerous cervical lesions due to HPV-6, -11, -16, and -18. This vaccine is given as three injections at zero, two, and six months, and is approved for use in females aged 9–26 years.

Cigarette Smoking

Cigarette smoking has been identified to be a significant risk factor for cervical cancer due to depression of the immune system, secondary to a systemic effect of cigarette smoke and its byproducts.

Oral Contraceptives

A higher incidence of cervical cancer, especially adenocarcinoma of the cervix, is observed in patients with prior oral contraceptive use.

Alterations in Immune System

Alterations of the immune system are associated with an increased incidence of cervical cancer, as exemplified by the fact that patients infected with human immunodeficiency virus (HIV) and those taking immunosuppressive medications are at an increased risk for developing both preinvasive and invasive cervical cancer.

Signs and Symptoms

The most common symptoms associated with cervical cancer are postcoital and intermenstrual bleeding. It can also present with postmenopausal bleeding, or may be asymptomatic until detected on routine cervical cancer screening. Less commonly, advanced cervical cancer presents with a foul-smelling vaginal discharge, pelvic pain and sciatica, or renal failure due to urinary tract obstruction.

Screening and Diagnosis

Papanicolaou (Pap) Smear

The cervical cytology, or Pap smear, is the paradigm for a cost-effective, easy-to-use, and reliable screening test for cervical cancer. The introduction of the Pap smear has resulted in a significant reduction in the incidence of invasive cervical carcinoma, as well as diagnosis at an earlier stage.

Current Screening Recommendations

The American College of Obstetricians and Gynecologists (ACOG) recommends that sexually active women aged 18 years or older be screened annually until three consecutive normal Pap smears, after which screening may be done less frequently, every two to three years. The American College of Surgeons (ACS) recommends that screening begin at least three years after the onset of vaginal intercourse, but no later than age 21, and should be performed every year with conventional cervical cytology smears, or every two years with liquid-based cytology until age 30. After age 30, HPV DNA testing may be added to cervical cytology for screening. Women older than 70 years with an intact cervix and three or more prior normal Pap smears within the past 10 years may elect to cease cervical cancer screening. Women with prior history of cervical cancer, in utero exposure to diethylstilbestrol (DES), and who are immunocompromised (including HIV positive) should continue cervical cancer screening for as long as they are in reasonably good health and do not have a life-limiting chronic condition. Women who have had a supracervical hysterectomy should continue cervical cancer screening as per the current guidelines.

Diagnosis

The diagnosis of invasive cervical cancer can be suggested by either an abnormal Pap smear or an abnormal physical finding. In the patient with an abnormal Pap smear but normal physical findings, colposcopy is indicated. Colposcopic findings of dense acetowhite epithelium, coarse punctuation and mosaic pattern, or atypical blood vessels are consistent with preinvasive or invasive cervical disease, and warrant biopsies for definitive diagnosis. If the biopsies demonstrate only precancerous changes, the patient should undergo an excisional biopsy of the cervix. The loop electrosurgical excision procedure (LEEP) is the most expedient method of performing an excisional biopsy. Patients with physical signs/symptoms of advanced invasive cervical cancer need a cervical biopsy for diagnosis and treatment planning.

Pathology

Squamous Cell Carcinoma

This accounts for 80% of all cervical carcinomas, and is the most common histology. Routine screening by Pap smears has resulted in a decline in the incidence of this histologic subtype.

Adenocarcinoma

This now accounts for about 20% of all cervical cancers. It has a similar prognosis to squamous cell carcinoma of the cervix when stratified by stage and size of tumor.

Aggressive Subtypes

Small cell or neuroendocrine tumors of the cervix are rare tumors that are very aggressive and have a poor prognosis, even when diagnosed at an early stage.

Rare Tumor Types

Lymphoma, sarcoma, and melanoma of the cervix are rare subtypes, which account for <1% of all cervical cancers.

Staging and Prognosis

Cervical cancer is staged clinically. After a histologic diagnosis of cervical carcinoma, an examination under anesthesia may determine whether the tumor is confined to the cervix or has extended to the adjacent vagina, parametrium, bladder, or rectum. Sometimes, the office examination gives enough information, and examination under anesthesia may not be necessary. According to the FIGO guidelines for clinical staging of cervical cancer (Table 20.5), diagnostic studies used for staging may include intravenous pyelography, cystoscopy, proctosigmoidoscopy, chest x-ray, and barium enema. Computed tomographic (CT) imaging and magnetic resonance imaging (MRI) are frequently used for pretreatment evaluation and treatment planning for

TABLE 20.5 *FIGO Staging for Carcinoma of the Uterine Cervix*	
STAGE	**DESCRIPTION**
0	Carcinoma in situ, intraepithelial carcinoma
I	Carcinoma strictly confined to the cervix (extension to the corpus should be disregarded)
IA	Invasive cancer identified only microscopically; invasion is limited to stromal invasion with maximum depth of 5 mm and no wider than 7 mm
IA1	Measured stromal invasion no greater than 3 mm deep and no wider than 7 mm
IA2	Measured stromal invasion greater than 3 mm but less than 5 mm deep and no wider than 7 mm
IB	Clinical lesions confined to the cervix or preclinical lesions greater than stage IA
IB1	Clinical lesions no greater than 4 cm
IB2	Clinical lesions greater than 4 cm
II	Carcinoma extends beyond the cervix but not onto the pelvic side wall Carcinoma involves the vagina but not the lower third
IIA	No obvious parametrial involvement
IIB	Obvious parametrial involvement
III	Carcinoma has extended onto the pelvic side wall; there is no cancer-free space between the tumor and pelvic wall; tumor involves lower third of vagina
IIIA	No extension onto pelvic side wall, but lower third of vagina involved
IIIB	Extension to the pelvic side wall or hydronephrosis or nonfunctioning kidney
IV	Carcinoma has extended beyond the true pelvis or has clinically involved the mucosa of the bladder or rectum
IVA	Spread to adjacent organs
IVB	Spread to distant organs

patients with advanced disease (stage IIB and greater), but findings on CT/MRI are not used to assign a stage for cervical cancer. Similarly, although the benefits of laparoscopic extraperitoneal surgical staging have been reported, this approach has not yet been incorporated into the FIGO staging system.

Prognosis

Clinical stage is the most important determinant of prognosis. For patients with early disease (stage IB), the size of the lesion, percentage of cervical stromal invasion, histology, tumor grade, and lymph-vascular space involvement (LVSI) are important prognostic factors. For patients with advanced disease (stages II–IV), histology and size of the primary lesion are important prognostic factors.

Treatment

Stage IA1

These patients have microinvasive disease with <3 mm depth of tumor invasion, <7 mm of lateral invasion, and no LVSI. Patients desiring preservation of fertility can be treated with a cone biopsy alone, provided that the margins of the cone are negative. For patients not desirous of further childbearing, a simple hysterectomy is the standard therapy. Vaginal, abdominal, and laparoscopic hysterectomies are equally effective.

Stages IA2, IB1, and Nonbulky IIA Disease

The standard treatment for patients with small-sized cervical carcinomas (<4 cm) confined to the uterine cervix or with minimal vaginal involvement (stage IIA) is radical hysterectomy (removal of uterus, cervix, and parametrial tissue), pelvic lymphadenectomy, and aortic lymph node sampling. There is no difference in survival between patients undergoing radical hysterectomy and those undergoing radiation therapy for early cervical cancer. Radical hysterectomy, however, provides an improved quality of life.

Laparoscopic-assisted radical vaginal hysterectomy and total laparoscopic radical hysterectomy are less invasive alternatives to traditional radical hysterectomy, and results from centers that have the necessary surgical expertise are promising (20,21). In patients desirous of preserving fertility, laparoscopic pelvic lymphadenectomy followed by radical vaginal trachelectomy (removal of uterine cervix and bilateral parametria) and radical abdominal trachelectomy are options offered at a few select centers (22,23). Successful pregnancies after this procedure have been reported. The

role of laparoscopic sentinel lymph node dissection in cervical cancer is an area of active investigation.

Adjuvant Therapy Following Radical Hysterectomy

Concurrent chemoradiation therapy (cisplatin + radiation) following radical hysterectomy has been shown to provide significant benefit in patients with positive nodes, margins, or parametria after radical hysterectomy for early-stage cervical cancer (24). Postoperative radiation therapy has been reported to be of benefit in patients with negative nodes but who are at risk for pelvic failure (primary tumor >4 cm, outer third cervical stromal invasion, LVSI, positive margins or parametria) (25).

Stages IB2 and Bulky IIA Disease

Patients with stage IB2 and bulky stage IIA cervical cancer are generally treated with either primary radical hysterectomy and bilateral pelvic lymphadenectomy, with adjuvant therapy based on risk factors, or primary concurrent radiotherapy and chemotherapy (26).

Stages IIB–IVA Disease

The standard therapy for patients with stage IIB–IVA cervical cancer is concurrent chemotherapy and radiation therapy. The chemotherapy is generally weekly cisplatin combined with external beam pelvic radiation.

Recurrent Disease

Pelvic exenteration is offered to patients whose disease recurs in the central pelvis after radiation therapy. Evidence of extrapelvic disease is a contraindication for pelvic exenteration. During surgery, careful exploration is carried out to confirm that there is no evidence of disease beyond the pelvis. In most cases, the operation involves removal of the bladder, uterus, cervix, vagina and rectum, with urinary and pelvic reconstruction. For patients undergoing successful pelvic exenteration, the five-year survival rates range from 25%–50%. For the rare patient who presents with a single isolated lung metastasis after treatment of invasive cervical carcinoma, pulmonary resection has been reported to be of benefit.

For patients with recurrent disease that is not confined to the pelvis or is thought to be unresectable, palliative chemotherapy is the only treatment that can be offered. A recent GOG study showed the combination of topotecan and cisplatin to have a significant survival advantage over single-agent cisplatin in this setting (27).

CONCLUSION

The three most common gynecologic cancers are carcinomas of the uterus, ovary, and cervix. Endometrial carcinoma is frequently diagnosed at an early stage when surgery alone or in conjunction with radiation therapy can be curative. Recent studies have demonstrated that chemotherapy may be more effective than radiation therapy for postoperative treatment of advanced-stage disease. The majority of women with ovarian carcinoma present with advanced-stage disease. These patients are best served by receiving their treatment in centers of excellence where comprehensive surgery and chemotherapy can be offered. The incidence of cervical carcinoma has decreased over the past 50 years and will most likely continue to decline due to the introduction of the HPV vaccine. Research is ongoing to develop innovative diagnostic, screening, surgical, and nonsurgical techniques for all of these malignancies. Significant advances have been made in our understanding of the molecular abnormalities associated with these diseases, and promising new drugs that target genetically defined abnormalities are being developed. Several such agents are undergoing phase 2 and 3 clinical trials, and offer new hope in the treatment of women with gynecologic cancers.

References

1. Jemal A, Siegel R, Ward E, et al. Cancer statistics, 2007. *CA Cancer J Clin.* 2007;57:43–66.
2. Creasman WT, Morrow CP, Bundy BN, et al. Surgical pathologic spread patterns of endometrial cancer. A Gynecologic Oncology Group study. *Cancer.* 1987;60(8 suppl.):2035–2041.
3. Morrow CP, Bundy BN, Kurman RJ, et al. Relationship between surgical pathologic risk factors and outcome in clinical stage I and II carcinoma of the endometrium. A Gynecologic Oncology Group study. *Gynecol Oncol.* 1991;40:55–65.
4. Barakat RR, Lev G, Hummer AJ, et al. Twelve-year experience in the management of endometrial cancer: a change in surgical and post operative radiation approaches. *Gynecol Oncol.* 2007;105:150–156.
5. Chi DS, Welshinger M, Venkatraman ES, Barakat RR. The role of surgical cytoreduction in stage IV endometrial carcinoma. *Gynecol Oncol.* 1997;67:56–60.
6. Bristow RE, Zahurak ML, Alexander CJ, Zellars RC, Montz FJ. FIGO stage IIIC endometrial carcinoma: resection of macroscopic nodal disease and other determinants of survival. *Int J Gynecol Cancer.* 2003;13:664–672.
7. Lambrou NC, Gomez-Marino, Mirhashemi R, et al. Optimal surgical cytoreduction in patients with stage III and stage IV endometrial carcinoma: a study of morbidity and survival. *Gynecol Oncol.* 2004;93:653–658.
8. Keys HM, Roberts JA, Brunetto VL, et al. A phase III trial of surgery with or without adjunctive external pelvic radiation therapy in intermediate risk endometrial adenocarcinoma: a Gynecologic Oncology Group study. *Gynecol Oncol.* 2004;92:744–751.
9. Randall ME, Filiaci VL, Muss H, et al. Randomized phase III trial of whole-abdominal irradiation versus doxorubicin and cisplatin chemotherapy in advanced endometrial carcinoma: a Gynecologic Oncology Group study. *J Clin Oncol.* 2006;24:36–44.
10. Morris M, Alvarez RD, Kinney WK, Wilson TO. Treatment of recurrent adenocarcinoma of the endometrium with pelvic exenteration. *Gynecol Oncol.* 1996;60:288–291.
11. Barakat RR, Goldman NA, Patel DA, Venkatraman ES, Curtin JP. Pelvic exenteration for recurrent endometrial cancer. *Gynecol Oncol.* 1999;75:99–102.
12. Risch HA, McLaughlin JR, Cole DE, et al. Prevalence and penetrance of germline BRCA1 and BRCA2 mutations in a population series of 649 women with ovarian cancer. *Am J Hum Genet.* 2001;68:700–710.
13. Pal T, Permuth-Wey J, Betts JA, et al. BRCA1 and BRCA2 mutations account for a large proportion of ovarian carcinoma cases. *Cancer.* 2005;104:2807–2816.
14. Bergfeldt K, Rydh B, Granath F, et al. Risk of ovarian cancer in breast cancer patients with a family history of breast or ovarian cancer: a population based cohort study. *Lancet.* 2002;360:891–894.
15. Chi DS, Abu-Rustum NR, Sonoda Y, et al. The safety and efficacy of laparoscopic surgical staging of apparent stage I ovarian and fallopian tube cancers. *Am J Obstet Gynecol.* 2005;192:1614–1619.
16. Chi DS, Eisenhauer EL, Lang J, et al. What is the optimal goal of primary cytoreductive surgery for bulky stage IIIC epithelial ovarian carcinoma? *Gynecol Oncol.* 2006;103:559–564.
17. Armstrong DK, Bundy B, Wenzel L, et al. Intraperitoneal cisplatin and paclitaxel in ovarian cancer. *N Engl J Med.* 2006;354:34–43.
18. Ozols RF, Bundy BN, Greer BE, et al. Phase III trial of carboplatin and paclitaxel compared with cisplatin and paclitaxel in patients with optimally resected stage III ovarian cancer: a Gynecologic Oncology Group study. *J Clin Oncol.* 2003;21:3194–3200.
19. Chi DS, McCaughty K, Diaz JP, et al. Guidelines and selection criteria for secondary cytoreductive surgery in patients with recurrent platinum sensitive epithelial ovarian carcinoma. *Cancer.* 2006;106:1933–1939.
20. Spirtos NM, Eisenkop SM, Schlaerth J, Ballon SC. Laparoscopic radical hysterectomy (type III) in patients with stage I cervical cancer: surgical morbidity and intermediate follow-up. *Am J Obstet Gynecol.* 2002;187:340–348.
21. Abu-Rustum NR, Gemignani ML, Moore K, et al. Total laparoscopic radical hysterectomy with pelvic lymphadenectomy using the argon-beam coagulator: pilot data and comparison to laparotomy. *Gynecol Oncol.* 2004;93:275.
22. Plante M, Renaud MC, Roy M. Radical vaginal trachelectomy: a fertility-preserving option for young women with early stage cervical cancer. *Gynecol Oncol.* 2005;99:S143–S146.
23. Abu-Rustum NR, Sonoda Y, Black D, et al. Fertility sparing radical abdominal trachelectomy for cervical carcinoma: technique and review of literature. *Gynecol Oncol.* 2007;105:830–831.
24. Peters WA 3rd, Liu PY, Barrett RJ 2nd, et al. Concurrent chemotherapy and pelvic radiation therapy compared with pelvic radiation therapy alone as adjuvant therapy after radical surgery in high-risk early-stage cancer of the cervix. *J Clin Oncol.* 2000;18:1606–1613.
25. Sedlis A, Bundy BN, Rotman MZ, et al. A randomized trial of pelvic radiation therapy versus no further therapy in selected patients with stage IB carcinoma of the cervix after radical hysterectomy and pelvic lymphadenectomy: a Gynecologic Oncology Group study. *Gynecol Oncol.* 1999;73:177–183.
26. Keys HM, Bundy BN, Stehman FB, et al. Cisplatin, radiation and adjuvant hysterectomy compared with radiation and adjuvant hysterectomy for bulky stage IB cervical carcinoma. *N Engl J Med.* 1999;340:1154–1161.
27. Long HJ III, Bundy BN, Grendys EC Jr., et al. Randomized phase III trial of cisplatin with or without topotecan in carcinoma of the uterine cervix. A gynecologic Oncology Group study. *J Clin Oncol.* 2005;23:4626–4633.

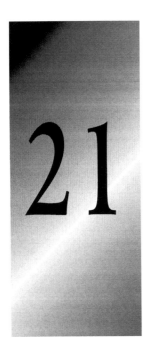

Evaluation and Treatment of Head and Neck Cancer

Laura Locati
Su Hsien Lim
Snehal Patel
David G. Pfister

Head and neck cancer (HNC) typically refers to malignant tumors arising from the mucosal lining of the upper aerodigestive tract, and encompasses primary sites within the oral cavity, larynx, and pharynx. Malignant tumors of the paranasal sinuses and nasal cavity are also sometimes included. Approximately 45,000 new cases of HNC (3% of all cancers) were diagnosed in the United States in 2007, with an associated 11,000 deaths (2% of all cancer deaths) (1). Worldwide, approximately 500,000 new cases of HNC are diagnosed annually, and the related mortality rate is over 50%. Squamous cell cancer or a variant is the histologic type in more than 90% of HNC. HNCs are associated with several challenges in their management, related to the direct involvement by these tumors of key anatomical areas involved with such vital functions as speech, breathing, chewing, and swallowing. Moreover, cosmesis can also be affected.

This chapter will provide a broad overview of the management of HNC with a focus on the anatomy, pathology, epidemiology, diagnostic evaluation, and treatment strategies. Salivary gland cancers will also be discussed, since these malignancies are unique to this body region. Thyroid cancers, also unique to this body region, are covered in another chapter of this text.

ANATOMIC SITES OF DISEASE

Knowledge of the related anatomy is critical to understanding the clinical presentation, patterns of spread, and management of HNCs.

The paranasal sinuses are air-filled spaces located within bones of the skull and face. The maxillary sinuses are the largest of the paranasal sinuses, and are located under the eyes. The frontal sinuses are located within the frontal bone above the eyes, while the ethmoid sinuses consist of several air cells within the ethmoid bones between the nose and the eyes. The sphenoid sinuses are positioned in the center of the skull base and lie superior to the nasopharynx and inferior-medial to the cavernous sinuses, which contain several important structures such as the internal carotid arteries and cranial nerves III (oculomotor nerve), IV (trochlear nerve), VI (abducens nerve), V_1 (ophthalmic nerve), and V_2 (maxillary nerve). Double vision is a typical symptom when a cavernous sinus is involved with tumor. The paranasal sinuses communicate with the nasal cavity.

The oral cavity is separated from the nasal cavity by the hard palate. It is bound anteriorly by the lips and posteriorly by the tonsillar pillars. The floor of the mouth is a U-shaped area bounded by the lower gum

KEY POINTS

- Head and neck cancer (HNC) typically refers to malignant tumors arising from the mucosal lining of the upper aerodigestive tract, and encompasses primary sites within the oral cavity, larynx, and pharynx.
- The vast majority of HNCs are of the squamous cell variety.
- Tobacco and alcohol use are the best established risk factors, and account for approximately 75% of all oral and pharyngeal cancers in the United States.
- Patients most commonly present with locoregional symptoms referable to the primary site or related spread to the neck and consistent with the anatomy of the region. A new ulcer that will not heal, pain, bleeding, dysphagia, odynophagia, changes in articulation, otalgia, hoarseness, nasal or ear congestion, epistaxis, diplopia, or a new lump in the neck are examples of common presenting symptoms.
- HNCs are associated with several challenges in their management, related to the direct involvement by these tumors of key anatomical areas with vital functions such as speech, breathing, chewing, and swallowing. Moreover, cosmesis can also be affected.
- Staging of HNC assesses the extent of disease, establishes prognosis, and guides management.

- Most commonly, the American Joint Committee on Cancer T (primary tumor) N (nodal disease) M (distant metastases) classification system (TNM system) is used for staging tumors of the head and neck.
- The aim of treatment for HNC is to maximize locoregional control and survival while minimizing functional and cosmetic alteration.
- Treatment plans are formulated optimally by a multidisciplinary team (ie, surgeon, radiation, and medical oncologist), particularly when more than one treatment option is available or when combined modality therapy is anticipated. Dental, speech, auditory, swallowing, and nutritional evaluations are commonly indicated before therapy.
- Surgery and radiation are both potentially curative treatments; chemotherapy by itself is generally considered a palliative modality.
- Comprehensive neck dissection involves removal of lymph node levels I–V; cranial nerve XI, the internal jugular vein, and the sternocleidomastoid muscle. A "modified" dissection spares some or all of these last three structures.
- Neck pain and shoulder dysfunction are potential sequelae to neck dissections, particularly comprehensive ones.

and the oral tongue. The mandible, the hard palate, the teeth, the anterior two-thirds of the tongue, and the retromolar trigone (located on the ascending portion of the mandible) are located in the oral cavity.

Posterior to the oral and nasal cavities is the pharynx. It is conventionally divided into three parts: nasopharynx, oropharynx, and hypopharynx. The nasopharynx lies behind the nasal cavity and extends from the skull base to the level of the junction of the hard and soft palates. Its lateral walls include the openings of the eustachian tubes within the fossae of Rosenmüller (pharyngeal recesses), which are located behind the torus tubari. Not surprisingly then, unilateral otitis media is a common presenting symptom for nasopharynx tumors. Inferiorly, the nasopharynx is continuous with the oropharynx and its inferior wall is formed, in part, by the superior surface of the soft palate.

The inferior surface of the soft palate and the uvula lie roughly at the level of C1, and they constitute the superior wall of oropharynx. The anterior wall consists of the base of the tongue, the vallecula, and glossoepiglottic folds, while the lateral wall is made up of the tonsil, tonsillar fossae, and tonsillar pillars. The surface of the base of the tongue appears irregular on exam due to scattered submucosal lymphoid follicles. This lingual tonsillar tissue may harbor a clinically

occult primary cancer. The musculature of the base of the tongue is continuous with that of the oral tongue. The posterior pharyngeal wall is continuous from the nasopharynx down to the hypopharynx. The plane of division between the posterior wall of the nasopharynx and the oropharynx is arbitrarily located at the Passavant ridge, a muscular ring that contracts to seal the nasopharynx from the oropharynx during swallowing. Lateral to the pharyngeal wall are the vessels, nerves, and muscles of the parapharyngeal space.

The oropharynx continues inferiorly into the hypopharynx and spans the area between C3 and C6, ending at the pharyngoesophageal junction. The hypopharynx comprises three subsites: the paired pyriform sinuses, the posterior pharyngeal wall, and the postcricoid area. The pyriform sinuses are grooves lateral to the larynx created by its intrusion into the anterior aspect of the pharynx. Each pyriform sinus has three walls—anterior, lateral, and medial—and communicates with the rest of the hypopharynx posteriorly. The medial wall of each pyriform sinus separates it from the larynx and is bordered superiorly by the aryepiglottic fold. The lateral walls of each pyriform sinus continue superiorly, with the lateral pharyngeal walls of the oropharynx behind the posterior tonsillar pillars. The transition from oropharynx to hypopharynx is located at the plane of the hyoid bone.

The larynx is divided into supraglottic, glottic, and subglottic regions. The supraglottic larynx consists of the epiglottis, false vocal cords, ventricles, aryepiglottic folds, and arytenoids. The glottis includes the true vocal cords and the anterior and posterior commissures. The subglottic larynx extends caudally from 5 mm below the free edge of the true vocal cords to the inferior border of the cricoid cartilage.

The lymphatic drainage of the mucosal surfaces of the head and neck is directed to the lymph nodes located within the fibroadipose tissues in the neck. These lymph nodes are grouped into levels I–VI (Fig. 21.1), corresponding to the submandibular and submental nodes (level I); upper, middle, and lower jugular nodes (levels II, III, and IV, respectively); posterior triangle nodes (level V); and the anterior or central compartment of the neck, located between the carotid arteries of the two sides (level VI). Lymph nodes at level VI receive lymphatics from the thyroid gland, subglottic larynx, cervical trachea, hypopharynx, and cervical esophagus.

With the exception of the glottic larynx and the paranasal sinuses, other sites within the head and neck have a sufficient lymphatic network such that spread to the neck lymph nodes is common. The previous classification of cervical lymph nodes into levels is useful to predict the lymph node groups that are most likely to be involved with metastatic disease for different locations of primary tumors (2). For example, oral cavity cancers typically spread to lymph node levels I and II, while levels II, III, and IV are common sites for the dissemination of laryngeal carcinomas. The classification system is also fundamental in standardizing the terminology used to describe the different types of neck dissections (3). In the case of comprehensive neck dissections (removal of lymph node levels I–V; cranial nerve XI, the internal jugular vein, and the sternocleidomastoid muscle may be all removed or be selectively spared in a "modified" dissection), at least 10 or more nodes are included in the dissected specimen for pathological review. For selective neck dissection in which fewer than five lymph node levels are removed, at least six or more nodes must be removed (4). Neck pain and shoulder dysfunction are potential sequelae to neck dissections, particularly comprehensive ones.

The arterial supply of the head and neck is complex. The principal arteries are the two common carotid arteries and their branches. The common carotid arteries ascend in the neck and each divides into two branches: the external carotid, supplying the exterior of the head, face, and greater part of the neck; and the internal carotid, supplying to a great extent the contents of the cranial and orbital cavities.

With regard to the salivary glands, paired sublingual glands lie immediately underneath the mucosa of the anterior floor of the mouth, while the submandibular glands lie in the upper neck, resting on the external surface of the mylohyoid muscle between the mandible and the insertion of the mylohyoid. The submandibular duct (Wharton duct) exits in the anterior floor of the mouth near the midline. In the subcutaneous tissue of the face, overlying the mandibular ramus and anterior-inferior to the external ear, lie the parotid glands. They secrete saliva through Stenson ducts, opening into the buccal mucosa opposite the second upper molars. Collectively, the sublingual, submandibular, and sublingual glands are known as the major salivary glands. In addition, numerous minor salivary glands are distributed along the submucosa of the entire upper aerodigestive tract. Salivary gland malignancies may also spread to lymph nodes within the neck.

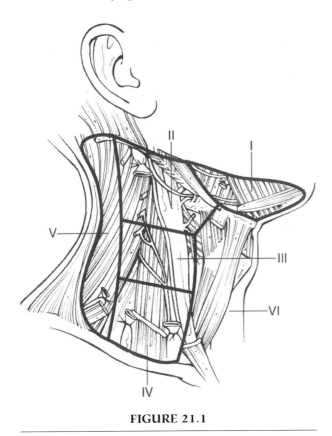

FIGURE 21.1

Superficial dissection of the right side of the neck, showing the carotid and subclavian arteries (Henry Gray, *Anatomy of the Human Body*, 20th ed, thoroughly revised and re-edited by Warren H. Lewis, Philadelphia: Lea & Febiger, 1918; New York: bartleby.com, 2000).

PATHOLOGY

Squamous Cell Cancer

As previously indicated, the vast majority of HNCs are of the squamous cell variety. Immunohistochemically, these tumors are positive for keratin. Carcinogenesis from normal epithelium starts with hyperplasia, with evolution to dysplasia, carcinoma in situ (restricted by the basement membrane and noninvasive) prior to invasive cancer. As such, squamous cell carcinomas may be preceded by various precancerous lesions. Erythroplakia (red, velvety plaque) and leukoplakia (a white plaque that does not rub off) are two widely appreciated premalignant entities. With erythroplakia, the incidence of dysplasia, carcinoma in situ, or invasive cancer is approximately 90%. Although overall, leukoplakia is less prognostically worrisome, a biopsy is recommended to evaluate the severity of dysplasia since the degree of atypia has a direct bearing on the prognosis and management (5).

The histologic grading of squamous cell carcinomas is based on the structure, degree of differentiation, nuclear polymorphism, and number of mitoses (6). Other parameters, such as mode and stage of invasion, presence of vascular invasion, and cellular response, are also assessed. Well-differentiated squamous cell carcinomas are easily recognizable. Epithelial pearls are commonly observed. Verrucous carcinoma, a variant of well-differentiated squamous cell carcinoma, is a low-grade tumor. The classic location of these lesions is the oral cavity (buccal mucosa and lower gingiva). Verrucous carcinomas are indolent neoplasms that may display malignant features such as basement membrane disruption without true signs of invasion. Regional lymph node metastases are rare, and the histology is not associated with distant metastases. Basaloid squamous cell carcinoma is an aggressive variant of squamous cell carcinoma. It is strongly associated with human papillomavirus (HPV) infection (7), and has a predilection for oral cavity, oropharynx, and larynx but can also occur in other sites outside the head and neck. Spindle cell carcinoma, adenoid squamous cell, adenosquamous, small cell, and lymphoepitheliomalike carcinoma are also derived from the surface epithelial tissue and are less frequently diagnosed variants of head and neck squamous cell carcinoma (HNSCC).

Nasopharynx Cancer (NPC)

Carcinomas account for about 85% of nasopharyngeal malignant tumors and are divided into three main histologic types according to the World Health Organization (WHO) classification: type I—keratinizing squamous cell carcinoma; type II—nonkeratinizing carcinoma; type III—undifferentiated, lymphoepithelioid carcinoma. Type I is identified in one-third to one-half of nasopharyngeal cancers, occurring in nonendemic areas of the world, such as North America, and has a more locoregional behavior not dissimilar to other squamous cell carcinomas of the head and neck. Types II and III predominate in endemic regions, such as southern China, North Africa, and the far north hemisphere.

These subtypes have a higher propensity for distant metastases. When a prominent lymphocytic infiltrate is present, the term lymphoepithelioma is applied, and the pathological distinction from lymphoma may be more difficult.

Nasal Cavity and Paranasal Sinus Cancer

Squamous cell carcinoma accounts for more than 50% of nasal cavity and paranasal sinus tumors, with the remainder consisting of minor salivary gland tumors, adenocarcinomas, and sinonasal neuroectodermal tumors (8–10). Squamous cell carcinoma comprises two basic histomorphologic subtypes: typical keratinizing and nonkeratinizing (cylindrical cell carcinoma, transitional-type carcinoma). Sinonasal neuroectodermal tumors include esthesioneuroblastomas, sinonasal neuroendocrine carcinomas (SNEC), and sinonasal undifferentiated carcinomas (SNUC) (11,12). This latter entity, possibly arising from the Schneiderian epithelium, has been recognized and clearly distinguished from esthesioneuroblastoma and undifferentiated nasopharyngeal carcinoma (13,14). Adenocarcinomas are relatively more common among ethmoidal sinus tumors and can be broadly classified into enteric and nonenteric subtypes based on their similarity to adenocarcinoma of the intestinal and seromucous glands, respectively.

Salivary Gland Cancer

Salivary gland cancers pose a particular challenge to the pathologist, primarily because of the complexity of the classification, which includes more than 20 different malignant histologies. The most commonly encountered are listed in Table 21.1. The situation is further compounded by the relative rarity of several entities and because there may be a broad spectrum of morphologic diversity within individual lesions.

TABLE 21.1
Histological Classification of Salivary Gland Carcinomas

Malignant Histology	Incidence (%)
Mucoepidermoid	15.7
Adenoid cystic carcinoma	10.0
Adenocarcinoma	8.0
Malignant mixed tumor	5.7
Acinic cell carcinoma	3.0
Epidermoid carcinoma	1.9
Other	1.3

Adapted from Spiro RH. Salivary neoplasms: overview of a 35-year experience with 2,807 *patients. Head Neck Surg.* 1986;8:177–184.

Mucoepidermoid carcinoma (MEC) is the most common malignant salivary gland neoplasm, and is the predominant subtype observed in the parotid gland (15). MEC is a malignant epithelial tumor that is composed of various proportions of mucous, epidermoid (squamous), intermediate, columnar, and clear cells, and often demonstrates prominent cystic growth. MECs are histologically classified as low grade, intermediate grade, and high grade. High-grade MEC is an aggressive malignancy that both metastasizes and recurs locally. Although tumor grade may be useful, stage appears to be a better indicator of prognosis (16,17).

Adenoid cystic carcinoma (ACC) is a slow-growing but aggressive neoplasm with a remarkable capacity for recurrence (17). It is the most common malignant histology found in the minor salivary glands. Morphologically, three growth patterns have been described: cribriform, or classic pattern; tubular; and solid, or basaloid, pattern. Solid ACC is a high-grade lesion with reported recurrence rates of as much as 100%, compared with 50%–80% for the tubular and cribriform variants (18). Regardless of histologic grade, ACCs, with their unusually slow biologic growth, tend to have a protracted course characterized by neurotropic as well as distant spread, and ultimately a poor outcome. The 10-year survival is <50% for all grades (15,19,20). However, due to its indolent growth and poor response to chemotherapy, asymptomatic metastases, especially to the lungs, are frequently observed and not immediately treated. Clinical stage, particularly tumor size, is more critical than histologic grade in determining the outcome of ACC (21).

EPIDEMIOLOGY AND RISK FACTORS

Squamous cell HNC is more common among men than women. The incidence increases with age, and the age-adjusted incidence and mortality rates are higher among African Americans than members of other ethnic groups (22). Tobacco and alcohol use are the best established risk factors, accounting for approximately 75% of all oral and pharyngeal cancers in the United States (23), and may explain much of the variation in incidence rates among different ethnic groups and genders (24). The use of tobacco and alcohol is associated with so-called "field cancerization" of the upper aerodigestive tract, with an associated increased risk for synchronous lesions as well as second primary cancers.

More specifically, squamous cell HNC is six times more frequent in smokers than nonsmokers (25); continued tobacco use after successful treatment of the initial HNC is associated with a fourfold increased risk

for a second primary cancer compared to those who stop smoking or never smoked (26). Smokeless tobacco and other chewed or ingested carcinogens, such as betel quid (Asia) and maté (South America), increase the risk of oral cancers (27,28). Alcohol appears to be a less potent carcinogen than tobacco (25); however, the combination of alcohol and tobacco is multiplicative not just additive (29). Of note, paranasal sinuses and the nasopharynx primary sites do not have a clear association with tobacco or alcohol usage.

There is a growing appreciation of the role of HPV infection as a risk factor for squamous cell HNC, particularly of the oropharynx in patients without a history of significant tobacco or alcohol use. The most commonly identified strains are HPV 16, -18, -31, -33, and -35, with HPV-16 being the most common. HPV genomic DNA has been detected in 26% of all squamous cell HNC and 50% of oropharyngeal cancer by polymerase chain reaction (PCR) methodology (7,30). HPV-positive HNC also seems to be a distinct entity in terms of epidemiologic, clinical, genomic, and histopathological characteristics when compared to the more common alcohol- and tobacco-related HNCs (7). HPV-positive HNSCC is more frequently seen in younger patients with high-risk sexual behavior, is characterized by poorly differentiated histology with basaloid histotype, and has a better overall prognosis compared to other HNCs related to more conventional risk factors (7).

Dietary factors may also contribute. The incidence of squamous cell HNC is highest among individuals with the lowest consumption of fruits and vegetables. Chronic nutritional deficiency as well as poor oral health may enhance the risk. Clinical findings consistent with poor oral hygiene (eg, mucosal irritation, dental caries, tartar) are associated with a two- to fourfold increase in the risk of oral cancer after adjustment for sex, age, diet, alcohol, and tobacco habits (31,32). The use of vitamin A and E supplementation may decrease the incidence of squamous cell HNC (33). Not surprisingly then, there has been keen interest in the use of certain vitamins and their analogues with chemopreventive intent.

With regard to other primary sites, certain occupational exposures, such as to nickel, wood, and leather dust, are associated with cancers of the sinonasal tract (25,34). Risk factors for salivary gland cancer are less well studied and established. However, prior exposure to ionizing radiation may increase the risk of salivary gland cancers, particularly MEC (35,36). An endemic form of nasopharyngeal cancer occurs in the Mediterranean basin and southern China, and appears linked to infection with the Epstein-Barr virus (EBV). EBV DNA levels seem to correlate with treatment response and may predict disease recurrence, suggesting that they may be an independent indicator of prognosis (37,38). In nonendemic regions in which WHO type I is more common, the connection with EBV is more controversial (39). Diets high in smoked foods are also associated with an increased risk for nasopharynx cancer.

PRESENTATION AND DIAGNOSIS

Patients most commonly present with locoregional symptoms referable to the primary site and consistent with the anatomy of the region. A new ulcer that will not heal, pain, bleeding, dysphagia, odynophagia, changes in articulation, otalgia, hoarseness, nasal or ear congestion, epistaxis, diplopia, or a new lump in the neck are examples of common presenting symptoms. Whether a patient will present early or late is affected by the anatomy of the primary site. For example, glottic cancers tend to present early because patients will seek attention for new hoarseness; however, supraglottic cancers tend to present later because symptoms of dysphagia or throat discomfort may be more vague and discounted as not serious by the patient. With the exception of nasopharynx and hypopharynx primaries, distant metastases at presentation are uncommon. The lung, bone, or liver are the most common distant metastatic sites. Of note, an isolated lung nodule is commonly a new lung primary, given the risk of second or synchronous cancers, as opposed to a metastatic lesion from the primary HNC.

There are no compelling data that screening for HNC improves health outcomes, and as such, the United States Preventive Services Task Force (USP-STF) (40) has no specific recommendations regarding screening for these diseases in the general population. Similarly, there are no tests of serum or saliva that are routinely utilized. Nonetheless, direct inspection and palpation during routine dental examination is commonly recommended and frequently applied as a screen for oral cancer.

As mentioned in the pathology section, leukoplakia and erythroplakia are widely appreciated for their premalignant potential for the development of HNC. Their presence heralds the presence or development of invasive cancer and should be carefully evaluated.

For patients who are disease-free after treatment for their HNC, follow-up is needed due to a risk of relapse, particularly during the first three years, and also an increased rate of second primary cancers (3%–5% per year) among those patients who had an initial squamous cell primary. Per National Comprehensive Cancer Network guidelines (41), history and physical exams are performed every 1–3 months during the first year, every 2–4 months during the second year, every 4–6 months during the third to fifth years, and

every 6–12 months thereafter. Thyroid function tests (if neck radiation was administered) are also recommended, as well as chest imaging as indicated. Once treatment is completed and the patient is felt to be disease-free, routine imaging of the primary site and neck are not routinely indicated in the absence of suspicious signs or symptoms.

Evaluation of a patient with suspected HNC is aimed at reaching a pathological diagnosis and ascertaining the stage of the disease. Tissue for pathological analysis can be obtained through biopsy performed on mucosal lesions during exam or endoscopy. Biopsies of tumors of the oral cavity and oropharynx can be obtained transorally under topical anesthetic; other tumors, such as those of the larynx and pharynx, that are not as easily accessible transorally require pharyngolaryngoscopy under general anesthesia. Fine-needle aspiration cytology (FNAC) is the least invasive and most expeditious method for investigating cervical lymph nodes (42). FNAC of smaller lymph nodes that are not definable on palpation can be performed using imaging guidance. Core biopsies of neck node/mass can be pursued when FNA yields equivocal or difficult to classify findings or lymphoma is suspected. Excisional biopsy of neck node may at times be necessary, but when squamous cell carcinoma is suspected and neck dissection is likely required, should be incorporated preferably into the definitive management plan.

STAGING OF HNC

Staging of HNC assesses the extent of disease, establishes prognosis, and guides management. Most commonly, the American Joint Committee on Cancer (AJCC, 2002) T (primary tumor) N (nodal disease) M (distant metastases) classification system (TNM system) is used for staging tumors of the head and neck. T staging is specific to different anatomical sites in the head and neck, while N staging is common to all head and neck sites (Table 21.2) except the nasopharynx. A final stage group (I–IV) is reached based on the aggregate TNM stage and is similar for all primary sites except NPC (Table 21.3). A detailed description of the TNM staging system for HNSCC is available elsewhere (43,44).

Clinical staging is assessed through physical exam, which often requires some type of endoscopic exam, and radiographic studies. Cross-sectional imaging with computed axial tomography (CAT) primary site and scan and/or magnetic resonance imaging (MRI) of the neck is routinely used to evaluate the locoregional extent of disease (T and N stages), except in case of T_1 laryngeal tumors confined to the vocal cords, where there is low likelihood that radiographic imaging improves the accuracy

TABLE 21.2

Neck Staging for All Head and Neck Sites Except for Nasopharynx Cancer

N Stage	Definition
NX	Regional lymph node cannot be assessed
N0	No regional lymph node metastasis
N1	Metastasis in a single ipsilateral lymph node, 3 cm or less in greatest dimension
N2a	Metastasis in a single ipsilateral lymph node more than 3 cm but no more than 6 cm in greatest dimension
N2b	Metastasis in multiple ipsilateral lymph nodes, none more than 6 cm in greatest dimension
N2c	Metastasis in bilateral or contralateral lymph nodes, none more than 6 cm in greatest dimension
N3	Metastasis in a lymph node more than 6 cm in greatest dimension

TABLE 21.3

Stage Grouping

Stage	T	N	M
0	Tis	N0	M0
I	T1	N0	M0
II	T2	N0	M0
III	T1-2/T3	N1/N0-1	M0
IVA	T1-3/T4a	N2/N0-2	M0
IVB	T4b	Nany	M0
	Tany	N3	
IVC	Tany	Nany	M1

Abbreviations: T, tumor; N, lymph node; M, metastasis.

of clinical staging (45). The lungs are the most common site of distant metastasis from squamous cell HNCs, and a chest x-ray is used to evaluate for distant metastases to the lung, a second lung primary cancer, or other cardiopulmonary disease because medical comorbidity is common among many of these patients. Patients who are at a higher risk of distant spread, such as patients with N_2 disease below the level of the thyroid notch or N_3 disease, should be considered for a more detailed evaluation with CAT scan of the chest. No routine imaging of the liver or bones is performed unless indicated by abnormal biochemical markers or suspicious symptoms, such as pain.

Fluorodeoxyglucose-positron emission tomography (FDG-PET) is not routinely performed, but is helpful in selected circumstances: the detection of occult lymph node disease, the detection of subtle recurrences, and the identification of an unknown primary site (46). The intent is to obtain PET when the information obtained may change management.

Stage IV includes a wide spectrum of locoregionally advanced as well as distantly metastatic disease. Treatment decisions need to be carefully individualized for each patient by an experienced multidisciplinary team. A stage IVA tumor by virtue of treatable N_2 neck disease in the presence of a T1, T2, or even T3 lesion is still considered eligible for curative treatment, whereas a stage IVB patient with an advanced unresectable primary cancer (T4B) or far-advanced neck disease (N3) or both would have a lower probability of cure. Patients with stage IVC disease, because of distant metastases, have exceedingly poor prognosis, with a median survival of less than one year.

TREATMENT

The aim of treatment for HNC is to maximize locoregional control and survival while minimizing functional and cosmetic alteration. Treatment plans are formulated optimally by a multidisciplinary team (ie, surgeon, radiation, and medical oncologist), particularly when more than one treatment option is available or when combined modality therapy is anticipated. Dental, speech, auditory, swallowing, and nutritional evaluations are commonly indicated before therapy.

Surgery and radiation are both potentially curative treatments; chemotherapy by itself is generally considered a palliative modality. In patients who undergo primary surgical therapy, an oncologically adequate resection that obtains pathologically negative margins is the goal. Simply debulking a tumor, or compromising surgical margins in hopes of preserving function, potentially increases the risk of local failure. The following features are suggestive of disease that is likely not resectable for cure: (1) massive skull base invasion, (2) involvement of the prevertebral fascia, (3) direct infiltration of the cervical vertebrae or brachial plexus, (4) carotid artery encasement, (5) skin infiltration, and (6) rapid recurrence after prior extensive surgery.

With regard to radiation therapy, a curative dose of ≥ 70 Gy is delivered to the primary and gross adenopathy, with ≥ 50 Gy delivered to low-risk nodal stations. When adjuvant radiation is applied after surgery, the dose to areas of prior resected gross disease is closer to 60 Gy. Conventional fractionation involves delivery of 2 Gy once daily, five times a week. Radiation-related side effects include dry mouth, mucositis, hypothyroidism (when the thyroid is within the portal) (47), loss of taste, dysphagia, and Lhermitte syndrome (a self-limited, shocklike sensation induced by neck flexion, extending down the spine to the extremities). Certain drugs may be beneficial with regard to the treatment (ie, pilocarpine) or prevention (ie, amifostine) of xerostomia (48–50). Altered fractionation radiation is sometimes utilized, such as hyperfractionation (more than one fraction daily), which has been shown to increase efficacy but at the expense of added acute toxicity. Concurrent chemotherapy similarly improves efficacy. More recently, intensity-modulated radiotherapy (IMRT) has become widely available and allows a more conformal dose distribution. By decreasing toxicity to normal adjacent tissue, it allows for dose escalation and may improve locoregional control.

To organize the subsequent discussion, treatment options will be reviewed based on disease extent.

Stage I or II Disease

One-third of patients with HNC present with limited disease at diagnosis (ie, stages I or II, without lymph node involvement). Five-year overall survival in cases of limited disease ranges from 60%–90% (51), varying with primary site, stage, and histology. These patients are generally treated with single-modality surgery or radiotherapy if possible. The choice of treatment is often determined by the anatomical site of disease, available expertise, and the side effect profiles that can be expected with different treatment approaches.

Radiotherapy is preferred for less advanced laryngeal and oro-/hypopharyngeal cancers to preserve voice and swallowing. Similarly, radiation is the primary approach for small nasopharynx cancers, as these tumors are sensitive to radiation and the location makes surgical resection difficult. Surgery is generally favored in treatment of localized lesions of the oral cavity. This approach avoids the acute and late sequelae of radiotherapy treatment such as xerostomia, dental damage, and osteoradionecrosis of the jaw.

Surgery is also the preferred option for salivary gland cancers in general and for limited-stage disease of paranasal sinus and nasal cavity.

Most patients with limited squamous cell HNC are cured of their disease. As such, second primary cancers related to prior tobacco or alcohol exposure are a particular concern. Counseling patients regarding the role of tobacco or alcohol in the genesis of their disease and the importance of eliminating or at least decreasing these behaviors is important. There has been keen interest in chemoprevention to reduce the incidence of these second primaries. Vitamin A analogs have been the most widely investigated. An initial trial using isotretinoin compared to placebo was found to decrease the rate of second primaries (52). However, subsequent studies were not able to corroborate these

results (53–55). Other agents are under investigation, but at present, the use of drugs with chemopreventive intent outside of a clinical trial after treatment is not recommended.

Stage III or IV, M0 Disease

Unfortunately, most patients with HNC present with locoregionally advanced disease at diagnosis and have an expected five-year overall survival of 30%–50% (51). Curative-intent treatment for patients with stage III or IVA-B disease requires a multimodality treatment strategy. As in patients with less advanced HNC, there is often more than one way to proceed with therapy, and the related side effects of different approaches are carefully considered.

In patients who undergo primary surgical treatment, in addition to surgical management of the primary site, surgical reconstruction is often necessary and neck dissection is frequently performed to address disease metastatic to neck lymph nodes. Although primary surgical management can be applied for resectable tumors at any primary site, it is arguably the preferred approach for advanced oral cavity and paranasal cancers, as good functional and cosmetic results after surgical removal can be obtained with flaps, grafts, and prostheses as indicated. Appropriate rehabilitation afterward remains nonetheless important. After surgical management of locoregionally advanced disease, adjuvant radiation is typically administered. The addition of concomitant chemotherapy (cisplatin) to postoperative radiotherapy has been demonstrated to improve locoregional disease control in patients with pathological features predicting high risk of failure, particularly: (1) microscopically involved resection margins and/or (2) extracapsular spread of tumor from neck nodes (56). The interval from surgery to completion of radiotherapy should be 10–11 weeks or less in the absence of any postoperative medical or surgical complications, since the cumulative time of combined therapy (from surgery to the completion of adjuvant radiotherapy) has been shown to affect locoregional control and survival in high-risk patients (57,58).

Primary chemoradiation, with surgery reserved for salvage, is preferred in settings where surgical treatment (eg, total laryngectomy) may lead to significant morbidity and available rehabilitative options (eg, esophageal speech, tracheoesophageal puncture [TEP]) may be viewed as not optimal by the patient. Under these circumstances, primary chemoradiation provides the benefit of possible organ and functional preservation without compromising survival. It is also pursued in patients with unresectable tumors. Radiation is the curative backbone of this treatment. In patients with advanced squamous cell head and neck cancer, concurrent chemotherapy with radiation appears to lead to superior disease control compared to the use of neoadjuvant (before radiation) or adjuvant (after radiation) chemotherapy (59,60). For example, concomitant chemoradiotherapy has resulted in better laryngectomy free-survival (organ preservation) compared to induction chemotherapy followed by radiotherapy or radiotherapy alone in a phase 3 trial in locally advanced laryngeal cancer (61). In patients with nasopharyngeal carcinoma, the addition of concomitant chemotherapy with cisplatin is also associated with therapeutic benefit, and for this site, adjuvant chemotherapy is also administered (62,63). Of note, newer triplet induction chemotherapy regimens appear superior to prior doublet ones (64–66), and the potential for integration of induction chemotherapy followed by concurrent chemoradiotherapy is being actively evaluated.

Cisplatin is the best established agent for concurrent use with radiation. Studies have found the most robust survival advantage using cisplatin, demonstrating an 11% absolute survival benefit at five years (59,60). Patients who are not optimal candidates for cisplatin therapy due to comorbidities such as preexisting renal insufficiency, neuropathy, or hearing loss can be considered for alternative concurrent options. One is cetuximab, a monoclonal antibody against the epidermal growth factor receptor (EGFR). In a recent phase 3 trial, concurrent administration of cetuximab resulted in a 10% improvement in overall survival at three years compared to radiotherapy alone without significantly increasing treatment-related local toxicities (67). However, cetuximab is not without its own side effects and can result in serious allergic reactions in a small minority of patients, and is also associated with an acneiform rash in the majority of patients.

It is important to appreciate that combined chemoradiotherapy is intense treatment and patients so treated often experience significant acute toxic effects. Mucositis, dysphagia, vomiting, dehydration, weight loss, anemia, and myelosuppression are commonly seen. The therapy is best done by an experienced multidisciplinary team with the availability of appropriate infrastructure to provide the necessary supportive care.

In patients who are treated with primary concurrent chemoradiation, persistent neck masses may require additional surgical management. Previously, studies found improved survival in patients with initial advanced nodal disease (N2–3) who underwent neck dissection following chemoradiation (68). However, more recently, the routine application of neck dissection under these circumstances independent of response has been questioned (69). Many centers will do such postchemoradiotherapy neck dissections more selectively based on observed response and radiographic imaging results.

Primary surgical management is preferred for advanced salivary gland cancers. Commonly applied indications for postoperative radiotherapy include: (1) microscopic (eg, R1 resection) or macroscopic (eg, R2 resection) residual disease after surgery; (2) multiple involved lymph nodes; (3) undifferentiated or high-grade tumors; (4) presence of perineural invasion; or (5) the presence of advance disease, for example, involvement of the deep lobe of the parotid (70). For unresectable salivary gland cancers, there are data to support the use of neutron therapy (71). Concomitant chemotherapy and radiation in this setting is less well studied.

Relapsed and/or Metastatic Disease

Most commonly, patients will have local or regional recurrent disease. If surgery or further radiotherapy (72) (possibly with concurrent chemotherapy) is feasible, these approaches offer the best chance for more durable disease control. Other patients with relapsed and/or metastatic disease are treated mainly with palliative chemotherapy and measures for best supportive care. The overall prognostic outlook for patients treated with the best available systemic therapies is worrisome. The expected major response rates to chemotherapy in this setting range between 10% and 40%, with median survivals consistently less than one year. Combination chemotherapy may improve the response rates, but at the expense of more toxicity and a disappointing impact on overall survival (73,74). Clinical trials evaluating new and promising agents are a particularly good option for many patients under these circumstances. There is keen interest in strategies that combine chemotherapy with newer targeted therapies. Preliminary results of a randomized trial comparing platinum-based chemotherapy with or without cetuximab in patients with recurrent or metastatic squamous cell HNC indicate a survival advantage with the addition of the cetuximab (75).

R*eferences*

1. Jemal A, Siegel R, Ward E, et al. Cancer statistics, 2007. *CA Cancer J Clin.* 2007;57(1):143–166.
2. Shah JP. Patterns of cervical lymph node metastasis from squamous carcinomas of the upper aerodigestive tract. *Am J Surg.* October 1990;160(4):405–409.
3. Shah JP, Patel SG. *Head and Neck Surgery and Oncology*, 3rd ed. Edinburgh: Mosby; 2003.
4. Sobin LH, Wittekind C, eds. *TNM Classification of Malignant Tumors*, 6th ed. New York: Wiley-Liss; 2000.
5. Hellquist H, Lundgren J, Olofsson J. Hyperplasia, keratosis, dysplasia and carcinoma in situ of the vocal cords—a follow-up study. *Clin Otolaryngol Allied Sci.* 1982;7:11–27.
6. Schanmugaratnam K, Sobin LH. The World Health Organization histological classification of tumours of the upper

respiratory tract and ear. A commentary on the second edition. *Cancer.* 1993;71:2689–2697.

7. Fakhry C, Gillison ML. Clinical implications of human papillomavirus in head and neck cancers. *J Clin Oncol.* June 10, 2006;24(17):2606–2611.

8. Katz TS, Mendenhall WM, Morris CG, et al. Malignant tumors of the nasal cavity and paranasal sinuses. *Head Neck.* September 2002;24(9):821–829.

9. Porceddu S, Martin J, Shanker G, et al. Paranasal sinus tumors: Peter MacCallum Cancer Institute experience. *Head Neck.* April 2004;26(4):322–330.

10. Dirix P, Nuyts S, Geussens Y, et al. Malignancies of the nasal cavity and paranasal sinuses: long-term outcome with conventional or three-dimensional conformal radiotherapy. *Int J Radiat Oncol Biol Phys.* November 15, 2007;69(4):1042–1050.

11. Silva EG, Butler JJ, Mac Kay B, et al. Neuroblastomas and neuroendocrine carcinomas of the nasal cavity: a proposed new classification. *Cancer.* 1982;50:2388–2405.

12. Haas I, Ganzer U. Does sophisticated diagnostic workup on neuroectodermal tumors have an impact on the treatment of esthesioneuroblastoma? *Onkologie.* 2003;26:261–267.

13. Frierson HF, Mills SE, Fechner RE, et al. Sinonasal undifferentiated carcinoma: an aggressive neoplasm derived from Schneiderian epithelium and distinct from olfactory neuroblastoma. *Am J Surg Pathol.* 1986;10:771–779.

14. Jeng J, Sung M, Fang C, et al. Sinonasal undifferentiated carcinoma and nasopharyngeal-type undifferentiated carcinoma: two clinically, biologically and histopathologically distinct entities. *Am J Surg Pathol.* 2002;26:371–376.

15. Speight PM, Barrett AW. Salivary gland tumours. *Oral Dis.* 2002;8(5):229–240.

16. Brandwein MS, Ivanov K, Wallace DI, et al. Mucoepidermoid carcinoma: a clinicopathologic study of 80 patients with special reference to histological grading. *Am J Surg Pathol.* 2001;25(7):835–845.

17. Ellis GL. Major and minor salivary glands. In: Rosai J, ed. *Ackerman's Surgical Pathology,* 8th ed. St. Louis: Mosby; 1996:815–856.

18. Tomich CE. Adenoid cystic carcinoma. In: Ellis GL, Auclair PL, Gnepp DR, eds. *Surgical Pathology of the Salivary Glands.* Philadelphia: Saunders; 1991:333–349.

19. Spiro RH. The controversial adenoid cystic carcinoma: clinical considerations. In: McGurk M, Renehan AG, eds. *Controversies in the Management of Salivary Gland Disease.* Oxford: Oxford University Press; 2001:207–211.

20. Friedrich RE, Bleckmann V. Adenoid cystic carcinoma of salivary and lacrimal gland origin: localization, classification, clinical pathological correlation, treatment results and long-term follow-up control in 84 patients. *Anticancer Res.* 2003;23(2A):931–940.

21. Spiro RH, Huvos AG. Stage means more than grade in adenoid cystic carcinoma. *Am J Surg.* 1992;164(6):623–628.

22. SEER registry. http://seer.cancer.gov, February 13, 2009.

23. Blot JW, McLaughlin JK, Winn DM, et al. Smoking and drinking in relation to oral and pharyngeal cancer. *Cancer Res.* June 1, 1988;46(11):3282–3287.

24. Day GL, Blot WJ, Austin DF, et al. Racial differences in risk of oral and pharyngeal cancer: alcohol, tobacco, and other determinants. *J Natl Cancer Inst.* March 17, 1993;85(6):465–473.

25. Decker J, Goldstein JC. Risk factors in head and neck cancer. *N Engl J Med.* 1982;306:1151–1155.

26. Day GL, Blot WL, Shore RE, et al. Second cancers following oral and pharyngeal cancers: role of tobacco and alcohol. *J Natl Cancer Inst.* January 19, 1994;82(2):131–137.

27. Ho PS, Ko YC, Yang YH, et al. The incidence of oropharyngeal cancer in Taiwan: an endemic betel quid chewing area. *J Oral Pathol Med.* 2002;31(4):213–219.

28. Goldenberg D, Golz A, Joachims HZ. The beverage maté: a risk factor for cancer of the head and neck. *Head Neck.* 2003;25(7):595–601.

29. Rothman K, Keller A. The effect of joint exposure to alcohol and tobacco on risk of cancer of the mouth and pharynx. *J Chronic Dis.* 1972;25:711–716.

30. Kreimer AR, Clifford GM, Boyle P, Franceschi S. Human papillomavirus types in head and neck squamous cell carcinomas worldwide: a systematic review. *Cancer Epidemiol Biomarkers Prev.* February 2005;14(2):467–475.

31. Talamini R, Vaccarella S, Barbone F, et al. Oral hygiene, dentition, sexual habits and risk of oral cancer. *Br J Cancer.* 2000;83:1238–1242.

32. Balaram P, Sridhar H, Rajkumar T, et al. Oral cancer in southern India: the influence of smoking, drinking, paan-chewing and oral hygiene. *Int J Cancer.* 2002;98:440–445.

33. Drigley G, McLaughlin JK, Block G, et al. Vitamin supplement use and reduced risk of oral and pharyngeal cancer. *Am J Epidemiol.* May 1992;135(10):1083–1092.

34. Barnes L. Intestinal-type adenocarcinoma of the nasal cavity and paranasal sinuses. *Am J Surg Pathol.* 1986;10: 192–202.

35. Ellis GL, Auclair PL. *Tumors of the Salivary Glands.* Washington, DC: Armed Forces Institute of Pathology; 1996. Atlas of Tumor Pathology

36. Guzzo M, Andreola S, Sirizzotti G, et al. Mucoepidermoid carcinoma of the salivary glands: clinicopathologic review of 108 patients treated at the National Cancer Institute of Milan. *Ann Surg Oncol.* 2002;9(7):688–695.

37. Lo YM, Chan LY, Chan AT, et al. Quantitative and temporal correlation between circulating cell-free Epstein-Barr virus DNA and tumor recurrence in nasopharyngeal carcinoma. *Cancer Res.* 1999;59:5452–5455.

38. Lin JC, Wang WY, Chen KY, et al. Quantification of plasma Epstein-Barr virus DNA in patients with advanced nasopharyngeal carcinoma. *N Engl J Med.* 2004;350:2461–2470.

39. Raab-Traub N. Epstein-Barr virus in the pathogenesis of NPC. *Semin Cancer Biol.* December 2002;12(6):431–441.

40. USPTF. http://www.ahrq.gov/clinic/uspstf/uspsoral.htm. (Accessed at February 13, 2009).

41. NCCN guidelines. http://www.nccn.org/professionals/physician_gls/default.asp. (Accessed at February 13, 2009).

42. el Hag IA, Chiedozi LC, al Reyees FA, Kollur SM. Fine needle aspiration cytology of head and neck masses. Seven years' experience in a secondary care hospital. *Acta Cytol.* May–June 2003;47(3):387–392.

43. Greene FL, Page DL, Fleming ID, et al. *AJCC Cancer Staging Manual,* 6th ed. New York: Springer; 2002.

44. Patel SG, Shah JP. TNM staging of cancers of the head and neck: striving for uniformity among diversity. *CA Cancer J Clin.* 2005;55(4):242–258.

45. Kaanders JH, Hordijk GJ. Dutch Cooperative Head and Neck Oncology Group. Carcinoma of the larynx: the Dutch national guideline for diagnostics, treatment, supportive care and rehabilitation. *Radiother Oncol.* June 2002;63(3):299–307.

46. Regelink G, Brouwer J, de Bree R, et al. Detection of unknown primary tumours and distant metastases in patients with cervical metastases: value of FDG-PET versus conventional modalities. *Eur J Nucl Med Mol Imaging.* August 2002;29(8):1024–1030.

47. Turner SL, Tiver KW, Boyages SC. Thyroid dysfunction following radiotherapy for head and neck cancer. *Int J Radiat Oncol Biol Phys.* 1995;31(2):279–283.

48. Johnson JT, Ferretti GA, Nethery WJ, et al. Oral pilocarpine for post-irradiation xerostomia in patients with head and neck cancer. *N Engl J Med.* August 5, 1993;329(6):390–395.

49. Chambers MS, Posner M, Jones CU, et al. Cevimeline for the treatment of postirradiation xerostomia in patients with head-and-neck cancer. *Int J Radiat Oncol Biol Phys.* 2007;68(40):1102–1109.

50. Brizel DM, Wasserman TH, Henke M, et al. Phase III randomized trial of amifostine as a radioprotector in head and neck cancer. *J Clin Oncol.* October 1, 2000;18(19):3339–3345.

51. Vokes EE. Head and neck cancer. In: Kasper DL, Braunwald E, Hauser S, et al., eds. *Harrison's Principles of Internal Medicine,* 16th ed. New York: McGraw-Hill; 2005;503–506.

52. Hong WK, Lippman SM, Itri LM, et al. Prevention of second primary tumors with isotretinoin in squamous-cell carcinoma of the head and neck. *N Engl J Med.* September 20, 1990;323(12):795–801.

53. Bolla M, Lefur R, Ton Van J, et al. Prevention of second primary tumours with etretinate in squamous cell carcinoma of the oral cavity and oropharynx. Results of a multicentric double-blind randomized study. *Eur J Cancer.* 1994;30A(6):767–772.

54. Khuri FR, Lee JJ, Lippman SM, et al. Randomized phase III trial of low-dose isotretinoin for prevention of second primary tumors in stage I and II head and neck cancer patients. *J Natl Cancer Inst.* April 5, 2006;98(7):426–427.

55. Van Zanwijk N, Dalesio O, Patorino U, et al. EUROSCAN, a randomized trial of vitamin A and N-acetylcysteine in patients with head and neck cancer or lung cancer: for the European Organization for Research and Treatment of Cancer Head and Neck and Lung Cancer Cooperative Groups. *J Natl Cancer Inst.* 2000;92:977–986.

56. Bernier J, Cooper JS, Pajak TF, et al. Defining risk levels in locally advanced head and neck cancers: a comparative analysis of concurrent postoperative radiation plus chemotherapy trials of the EORTC (#22931) and RTOG (# 9501). *Head Neck.* October 2005;27(10):843–850.

57. Ang KK, Trotti A, Brown BW, et al. Randomized trial addressing risk features and time factors of surgery plus radiotherapy in advanced head-and-neck cancer. *Int J Radiat Oncol Biol Phys.* November 1, 2001;51(3):571–578.

58. Awwad HK, Lotayef M, Shouman T, et al. Accelerated hyperfractionation (AHF) compared to conventional fractionation (CF) in the postoperative radiotherapy of locally advanced head and neck cancer: influence of proliferation. *Br J Cancer.* February 12, 2002;86(4):517–523.

59. Pignon JP, Bourhis J, Domenge C, Designe L. Chemotherapy added to locoregional treatment for head and neck squamous-cell carcinoma: three meta-analyses of updated individual data. MACH-NC Collaborative Group. Meta-Analysis of Chemotherapy on Head and Neck Cancer. *Lancet.* March 18, 2000;355(9208):949–955.

60. Bouhris J, Amand C, Pignon JP. Update of MACH-NC (Meta-analysis of chemotherapy in Head & Neck cancer) database focused on concomitant chemoradiotherapy: 5505. *J Clin Oncol,* ASCO Annual Meeting Proceedings (Post-Meeting edition) 2004; 22 (145 (July 15 Supplement).

61. Forastiere AA, Goepfert H, Maor M, et al. Concurrent chemotherapy and radiotherapy for organ preservation in advanced laryngeal cancer. *N Engl J Med.* November 27, 2003;349(22):2091–2098.

62. Al-Sarraf M, LeBlanc M, Giri PG, et al. Chemoradiotherapy versus radiotherapy in patients with advanced nasopharyngeal cancer: phase III randomized Intergroup study 0099. *J Clin Oncol.* April 1998; 16(4):1310–1317.

63. Langendijk JA, Leemans CR, Buter J, et al. The additional value of chemotherapy to radiotherapy in locally advanced nasopharyngeal carcinoma: a meta-analysis of the published literature. *J Clin Oncol.* November 15, 2004;22(22):4604–4612.

64. Posner MR, Hershock DM, Blajman CR, et al. Cisplatin and fluorouracil alone or with docetaxel in head and neck cancer. *N Engl J Med.* 2007;357:1705–1715.

65. Vermorken JB, Remenar E, van Herpen C, et al. Cisplatin, fluorouracil, and docetaxel in unresectable head and neck cancer. *N Engl J Med.* 2007;357:1695–1704.

66. Hitt R, Lopez-Pousa A, Martinez-Trufero J, et al. Phase III study comparing cisplatin plus fluorouracil to paclitaxel, cisplatin, and fluorouracil induction chemotherapy followed by chemoradiotherapy in locally advanced head and neck cancer. *J Clin Oncol.* 2005;23:8636–8645.

67. Bonner JA, Harari PM, Giralt J, et al. Radiotherapy plus cetuximab for squamous-cell carcinoma of the head and neck. *N Engl J Med.* February 9, 2006;354(6):567–578.

68. Brizel DM, Prosnitz RG, Hunter S, et al. Necessity for adjuvant neck dissection in setting of concurrent chemoradiation for advanced head-and-neck cancer. *Int J Radiat Oncol Biol Phys.* April 1, 2004;58(5):1418–1423.

69. Goguen LA, Posner MR, Tishler RB, et al. Examining the need for neck dissection in the era of chemoradiation therapy for advanced head and neck cancer. *Arch Otolaryngol Head Neck Surg.* May 2006;132(5):526–531.

70. Licitra L, Locati LD, Bossi P, Cantu G. Head and neck tumors other than squamous cell carcinoma. *Curr Opin Oncol.* May 2004;16(3):236–241.

71. Laramore GE, Krall JM, Griffin BR, et al. Neutron versus photon irradiation for unresectable salivary gland tumors: final report of an RTOG-MRC randomized clinical trial. *Int J Radiol Oncol Bio Phys.* 1993;27:235–240.

72. De Crevoisier R, Bourhis J, Domenge C, et al. Full-dose reirradiation for unresectable head and neck carcinoma: experience of the Gustave-Roussy Institute in a series of 169 patients. *J Clin Oncol.* November 1998; 6(11):3556–3562.

73. Jacobs C, Lyman G, Velez-Garcia E, et al. A phase III randomized study comparing cisplatin and fluorouracil as single-agents and in combination for advanced squamous cell carcinoma of the head and neck. *J Clin Oncol.* 1992;10:257–263.

74. Forastiere AA, Metch B, Schuller DE, et al. Randomized comparison of cisplatin plus fluorouracil and carboplatin plus fluorouracil versus methotrexate in advanced squamous-cell carcinoma of the head and neck: a Southwest Oncology Group study. *J Clin Oncol.* 1992;10:1245–1251.

75. Vermorken JB, Mesia R, Rivera F., et al. Platinum–based chemotherapy plus cetuximab in head and neck cancer. *NEJM.* 2008;359:1116–1127.

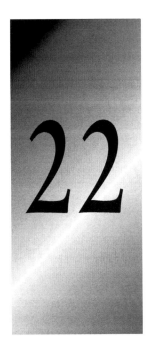

Evaluation and Treatment of Thyroid Cancer

Robert Michael Tuttle
Rebecca Leboeuf

Accounting for more than 90% of all endocrine malignancies, thyroid cancer represents only about 1% of all human cancers. While there are five principal histological forms of thyroid cancer, more than 95% arise from thyroid follicular cells which, in the normal thyroid, concentrate iodine and synthesize thyroid hormone in response to TSH stimulation (1,2) (Table 22.1).

Although the incidence of very low disease-specific mortality for thyroid cancer has remained rather stable over the last 25 years, a dramatic rise in papillary thyroid cancer incidence has been seen over the last 20 years. In women, the incidence of thyroid cancer has risen from approximately 6 per 100,000 in the early 1970s to more than 12 per 100,000 by 2000–2003. A smaller, although statistically significant, rise has been seen in men over the same time frame (2.1 per 100,000 to 4.2 per 100,000) (3,4). Data from the same time period demonstrate no such rise in incidence in the other primary types of thyroid cancer.

It remains unclear whether this rise in thyroid cancer incidence is secondary to an unidentified environmental risk factor (5) or a product of more aggressive detection with more widespread use of neck ultrasound and other cross-sectional imaging over the last 20 years (3). While exposure to ionizing radiation is the best known risk factor for subsequent development of thyroid cancer after a 5–20 year latency period (6), it seems unlikely that most patients currently being diagnosed were exposed to significant radiation exposures during their lifetime.

TABLE 22.1 *Histology: disease specific survival*			
	CELL OF ORIGIN	**% OF ALL THYROID CANCERS**	**10-YR DISEASE-SPECIFIC SURVIVAL (%)**
Papillary	Thyroid follicular cell	90	98
Follicular	Thyroid follicular cell	5	92
Anaplastic	Thyroid follicular cell	1	1–13
Medullary	C-cell (neuroendocrine)	3	80
Lymphoma	Lymphocytes	1	50–90

DIFFERENTIATED THYROID CANCER

Initial Presentation

Because the presentation, initial evaluation, and initial therapy of papillary and follicular thyroid cancer are quite similar, and because until the last 10–15 years these tumors were often lumped together by pathologists, they are often considered together as a group of malignancies knows as differentiated thyroid cancers.

In the past, differentiated thyroid cancer usually presented as a painless thyroid nodule detected either

KEY POINTS

- Thyroid cancer represents only about 1% of all human cancers, but 90% of all endocrine malignancies.
- There are five principal histological forms of thyroid cancer: papillary, follicular, anaplastic, medullary, and lymphoma.
- Most (95%) thyroid cancers arise from thyroid follicular cells.
- Because the presentation, initial evaluation, and initial therapy of papillary and follicular thyroid cancer are quite similar, they are often considered together as a group of malignancies knows as differentiated thyroid cancers.
- While the very low disease-specific mortality for thyroid cancer has remained rather stable over the last 25 years, a dramatic rise in papillary thyroid cancer incidence has been seen over the last 20 years.
- In the past, differentiated thyroid cancer usually presented as a painless thyroid nodule detected either by the patient, or a health care provider. With more widespread use of cross sectional radiologic imaging, thyroid cancer is now frequently detected as an asymptomatic incidental finding for unrelated medical conditions.
- Routine thyroid function tests (TSH, T4) are almost uniformly normal and are not used to confirm, nor can they rule out, the presence of thyroid cancer.
- Differentiated thyroid cancer usually responds very well to the standard initial therapy of thyroidectomy, lymph node dissection, and radioactive iodine (RAI) therapy. Tumor recurrence rates over a 20–30 year follow-up period remain as high as 15%–30%, particularly at both extremes of age.
- Clinically evident recurrences are not a trivial event, with as many as 8% of patients with local recurrence and 50% of patients with distant recurrence dying of the disease.
- The primary tool for detection of recurrent or persistent thyroid cancer is serum thyroglobulin (Tg).
- Since the vast majority of recurrent thyroid cancer occurs in cervical lymph nodes, and since they usually produce Tg very well, a combination of TSH stimulated Tg and careful neck ultrasonography has a very high sensitivity for detection of recurrent disease.
- RAI is often a very effective therapy for distant metastases.
- Unlike well-differentiated thyroid cancers, anaplastic thyroid cancer is a locally aggressive, poorly differentiated thyroid cancer that develops in older patients and has a disease specific mortality rate of more than 95% over 6–12 months after diagnosis.
- Primary thyroid lymphomas make up less than 2% of extranodal lymphomas, and are generally classified as either mucosa-associated lymphoid tissue (MALT) or diffuse large B-cell or mixed subtype lymphomas.
- Medullary thyroid cancer (MTC) is a neuroendocrine tumor arising from parafollicular C-cells within the thyroid gland.

by the patient or a health care provider. With more widespread use of cross-sectional radiologic imaging, thyroid cancer is now frequently detected as an asymptomatic incidental finding for unrelated medical conditions. With an average age at diagnosis of between 35 and 45, women are affected two to three times more commonly than men (7). Since more than 90% of all thyroid nodules are benign, fine-needle aspiration, often with ultrasound guidance, is used to establish a cytologic diagnosis and identify those malignant thyroid nodules that will require surgical resection (8). It is important to note that routine thyroid function tests (TSH, T4) are almost uniformly normal and are not used to rule in or cannot be used to rule out the presence of thyroid cancer.

At the time of diagnosis, differentiated thyroid cancer has metastasized to local cervical lymph nodes in at least 20%–50% of patients, but distant metastatic spread is seen in only about 2%–5% of all cases (4,9,10). Even though differentiated thyroid cancer usually responds very well to the standard initial therapy of thyroidectomy, lymph node dissection, and radioactive iodine (RAI) therapy, tumor recurrence rates over a 20–30 year follow-up period remain as high as 15%–30%, particularly at both extremes of age (9,10). Clinically evident recurrences are not a trivial event, with as many as 8% of patients with local recurrence and 50% of patients with distant recurrence dying of the disease (10).

Initial Therapy

The mainstay of thyroid cancer therapy is surgical resection of all gross evidence of disease with appropriate compartmental resection of involved cervical lymph node chains (11). Thyroid cancer patients who are at low risk of recurrence can be adequately treated with hemithyroidectomy while high risk patients usually require total thyroidectomy, resection of involved lymph node chains, and radioactive iodine ablation in the postoperative setting (8,12–15).

RAI is one of the oldest examples of targeted therapy. Because the thyroid follicular cells require iodine to synthesize thyroid hormone, they express a sodium iodine symporter in the cell membrane that very effectively transports iodine from the blood stream into the thyroid cell. Fortunately, at least 75% of malignant thyroid cells retain the function of this sodium iodine symporter and are therefore potential targets for RAI therapy. Since this transporter cannot differentiate stable iodine from RAI, we can effectively deliver a significant radiation dose to metastatic thyroid cancer cells while exposing the rest of the body to minimal radiation exposure. Low doses of RAI can be used for diagnostic whole-body scanning, whereas larger doses can be used for tumoricidal effects.

Maximal targeting of RAI to thyroid cells requires TSH stimulation (either thyroid hormone withdrawal or administration of recombinant human TSH) and depletion of stable iodine stores from the body, along with a low iodine diet for several days prior to treatment. It is necessary to avoid iodinated contrast (such as that used in CT scans) for several months before RAI treatment. If the whole body iodine stores are elevated, the relatively small amount of RAI is diluted out and will not effectively reach the metastatic thyroid cancer cells in sufficient quantity to result in cell death.

In the setting of initial therapy, external beam radiation therapy (EBRT) is seldom necessary in patients with differentiated thyroid cancer (16). EBRT is most often used for unresectable tumors that do not concentrate RAI, or older patients (older than aged 45 years) with evidence of gross extrathyroidal extension of the tumor into surrounding structures that are very likely to have microscopic or small volume macroscopic disease that is not amenable to RAI therapy. Similarly, traditional cytotoxic chemotherapy has a poor track record in differentiated thyroid cancer, and is seldom recommended in the initial management of all but the most aggressive thyroid cancers.

Since TSH is a growth factor to both normal and malignant thyroid cells, it is not surprising that retrospective studies demonstrate that TSH suppression with supraphysiologic doses of levothyroxine is associated with decreased recurrence rates. Therefore, following initial thyroid surgery and RAI treatment, TSH suppression has become a cornerstone of treatment for more than 40 years (17,18). In general, the TSH should be kept just below the reference range in most patients with differentiated thyroid cancer,

reserving high level suppression (undetectable TSH) for patients with advanced, progressive, or metastatic disease (8).

Detection of Recurrent Disease

Serum Tumor Marker

The primary tool for detection of recurrent or persistent thyroid cancer is serum thyroglobulin (Tg) (19,20). Tg is a protein synthesized and secreted by both normal and malignant thyroid cells into the peripheral circulation. The production of thyroglobulin by normal thyroid cells precludes the use of Tg as a diagnostic tool for thyroid cancer prior to FNA or surgery.

Since our initial therapies of total thyroidectomy and RAI ablation are designed to destroy all normal and malignant thyroid cells, patients cured of thyroid cancer should have nearly undetectable serum levels of Tg within 12–18 months of initial therapy. To improve the sensitivity for detection of low level thyroid cancer, serum Tg levels are often measured following TSH stimulation.

From a practical standpoint, it is critical that the Tg be measured serially in the same laboratory. Marked variations in serum Tg values are reported when the same blood samples are analyzed using different Tg assays (20). Additionally, the presence of anti-Tg antibodies in as many as 20% of thyroid cancer patients interferes with the sensitivity of Tg testing. Anti-Tg antibodies often result in falsely low Tg values through assay interference in patients that have persistent thyroid cancer.

Imaging Modalities

For many years, diagnostic RAI scanning was the primary follow up modality for patients with differentiated thyroid cancer. However, the last 15 years has seen a major paradigm shift away from routine RAI scanning and toward routine use of serum Tg and neck ultrasonography in the follow up of most of these patients (8,21). Because the vast majority of recurrent thyroid cancer is in cervical lymph nodes, which usually produce Tg very well, a combination of TSH-stimulated Tg and careful neck ultrasonography has a very high sensitivity for detection of recurrent disease.

Other imaging modalities such as CT, MRI, and 18 fluorodeoxyglucose positron emission tomography (FDG PET) scanning are generally reserved either for patients with aggressive thyroid cancers and very high risk, or patients in whom the serum Tg is elevated, but in whom the source of disease cannot be localized by physical examination or neck ultrasonography (22,23).

Treatment Options for Persistent/ Recurrent Disease

Locally Recurrent Disease

For structurally progressive, locally recurrent disease that is 1 cm or greater in size, surgical resection is generally considered the preferred treatment option. Recurrent disease less than 1 cm, or detected only on RAI scanning without associated structural disease, is often treated with additional RAI therapy (8,13). With the dramatic improvement in sensitivity for detecting persistent/recurrent disease using neck ultrasonography, and highly sensitive Tg assays, we are often finding small volume disease in cervical lymph nodes that progresses slowly, if at all. Often, these patients are carefully watched with serial ultrasounds with intervention reserved for only those documented disease progression.

In patients with a structurally significant local disease recurrence in which surgical resection would be associated with unacceptable morbidity or mortality, consideration is given to external beam irradiation. Unlike many other malignancies, surgical resection of locally recurrent disease for palliation and prevention of gross invasion into the aerodigestive tract is often considered even in the presence of untreatable distant metastases (8).

Distant Metastases

RAI is often a very effective therapy for distant metastases. Unfortunately, RAI is much less effective at destroying macroscopic pulmonary metastases, particularly when they arise in older patients with less-differentiated disease. While resection or EBRT to individual metastatic lesion in critical locations will not be curative, appropriate treatment can avert serious neurovascular symptoms or prevent seriously morbid complications. Patients with structurally progressive macroscopic metastatic disease that is not responsive to RAI should be referred for consideration of a clinical trial or other systemic therapy (24).

ANAPLASTIC THYROID CANCER

Unlike well-differentiated thyroid cancers, anaplastic thyroid cancer is a locally aggressive, poorly differentiated thyroid cancer that develops in older patients (mean age at diagnosis approximately 65 years) (25). In the vast majority of cases, the tumor is not resectable, does not concentrate RAI, and responds poorly to chemotherapy. Unfortunately, the disease specific mortality rate is more than 95% over 6–12 months after diagnosis. While unlikely to be curative, combination chemotherapy and external beam irradiation may result in a modest increase in progression-free survival from just a few days to at least a few months.

THYROID LYMPHOMA

Primary thyroid lymphomas make up less than 2% of extranodal lymphomas and are generally classified as either mucosa-associated lymphoid tissue (MALT) or diffuse large B-cell or mixed subtype lymphomas (26). They often present as a rapidly increasing thyroid mass in older patients with preexisting chronic lymphocytic thyroiditis.

While MALT lymphomas may follow a more indolent course and be amenable to single modality radiation therapy or total thyroidectomy diagnosed at an early stage, both the large B-cell and mixed subtype lymphomas are generally treated with multimodality therapy consisting of chemotherapy and hyperfractionated EBRT (25).

MEDULLARY THYROID CANCER

MTC is a neuroendocrine tumor arising from parafollicular C cells within the thyroid gland (27). Although these C cells cannot concentrate iodine nor produce thyroid hormones, they do synthesize calcitonin and CEA, which are commonly used as serum tumor markers in patients with MTC. In 75% of the cases, MTC presents as a sporadic (nonfamilial), unilateral thyroid mass, usually in the fourth to sixth decade of life, often with associated cervical lymphadenopathy (50% of patients), with no other associated endocrinopathies.

However, 25% of patients present with MTC as part of a well-defined clinical syndrome caused by germline mutation in the RET proto-oncogene. Although MTC is often the initial presentation in these clinical syndromes, patients may also present with hypertension associated with pheochromocytoma or with hypercalcemia associated with hyperparathyroidism. Therefore, screening for these diagnoses is essential in order to appropriately plan and sequence necessary surgical procedures. In addition, with the aid of commercially available genetic testing for carriers of the RET proto-oncogene, early detection of asymptomatic disease can be found in affected family members of patients with hereditary MTC.

After assessment for possible concurrent hyperparathyroidism and/or pheochromocytoma, the usual initial therapy for MTC is total thyroidectomy with compartmental dissection of potentially affected cervical lymph node chains. MTC is often a slow growing tumor with an indolent clinical course. The overall survival of patients with sporadic MTC ranges from 80%–85% at five years, 55%–65% at 10 years, and 45%–50% at 20 years.

CONCLUSIONS

Although generally considered a rare tumor, the incidence of thyroid cancer has dramatically increased over the last 20 years. The etiology of this rise in incidence remains elusive. While the 30-year disease-specific survival in thyroid cancer exceeds 90% in most patients, the risk of recurrent disease is as high as 30% over the same time period. Over the last 10–15 years, more widespread use of serum Tg and neck ultrasonography has resulted in earlier detection of locally recurrent disease, allowing more effective treatment of these recurrences. Unfortunately, treatment options for non-RAI avid, progressive, distant metastases are much less effective, resulting in a resurging interest in the development of novel systemic therapies.

References

1. Gilliland FD, Hunt WC, Morris DM, et al. Prognostic factors for thyroid carcinoma. A population-based study of 15,698 cases from the Surveillance, Epidemiology and End Results (SEER) program 1973–1991. *Cancer.* 1997;79(3):564–573.

2. Hundahl SA, Cady B, Cunningham MP, et al. Initial results from a prospective cohort study of 5583 cases of thyroid carcinoma treated in the United States during 1996. U.S. and German Thyroid Cancer Study Group. An American College of Surgeons Commission on Cancer Patient Care Evaluation study. *Cancer.* 2000;89(1):202–217.

3. Davies L, Welch HG. Increasing incidence of thyroid cancer in the United States, 1973–2002. *JAMA.* 2006;295(18):2164–2167.

4. Ries LA, Harkins D, Krapcho M, et al. *SEER Cancer Statistics Review, 1975-2003, based on November 2005 SEER data submission.* 2006 [cited 2006 November 1]; Available from: http://seer.cancer.gov/csr/1975_2003/.

5. Nagataki S, Nystrom E. Epidemiology and primary prevention of thyroid cancer. *Thyroid.* 2002;12(10):889–896.

6. Schneider AB, Sarne DH. Long-term risks for thyroid cancer and other neoplasms after exposure to radiation. *Nat Clin Pract Endocrinol Metab.* 2005;1(2):82–91.

7. Sherman SI. Thyroid carcinoma. *Lancet.* 2003;361(9356):501–511.

8. Cooper DS, Doherty GM, Haugen BR, et al. Management guidelines for patients with thyroid nodules and differentiated thyroid cancer. *Thyroid.* 2006;16(2):109–142.

9. Hay ID, Thompson GB, Grant CS, et al. Papillary thyroid carcinoma managed at the Mayo Clinic during six decades (1940–1999): temporal trends in initial therapy and long-term outcome in 2444 consecutively treated patients. *World J Surg.* 2002;26(8):879–885.

10. Mazzaferri EL, Kloos RT. Clinical review 128: current approaches to primary therapy for papillary and follicular thyroid cancer. *J Clin Endocrinol Metab.* 2001;86(4):1447–1463.

11. Tuttle RM, Leboeuf R, Martorella AJ. Papillary thyroid cancer: monitoring and therapy. *Endocrinol Metab Clin North Am.* 2007;36(3):753–778, vii.

12. BTA. *British Thyroid Association and Royal College of Physicians: Guidelines for the Management of Thyroid Cancer in Adults.* 2002 [cited 2006 November 1]; Available from: british-thyroid-association.org.

13. Pacini F, Schlumberger M, Dralle H, et al. European consensus for the management of patients with differentiated thyroid carcinoma of the follicular epithelium. *Eur J Endocrinol.* 2006;154(6):787–803.

14. Sherman SI. *National Comprehensive Cancer Network, Clinical Practice Guidelines in Oncology, Thyroid Cancer V.2.2006.* 2006 [cited 2006 November 1]; Available from: http://www.nccn.org/professionals/physician_gls/PDF/thyroid.pdf.

15. ThyroidCarcinomaTaskForce. AACE/AAES medical/surgical guidelines for clinical practice: management of thyroid carcinoma. American Association of Clinical Endocrinologists. American College of Endocrinology. *Endocr Pract.* 2001;7(3):202–220.

16. Lee N, Tuttle RM. External beam radiation for differentiated thyroid cancer. *Endocrine Related Cancers,* 2006;13(4):971–977.

17. Biondi B, Filetti S, Schlumberger M. Thyroid-hormone therapy and thyroid cancer: a reassessment. *Nat Clin Pract Endocrinol Metab.* 2005;1(1):32–40.

18. McGriff NJ, Csako G, Gourgiotis L, et al. Effects of thyroid hormone suppression therapy on adverse clinical outcomes in thyroid cancer. *Ann Med.* 2002;34(7–8):554–564.

19. Spencer CA. Serum thyroglobulin measurements: clinical utility and technical limitations in the management of patients with differentiated thyroid carcinomas. *Endocr Pract.* 2000;6(6):481–484.

20. Spencer CA, Bergoglio LM, Kazarosyan M, et al. Clinical impact of thyroglobulin (Tg) and Tg autoantibody method differences on the management of patients with differentiated thyroid carcinomas. *J Clin Endocrinol Metab.* 2005;90(10):5566–5575.

21. Wong KT, Ahuja AT. Ultrasound of thyroid cancer. *Cancer Imaging.* 2005;5:157–166.

22. Larson SM, Robbins R. Positron emission tomography in thyroid cancer management. *Semin Roentgenol.* 2002;37(2):169–174.

23. Stokkel MP, Duchateau CS, Dragoiescu C. The value of FDG-PET in the follow-up of differentiated thyroid cancer: a review of the literature. *Q J Nucl Med Mol Imaging.* 2006;50(1):78–87.

24. Tuttle RM, Leboeuf R. Investigational therapies for metastatic thyroid carcinoma. *J Natl Compr Canc Netw.* 2007;5(6):641–646.

25. Green LD, Mack L, Pasieka JL. Anaplastic thyroid cancer and primary thyroid lymphoma: a review of these rare thyroid malignancies. *J Surg Oncol.* 2006;94(8):725–736.

26. Mack LA, Pasieka JL. An evidence-based approach to the treatment of thyroid lymphoma. *World J Surg.* 2007;31(5):978–986.

27. Ball DW. Medullary thyroid cancer: monitoring and therapy. *Endocrinol Metab Clin North Am.* 2007;36(3):823–837, viii.

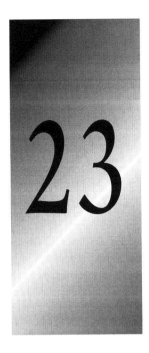

Evaluation and Treatment of Sarcoma

Robert G. Maki

Sarcomas constitute less than 1% of all cancers diagnosed annually, with ~12,000 people developing a sarcoma this year in the United States (census of 300 million people in 2006) (1). Approximately half of patients with newly diagnosed sarcoma will die of disease (2). The small number of cases seen and the diversity of histology (more than 50 histologies, the most common of which are shown in Table 23.1), anatomical site, and biologic behavior have made study of this family of tumors difficult. However, some features regarding treatment stand out, and those will be highlighted in this section. Loss of muscle or bone and its ability to heal will affect rehabilitation of the patient. The nature of the local therapy, whether radiation is involved, and whether periosteal stripping is employed can also make a difference in terms of risk to the limb of fracture, points that require discussion between treating physicians in a multidisciplinary setting.

ETIOLOGY

There is no clear cause for most sarcomas, the exception being those associated with radiation therapy (3,4). Radiation-associated sarcomas, often of the malignant fibrous histiocytoma (MFH) variety or "sarcoma not otherwise specified" are associated with diseases that are commonly treated with radiotherapy and in those in which a long survival period

TABLE 23.1
Common Soft-Tissue and Bone Sarcomas

Common Soft-Tissue Sarcomas
Gastrointestinal stromal tumor (GIST)
Liposarcoma
   Well-differentiated/dedifferentiated
   Myxoid/round cell
   Pleomorphic
Leiomyosarcoma
High-grade undifferentiated pleomorphic sarcoma (formerly termed MFH, malignant fibrous histiocytoma)
Synovial sarcoma
Fibrosarcoma
Malignant peripheral nerve sheath tumor (MPNST) also called malignant schwannoma
Common sarcomas of bone and cartilage
Osteogenic sarcoma (osteosarcoma)
   Osteoblastic
   Chondroblastic
   Fibroblastic
Ewing sarcoma
Chondrosarcoma
Malignant fibrous histiocytoma of bone
Leiomyosarcoma of bone
Chordoma

KEY POINTS

- Sarcomas constitute less than 1% of all cancers diagnosed annually, with ~12,000 people developing a sarcoma this year in the United States.
- Approximately half of patients with newly diagnosed sarcoma will die of disease.
- There are at least 50 soft-tissue sarcoma subclasses, many with distinctive features regarding anatomical distribution or responses to various chemotherapy agents.
- The small number of cases seen and the diversity of histology, anatomical site, and biologic behavior have made study of this family of tumors difficult.
- There is no clear cause for most sarcomas, the exception being those associated with radiation therapy.
- Radiation-associated sarcomas are associated with diseases that are commonly treated with radiother-

apy and in those in which a long survival period is expected, such as Hodgkin lymphoma and breast carcinoma.
- Surgery is the only curative modality for most sarcomas.
- Long-term sequelae resulting from larger radiotherapy doses and volumes are associated with increased fibrosis and edema, and possibly an increased rate of bone fractures.
- The orthopedic implications for primary bone sarcomas are often greater than those of soft-tissue sarcomas, due to extensive operations, such as those on the spine, internal or complete hemipelvectomies, and forequarter amputations.
- As with soft-tissue sarcomas, amputation is now uncommon for primary bone tumors, with allografts and increasingly sophisticated prostheses used for reconstruction.

is expected, such as Hodgkin lymphoma and breast carcinoma. Data regarding exposure to chemical compounds such as dioxins or herbicides, including Agent Orange, have not been conclusive (5). Other associations between patient exposures and subsequent sarcoma development include that of Kaposi sarcoma with human herpesvirus 8 (HHV-8, also termed Kaposi sarcoma herpesvirus, KSHV), whether in epidemic form associated with human immunodeficiency virus (HIV) infection or those endemic cases typically found in octogenarians of Mediterranean descent (6).

Familial syndromes associated with sarcomas give insight into the key genetic mediators. There is a high incidence of sarcomas, sometimes multiple asynchronous tumors, in patients with Li-Fraumeni syndrome (7). Li-Fraumeni syndrome is characterized by p53 genetic alterations and in second cancers in patients with retinoblastoma (Rb) who develop unilateral and oftentimes bilateral primary retinoblastomas. A genetic predisposition to soft-tissue sarcoma has also been associated with neurofibromatosis (8) (with germline NF1 alterations). What is perhaps surprising is that only ~5% of patients with neurofibromatosis (NF) develop malignant peripheral nerve sheath tumors (MPNSTs); primary tumors in the central nervous system, including acoustic neuromas and low-grade astrocytomas, are more typical of this syndrome. Familial adenomatous polyposis (FAP), a subset of which is termed Gardner syndrome, is associated with the development of intra-abdominal deep fibromatoses, also termed desmoid tumors, tumors that are technically benign but that

can kill patients through involvement of local structures (9,10), as noted in a following section.

Finally, a familial gastrointestinal stromal tumor (GIST) syndrome has now been identified in fewer than 20 families worldwide to date (11,12). They often have multifocal and relatively indolent disease, though some can succumb to progression of one or many of the primary tumors. The syndrome, with a mutation in c-kit, is associated with pigment changes in the hands and feet as well as bowel dysmotility issues, in comparison to unaffected siblings, consistent with effect on the interstitial cells of Cajal, the pacemaker cells of the gut thought to be the origin of GISTs (13).

CYTOGENETIC ABNORMALITIES

While there have been associations between genetic syndromes and sarcomas, an entirely different group of sarcomas are interesting for the involvement of specific translocations, making sarcomas a solid tumor relative of hematalogic malignancies. The best examples include the Ewing sarcoma/primitive neuroectodermal tumor translocation t(11;22)(q24;q11.2-12) and the synovial sarcoma translocation t(X;18)(p11.2;q11.2) (Table 23.2). These genetic abnormalities can be used as a diagnostic tool. Multiple studies of genetic abnormalities have been published (14). For example, myxoid-round cell liposarcomas contain the translocation t(12;16)(q13;p11) FUS-DDIT3 (formerly called TLS-CHOP), which links these two morphologically distinct liposarcoma subtypes.

TABLE 23.2
Common Translocation-Associated Sarcomas

HISTOLOGY	CHROMOSOMAL ALTERATION	INVOLVED GENES	APPROXIMATE FREQUENCY (%)
Synovial sarcoma	t(X;18)(p11;q11)	SYT-SSX1, SYT-SSX2, SYT-SSX4	95
Myxoid—round cell liposarcoma	t(12;16)(q13;p11)	FUS(TLS)-DDIT3 (CHOP)	75
Ewing sarcoma	t(11;22)(q24;q12)	EWS-FLI1	85
Alveolar rhabdomyosarcoma	t(2;13)(q35;q14)	PAX3-FKHR	70
	t(1;13)(p36;q14)	PAX7-FKHR	20
Desmoplastic small round cell tumor	t(11;22)(p13;q12)	EWS-WT1	>90
Endometrial stromal sarcoma	t(X;17)(p15;q21)	JAZF1-JJAZ1	65

PATHOLOGIC CLASSIFICATION

There are at least 50 soft-tissue sarcoma subclasses, many with distinctive features regarding anatomical distribution or responses to various chemotherapy agents (15). Sarcoma histologic subtype is an important determinant of prognosis and an important predictor of distinctive patterns of behavior. For example, liposarcoma is characterized by five histologic subtypes (well differentiated, dedifferentiated, myxoid, round cell, and pleomorphic), each with its own biology, patterns of metastasis, and responsiveness to chemotherapy. The pattern of metastasis of most sarcomas is hematogenous. Some sarcomas, in particular extraskeletal myxoid chondrosarcoma and alveolar soft part sarcoma, spread in a characteristic fashion early in their course as innumerable small, round metastatic deposits that grow slowly over years. Patients with such diseases can live a surprisingly long time with a great burden of disease (Fig. 23.1). Lymph node metastases are uncommon, except for selected cell types most commonly associated with childhood sarcoma.

CLINICAL PRESENTATION

Soft-tissue sarcomas present as an enlarging mass, keeping in mind that benign tumors are at least 100 times more common than sarcomas. The mass is often large and painless, only coming to attention when more than 5 cm in maximum dimension (Fig. 23.2). A core-needle biopsy usually clinches the diagnosis, and when it does not, an incisional biopsy or planned resection of the entire mass en bloc is usually pursued next (16). Fine-needle aspiration is not often used for primary diagnosis in the United States; however, it is useful in defining recurrence of disease.

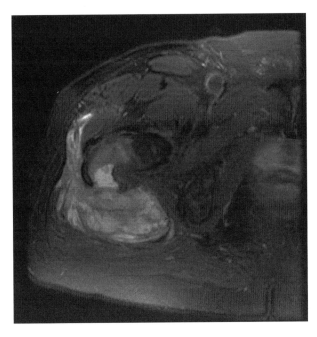

FIGURE 23.1

Axial T2 fat saturation Magnetic Resonance Imaging scan of a myxofibrosarcoma affecting the right hip. Deep tumors such as this can present late in their course.

IMAGING STUDIES

Magnetic resonance imaging (MRI) or computed tomography (CT) scans are the usual way to define the primary tumor and a means to examine for metastatic disease, seen in as many as 20% of patients at time of presentation. Imaging with multiple modalities, all focusing on the same entity, is not required. Positron emission tomography (PET) is occasionally employed

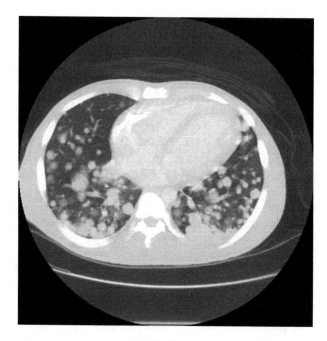

FIGURE 23.2

Chest Computed Tomograph scan from a young male patient with widespread lung metastases from alveolar soft part sarcoma. This is a characteristic pattern for this diagnosis.

to examine patients for evidence of distant disease at time of presentation prior to resection, but is not yet Food and Drug Administration (FDA)-approved for this indication (17). PET may also be helpful in following the development of GIST, but it is not yet clear if it is superior in detecting disease progression on imatinib or sunitinib than contrast-enhanced CT scans (18,19).

PATHOLOGICAL GRADE

After establishing the diagnosis of sarcoma, the most important piece of information the pathologist can provide is histologic grade. Grade comprises the overall assessment of cellularity, differentiation, pleomorphism, necrosis, and number of mitoses. Several grading scales and systems are used. Despite the presence of such criteria, the specific criteria that define a particular grade are not well defined. A four-grade system (Broders); a three-grade system, such as that of the French Federation of Cancer Centers Sarcoma Group; and a binary system (high- vs low-grade) are in use simultaneously at different institutions. Implications for the definition of grade, which heavily influences tumor staging, are clear. If "high grade" is defined differently at different centers, comparison of results between trials becomes difficult.

TABLE 23.3 AJCC Sixth Edition Staging System for Soft-Tissue Sarcoma			
STAGE	GRADE	T SIZE	METASTASES
I	Low (1–2)	Any	M0
II	High (3–4)	T1a—b, T2a	M0
III	High (3–4)	T2b	M0
IV	Any	Any	N1 or M1

T1 ≤5 cm; T2 >5 cm; a, superficial to investing fascia; b, deep
Abbreviation: AJCC, American Joint Committee on Cancer.

STAGING

It is now clear that survival is defined by tumor grade, size, and location of tumor relative to a site's investing fascia (deep or superficial), and each factor helps define the risk of tumor spread to distant metastatic sites. New modalities, such as the presence of a specific genetic signature, may help stratify patient risk for recurrence in the future, but remain investigational.

Stage determines outcome in each commonly used staging system. In the United States, the American Joint Committee on Cancer (AJCC) version 6 staging system is most commonly used (20). This staging system is noted in Table 23.3. Risk is stratified first by grade of tumor, then by location (deep or superficial to the most superficial investing fascia of that site), size (cutoff of 5 cm), and presence or absence of metastatic disease. Lymph node metastasis carries a prognosis as poor or nearly as poor as that of bloodborne metastasis, and is included in stage IV disease.

SURGERY AS PRIMARY THERAPY

Surgery is the only curative modality for most sarcomas. In situations where surgery for en bloc resection is not feasible, such as the spine, some combination of local therapy employing definitive radiation is occasionally used. The idea of surgery is to perform an en bloc resection when feasible, which has now lowered the need for amputation for primary therapy of sarcomas to less than 10% (21). Importantly, local recurrence after a limb-sparing operation is nearly always feasible without affecting overall survival. For small primary lesions (under 5 cm), excision with wide margins is feasible and usually sufficient, with radiation reserved for local disease recurrence (after a repeat resection) (22,23).

Conversely, since high-grade, soft-tissue sarcomas more than 10 cm have a high risk of both local and distant recurrence, patients are good candidates for investigational approaches, such as neoadjuvant chemotherapy. Of note, all patients with primary soft-tissue sarcomas over 5 cm in size, high or low grade, should be considered for adjuvant radiation therapy, since it is proved to decrease the risk of local recurrence (24–27).

RADIATION THERAPY

Radiation therapy is used in the primary treatment of sarcomas to decrease the risk of local relapse, enhancing the effect of a definitive operation. Limb conservation using adjuvant external beam radiation therapy was shown to give local control similar to that of amputation in a randomized trial at the National Cancer Institute (NCI) (28). It is also worth noting that radiation should not be considered an acceptable option to make up for grossly positive tumor margins at time of primary resection.

External beam radiation therapy (EBRT) is the most commonly used form of radiation, since it is easy to perform relative to brachytherapy (temporary implants of radioactive seeds in the tumor bed) or more sophisticated planning techniques. Both EBRT and brachytherapy have been shown to decrease the risk of local recurrence for patients with high-grade sarcomas, but only EBRT provides improved local tumor control for low-grade sarcomas (25). Careful planning to ensure coverage of tumor margins and drain sites is paramount in maximizing the potential benefit of radiation therapy to a patient, while at the same time avoiding irradiation of such a large proportion of the cross-sectional area of the extremity that lymphedema becomes a more significant issue.

Few data are available to determine whether to give radiation before or after primary surgery. Radiation therapy before surgery employs a smaller radiation field and lower doses than postoperative radiation therapy, which often also employs a boost to the tumor bed. Radiation therapy before surgery is associated with a higher risk of wound complications than postoperative radiation therapy, nearly completely limited to lower extremity lesions (29–31). However, since higher doses and a larger volume of tissue is irradiated in the postoperative setting, the risk of chronic cicatricial and other wound changes was higher in the only randomized study of preoperative vs postoperative external beam irradiation for extremity sarcomas performed to date (29). There may also be a higher risk of bone fracture in patients receiving (higher dose, larger volume) postoperative irradiation therapy. This is of concern since this could affect the rehabilitation plan.

Special techniques for radiation therapy, including brachytherapy, intensity-modulated radiation therapy, combinations of chemotherapy and radiation, and investigational schedules of therapy, hold promise for the treatment of sarcoma but are beyond the scope of this chapter. One of the key complications of radiation therapy is the injury suffered by normal tissues that may reduce function in the long term.

ADJUVANT CHEMOTHERAPY

Despite good local control of disease, as many as half of patients with adequate local control of disease develop distant metastasis, usually to the lungs (extremity sarcomas) or liver (abdominal primary). It was the hope that adjuvant chemotherapy would decrease the frequency of distant metastases and thus increase overall survival. At least 15 randomized studies have examined adjuvant chemotherapy for soft-tissue sarcomas. Because anthracyclines are the most active agents in sarcoma therapy in the metastatic setting, they have been used in nearly all of the adjuvant trials, alone or in combination. Most of the studies are small and lack statistical power to detect small changes in overall survival.

Meta-analyses and more recent studies provide more data on the utility of chemotherapy combinations using the most active types of agents for most sarcomas, that is, anthracyclines and ifosfamide. The most rigorous meta-analysis regarding adjuvant doxorubicin-based chemotherapy is that published in 1997 (32). Median follow-up was 9.4 years. Analyses were stratified by trial, and hazard ratios were calculated for each trial and combined for each of the 14 trials, which allowed for an assessment of the risk of death or recurrence in comparison to control patients. Disease-free survival at 10 years was improved from 45% to 55% ($p = 0.0001$). Local disease-free survival at 10 years also favored chemotherapy, 81% versus 75% ($p < 0.02$). Although overall survival improved at 10 years from 50% to 54%, the difference was not statistically significant ($p = 0.12$). In an unplanned analysis, overall survival was shown to increase 7% in the subset of patients with extremity sarcomas receiving chemotherapy ($p = 0.029$).

Newer studies have examined ifosfamide combined with an anthracycline in the adjuvant or neoadjuvant setting. The largest of these studies (from Italy) showed a statistically significant overall survival advantage at five years, with borderline significance ($p = 0.07$) survival advantage overall (33,34). Two smaller studies, one of adjuvant and one of neoadjuvant chemotherapy, showed no survival advantage to the chemotherapy (35,36). Hence, based on these data, even if there is a benefit for the adjuvant use of chemotherapy, it appears a small one. The risks and benefits of adjuvant chemotherapy for any specific person should be discussed on a case-by-case basis.

COMPLICATIONS OF PRIMARY TREATMENT

Wound Complications

Assessment of the influence of preoperative chemotherapy on wound complications is difficult. The University of Texas M.D. Anderson Cancer Center compared morbidity of radical surgery for soft-tissue sarcoma in 104 patients receiving preoperative chemotherapy and 204 patients who had surgery first (37). The most common complications were wound infections and other wound complications, but the incidence of surgical complications was no different for patients who received chemotherapy or not.

One of the key features of the preoperative vs postoperative radiation study from Canada was inclusion of acute wound complication assessment in the study design from the outset and at defined time points for the initial four months after surgery (31). Using these criteria, postoperative radiotherapy also showed a significant risk of wound complications (17%). Furthermore, the wound complication rate after preoperative radiotherapy and primary direct wound closure was 16%, apparently lower than patients treated with a vascularized graft. Thus, in situations in which wound complications may be an issue, transpositional or free grafts should be considered before radiation therapy to attempt to decrease the local complication rate. It is notable that the risk of wound complication in the Canadian study appeared to be limited to lower extremity lesions.

Fracture

The question of weight bearing and the potential risk of fracture is common in the rehabilitation setting. A study of 145 patients with soft-tissue sarcoma undergoing limb-sparing surgery and postoperative radiation with or without chemotherapy demonstrated a 6% fracture rate (38). Patients treated with adjuvant beam radiation therapy (BRT) in a randomized trial from Memorial Sloan-Kettering Cancer Center (MSKCC) had a fracture rate of 4% versus 0% in the control arm, though this difference was not statistically significant (26).

One study highlighted the fracture risk associated with peritoneal stripping (39). Two hundred five patients with soft-tissue sarcoma of the thigh were examined for factors contributing to pathologic femur fracture after adjuvant radiation. One hundred fifteen patients were treated with BRT, 59 received EBRT, and 31 received a combination of EBRT and BRT. The five-year actuarial risk was 8.6%. On multivariate analysis of risk factors associated with fracture, only periosteal stripping was significant. Thus, while

rehabilitation is crucial to a patient's recovery after limb salvage surgery, particular attention should be paid to those patients who have periosteal stripping as part of their primary therapy.

QUALITY OF LIFE AND FUNCTIONAL OUTCOME

Quality of life (QOL) evaluations highlight the potential pitfalls of local therapy as it pertains to functional outcome. Obvious factors affecting QOL include those features associated with the primary tumor resection. Not surprisingly, there is a higher level of handicap in amputated patients compared to those treated with conservative surgery (40). Resection involving nerves was associated with poorer outcome on multivariate analysis ($p < 0.02$) in a separate study (41). Conventional chemotherapy has not had an impact on the functional outcome of patients with extremity sarcoma.

The best data regarding effects of radiation on functional outcome are again from the Canadian preoperative versus postoperative radiation therapy study, using well-examined instruments of outcome (29,31). Validated instruments, including the Musculoskeletal Tumor Society Rating Scale, Toronto Extremity Salvage Score, and the Short Form-36 Health Survey QOL instruments were used to evaluate patient outcomes and QOL. The preoperative group had inferior function, with lower bodily pain scores on all three rating instruments at six weeks. However, at later times up to one year after surgery, there were no differences in these scores. Thus, it appears that the timing of radiotherapy has little impact on the ultimate function of soft-tissue sarcoma patients. However, longer follow-up now indicates that late tissue sequelae resulting from larger radiotherapy doses and volumes are associated with increased fibrosis and edema, and possibly an increased rate of bone fractures. These late outcomes may ultimately override the influence of acute wound complications, although patients with acute wound complications can experience long-term functional impairment (29).

SURGERY FOR METASTATIC DISEASE

Median survival from the time metastases are recognized is 12–18 months, though the situation for patients with metastatic GIST has changed radically with the introduction of imatinib; for patients with non-GIST sarcomas, only 20%–25% of patients are expected to live more than two years, another factor in determining the appropriateness of patients for rehabilitation. Surgical resection can provide selected patients with prolonged periods of freedom from disease, and radiation therapy provides palliation for individual patients who have localized symptomatic metastases. Optimal treatment of patients with unresectable or metastatic soft-tissue sarcoma requires an appreciation for the natural history of the disease, close attention to the individual patient, and an understanding of the benefits and limitations of the therapeutic options. One such challenge, that of local-regionally recurrent angiosarcoma, can give surgeons fits (Fig. 23.3). The tumor, cleanly resected previously, recurred aggressively well clear of the negative margin, a frequent characteristic of angiosarcomas.

The MSKCC experience is emblematic of the situation for patients with lung-only metastatic disease. In their database of 716 patients with primary extremity sarcoma, pulmonary-only metastases occurred in 19%, or 135 patients. Of these 135 patients, 58% underwent thoracotomy, and 83% of those had a complete resection of their tumor. In the 65 patients who had a complete resection of their tumor, 69% had recurrence, with pulmonary metastases as their only site of disease. Median survival time from complete resection was 19 months, and three-year survival was 23% of those undergoing resection and 11% of those presenting with lung metastasis only. Patients who did not undergo thoracotomy all died within three years (42,43). Chemotherapy had no obvious impact on survival in either the patients who did or those who did not undergo resection. Thus, resection of limited metastatic disease, where feasible, remains a good standard of care for recurrent soft-tissue sarcoma. Not discussed here further are the equally important data that resection of

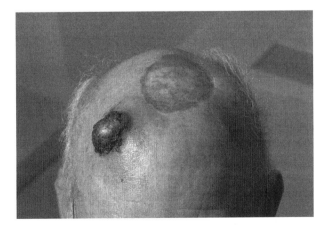

FIGURE 23.3

Regional recurrence of a scalp angiosarcoma following resection and skin graft of the primary site. Note the heaped-up nature of the tumor in this image, which is surrounded by tissue infiltrated with angiosarcoma.

metastatic disease of osteogenic sarcomas can also be associated with cure.

SYSTEMIC THERAPY FOR METASTATIC DISEASE

Table 23.4 documents the expected response rate for selected systemic chemotherapy agents or combinations. Doxorubicin has been the workhorse of chemotherapy for advanced sarcoma. Liposomal forms of doxorubicin may have fewer side effects than doxorubicin itself. Response rates have been low, however, and in one randomized phase 2 study, the response rate to doxorubicin was as low as that of liposomal doxorubicin, perhaps owing to sarcoma subtypes enrolled on the study (44).

Ifosfamide has approximately the same efficacy as doxorubicin. During its development, ifosfamide administration was limited by hemorrhagic cystitis. The uroprotective agent mesna has markedly changed the ability to give both ifosfamide and cyclophosphamide, and ifosfamide doses as large as 14–18 g/m² or more have been given over one to two weeks (45). A third drug with modest activity in sarcoma is dacarbazine (DTIC) (46), whose activity was recognized more than 20 years ago. Temozolomide, an orally available version of dacarbazine, has demonstrated activity against leiomyosarcomas (47,48).

Combinations of doxorubicin and ifosfamide [and mesna, (AIM)] and of [mesna], doxorubicin, ifosfamide and dacarbazine (MAID) are used most frequently in patients in need of a response; the drugs appear to have additive benefit, but do not appear to synergize with one another. As for other single agents, excluding the remarkable story of the sensitivity of GIST to imatinib, the most significant investigational agent in soft-tissue sarcomas is presently ecteinascidin (ET-743), with an 8%–10% response rate in sarcomas (49,50), but striking activity against myxoid-round liposarcoma. mTOR inhibitors, such as temsirolimus, sirolimus, everolimus (RAD001), and deforolimus, have shown minor activity in sarcomas, as have sorafenib and other multi-targeted tyrosine kinase inhibitors; these new orally available agents remain investigational.

SARCOMAS OF BONE

Sarcomas of bone, mostly osteogenic sarcoma, Ewing sarcoma in children, and chondrosarcoma in adults, are only approximately one-fourth as common as soft-tissue sarcomas. Furthermore, primary bone tumors are, as a whole, much less common than metastatic carcinomas to bone, with their attendant complications.

TABLE 23.4
*Selected Systemic Chemotherapeutic Agents
for Soft-Tissue Sarcoma and Approximate Response Rates*

REGIMEN	DOSE	RESPONSE RATE (%)
Doxorubicin	60–75 mg/m^2	10–25
Ifosfamide	5–16 g/m^2	10–25
Dacarbazine	1000–1250 mg/m^2	10
AIM: (mesna) + Doxorubicin + Ifosfamide	varies	20–40
MAID: (mesna) + Doxorubicin + Ifosfamide + Dacarbazine	varies	20–40
Gemcitabine/Docetaxel	varies	15–20
Trabectedin (ET-743)	1.5 mg/m^2 over 24 h	10
Imatinib (for GIST only)	400–800 mg daily	50

Note: All drugs listed here except imatinib are given intravenously, typically on a 3-week repeating schedule. Imatinib is given daily by mouth.

However, like metastatic carcinoma to bone, the orthopedic implications for primary bone sarcomas are oftentimes greater than that of soft-tissue sarcomas, especially when factoring in extensive operations, such as those on the spine, internal or complete hemipelvectomies, and forequarter amputations. Functional loss with resection of a humeral osteogenic sarcoma oftentimes is greater than that of resection of a soft-tissue sarcoma affecting the shoulder girdle, and thus a few key points of management of these challenging tumors is warranted.

While not all bone tumors (eg, aneurysmal bone cyst, eosinophilic granuloma, and osteoid osteoma) require excision, surgery is the standard of care for more aggressive tumors, such as osteogenic sarcoma (osteosarcoma), chondrosarcoma, and Ewing sarcoma of bone. As a result, the reconstruction and its consequences have profound effects on the rehabilitation potential of patients. There are particularly important issues pertaining to children with osteogenic sarcoma. As with soft-tissue sarcomas, amputation is now uncommon for primary bone tumors, with allografts and increasingly sophisticated prostheses used for reconstruction, including those that can be extended at time of a followup surgery, or even via even newer devices that can extend themselves using strong external magnetic fields to drive an internal motor to extend the prosthesis (51).

Bone sarcomas are staged using a system similar to that for soft-tissue sarcomas (Table 23.5) (20). In comparison to soft-tissue sarcomas, the size cutoff for staging is 8 cm, not 5 cm, between small (A) and large (B) primary tumors. Stage IV is divided into two subsets: IVA (lung metastasis) and IVB (other metastatic disease), since patients with lung metastases can still be resected with curative intent.

TABLE 23.5
*AJCC Sixth Edition Bone Sarcoma
Staging System*

STAGE	GRADE	T SIZE	METS
IA	Low (1,2)	T1	M0
IB	Low (1,2)	T2	M0
IIA	High (3,4)	T1	M0
IIB	High (3,4)	T2	M0
III	Any	T3	M0
IVA	Any	Any	M1a
IVB	Any	Any	N1
	Any	Any	M1b

T1 ≤8 cm; T2 >8 cm; T3, discontiguous disease in one bone; M1a, lung; M1b other.

Abbreviation: AJCC, American Joint Committee on Cancer.

With the finding that tumor necrosis can serve as an indicator of responsiveness at the time of surgery, neoadjuvant chemotherapy is the standard of care for osteogenic sarcoma and for Ewing sarcoma of bone. Since chondrosarcomas are chemotherapy-insensitive, by and large, they are treated with surgery alone and occasionally with radiation as well. In the cases of osteogenic sarcoma and Ewing sarcoma, a period of chemotherapy is followed by definitive surgery, and then chemotherapy is continued to complete what is typically a 6-month (osteosarcoma) or nearly 12-month (Ewing sarcoma) course of therapy. Radiation is typically given during chemotherapy after the definitive surgery.

The standard of care for neoadjuvant chemotherapy for younger patients is doxorubicin, cisplatin, and methotrexate (52), although there is not particularly strong evidence that to support the contention that methotrexate is useful in the adjuvant setting (53). In older patients, cisplatin and doxorubicin form a reasonable combination for neoadjuvant/adjuvant therapy (54), although even this combination is difficult to administer to patients who develop osteosarcoma during the second peak of diagnosis of the disease in the eighth decade. Dose intensification of a standard doxorubicin-cisplatin backbone does not appear to improve survival (55). Ifosfamide is also active in osteosarcoma, though its use in a nonprotocol setting was called into question in the recent study from Meyers et al. in which ifosfamide and nonspecific immune-stimulate muramyl tripeptide were added to a standard doxorubicin-cisplatin-methotrexate backbone. Ifosfamide increased the cure rate in patients receiving chemotherapy, but only when given in conjunction with muramyl tripeptide (MTP), a bacterial cell wall component that is proinflammatory. In fact, survival in patients receiving ifosfamide was inferior to that of patients receiving the standard three-drug combination. Since MTP is not commercially available, the role of ifosfamide in the adjuvant setting is unclear, and remains investigational (52). Ifosfamide is active in metastatic disease and is often given in that setting. Other standard cytotoxic chemotherapy agents have little activity in osteogenic sarcoma, making this a ripe target for newer targeted therapeutics that may affect the ability of osteogenic sarcoma to metastasize.

Ewing sarcoma is most commonly treated with neoadjuvant chemotherapy, surgery, and postoperative radiation. It tends to spread locally without regard to tissue planes, so en bloc resection and adjuvant radiation must be carefully planned to involve a wide enough field. The standard of care for Ewing sarcoma is a five-drug regimen of vincristine, doxorubicin, cyclophosphamide (VAC), alternating with a combination of ifosfamide (with mesna) and etoposide (I/E) (56). The five-drug combination was shown superior to VAC in a large clinical trial and represents the best standard of care off-protocol. Topoisomerase I inhibitor combinations and cisplatin are somewhat active against Ewing sarcoma in the metastatic setting (57,58), and recent anecdotes of responses to insulinlike growth factor receptor inhibitors may form the basis for a new generation of studies combining targeted and standard cytotoxic agents in the near future.

Since both osteogenic sarcoma and Ewing sarcoma are common in younger patients, with peak age of incidence of both during adolescence, rehabilitation is a particularly important part of the multidisciplinary effort, especially in children without closure of their growth plates. Expandable prostheses and allograft reconstructions have helped minimize the residual dysfunction of the limb, but are still associated with episodes of nonunion, prosthesis failure, fracture, or wear and tear to the plastic parts of the prosthesis, requiring replacement (51). In some cases, poor local reconstruction options remain an inferior treatment to simple below-the-knee amputation, in which the rehabilitation potential ends up being greater with a good prosthesis, rather than a destabilizing operation, even if local control can be achieved.

DESMOID TUMORS (AGGRESSIVE FIBROMATOSES)

It is worth mentioning this soft-tissue neoplasm, as it can cause a great deal of morbidity, either from the primary tumor itself or from its treatment. Desmoid tumors are not quite sarcomas, belonging to a family of myofibroblastic tumors that are unusual in their bland histology and slow progression (15). Surgery remains the treatment of choice for these lesions, which cannot truly be called sarcomas due to their lack of metastatic potential. However, deaths have still been seen in patients with locally advanced disease, in particular in patients with desmoids associated with familial adenomatous polyposis (9). The complications of surgery can outweigh any perceived benefit from resection, however, and deaths in the series of patients treated at MSKCC have more frequently been iatrogenic rather than due to tumor per se. Whether this reflects the more aggressive nature of some desmoids versus others, these data indicate that one must proceed with great caution in the management of these lesions, which are occasionally seen to regress spontaneously. For truly resectable disease, surgery alone appears to be the optimal approach, especially in patients with negative microscopic margins. In advanced cases, a trial of nonsteroidal antiinflammatory drugs or hormonal therapy can be considered in most patients before moving to chemotherapy; those patients who are symptomatic and not a candidate for surgery should be given to radiation or chemotherapy.

CONCLUSION

A number of approaches will affect patient survival in the present and near future. Surgical approaches have benefitted from improvements in tumor imaging, which now make limb-sparing surgeries more routine. Improved techniques in tissue transfer make reconstruction of very large tissue defects feasible. Perhaps we will see in the next generation development of tissues in vitro to help with reconstruction of patients' wounds. Radiation therapy techniques have shown rapid increases in sophistication with the application of intensity-modulated external beam techniques to extremity tumors, minimizing toxicity while maintaining or improving local control (30). However, systemic therapy outside of GIST remains somewhat in a rut. Though there have been some particular success with synovial sarcoma and ifosfamide, angiosarcoma and paclitaxel, and trabectedin and myxoid-round cell liposarcoma, the truth is we still need better systemic agents to treat the bulk of sarcomas encountered in practice. Advances in the most important area of research, that is, basic and translational research, will hopefully have an impact on the treatment of a number of sarcoma subtypes in the near future.

References

1. Jemal A, Siegel R, Ward E, Murray T, Xu J, Thun MJ. Cancer statistics, 2007. *CA Cancer J Clin.* 2007;57(1):43–66.
2. Weitz J, Antonescu CR, Brennan MF. Localized extremity soft tissue sarcoma: improved knowledge with unchanged survival over time. *J Clin Oncol.* 2003;21(14):2719–2725.
3. Brady MS, Gaynor JJ, Brennan MF. Radiation-associated sarcoma of bone and soft tissue. *Arch Surg.* 1992;127(12): 1379–1385.
4. Spiro IJ, Suit HD. Radiation-induced bone and soft tissue sarcomas: clinical aspects and molecular biology. *Cancer Treat Res.* 1997;91:143–155.
5. Fingerhut MA, Halperin WE, Marlow DA, et al. Cancer mortality in workers exposed to 2,3,7,8-tetrachlorodibenzo-p-dioxin. *N Engl J Med.* 1991;324(4):212–218.
6. Schwartz RA. Kaposi's sarcoma: an update. *J Surg Oncol.* 2004;87(3):146–151.
7. Li FP, Fraumeni JF, Jr. Soft-tissue sarcomas, breast cancer, and other neoplasms. A familial syndrome? *Ann Intern Med.* 1969;71(4):747–752.
8. D'Agostino AN, Soule EH, Miller RH. Sarcomas of the peripheral nerves and somatic soft tissues associated with multiple neurofibromatosis (Von Recklinghausen's disease). *Cancer.* 1963;16:1015–1027.
9. Lewis JJ, Boland PJ, Leung DH, Woodruff JM, Brennan MF. The enigma of desmoid tumors. *Ann Surg.* 1999;229(6):866–872; discussion 72–73.
10. Lotfi AM, Dozois RR, Gordon H, et al. Mesenteric fibromatosis complicating familial adenomatous polyposis: predisposing factors and results of treatment. *Int J Colorectal Dis.* 1989;4(1):30–36.
11. Maeyama H, Hidaka E, Ota H, et al. Familial gastrointestinal stromal tumor with hyperpigmentation: association with a germline mutation of the c-kit gene. *Gastroenterology.* 2001;120(1):210–215.
12. Robson ME, Glogowski E, Sommer G, et al. Pleomorphic characteristics of a germ-line KIT mutation in a large kindred with gastrointestinal stromal tumors, hyperpigmentation, and dysphagia. *Clin Cancer Res.* 2004;10(4):1250–1254.
13. Hirota S, Isozaki K, Moriyama Y, et al. Gain-of-function mutations of c-kit in human gastrointestinal stromal tumors. *Science.* 1998;279(5350):577–580.
14. Antonescu CR. The role of genetic testing in soft tissue sarcoma. *Histopathology.* 2006;48(1):13–21.
15. Fletcher CDM, Unni KK, Mertens F. *Pathology and Genetics of Tumours of Soft Tissue and Bone.* Lyon: IARC Press; 2002.
16. Heslin MJ, Lewis JJ, Woodruff JM, Brennan MF. Core needle biopsy for diagnosis of extremity soft tissue sarcoma. *Ann Surg Oncol.* 1997;4(5):425–431.
17. Schuetze SM. Imaging and response in soft tissue sarcomas. *Hematol Oncol Clin North Am.* 2005;19(3):471–487, vi.
18. Choi H, Charnsangavej C, de Castro Faria S, et al. CT evaluation of the response of gastrointestinal stromal tumors after

19. imatinib mesylate treatment: a quantitative analysis correlated with FDG PET findings. *AJR.* 2004;183(6):1619–1628.
19. Van den Abbeele AD, Badawi RD. Use of positron emission tomography in oncology and its potential role to assess response to imatinib mesylate therapy in gastrointestinal stromal tumors (GISTs). *Eur J Cancer.* 2002;38(Suppl 5):S60–S65.
20. Greene FL, Page DL, Fleming ID, et al. *AJCC Cancer Staging Handbook,* 6th ed. New York: Springer; 2002.
21. Brennan MF. The management of soft tissue sarcomas. *Br J Surg.* 1984;71(12):964–967.
22. Lewis JJ, Leung D, Espat J, Woodruff JM, Brennan MF. Effect of reresection in extremity soft tissue sarcoma. *Ann Surg.* 2000;231(5):655–663.
23. Pisters PW, Leung DH, Woodruff J, Shi W, Brennan MF. Analysis of prognostic factors in 1,041 patients with localized soft tissue sarcomas of the extremities. *J Clin Oncol.* 1996;14(5):1679–1689.
24. Alekhteyar KM, Leung DH, Brennan MF, Harrison LB. The effect of combined external beam radiotherapy and brachytherapy on local control and wound complications in patients with high-grade soft tissue sarcomas of the extremity with positive microscopic margin. *Int J Rad Oncol Biol Phys.* 1996;36(2):321–324.
25. Alektiar KM, Leung D, Zelefsky MJ, Brennan MF. Adjuvant radiation for stage II-B soft tissue sarcoma of the extremity. *J Clin Oncol.* 2002;20(6):1643–1650.
26. Alektiar KM, Zelefsky MJ, Brennan MF. Morbidity of adjuvant brachytherapy in soft tissue sarcoma of the extremity and superficial trunk. *Int J Rad Oncol Biol Phys.* 2000;47(5):1273–1279.
27. Casper ES, Gaynor JJ, Harrison LB, Panicek DM, Hajdu SI, Brennan MF. Preoperative and postoperative adjuvant combination chemotherapy for adults with high grade soft tissue sarcoma. *Cancer.* 1994;73(6):1644–1651.
28. Rosenberg SA, Kent H, Costa J, et al. Prospective randomized evaluation of the role of limb-sparing surgery, radiation therapy, and adjuvant chemoimmunotherapy in the treatment of adult soft-tissue sarcomas. *Surgery.* 1978;84(1):62–69.
29. Davis AM, O'Sullivan B, Turcotte R, et al. Late radiation morbidity following randomization to preoperative versus postoperative radiotherapy in extremity soft tissue sarcoma. *Radiother Oncol.* 2005;75(1):48–53.
30. O'Sullivan B, Ward I, Catton C. Recent advances in radiotherapy for soft-tissue sarcoma. *Curr Oncol Rep.* 2003;5(4):274–281.
31. O'Sullivan B, Davis AM, Turcotte R, et al. Preoperative versus postoperative radiotherapy in soft-tissue sarcoma of the limbs: a randomised trial. *Lancet.* 2002;359(9325):2235–2241.
32. Sarcoma Meta-analysis Collaboration. Adjuvant chemotherapy for localised resectable soft-tissue sarcoma of adults: meta-analysis of individual data. *Lancet.* 1997;350(9092):1647–1654.
33. Frustaci S, De Paoli A, Bidoli E, et al. Ifosfamide in the adjuvant therapy of soft tissue sarcomas. *Oncology.* 2003;65(Suppl 2):80–84.
34. Frustaci S, Gherlinzoni F, De Paoli A, et al. Adjuvant chemotherapy for adult soft tissue sarcomas of the extremities and girdles: results of the Italian randomized cooperative trial. *J Clin Oncol.* 2001;19(5):1238–1247.
35. Brodowicz T, Schwameis E, Widder J, et al. Intensified adjuvant IFADIC chemotherapy for adult soft tissue sarcoma: a prospective randomized feasibility trial. *Sarcoma.* 2000;4:151–160.
36. Gortzak E, Azzarelli A, Buesa J, et al. A randomised phase II study on neo-adjuvant chemotherapy for "high-risk" adult soft-tissue sarcoma. *Eur J Cancer.* 2001;37(9):1096–1103.
37. Meric F, Milas M, Hunt KK, et al. Impact of neoadjuvant chemotherapy on postoperative morbidity in soft tissue sarcomas. *J Clin Oncol.* 2000;18(19):3378–3383.
38. Stinson SF, DeLaney TF, Greenberg J, et al. Acute and long-term effects on limb function of combined modality limb sparing therapy for extremity soft tissue sarcoma. *Int J Rad Oncol Biol Phys.* 1991;21(6):1493–1499.
39. Lin PP, Schupak KD, Boland PJ, Brennan MF, Healey JH. Pathologic femoral fracture after periosteal excision and

radiation for the treatment of soft tissue sarcoma. *Cancer.* 1998;82(12):2356–2365.

40. Davis AM, Devlin M, Griffin AM, Wunder JS, Bell RS. Functional outcome in amputation versus limb sparing of patients with lower extremity sarcoma: a matched case-control study. *Arch Phys Med Rehabil.* 1999;80(6):615–618.

41. Bell RS, O'Sullivan B, Davis A, Langer F, Cummings B, Fornasier VL. Functional outcome in patients treated with surgery and irradiation for soft tissue tumours. *J Surg Oncol.* 1991;48(4):224–231.

42. Billingsley KG, Burt ME, Jara E, et al. Pulmonary metastases from soft tissue sarcoma: analysis of patterns of diseases and postmetastasis survival. *Ann Surg.* 1999;229(5):602–610; discussion 10–12.

43. Billingsley KG, Lewis JJ, Leung DH, Casper ES, Woodruff JM, Brennan MF. Multifactorial analysis of the survival of patients with distant metastasis arising from primary extremity sarcoma. *Cancer.* 1999;85(2):389–395.

44. Judson I, Radford JA, Harris M, et al. Randomised phase II trial of pegylated liposomal doxorubicin (DOXIL/CAELYX) versus doxorubicin in the treatment of advanced or metastatic soft tissue sarcoma: a study by the EORTC Soft Tissue and Bone Sarcoma Group. *Eur J Cancer.* 2001;37(7):870–877.

45. Patel SR, Vadhan-Raj S, Papadopolous N, et al. High-dose ifosfamide in bone and soft tissue sarcomas: results of phase II and pilot studies—dose-response and schedule dependence. *J Clin Oncol.* 1997;15(6):2378–2384.

46. Buesa JM, Mouridsen HT, van Oosterom AT, et al. High-dose DTIC in advanced soft-tissue sarcomas in the adult. A phase II study of the E.O.R.T.C. Soft Tissue and Bone Sarcoma Group. *Ann Oncol.* 1991;2(4):307–309.

47. Anderson S, Aghajanian C. Temozolomide in uterine leiomyosarcomas. *Gynecol Oncol.* 2005;98(1):99–103.

48. Garcia del Muro X, Lopez-Pousa A, Martin J, et al. A phase II trial of temozolomide as a 6-week, continuous, oral schedule in patients with advanced soft tissue sarcoma: a study by the Spanish Group for Research on Sarcomas. *Cancer.* 2005;104(8):1706–1712.

49. Garcia-Carbonero R, Supko JG, Maki RG, et al. Ecteinascidin-743 (ET-743) for chemotherapy-naive patients with advanced soft tissue sarcomas: multicenter phase II and pharmacokinetic study. *J Clin Oncol.* 2005;23(24):5484–5492.

50. Verweij J. Ecteinascidin-743 (ET-743): early test or effective treatment in soft tissue sarcomas? *J Clin Oncol.* 2005;23(24):5420–5423.

51. Cheng EY. Surgical management of sarcomas. *Hematol Oncol Clin North Am.* 2005;19(3):451–470, v.

52. Meyers PA, Schwartz CL, Krailo M, et al. Osteosarcoma: a randomized, prospective trial of the addition of ifosfamide and/or muramyl tripeptide to cisplatin, doxorubicin, and high-dose methotrexate. *J Clin Oncol.* 2005;23(9):2004–2011.

53. Bacci G, Gherlinzoni F, Picci P, et al. Adriamycin-methotrexate high dose versus adriamycin-methotrexate moderate dose as adjuvant chemotherapy for osteosarcoma of the extremities: a randomized study. *Eur J Cancer Clin Oncol.* 1986;22(11):1337–1345.

54. Souhami RL, Craft AW, Van der Eijken JW, et al. Randomised trial of two regimens of chemotherapy in operable osteosarcoma: a study of the European Osteosarcoma Intergroup. *Lancet.* 1997;350(9082):911–917.

55. Lewis IJ, Nooij MA, Whelan J, et al. Improvement in Histologic Response But Not Survival in Osteosarcoma Patients Treated With Intensified Chemotherapy: A Randomized Phase III Trial of the European Osteosarcoma Intergroup. In; 2007:112–128.

56. Grier HE, Krailo MD, Tarbell NJ, et al. Addition of ifosfamide and etoposide to standard chemotherapy for Ewing's sarcoma and primitive neuroectodermal tumor of bone. *N Engl J Med.* 2003;348(8):694–701.

57. Wagner LM, Crews KR, Iacono LC, et al. Phase I trial of temozolomide and protracted irinotecan in pediatric patients with refractory solid tumors. *Clin Cancer Res.* 2004;10(3):840–848.

58. Wagner LM, McAllister N, Goldsby RE, et al. Temozolomide and intravenous irinotecan for treatment of advanced Ewing sarcoma. *Pediatr Blood Cancer.* 2007;48(2):132–139.

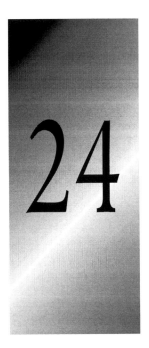

Evaluation and Treatment of Primary Bone Tumors

Gary C. O'Toole
Patrick J. Boland

Primary bone tumors are rare, with approximately 2,600 new malignant tumors of bone being diagnosed each year in the United States (1). The majority of these tumors arise in the lower limb, and the survival rate for children younger than 15 years with localized extremity disease is between 64% and 80%, as observed in specialized centers or multicentric groups (2,3).

There is a wide variety in histological subtype for primary bone tumors (Table 24.1). Osteogenic sarcoma is the most common of these tumors and represents the greatest paradigm of oncologic advancement in the 20th century. Historically, survival rates were 21% (4,5), and it was not until the 1970s, when chemotherapy was introduced into the treatment protocol, that survival rates improved (6). The advances in chemotherapy, coupled with improved radiological imaging techniques and surgical understanding of the disease behavior, have further helped improve survival rates. Despite this, the management of these patients from the initial biopsy through to the definitive resection is labor intensive and demanding, and should only be undertaken in a specialized center.

SURGICAL STAGING

The development of a staging system requires systematic accumulation and specialist interpretation of clinicopathologic data. Enneking (7) was the first to develop a universally accepted surgical staging system

TABLE 24.1 *Primary Bone Tumors*		
HISTOLOGIC TYPE	**BENIGN**	**MALIGNANT**
Hematopoietic		Myeloma
Chondrogenic	Osteochondroma	Primary chondrosarcoma
	Chondroma	Secondary chondrosarcoma
	Chondroblastoma	Dedifferentiated chondrosarcoma
	Chondromyxoid fibroma	Mesenchymal chondrosarcoma
Osteogenic	Osteoid osteoma	Osteosarcoma
	Benign osteoblastoma	Parosteal osteogenic sarcoma
Unknown origin	Giant cell tumor	Ewing's tumor
		Malignant giant cell tumor
		Adamantinoma
Fibrogenic	Fibroma	Fibrosarcoma
	Desmoplastic fibroma	
Notochordal		Chordoma
Vascular	Hemangioma	Hemangioendothelioma
		Hemangiopericytoma
Lipogenic	Lipoma	

KEY POINTS

- Primary bone tumors are rare, with approximately 2,600 new malignant tumors of bone being diagnosed each year in the United States.
- Osteogenic sarcoma is the most common primary bone tumor.
- Biopsy is often the most important procedure performed in the patient's management. Over 4% of cases required an amputation as a direct consequence of a poorly performed biopsy. Furthermore 8.5% of patients had their prognosis or outcome adversely affected as a result of a poorly planned biopsy.

- High dose methotrexate, adriamycin, cisplatin, and ifosfamide are the most commonly used as chemotherapeutic agents in osteogenic sarcoma and most other chemotherapy sensitive primary bone tumors.
- Radiation therapy has a limited role in the management of primary bone sarcomas.
- There are several reconstructive choices for the surgical management of malignant bone sarcomas including intercalary allografts, alloprosthetic composites, osteoarticular allografts, and endoprostheses. Other choices include rotationplasty and amputation.

for sarcomas of both bone and soft tissue lesions (Table 24.2). It was shown that the preoperative Enneking stage directly corresponds to five-year survival rates (8) (Fig. 24.1).

The Enneking staging system has been modified by the Musculoskeletal Tumor Society, and this newer system is accepted by most musculoskeletal oncologists (9) (Table 24.3).

The surgical staging system classifies bone and soft tissue tumors by a combination of grade (G0, G1, and G2), anatomic setting (T1 or T2), and the absence or presence of metastases (M0 or M1). The grade is determined by biopsy; the anatomic setting and metastases are determined by radiologic evaluation.

This staging system is used when planning definitive surgical resection. The primary aim of surgical intervention is to resect the tumor with wide negative margins, but benign bone tumors may be treated with intralesional therapy such as curettage, with or without cryotherapy as an adjunct. Wide negative margins remain the aim when intervening surgically in primary malignant bone sarcomas.

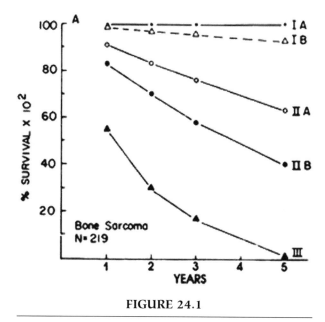

FIGURE 24.1

Preoperative Enneking stage, corresponds to five year survival rate.

TABLE 24.2 *Enneking Surgical Classification System*			
STAGE	GRADE	SITE	META-STASIS
IA	Low (G1)	Intracompartmental (T1)	M0
IB	Low (G1)	Extracompartmental (T2)	M0
IIA	High (G2)	Intracompartmental (T1)	M0
IIB	High (G2)	Extracompartmental (T2)	M0
III	Any G	Any T	M1

TABLE 24.3 *The AJCC Classification System*				
STAGE	GRADE	TUMOR	NODES	METASTASES
IA	Low	T1	N0	M0
IB	Low	T2	N0	M0
IIA	High	T1	N0	M0
IIB	High	T2	N0	M0
III	Any grade	T3	N0	M0
IVA	Any grade	Any T	N0	M1a
IVB	Any grade	Any T	N0/N1	M1b

Radiologic Evaluation

Conventional bone radiography remains the mainstay investigation in the evaluation of primary bone tumors (Fig. 24.2). However, primary bone tumors require further radiological investigations, such as magnetic resonance imaging (MRI) of the lesion. This MRI evaluates the proximity or involvement of the vascular structures of the limb and helps determine whether the lesion is suitable for limb salvage surgery (10). A bone scan and computed tomography (CT) scan of the thorax are helpful when looking for metastases (11,12) (Fig. 24.3).

The Biopsy

The biopsy of a primary bone tumor is not the easy operation many surgeons believe, but it is often the most important procedure performed in the patient's management. Members of the American Musculoskeletal Tumor Society (MSTS) assessed the hazards of biopsy in patients with malignant primary extremity bone and soft tissue tumors (13). For patients who had a biopsy prior to referral, there was an incidence of 18.2% major errors in diagnosis and a 17.3% incidence of skin, soft tissue, or wound problems. Over 4% of cases required an amputation as a direct consequence of a poorly performed biopsy. Furthermore, 8.5% of patients had their prognosis or outcome adversely affected as a result of a poorly planned biopsy. The authors recommended careful biopsy planning and execution, and advocated referral to a tumor center prior to biopsy when the surgeon was not prepared to proceed with definitive tumor treatment.

In 1996, the MSTS published a follow-up paper (14). Despite exhaustive educational efforts in the 10-year intervening period, the results were essentially the same. Furthermore, despite significant advances in radiological technology during this interval, the often innocuous clinical appearance of these tumors continued to deceive surgeons, and patients were often treated without any imaging studies. The findings prompted an editorial comment, "Has anyone been listening?" (15).

There are several simple rules for the surgical technique of carrying out a biopsy. For lesions of the periphery, where they allow for application of a tourniquet, only gravity exsanguination is permitted in order to avoid compression of the tumor. Fine-needle aspiration biopsy has been shown to be safe and an acceptable method for sampling pathological tissue (16).

When performing an open biopsy, biopsy tracts should be along the line with the definitive limb salvage surgical incision, so the biopsy tract can be later excised. Transverse incisions should be avoided because they compromise the definitive surgical procedure (Fig. 24.4). The incision should traverse the fewest possible

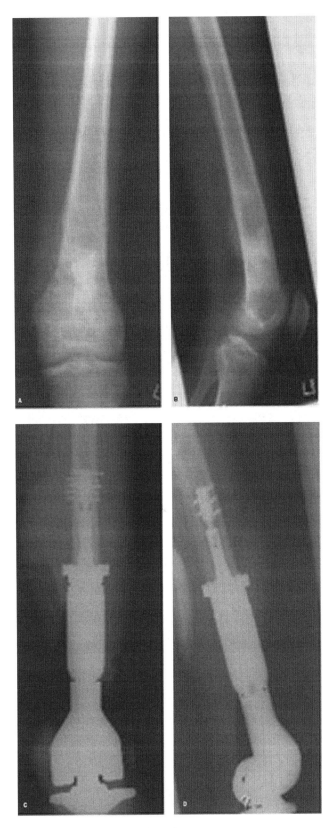

FIGURE 24.2

Conventional x-rays; preoperative anteroposterior (A); lateral (B); postresection anteroposterior (C); and lateral (D) of a malignant osteogenic sarcoma of the distal left femur.

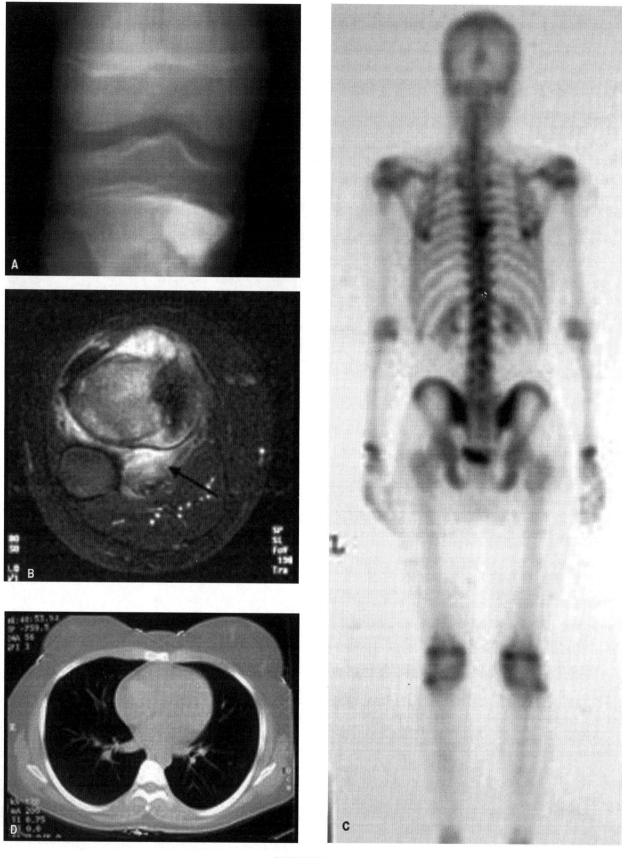

FIGURE 24.3

Preoperative radiologic studies for the investigation of a primary bone sarcoma of the proximal right tibia. In addition to plain radiographs (A), the patient underwent an MRI of the lesion (B), a whole body bone scan (C), and a CT scan of the chest (D).

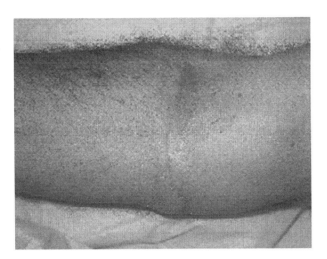

FIGURE 24.4

A biopsy of a lesion through a transverse incision, compromising future surgical intervention.

fascial compartments, and nerves and vessels should not be dissected or identified because this causes contamination and may necessitate amputation. Contamination of any joint should be avoided; where facilities allow, the biopsy should be sent for frozen section to ensure that it contains representative tissue. Biopsy material should be sent for culture and sensitivity to rule out infection. Meticulous hemostasis should be achieved prior to closing the skin to avoid a postoperative hematoma.

In addition to the above rules, bone biopsies necessitate that the defect created by the biopsy should be small and rounded in order to avoid a stress riser that could result in a postoperative fracture. Patients who undergo lower limb biopsies should be protected with crutches to avoid torsional stresses at the biopsy site.

TREATMENT PROTOCOL

Osteogenic sarcoma is the most common of the primary bone tumors and the tumor upon which the treatment protocol for primary bone tumors is based. Classically, once the tumor is confirmed by biopsy, the patient undergoes preoperative chemotherapy (17). No difference in survival has been demonstrated if preoperative chemotherapy is deferred in favor of surgery and only postoperative chemotherapy is given (18). High dose methotrexate (Trexall), doxorubicin (Adriamycin), cisplatin (Platinol), and ifosfamide (Mitoxana) are the most commonly used as chemotherapeutic agents.

Usually, after three cycles of preoperative chemotherapy the definitive surgery is undertaken, with chemotherapy being revisited again postoperatively. The resected specimen is then analyzed microscopically and can be compared to the biopsy specimen to evaluate the effect of the preoperative chemotherapy on the tumor. The percentage necrosis is graded according to the Huvos Classification (Table 24.3 and Fig. 24.5). A poor response to preoperative chemotherapy is predictive of a poor outcome, as is an elevated serum alkaline phosphatase at presentation, central (pelvic) location, older age, African American race, and radiation-induced bone sarcomas (19).

Such a protocol is acceptable for all chemotherapy-sensitive bone tumors and results similar to those demonstrated for osteogenic sarcomas have been demonstrated for Ewing sarcoma of bone (20). Chondrosarcomas are not chemosensitive, and there is no role for chemotherapy in primary malignant chondrosarcomas of bone (21); wide excision is the treatment of choice.

Radiation therapy has a limited role in the management of primary bone sarcomas. When surgery is not possible, radiotherapy has been used to help provide local control although results are not comparable to the gold standard chemotherapy and surgical combination (22,23).

Surgical Management

There are several reconstructive choices for the surgical management of malignant bone sarcomas. These choices include intercalary allografts (Fig. 24.6); alloprosthetic composites (Fig. 24.7); osteoarticular allografts (Fig. 24.8); and endoprostheses (Fig. 24.2). Other choices include rotationplasty (Fig. 24.9) and amputation. The choice depends on patient factors such as age, and tumor characteristics, such as size and position in bone and the presence or absence of a soft-tissue mass. The single most important factor is the ability to achieve negative margins at the time of surgery.

TABLE 24.4 *The Huvos Classification System of Tumor Necrosis*	
GRADE	**NECROSIS**
I	Little or no effect
II	Areas of viable tumor, 60%–89% necrosis
III	Scattered foci, 90%–99% tumor necrosis
IV	No histological evidence of viable tumor—100%

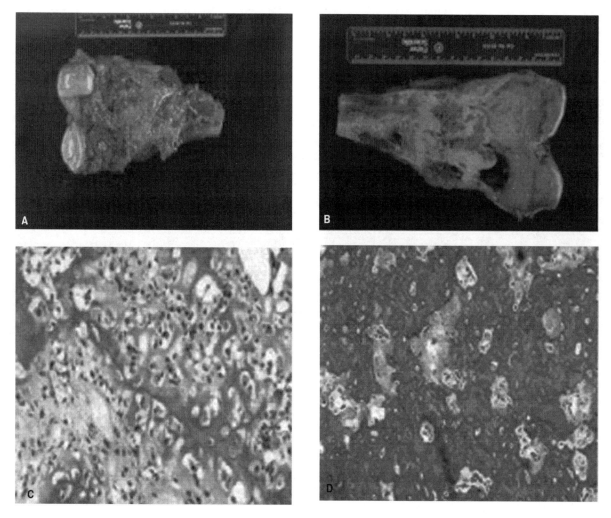

FIGURE 24.5

A typical resection specimen of a distal femoral osteogenic sarcoma. (A) and (B) show the gross resected specimen, (C) demonstrates the preoperative histological appearance, and (D) demonstrates a 40% necrosis rate as a result of the preoperative chemotherapy—a poor response to chemotherapy.

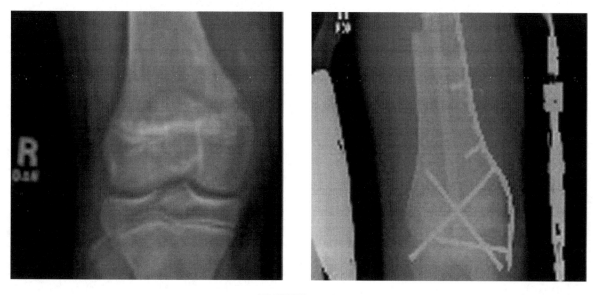

FIGURE 24.6

Physis sparing resection of osteogenic sarcoma of distal femur; preoperative picture (A) and postoperative picture (B). Reconstruction was achieved with intercalary bone graft, stabilized with a distal femur locking plate. The resection was achieved with negative margins and good knee function was achieved postoperatively.

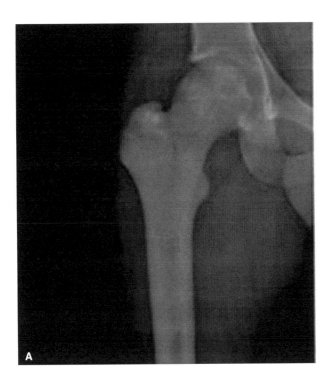
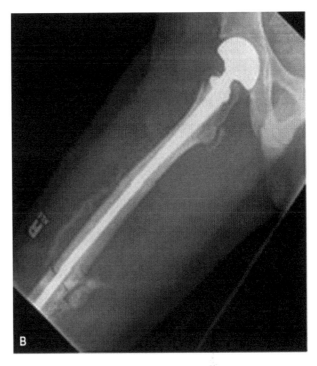

FIGURE 24.7

Osteogenic sarcoma proximal femur, resected with negative margins and reconstructed using an implant allograft (allo-prosthetic) composite.

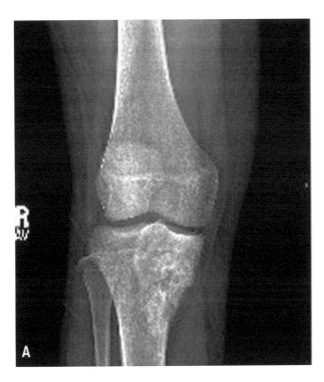
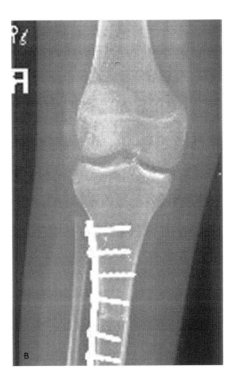

FIGURE 24.8

Primary osteogenic sarcoma of proximal tibia; negative resection margins were achieved and reconstruction was achieved using an osteoarticular allograft.

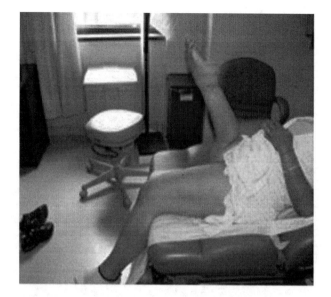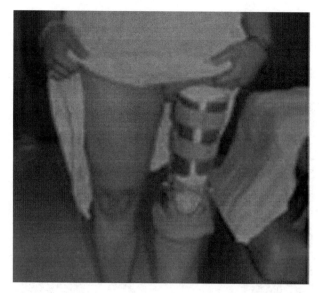

FIGURE 24.9

Postoperative rotationplasty patient.

References

1. Cancer Facts and Figures. 2007. American Cancer Society (ACS). Atlanta Georgia 2007.
2. Bielack SS, Kempf-Bielack B, Delling G, et al. Prognostic factors in high-grade osteosarcoma of extremities or trunk: an analysis of 1,702 patients treated on neoadjuvant cooperative osteosarcoma study group protocols. *J Clin Oncol.* 2002;20(3):776–790.
3. Landis S, Murray T, Boldern S, Wingo P. Cancer statistics, 1999. *CA Cancer J Clin.* 1999;49:31.
4. Cade S. Osteogenic sarcoma: a study based on 33 patients. *J R Coll Surg Edinb.* 1955;1:79.
5. Friedman MA, Carter SK. The therapy of osteogenic sarcoma: current status and thoughts for the future. *J Surg Oncol.* 1972;4:482.
6. Rosen G, Murphy ML, Huvos AG, Gutierrez M, Marcove RC. Chemotherapy, en bloc resection, and prosthetic bone replacement in the treatment of osteogenic sarcoma. *Cancer.* January 1976;37(1):1–11.
7. Enneking W, Spanier S, Goodman M. Current concepts review. The surgical staging of musculoskeletal sarcoma. *J Bone Joint Surg.* 1980;62A:1027.
8. Enneking W, Spanier S, Malawer M. The effect of the anatomic setting on the results of surgical procedures for soft parts sarcoma of the thigh. *Cancer.* 1981;47:1005.
9. Enneking W. A system of staging musculoskeletal neoplasms. *Clin Orthop.* 1986;204:9.
10. Exner G, von Hochstetter A, Augustiny N, von Schulthess G. Magnetic resonance imaging in malignant bone tumors. *Int Orthop.* 1990;14:49.
11. Gosfield E, Alvai A, Kneeland B. Comparison of radionuclide bone scans and magnetic imaging in detecting spinal metastases. *J Nucl Med.* 1993;34:2191.
12. Simon M, Finn H. Diagnostic strategy for bone and soft tissue tumors. *J Bone Joint Surg.* 1993;75A:622.
13. Mankin HJ, Lange TA, Spanier SS. The hazards of biopsy in patients with malignant primary bone and soft tissue tumours. *J Bone Joint Surg Am.* 1982;64:1121.
14. Mankin HJ, Mankin CJ, Simon MA. The hazards of the biopsy, revisited. *J Bone Joint Surg Am.* May 1996;78(5):656–663.
15. Springfield DS, Rosenberg A. Biopsy: complicated and risky (an editorial). *J Bone Joint Surg (Am).* 1996;78(5):639–643.
16. Jelinek JS, Murphey MD, Welker JA, et al. Diagnosis of primary bone tumors with image-guided percutaneous biopsy: experience with 110 tumors. *Radiology.* 2002;223:731.
17. Goorin AM, Schwartzentruber DJ, Devidas M, et al. Presurgical chemotherapy compared with immediate surgery and adjuvant chemotherapy for nonmetastatic osteosarcoma: Pediatric Oncology Group Study POG-8651. *J Clin Oncol.* 2003;21:1574.
18. Link M, Goorin A, Miser A, et al. Adjuvant chemotherapy of high-grade osteosarcoma of the extremity. Updated results of the multi-institutional osteosarcoma study. *Clin Orthop.* 1991;270:8.
19. Myers PA, Heller G, Healey J, et al. Chemotherapy for nonmetastatic osteogenic sarcoma: the memorial Sloan-Kettering experience. *J Clin Oncol.* 1992;10:5.
20. Wunder JS, Paulian G, Huvos AG, Heller G, Myers PA, Healey JH. The histological response to chemotherapy as a predictor of the oncological outcome of operative treatment of ewing sarcoma. *J Bone Joint Surg.* 1998;80(A):7, 1020.
21. Marco RAW, Gitelis S, Brebach GT, Healey JH. Cartilage tumors: evaluation and treatment. *J Am Acad Orthop Surg.* 2000;8:292.
22. DeLaney TF, Park L, Goldberg SI, et al. Radiotherapy for local control of osteosarcoma. *Int J Radiation Oncology Biol Phys.* 2005;61(2):492.
23. La TH, Meyers PA, Wexler LH, et al. Radiation therapy for Ewing's sarcoma: results from memorial Sloan-Kettering in the modern era. *Int J Radiation Oncology Biol Phys.* 2006;64(2):544.

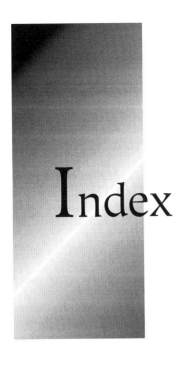

Index